Pulmonary Diseases and Disorders

Pulmonary Diseases and Disorders

Edited by Beatrice Gunther

AMERICAN
MEDICAL PUBLISHERS
www.americanmedicalpublishers.com

American Medical Publishers,
41 Flatbush Avenue,
1st Floor, New York,
NY 11217, USA

Visit us on the World Wide Web at:
www.americanmedicalpublishers.com

ISBN: 978-1-63927-462-8

Cataloging-in-Publication Data

Pulmonary diseases and disorders / edited by Beatrice Gunther.
p. cm.
Includes bibliographical references and index.
ISBN 978-1-63927-462-8
1. Lungs--Diseases. 2. Lungs--Diseases, Fungal. 3. Lungs--Diseases, Obstructive.
4. Lungs--Blood-vessels--Diseases. 5. Pulmonary manifestations of general diseases.
6. Respiratory organs--Diseases. I. Gunther, Beatrice.

RC756 .P85 2022

616.24--dc23

Table of Contents

Preface

The lungs can be affected adversely by exposure to toxins and infectious agents. Some individuals may have hereditary diseases which affect the lungs such as cystic fibrosis or alpha 1-antitrypsin deficiency. There can also be a constitutional or genetic predisposition towards lung conditions like pulmonary hypertension or pulmonary fibrosis. The field of pulmonology is concerned with the diagnosis and management of pulmonary diseases. It is also involved in the management of patient's requiring mechanical ventilation and life support. Interventional pulmonology is an emerging specialty within pulmonary medicine which employs procedures like pleuroscopy and bronchoscopy for the treatment of pulmonary diseases. While lung conditions like asthma or chronic obstructive pulmonary disease can be treated with inhalers, oxygen therapy and mechanical ventilation are required in cases of severe respiratory disease. From theories to research, case studies related to all contemporary topics of relevance to pulmonology have been included in this book. The topics covered herein deal with diverse pulmonology diseases and disorders. This book is meant for students who are looking for an elaborate reference text on pulmonology.

All of the data presented henceforth, was collaborated in the wake of recent advancements in the field. The aim of this book is to present the diversified developments from across the globe in a comprehensible manner. The opinions expressed in each chapter belong solely to the contributing authors. Their interpretations of the topics are the integral part of this book, which I have carefully compiled for a better understanding of the readers.

At the end, I would like to thank all those who dedicated their time and efforts for the successful completion of this book. I also wish to convey my gratitude towards my friends and family who supported me at every step.

Editor

1

Incidence and prevalence of neuroendocrine tumors of the lung: analysis of a US commercial insurance claims database

Michael S. Broder[1*], Beilei Cai[2], Eunice Chang[1] and Maureen P. Neary[2]

Abstract

Background: As reported in Surveillance, Epidemiology, and End Results (SEER) data, US incidence and prevalence of neuroendocrine tumors (NET) has increased over recent years. The study objective was to update incidence and prevalence information for lung NET using administrative claims.

Methods: This descriptive epidemiological study used 2009–2014 data from 2 US claims databases: MarketScan and PharMetrics. Patients (18–64 years old) had ≥1 inpatient or ≥ 2 outpatient claims with NET of bronchus or lung, identified by International Classification of Diseases, 9th Revision, Clinical Modification diagnosis codes. Prevalence was number of lung NET patients divided by number of enrollees/year. Incidence was number of patients with a first observed NET diagnosis who were disease-free for 2 years prior, divided by number of enrollees. Age and gender adjustments performed.

Results: The annual number of patients with lung NET identified from 2009 to 2014 ranged from 435 to 796 (MarketScan) and 419–648 (PharMetrics). In MarketScan, there was a 7.4% (95%CI 2.1–13.0; $p = 0.027$) annual percent change (APC) in the age-adjusted incidence for males and 6.8% (− 0.2–14.3; 0.052) for females. In PharMetrics, APC was − 2.9% (− 13.8–9.4; 0.395) for males; 14.7% (− 12.9–51.2; 0.165) for females. In MarketScan, APC in age-adjusted prevalence for males was 9.9% (4.7–15.3; 0.006); 16.2% (11.4-21.1; <.001) for females. For PharMetrics, APCs were 9.5% (2.3–17.2; 0.021) for males; 16.3% (9.6–23.5; 0.002) for females.

Conclusions: From 2009 to 2014 there was a statistically significant increase in age-adjusted lung NET incidence for males in MarketScan, and a statistically significant increase in age-adjusted prevalence for both genders in PharMetrics. Incidence and prevalence changes, to the extent they exist, may be due to better diagnostic methods, increased awareness of NET among clinicians and pathologists, and/or an actual increase in US disease occurrence. Differences in rates across databases are difficult to explain. These results suggest the need for awareness of the clinically effective and safe treatment options available for lung NET patients among healthcare providers.

Keywords: Lung neuroendocrine tumors, Epidemiology, Prevalence, Incidence, Insurance claims

* Correspondence: mbroder@pharllc.com
[1]Partnership for Health Analytic Research, LLC, 280 S. Beverly Dr. Ste. 404, Beverly Hills, CA, USA
Full list of author information is available at the end of the article

Background

Neuroendocrine tumors (NET) comprise a broad family of rare and often slow growing malignancies. NET can develop anywhere in the body and arise from neuroendocrine cells throughout the endocrine system [1, 2]. Approximately one-quarter to one-third of NET occur in the lung [3, 4]. NET secrete peptides and neuroamines that may cause distinct syndromes (e.g., carcinoid syndrome, glucagonoma), in which case they are referred to as "functional" tumors. Clinical presentation depends on the site of the primary tumor and whether or not they are functional. Research on risk factors for lung NET is limited, although the authors of a recent meta-analysis concluded, "family history of cancer is the most relevant risk factor for [NET] development at all investigated sites, followed by BMI and diabetes. Cigarette smoking and alcohol consumption are potential risk factors for selected anatomical sites" [5]. Surgery may be curative in the early stages, but delayed diagnosis is typical.

While rare, the incidence and prevalence of NET appear to be increasing worldwide [4–10]. In a 2008 study using the US Surveillance, Epidemiology, and End Results (SEER) database, the incidence of NET in the US increased from 10.9 cases per million person-years (PMPY) in 1973 to 52.5 PMPY in 2004 [4] and in a 2017 study to 69.8 PMPY in 2012 [10]. Overall NET prevalence was 350 per 1 million in 2004 [4] and 480 per 1 million in 2012 [10]. Only patients with malignant cancers are included in the SEER registries, and the separation of NET into clear-cut benign and malignant categories is not as straightforward as it is for most epithelial malignancies [11]. NET that have not invaded adjacent organs or metastasized may not be immediately labeled as malignant. Thus, many small, benign-appearing tumors may not get included in SEER [4].

The objective of this study was to update incidence and prevalence information for lung NET with non-registry-based data, specifically insurance claims, using additional data beyond what had previously been reported.

Methods

Design and data source

This was a descriptive epidemiological study using insurance claims data from January 1, 2009 to December 31, 2014. The data were from two large US commercial claims databases: Truven Health MarketScan Commercial Claims and Encounters Database, and IMS Health PharMetrics. The MarketScan database has information from more than 100 payers of private health insurance for employees and their dependents, covering more than 25 million lives annually. The PharMetrics database is a nonpayer owned integrated claims database of commercial insurers that includes medical and pharmacy claims for more than 70 million unique individuals across the US. Both databases contain de-identified adjudicated medical claims (e.g., inpatient and outpatient services) and pharmacy claims (e.g., outpatient prescriptions).

Payments to providers, healthcare facilities, and pharmacies for the 66% of the US population with commercial insurance are contingent on submission of claims for services [12]. These insurance claims contain information about diagnoses (International Classification of Diseases, 9th Revision, Clinical Modification [ICD-9-CM] diagnosis codes) and procedures (Current Procedural Terminology 4 [CPT-4] and ICD-9-CM procedure codes). Information on each physician visit, medical procedure, hospitalization, drug dispensed, date of service, number of days of medication supplied, test performed, as well as complete payment information, is available for covered individuals from their insurance claims. Available patient demographic information is limited to age, gender, and broad geographic region. An "enrollment" file provides information on each individuals' dates of coverage—the dates for which we can find their insurance claims. No information is available about individuals for dates outside their dates of enrollment. Information about death, including date or cause, is not available. Privacy restrictions make it impossible to contact patients or review their detailed medical records to obtain additional clinical or demographic information such as health behaviors, tumor size/stage, or race/ethnicity. In the US, individuals may change their insurance coverage over time, and thus the number of individuals enrolled in a given plan changes from year to year. For this study, we were provided the total number of individuals in each database each year, broken down by age and gender. Both databases contain a limited number of individuals ≥65 years old. US individuals ≥65 who have commercial insurance are not representative of the broader age group, a large majority of whom are insured through the Federal Medicare program. Therefore, the analysis was restricted to individuals < 65. Analyses were performed separately using each database and results were compared to check consistency. As the data were de-identified, this study was considered exempt from approval by the Institutional Review Board.

Cohort selection

Individuals at least 18 years of age were identified as having lung NET if, during a single calendar year, they had at least 1 claim from a hospital setting, or at least 2 claims from the outpatient setting, that included an ICD-9-CM diagnosis code for lung NET (that is, either 209.21 malignant carcinoid tumor of bronchus and lung, or 209.61 benign carcinoid tumor of bronchus and lung). Coding of inpatient claims in the US is usually performed by professional coders and is thus more reliable than claims from the outpatient setting, which may be recorded by a variety of staff with limited clinical training. A limitation of using claims data to estimate disease incidence is the inability to know with certainty that the first diagnosis seen in the data represents the first clinical diagnosis of the condition. Therefore, for incident cases, we required individuals to have been continuously enrolled for 3 years: the specific calendar year of diagnosis and 2 years prior, with no evidence of disease in the prior 2 years. For example, a cohort of individuals identified with lung NET in 2011 must have been enrolled during the entire 2009 to 2011 period, with their lung NET diagnosis in 2011.

Statistical analysis

For each calendar year, we reported the distribution of patient demographics, summarizing continuous variables with means, and categorical variables with patient counts and percentages. Incidence rate was calculated as the number of individuals with lung NET in a particular year divided by the number of all individuals who were continuously enrolled (that is, for whom we had data for the entire year) across the three-year period (year of diagnosis and 2 prior disease-free years) and reported as per million person-years (PMPY). Prevalence was calculated as the number of lung NET patients in a particular year divided by the total number of individuals continuously enrolled for that calendar year and reported as patients per million. For both incidence and prevalence, rates were reported overall and by sex and age categories (18–24, 25–34, 35–44, 45–54, and 55–64 years). To allow comparisons within genders and between databases over time, we calculated adjusted (gender-specific) rates by standardizing the age distribution for each gender based on the distribution of ages (in those same 4 age categories) from both databases in 2014. Similarly, we calculated overall adjusted rates by standardizing to the age and gender distribution from both databases in 2014. The enrollment requirements for inclusion in the incidence and prevalence denominators differed (3 years of enrollment for incidence and a single calendar year for prevalence), and the denominator drops substantially when the continuous enrollment criteria is added. We believe the underlying US commercially insured population is more similar to the one used for calculating prevalence; therefore, to calculate standardized rates for both incidence and prevalence, we used the age and gender distribution from the prevalent population in 2014.

We used annual percent change (APC) to study trends over time [13, 14]. APC was calculated by least-squares linear regression on a log-linear model to characterize trends in rates over calendar year. With this approach, each rate is assumed to change at a constant percentage of the previous year's rate. Because each database had a different denominator, results are reported separately by database. All data transformations and statistical analysis were performed using SAS® version 9.4 (SAS Institute, Cary, NC).

Results

On average, in each year from 2009 to 2014, 631 patients were identified as having lung NET in the MarketScan database. The annual number ranged from 435 in 2009 to low of 435 in 2009 to a high of 796 in 2012. In the PharMetrics database, the range was 419 in 2009 to 648 in 2014, with a mean of 559. In the MarketScan and PharMetrics databases, 65.2 and 64.0% of cases were female, respectively (ranging from 59.8 to 69.4%). More than half of the cases (53.0 to 61.7%) were patients between 55 and 64 years old (Table 1).

Generally, in every year and for both databases, unadjusted incidence was higher for each successive age group. Incidence was highest in the two oldest groups: 12.2–27.8 PMPY (depending on year and gender) in individuals aged 45–54, compared to 25.7–53.6 PMPY in individuals aged 55–64 in MarketScan; and 8.2–19.5 PMPY in individuals 45–54 compared to 20.6–55.4 in 55–64 year olds in PharMetrics (Tables 2 and 3).

After adjustment for age and gender, in the MarketScan database combined (males and females) incidence increased from 14.4 PMPY in 2011 and to 17.5 in 2014, an annual percent change (APC) (95% CI; P value) of 7.0% (4.3–9.8; 0.008). The gender-specific incidence (adjusted for age) showed a statistically significant change for males: 7.4% (2.1–13.0; 0.027); and a similar (but not statistically significant) change for females: 6.8% (− 0.2–14.3; 0.052). In the PharMetrics database, the overall age and gender-adjusted incidence was 11.7 PMPY in 2011, 13.8 in 2012, 15.2 in 2013 and 14.6 in 2014, an APC of 7.8% (− 5.7–23.4; 0.137) (Fig. 1, Tables 2 and 3). The APC was not statistically significant for males (− 2.9% [− 13.8–9.4; 0.395]) or females (14.7% [− 12.9–51.2; 0.165]) individually. When data from MarketScan and PharMetrics were combined and adjusted to the age-gender distribution for 2014, incidence rose from 13.0 PMPY in 2011 to 16.2 PMPY in 2014, an overall APC of 7.7% (1.3–14.4; 0.035). However, the combined result masks differences in results across the 2 databases, as described above.

With few exceptions, in each year and for both databases, unadjusted prevalence was higher for each successive age group. Prevalence was highest in 55–64 year olds (between 25.1 and 102.3 per million, depending on year, gender, and database). With few exceptions, unadjusted prevalence was higher in females than in males in every age category (Tables 4 and 5). After age and gender adjustment, prevalence for males and females combined rose from 16.0 per million in 2009 to 30.7 in 2014 in the MarketScan database, an APC of 14.0% (10.2–17.9; <.001). The age-adjusted APC in

Table 1 Patients with lung NET, N[a]

	MarketScan						PharMetrics					
	2009	2010	2011	2012	2013	2014	2009	2010	2011	2012	2013	2014
N	435	521	681	796	667	687	419	510	563	598	616	648
Age, year, no. (%)												
18–24	9 (2.1)	6 (1.2)	9 (1.3)	9 (1.1)	7 (1.0)	2 (0.3)	7 (1.7)	5 (1.0)	10 (1.8)	10 (1.7)	7 (1.1)	9 (1.4)
25–34	16 (3.7)	27 (5.2)	26 (3.8)	37 (4.6)	26 (3.9)	30 (4.4)	29 (6.9)	18 (3.5)	23 (4.1)	19 (3.2)	27 (4.4)	17 (2.6)
35–44	44 (10.1)	57 (10.9)	67 (9.8)	75 (9.4)	68 (10.2)	79 (11.5)	38 (9.1)	59 (11.6)	46 (8.2)	61 (10.2)	65 (10.6)	60 (9.3)
45–54	117 (26.9)	152 (29.2)	205 (30.1)	217 (27.3)	182 (27.3)	198 (28.8)	123 (29.4)	136 (26.7)	156 (27.7)	166 (27.8)	165 (26.8)	162 (25.0)
55–64	249 (57.2)	279 (53.6)	374 (54.9)	458 (57.5)	384 (57.6)	378 (55.0)	222 (53.0)	292 (57.3)	328 (58.3)	342 (57.2)	352 (57.1)	400 (61.7)
Female	260 (59.8)	340 (65.3)	445 (65.3)	515 (64.7)	463 (69.4)	459 (66.8)	258 (61.6)	315 (61.8)	352 (62.5)	392 (65.6)	403 (65.4)	435 (67.1)

[a] Adult patients (age 18 years or older) with ≥1 inpatient or ≥ 2 outpatient claims for lung NET in a calendar year. Patients may have been identified in multiple calendar years. Continuous enrollment not required

Table 2 MarketScan Database: Lung NET Incidence Rate, Cases per Million Person-Years[a]

		No. Of Cases Per Million Person-Years (Numerator/Denominator)											
		2011			2012			2013			2014		
Gender	Age												
Female	18–24	0.0	(0	/629,902)	2.6	(2	/761,959)	2.5	(2	/806,972)	0.0	(0	/791,556)
	25–34	5.8	(5	/857,782)	4.4	(4	/905,705)	2.7	(2	/751,148)	1.4	(1	/711,916)
	35–44	10.3	(14	/1,361,165)	7.5	(11	/1,460,802)	12.7	(16	/1,264,584)	11.6	(14	/1,203,355)
	45–54	15.8	(28	/1,767,104)	23.3	(44	/1,889,625)	26.7	(44	/1,645,900)	27.8	(43	/1,547,477)
	55–64	49.2	(76	/1,545,517)	44.5	(75	/1,687,254)	49.0	(75	/1,531,896)	53.6	(78	/1,454,099)
	All Female	20.0	(123	/6,161,470)	20.3	(136	/6,705,345)	23.2	(139	/6,000,500)	23.8	(136	/5,708,403)
Male	18–24	1.6	(1	/632,342)	0.0	(0	/768,240)	0.0	(0	/829,650)	0.0	(0	/813,048)
	25–34	1.3	(1	/741,337)	2.6	(2	/775,911)	6.2	(4	/648,646)	1.6	(1	/626,307)
	35–44	5.7	(7	/1,221,845)	6.2	(8	/1,294,055)	5.4	(6	/1,120,973)	7.5	(8	/1,066,055)
	45–54	12.2	(19	/1,562,471)	13.9	(23	/1,656,616)	14.5	(21	/1,446,886)	16.8	(23	/1,365,158)
	55–64	25.7	(35	/1,363,927)	28.8	(42	/1,458,077)	27.2	(36	/1,323,391)	31.8	(40	/1,256,884)
	All Male	11.4	(63	/5,521,922)	12.6	(75	/5,952,899)	12.5	(67	/5,369,546)	14.0	(72	/5,127,452)
All Gender	18–24	0.8	(1	/1,262,244)	1.3	(2	/1,530,199)	1.2	(2	/1,636,622)	0.0	(0	/1,604,604)
	25–34	3.8	(6	/1,599,119)	3.6	(6	/1,681,616)	4.3	(6	/1,399,794)	1.5	(2	/1,338,223)
	35–44	8.1	(21	/2,583,010)	6.9	(19	/2,754,857)	9.2	(22	/2,385,557)	9.7	(22	/2,269,410)
	45–54	14.1	(47	/3,329,575)	18.9	(67	/3,546,241)	21.0	(65	/3,092,786)	22.7	(66	/2,912,635)
	55–64	38.2	(111	/2,909,444)	37.2	(117	/3,145,331)	38.9	(111	/2,855,287)	43.5	(118	/2,710,983)
	All Patients	15.9	(186	/11,683,392)	16.7	(211	/12,658,244)	18.1	(206	/11,370,046)	19.2	(208	/10,835,855)
		Adjusted Rate (No. Of Cases Per Million Person-Years)[b]											
All Female[c]		18.3			18.6			21.3			21.8		
All Male[d]		10.3			11.4			11.7			12.9		
All Patients[e]		14.4			15.2			16.6			17.5		

[a] Cases (adults with ≥1 inpatient or ≥ 2 outpatient claims for lung NET in listed year and continuous enrollment in year listed and two years prior) ÷ number of members with continuous enrollment in same period

[b]APC (95% CI; P value): female 6.8% (−0.2–14.3; 0.052); male 7.4% (2.1–13.0; 0.027); all patients 7.0% (4.3–9.8; 0.008)

[c]Adjusted based on distribution of age among male from both databases in 2014

[d]Adjusted based on distribution of age among female from both databases in 2014

[e]Adjusted based on combined distribution of age among male from both databases in 2014

Table 3 PharMetrics Database: Lung NET Incidence Rate, Cases per Million Person-Years[a]

		No. Of Cases Per Million Person-Years (Numerator/Denominator)			
		2011	2012	2013	2014
Gender	Age				
Female	18–24	2.5 (2/809,900)	1.2 (1/803,203)	0.0 (0/844,220)	1.5 (1/670,429)
	25–34	5.5 (5/915,829)	4.7 (4/846,136)	3.5 (3/851,694)	1.5 (1/659,964)
	35–44	2.2 (3/1,387,525)	7.0 (9/1,280,702)	12.8 (16/1,249,676)	10.3 (10/972,515)
	45–54	10.0 (19/1,902,036)	18.9 (33/1,747,518)	18.9 (32/1,688,747)	19.5 (25/1,282,436)
	55–64	37.6 (68/1,809,406)	47.4 (81/1,708,362)	55.4 (94/1,697,399)	51.9 (67/1,290,342)
	All Female	14.2 (97/6,824,696)	20.0 (128/6,385,921)	22.9 (145/6,331,736)	21.3 (104/4,875,686)
Male	18–24	1.2 (1/828,261)	3.6 (3/823,432)	2.3 (2/875,326)	1.4 (1/698,342)
	25–34	2.4 (2/839,247)	1.2 (1/800,680)	0.0 (0/818,984)	1.5 (1/662,957)
	35–44	5.5 (7/1,266,850)	5.1 (6/1,185,774)	3.4 (4/1,164,816)	6.4 (6/935,200)
	45–54	10.5 (18/1,713,588)	11.9 (19/1,599,135)	12.8 (20/1,556,840)	8.2 (10/1,218,043)
	55–64	28.7 (47/1,637,294)	20.6 (32/1,552,538)	23.2 (36/1,551,338)	26.3 (32/1,216,691)
	All Male	11.9 (75/6,285,240)	10.2 (61/5,961,559)	10.4 (62/5,967,304)	10.6 (50/4,731,233)
All Gender	18–24	1.8 (3/1,638,161)	2.5 (4/1,626,635)	1.2 (2/1,719,546)	1.5 (2/1,368,771)
	25–34	4.0 (7/1,755,076)	3.0 (5/1,646,816)	1.8 (3/1,670,678)	1.5 (2/1,322,921)
	35–44	3.8 (10/2,654,375)	6.1 (15/2,466,476)	8.3 (20/2,414,492)	8.4 (16/1,907,715)
	45–54	10.2 (37/3,615,624)	15.5 (52/3,346,653)	16.0 (52/3,245,587)	14.0 (35/2,500,479)
	55–64	33.4 (115/3,446,700)	34.7 (113/3,260,900)	40.0 (130/3,248,737)	39.5 (99/2,507,033)
	All Patients	13.1 (172/13,109,936)	15.3 (189/12,347,480)	16.8 (207/12,299,040)	16.0 (154/9,606,919)
		Adjusted Rate (No. Of Cases Per Million Person-Years)[b]			
All Female[c]		12.8	18.0	20.6	19.3
All Male[d]		10.6	9.3	9.3	9.6
All Patients[e]		11.7	13.8	15.2	14.6

[a] Cases (adults with ≥1 inpatient or ≥ 2 outpatient claims for lung NET in listed year and continuous enrollment in year listed and two years prior) ÷ number of members with continuous enrollment in same period

[b] APC (95% CI; P value): female 14.7% (−12.9–51.2; 0.165); male −2.9% (−13.8–9.4; 0.395); all patients 7.8% (−5.7–23.4; 0.137)

[c] Adjusted based on distribution of age among male from both databases in 2014

[d] Adjusted based on distribution of age among female from both databases in 2014

[e] Adjusted based on combined distribution of age among male from both databases in 2014

prevalence for females was 16.2% (11.4–21.1; <.001) and for males was 9.9% (4.7–15.3; 0.006). The age- and gender-adjusted APC in the PharMetrics database was 13.9% (7.4–20.9; 0.004); 16.3% (9.6–23.5; 0.002) for females and 9.5% (2.3–17.2; 0.021) for males. (Fig. 2, Tables 4 and 5). When both datasets were combined and adjusted for age and gender, prevalence rose from 14.6 cases per million in 2009 to 28.5 per million in 2014, an APC of 14.2% (9.5–19.0; <.001) overall (16.5% [10.9–22.3; 0.001] for females and 9.9% (5.6–14.3; 0.003) for males.

Discussion

From 2009 to 2014 there was a statistically significant increase in age-adjusted lung NET incidence for males in the MarketScan database. Incidence increased at an annual age and gender-adjusted rate of 7.0% per year, reaching an overall 17.5 PMPY by 2014. In the same database, prevalence rose at an annual age- and gender-adjusted rate of 14.0% per year, reaching 30.7 cases per million per year. The number of cases identified, incidence, and prevalence were all higher in the MarketScan database than in the PharMetrics database. In the PharMetrics database, incidence increased 7.8% per year, but this change was not statistically significant, while age- and gender-adjusted prevalence increased 13.9% per year ($p < .001$). A study using older data recently reported the incidence of NET in the US increased from 3 cases PMPY in 1973 to 16 PMPY in 2012 [10]. The preponderance of female cases has been observed in prior studies using these and other data sources [4, 9, 15].

There are many possible reasons for the observed changes in incidence and prevalence, although determining which reason or reasons are most important was beyond the scope of this study. First, more tumors may be found incidentally over time. Rates of both CT and MRI use in the general population have been steadily

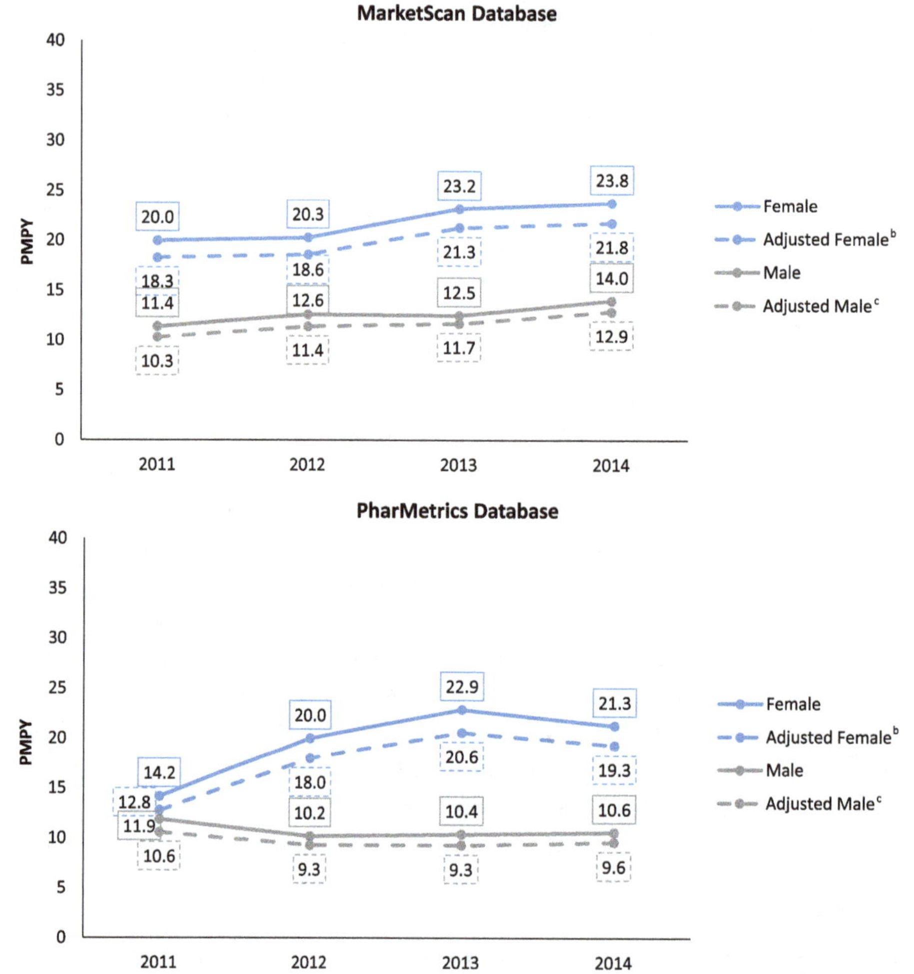

Fig. 1 Lung NET Incidence Rate, Cases per Million Person-Years[a]. [a] In the combined database (adjusted for age and gender) the no. of cases per million person-years was 13.0 (2011), 14.5 (2012), 15.9 (2013), and 16.2 (2014) for all patients. [b] Adjusted based on distribution of age among males from both databases in 2014. [c] Adjusted based on distribution of age among females from both databases in 2014

increasing, as has the accuracy of these tests [16]. Some patients may have their tumors detected simply because they have a chest imaging study for another reason. Second, screening for lung cancer appears to be rising [17]. As screening rates increase, more lung NET may be detected. Third, in the last decade, high sensitivity assays for 5-hydroxyindoleacetic acid (5-HIAA) and chromogranin A, both markers for certain NET, have come into more common use. Increased use of these tests may have improved identification of previously undetected tumors [18]. Fourth, pathologists may be improving their ability to identify NET. Finally, the underlying rate of the development of NET may be increasing. The increased prevalence would be expected from the combination of increasing incidence [4, 10] and improved survival [19, 20]. Incidental identification of lung NET might also partially explain the finding that prevalence increased more than incidence during the period studied. If earlier tumors were being identified, survival would appear to increase, which in turn would increase prevalence. We could not test this theory in the current study, as data on disease stage is lacking. A recent analysis of pancreatic NET using the SEER database found increases in both incidence and survival and concluded that stage migration, or an increased detection of localized disease, explained at least part of these observations [21]. In the current study, although the adjusted annual percent change differed between the PharMetrics and MarketScan databases, these between-database differences were not statistically significant (e.g., the 95% CI overlapped) and the estimate from the combined databases was consistent with the individual ones. Both databases are derived from wide geographic regions, encompass diverse practice types, and represent multiple insurance plan types, between-database differences on any of these individual factors may explain why the estimates are numerically different between PharMetrics and MarketScan.

Table 4 MarketScan Database: Lung NET Prevalence, Cases per Million per Year[a]

		No. Of Cases Per Million Per Year (Numerator/Denominator)																	
		2009			2010			2011			2012			2013			2014		
Gender	Age																		
Female	18–24	1.7	(2	/1,200,214)	1.7	(2	/1,179,801)	0.7	(1	/1,535,683)	3.0	(5	/1,668,409)	3.6	(5	/1,404,034)	0.7	(1	/1,342,845)
	25–34	4.9	(10	/2,032,535)	8.2	(16	/1,962,108)	5.8	(12	/2,052,889)	10.5	(22	/2,089,096)	9.8	(16	/1,640,542)	8.3	(13	/1,562,298)
	35–44	7.6	(20	/2,616,976)	9.9	(25	/2,533,283)	12.9	(34	/2,643,239)	14.7	(39	/2,660,474)	18.8	(40	/2,123,456)	21.0	(42	/1,996,743)
	45–54	18.1	(56	/3,090,478)	24.7	(75	/3,031,223)	31.0	(99	/3,190,617)	36.8	(118	/3,204,967)	40.3	(102	/2,529,219)	42.4	(99	/2,336,993)
	55–64	52.8	(124	/2,349,482)	59.7	(144	/2,411,232)	75.1	(197	/2,624,303)	85.9	(231	/2,688,474)	95.2	(209	/2,194,982)	102.3	(210	/2,053,379)
	All Female	18.8	(212	/11,289,685)	23.6	(262	/11,117,647)	28.5	(343	/12,046,731)	33.7	(415	/12,311,420)	37.6	(372	/9,892,233)	39.3	(365	/9,292,258)
Male	18–24	5.2	(6	/1,147,214)	3.5	(4	/1,129,804)	2.6	(4	/1,549,206)	2.3	(4	/1,705,487)	1.4	(2	/1,431,673)	0.0	(0	/1,365,613)
	25–34	2.3	(4	/1,760,823)	4.8	(8	/1,669,422)	3.9	(7	/1,788,710)	4.9	(9	/1,850,139)	4.2	(6	/1,436,317)	5.8	(8	/1,388,742)
	35–44	7.2	(17	/2,359,613)	7.1	(16	/2,250,466)	11.3	(27	/2,381,647)	9.2	(22	/2,403,534)	8.9	(17	/1,900,182)	12.3	(22	/1,791,028)
	45–54	10.3	(28	/2,731,422)	15.9	(42	/2,636,290)	16.7	(47	/2,817,734)	21.1	(60	/2,841,640)	18.4	(41	/2,223,287)	24.2	(50	/2,066,977)
	55–64	33.7	(71	/2,104,573)	30.8	(65	/2,107,551)	38.3	(88	/2,296,348)	45.7	(107	/2,342,101)	42.7	(81	/1,897,684)	52.1	(93	/1,783,325)
	All Male	12.5	(126	/10,103,645)	13.8	(135	/9,793,533)	16.0	(173	/10,833,645)	18.1	(202	/11,142,901)	16.5	(147	/8,889,143)	20.6	(173	/8,395,685)
All Gender	18–24	3.4	(8	/2,347,428)	2.6	(6	/2,309,605)	1.6	(5	/3,084,889)	2.7	(9	/3,373,896)	2.5	(7	/2,835,707)	0.4	(1	/2,708,458)
	25–34	3.7	(14	/3,793,358)	6.6	(24	/3,631,530)	4.9	(19	/3,841,599)	7.9	(31	/3,939,235)	7.2	(22	/3,076,859)	7.1	(21	/2,951,040)
	35–44	7.4	(37	/4,976,589)	8.6	(41	/4,783,749)	12.1	(61	/5,024,886)	12.0	(61	/5,064,008)	14.2	(57	/4,023,638)	16.9	(64	/3,787,771)
	45–54	14.4	(84	/5,821,900)	20.6	(117	/5,667,513)	24.3	(146	/6,008,351)	29.4	(178	/6,046,607)	30.1	(143	/4,752,506)	33.8	(149	/4,403,970)
	55–64	43.8	(195	/4,454,055)	46.3	(209	/4,518,783)	57.9	(285	/4,920,651)	67.2	(338	/5,030,575)	70.9	(290	/4,092,666)	79.0	(303	/3,836,704)
	All Patients	15.8	(338	/21,393,330)	19.0	(397	/20,911,180)	22.6	(516	/22,880,376)	26.3	(617	/23,454,321)	27.6	(519	/18,781,376)	30.4	(538	/17,687,943)
		Adjusted Rate (No. Of Cases Per Million Per Year)[b]																	
All Female[c]		19.2			23.5			28.6			34.0			37.9			39.8		
All Male[d]		12.6			13.5			15.9			18.3			16.7			20.9		
All Patients[e]		16.0			18.7			22.5			26.4			27.6			30.7		

[a] Cases of adults with ≥1 inpatient or ≥ 2 outpatient claims for Lung NET in listed year and continuous enrollment in year listed ÷ number of members with continuous enrollment in same period

[b] APC (95% CI; P value): female 16.2% (11.4–21.1; <.001); male 9.9% (4.7–15.3; 0.006); all patients: 14.0% (10.2–17.9; <.001)

[c] Adjusted based on distribution of age among males from both databases in 2014

[d] Adjusted based on distribution of age among females from both databases in 2014

[e] Adjusted based on combined distribution of age among males from both databases in 2014

Table 5 PharMetrics Database: Lung NET Prevalence, Cases per Million per Year[a]

		No. Of Cases Per Million Per Year (Numerator/Denominator)																	
		2009			2010			2011			2012			2013			2014		
Gender	Age																		
Female	18–24	2.9	(4	/1,388,059)	2.3	(3	/1,318,141)	3.5	(5	/1,431,236)	4.4	(6	/1,360,555)	2.2	(3	/1,335,252)	1.9	(2	/1,048,351)
	25–34	6.6	(13	/1,960,213)	3.8	(7	/1,849,997)	8.1	(15	/1,851,913)	4.7	(8	/1,708,390)	7.1	(12	/1,684,490)	3.7	(5	/1,341,604)
	35–44	6.0	(15	/2,508,808)	10.7	(25	/2,335,199)	6.6	(15	/2,269,096)	12.2	(25	/2,055,088)	20.3	(40	/1,969,715)	16.1	(25	/1,553,850)
	45–54	18.7	(59	/3,149,529)	24.0	(71	/2,959,455)	26.5	(76	/2,867,408)	31.9	(82	/2,574,529)	32.8	(80	/2,436,504)	35.2	(66	/1,875,797)
	55–64	38.2	(101	/2,643,692)	55.5	(143	/2,576,843)	65.6	(169	/2,575,456)	77.4	(184	/2,377,377)	92.0	(212	/2,305,347)	91.9	(165	/1,796,085)
	All Female[b]	16.5	(192	/11,650,301)	22.6	(249	/11,039,635)	25.5	(280	/10,995,109)	30.3	(305	/10,075,939)	35.7	(347	/9,731,308)	34.5	(263	/7,615,687)
Male	18–24	1.4	(2	/1,387,054)	1.5	(2	/1,322,440)	1.4	(2	/1,462,310)	2.8	(4	/1,406,293)	2.9	(4	/1,386,541)	3.6	(4	/1,097,662)
	25–34	4.5	(8	/1,759,919)	3.0	(5	/1,671,459)	3.0	(5	/1,687,428)	1.9	(3	/1,609,181)	6.2	(10	/1,604,977)	2.3	(3	/1,323,432)
	35–44	4.3	(10	/2,300,612)	12.6	(27	/2,147,076)	10.5	(22	/2,093,812)	9.3	(18	/1,928,820)	10.2	(19	/1,864,293)	10.6	(16	/1,505,314)
	45–54	11.2	(32	/2,850,321)	14.9	(40	/2,681,967)	16.1	(42	/2,602,786)	20.2	(48	/2,375,529)	19.4	(44	/2,267,225)	17.9	(32	/1,786,707)
	55–64	25.1	(60	/2,392,616)	33.5	(78	/2,331,410)	37.4	(87	/2,325,581)	33.8	(73	/2,158,306)	39.3	(83	/2,110,883)	44.5	(75	/1,684,375)
	All Male[c]	10.5	(112	/10,690,522)	15.0	(152	/10,154,352)	15.5	(158	/10,171,917)	15.4	(146	/9,478,129)	17.3	(160	/9,233,919)	17.6	(130	/7,397,490)
All Gender	18–24	2.2	(6	/2,775,113)	1.9	(5	/2,640,581)	2.4	(7	/2,893,546)	3.6	(10	/2,766,848)	2.6	(7	/2,721,793)	2.8	(6	/2,146,013)
	25–34	5.6	(21	/3,720,132)	3.4	(12	/3,521,456)	5.7	(20	/3,539,341)	3.3	(11	/3,317,571)	6.7	(22	/3,289,467)	3.0	(8	/2,665,036)
	35–44	5.2	(25	/4,809,420)	11.6	(52	/4,482,275)	8.5	(37	/4,362,908)	10.8	(43	/3,983,908)	15.4	(59	/3,834,008)	13.4	(41	/3,059,164)
	45–54	15.2	(91	/5,999,850)	19.7	(111	/5,641,422)	21.6	(118	/5,470,194)	26.3	(130	/4,950,058)	26.4	(124	/4,703,729)	26.8	(98	/3,662,504)
	55–64	32.0	(161	/5,036,308)	45.0	(221	/4,908,253)	52.2	(256	/4,901,037)	56.7	(257	/4,535,683)	66.8	(295	/4,416,230)	69.0	(240	/3,480,460)
	All Patients[d]	13.6	(304	/22,340,823)	18.9	(401	/21,193,987)	20.7	(438	/21,167,026)	23.1	(451	/19,554,068)	26.7	(507	/18,965,227)	26.2	(393	/15,013,177)
		Adjusted Rate (No. Of Cases Per Million Per Year)[b]																	
All Female[c]		16.2			21.8			24.8			29.5			34.9			34.0		
All Male[d]		10.2			14.4			15.1			15.1			17.0			17.3		
All Patients[e]		13.3			18.2			20.1			22.6			26.3			25.9		

[a] Cases of adults with ≥1 inpatient or ≥ 2 outpatient claims for Lung NET in listed year and continuous enrollment in year listed ÷ number of members with continuous enrollment in same period

[b] APC (95% CI; P value): female 16.3% (9.6–23.5; 0.002); male 9.5% (2.3–17.2; 0.021); all patients: 13.9% (7.4–20.9; 0.004)

[c] Adjusted based on distribution of age among males from both databases in 2014

[d] Adjusted based on distribution of age among females from both databases in 2014

[e] Adjusted based on combined distribution of age among males from both databases in 2014

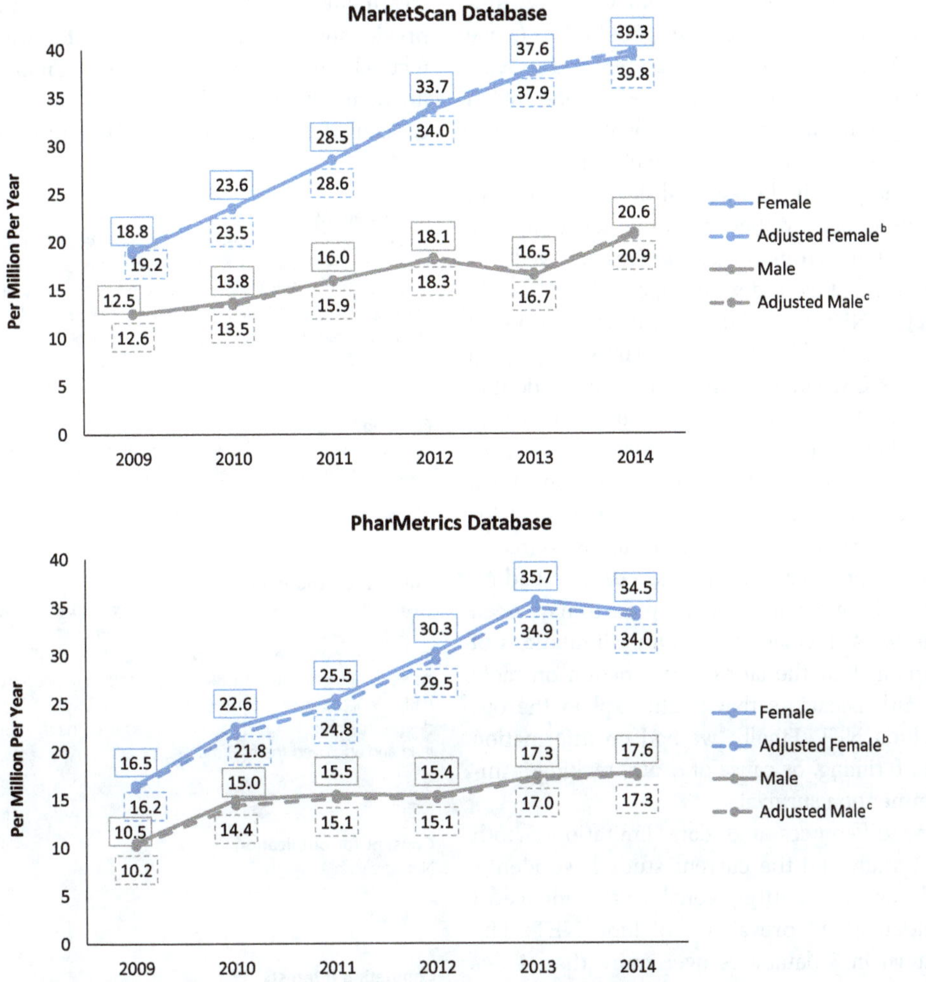

Fig. 2 Lung NET Prevalence, Cases per Million/Year[a]. [a] In the combined database (adjusted for age and gender) the no. of cases per million per year was 14.6 (2009), 18.4 (2010), 21.3 (2011), 24.6 (2012), 26.9 (2013), and 28.5 (2014) for all patients. [b] Adjusted based on distribution of age among males from both databases in 2014. [c] Adjusted based on distribution of age among females from both databases in 2014

Estimates from the current study are consistent with that reported from SEER for 2012 [10]. The incidence of all NET was reported as 69.8 PMPY for 2012 and lung NET as 16.3, and our combined, adjusted estimate was 16.2 PMPY in 2014 (although this rate from the combined databases should be interpreted with caution since it obscures differences between different sources). Although these numbers are quite similar, comparing our results directly to prior estimates presents several challenges. First, we were able to use data through 2014, 2 years more recent than SEER. Second, SEER, the source of data for the 2008 and 2017 studies, is a coordinated system of population-based cancer registries located across the US. The SEER Program collects cancer incidence and survival data from 18 geographic areas, together representing about 1/4 of the US population [22]. The insurance claims used in the present study, in contrast, are a convenience sample, albeit an extremely large one. Based on information provided by MarketScan and PharMetrics, the combined databases have claims for a geographically dispersed sample representing about 1/3 of the US population. Third, SEER includes patients of all ages; the current study only included individuals 18–64 years of age. About 95% of individuals ≥65 are covered by Medicare [12]. A small number of individuals in this age group would have been available for inclusion in our study (e.g. they had commercial insurance as the primary payer, and therefore, their data were included in our databases), but they do not represent typical Medicare-age individuals, and thus were excluded from analysis. The incidence of NET is twice as high in individuals ≥65 compared to those 50–64 [10]. Our estimates are thus likely to understate the actual incidence and prevalence. Fourth, SEER registrars are trained and provided with software to improve their ability to accurately code reportable cancers. Claims coding is performed by a mix of care providers and professional coders. Fourth, the coding systems differ between SEER and insurance claims. SEER currently uses the

International Classification of Diseases for Oncology system (ICD-O-3), whereas claims use ICD-9-CM (since 2015, ICD-10). While the systems can be mapped to each other, the mapping is not one-to-one. NET represent an unusual tumor type for which the traditional labels of benign and malignant are a poor fit. While classification has evolved considerably in the last several decades, NET are now generally described by their anatomic location (e.g., GI or lung), degree of differentiation (either "well" or "poorly"), and proliferative index (mitotic activity). Small, well differentiated NET may thus have been overlooked for inclusion into SEER [4]. Insurance claims, relying as they do on ICD-9-CM codes, cannot be used to identify stage or tumor size. Claims data cannot be used to identify with certainty whether a case is truly incident or represents a patient who simply did not present for care for a prolonged period. We required continuous enrollment for 2 years before the first NET claim to reduce this source of uncertainty. Prevalent patients would have to have had no care for their condition for more than 2 years to have been incorrectly counted as incident cases. Other limitations of insurance claims include the lack of information on race/ethnicity or health behaviors that might explain the observed rise in lung NET. Finally, we had no information on occurrence of, timing, or cause of death, making it impossible to comment on survival.

Despite these differences and data limitations, both the prior SEER study and the current study have identified some, although not entirely consistent, evidence of increasing incidence and prevalence of lung NET. The consistent pattern in 3 databases over more than 4 decades strongly suggests the increase in lung NET cases is not an artifact of the database chosen, the method used, or changes in patient enrollment over time. Recent increases in other cancer types have a variety of explanations. At least some portion of the recent increases in thyroid cancer appears to result from improved screening [23], but there also appears to be an underlying increase in disease incidence as well [24]. In NET, multiple mechanisms may be operating, and studies using other sources of data will be required to determine the extent to which each contributes to the observed rise.

Conclusions

The incidence and prevalence of lung NET appears to be increasing over time, although in the current study the gender- and database-specific findings are inconsistent. Although lung cancer overall appears to be on the decline in the US [25], an increase in NET in multiple anatomic locations, including lung NET, has been observed [10]. Pulmonologists, gastroenterologists, oncologists, and other physicians may see patients with these tumors with increasing frequency in years to come and may thus need to become more familiar with its presentation and treatment. Health plans will also see an increase in this previously rare disease and should consider ways to effectively manage this population. Finally, because higher incidence brings higher costs, studies assessing the increasing economic burden of this disease are warranted.

Abbreviations

5-HIAA: 5-hydroxyindoleacetic acid; APC: annual percent change; CPT-4: Current Procedural Terminology 4; ICD-9-CM: International Classification of Diseases, 9th Revision, Clinical Modification; ICD-O-3: International Classification of Diseases for Oncology system; NET: Neuroendocrine tumors; PMPY: Per million person-years; SEER: Surveillance Epidemiology, and End Results

Funding

This study was funded by Novartis Pharmaceuticals. The sponsor was involved in the study design, interpretation, and manuscript writing.

Authors' contributions

All authors meet the ICMJE criteria for authorship. MSB was involved in the conception, design, interpretation and writing of the manuscript. EC was involved in the conception, design, interpretation and statistical analyses and had final approval of the manuscript. BC was involved in the design, interpretation and had final approval of the manuscript. MN was involved in the conception, design, interpretation and had final approval of the manuscript. All authors read and approved the final manuscript.

Consent for publication

Not applicable

Competing interests

BC and MPN are employees of Novartis. MB and EC are employees of Partnership for Health Analytic Research, a health services research firm paid by Novartis to conduct this research.

Author details

[1]Partnership for Health Analytic Research, LLC, 280 S. Beverly Dr. Ste. 404, Beverly Hills, CA, USA. [2]Novartis Pharmaceuticals Corporation, One Health Plaza, East Hanover, New Jersey, USA.

References

1. Korse CM, Taal BG, van Velthuysen M-LF, Visser O. Incidence and survival of neuroendocrine tumours in the Netherlands according to histological grade: experience of two decades of cancer registry. Eur J Cancer. 2013;49:1975–83.
2. Modlin IM, Oberg K, Chung DC, Jensen RT, de Herder WW, Thakker RV, et al. Gastroenteropancreatic neuroendocrine tumours. Lancet Oncol. 2008;9:61–72.
3. Gustafsson BI, Kidd M, Modlin IM. Neuroendocrine tumors of the diffuse neuroendocrine system. Curr Opin Oncol. 2008;20:1–12.
4. Yao JC, Hassan M, Phan A, Dagohoy C, Leary C, Mares JE, et al. One hundred years after "carcinoid": epidemiology of and prognostic factors for neuroendocrine tumors in 35,825 cases in the United States. J Clin Oncol. 2008;26:3063–72.
5. Leoncini E, Carioli G, La Vecchia C, Boccia S, Rindi G. Risk factors for neuroendocrine neoplasms: a systematic review and meta-analysis. Ann Oncol. 2016;27:68–81.

6. Tsai H-J, Wu C-C, Tsai C-R, Lin S-F, Chen L-T, Chang JS. The epidemiology of neuroendocrine tumors in Taiwan: a nation-wide cancer registry-based study. PLoS One. 2013;8:e62487. Gorlova OY, editor
7. Fraenkel M, Kim M, Faggiano A, de Herder WW, Valk GD. On behalf of the knowledge NETwork. Incidence of gastroenteropancreatic neuroendocrine tumours: a systematic review of the literature. Endocr Relat Cancer. 2014;21: R153–63.
8. Ito T, Igarashi H, Nakamura K, Sasano H, Okusaka T, Takano K, et al. Epidemiological trends of pancreatic and gastrointestinal neuroendocrine tumors in Japan: a nationwide survey analysis. J Gastroenterol. 2015;50:58–64.
9. Hallet J, Law CHL, Cukier M, Saskin R, Liu N, Singh S. Exploring the rising incidence of neuroendocrine tumors: a population-based analysis of epidemiology, metastatic presentation, and outcomes. Cancer. 2015;121:589–97.
10. Dasari A, Shen C, Halperin D, Zhao B, Zhou S, Xu Y, et al. Trends in the incidence, prevalence, and survival outcomes in patients with neuroendocrine tumors in the United States. JAMA Oncol. 2017;3:1335.
11. Boudreaux JP, Klimstra DS, Hassan MM, Woltering EA, Jensen RT, Goldsmith SJ, et al. The NANETS consensus guideline for the diagnosis and management of neuroendocrine tumors: well-differentiated neuroendocrine tumors of the jejunum, ileum, appendix, and Cecum. Pancreas. 2010;39:753–66.
12. Smith JC, Medalia C. Health insurance coverage in the United States: 2014. In: U.S. Census Bureau current population reports. U.S. government printing office; 2015. https://www.census.gov/content/dam/Census/library/publications/2015/demo/p60-253.pdf. Accessed 24 Jan 2017.
13. Kleinbaum DG, Kupper LL, Muller KE. Applied regression analysis and other multivariable methods. 2nd ed. Boston: Duxbury Press; 1987.
14. Clegg LX, Hankey BF, Tiwari R, Feuer EJ, Edwards BK. Estimating average annual per cent change in trend analysis. Stat Med. 2009;28:3670–82.
15. Hassan MM, Phan A, Li D, Dagohoy CG, Leary C, Yao JC. Risk factors associated with neuroendocrine tumors: a U.S.-based case-control study. Int J Cancer. 2008;123:867–73.
16. Smith-Bindman R, Miglioretti DL, Johnson E, Lee C, Feigelson HS, Flynn M, et al. Use of diagnostic imaging studies and associated radiation exposure for patients enrolled in large integrated health care systems, 1996-2010. JAMA. 2012;307:2400–9.
17. Eberth JM, Sercy E. Implementation of lung Cancer screening in the United States: changing trends based on a survey of Society of Thoracic Radiology Members. J Thorac Imaging. 2015;30:W60–2.
18. Bajetta E, Ferrari L, Martinetti A, Celio L, Procopio G, Artale S, et al. Chromogranin a, neuron specific enolase, carcinoembryonic antigen, and hydroxyindole acetic acid evaluation in patients with neuroendocrine tumors. Cancer. 1999;86:858–65.
19. Modlin IM, Lye KD, Kidd M. A 5-decade analysis of 13,715 carcinoid tumors. Cancer. 2003;97:934–59.
20. Modlin IM, Lye KD, Kidd M. A 50-year analysis of 562 gastric carcinoids: small tumor or larger problem? Am J Gastroenterol. 2004;99:23–32.
21. Alsidawi S, Westin G, Hobday T, Halfdanarson T. Pancreatic neuroendocrine tumors: a population-based analysis of epidemiology and outcomes. 2017.
22. National Cancer Institute. SEER Program Overview. 2010. https://seer.cancer.gov/about/factsheets/SEER_Overview.pdf. Accessed 27 Jan 2017.
23. Davies L, Welch HG. Increasing incidence of thyroid cancer in the United States, 1973-2002. JAMA. 2006;295:2164–7.
24. National Cancer Institute. A snapshot of thyroid cancer. 2014. https://www.cancer.gov/research/progress/snapshots/thyroid. Accessed 27 Jan 2017.
25. Meza R, Meernik C, Jeon J, Cote ML. Lung cancer incidence trends by gender, race and histology in the United States, 1973-2010. PLoS One. 2015; 10:e0121323.

2

Disease progression in idiopathic pulmonary fibrosis with mild physiological impairment: analysis from the Australian IPF registry

Helen E. Jo[1,2*], Ian Glaspole[3], Yuben Moodley[4], Sally Chapman[5], Samantha Ellis[3], Nicole Goh[3,6], Peter Hopkins[7], Greg Keir[8], Annabelle Mahar[1], Wendy Cooper[1,2,9], Paul Reynolds[5], E. Haydn Walters[10,11], Christopher Zappala[12], Christopher Grainge[13], Heather Allan[14], Sacha Macansh[14] and Tamera J. Corte[1,2]

Abstract

Background: Idiopathic pulmonary fibrosis (IPF) is a progressive and fatal fibrosing lung disease of unknown cause. The advent of anti-fibrotic medications known to slow disease progression has revolutionised IPF management in recent years. However, little is known about the natural history of IPF patients with mild physiological impairment. We aimed to assess the natural history of these patients using data from the Australian IPF Registry (AIPFR).

Methods: Using our cohort of real-world IPF patients, we compared FVC criteria for mild physiological impairment (FVC ≥ 80%) against other proposed criteria: DLco ≥ 55%; CPI ≤40 and GAP stage 1 with regards agreement in classification and relationship with disease outcomes. Within the mild cohort (FVC ≥ 80%), we also explored markers associated with poorer prognosis at 12 months.

Results: Of the 416 AIPFR patients (mean age 70.4 years, 70% male), 216 (52%) were classified as 'mild' using FVC ≥ 80%. There was only modest agreement between FVC and DLco (k = 0.30), with better agreement with GAP (k = 0.50) and CPI (k = 0.48). Patients who were mild had longer survival, regardless of how mild physiologic impairment was defined. There was, however, no difference in the annual decline in FVC% predicted between mild and moderate-severe groups (for all proposed criteria). For patients with mild impairment (*n* = 216, FVC ≥ 80%), the strongest predictor of outcomes at 12 months was oxygen desaturation on a 6 min walk test.

Conclusion: IPF patients with mild physiological impairment have better survival than patients with moderate-severe disease. Their overall rate of disease progression however, is comparable, suggesting that they are simply at different points in the natural history of IPF disease.

Keywords: Idiopathic pulmonary fibrosis, Interstitial lung disease, Disease severity

Background

Idiopathic pulmonary fibrosis (IPF), a progressive fibrosing interstitial lung disease (ILD) of unknown cause, results in respiratory failure and ultimately death. Historically the median survival is thought to be only 2-5 years [1], and the incidence of IPF appears to be increasing globally [2]. Recently, two agents – nintedanib and pirfenidone – have demonstrated efficacy in slowing the rate of FVC decline as well as impacting on a number of other important disease outcomes [3–6]. However, each trial focused on cohorts with moderate physiologic impairment and the ASCEND trial excluded subjects with a forced vital capacity (FVC) above 90% predicted [3]. Although post-hoc analyses demonstrate comparable responses to anti-fibrotic therapy between participants with preserved lung volumes and those with more significant impairment, access to anti-fibrotic

* Correspondence: helen.jo@sydney.edu.au
[1]Royal Prince Alfred Hospital, Missenden Road, Camperdown, NSW 2050, Australia
[2]University of Sydney, Camperdown, NSW, Australia
Full list of author information is available at the end of the article

medications has been excluded from patients with lesser physiological impairment in several drug jurisdictions due to the limited nature of efficacy data for this cohort [7, 8].

There have been various attempts to define severity of IPF [9–11]. Physiologic measurements, such as FVC or diffusion capacity for carbon monoxide (DLco) have been commonly used [12, 13], as have composite measures of several physiologic values or demographic features [14, 15]. The two most commonly used composite scores are the composite physiological index (CPI) [14] and the GAP (gender, age and physiology) stage [15]. While both individual physiologic measurements and composite scores predict mortality, the ability of each to distinguish differences in disease progression among those with mild disease from those more significantly affected remains unknown. Clinically, the FVC has been used not only as a clinical trial endpoint, but also by funding authorities worldwide to limit access to anti-fibrotic medications.

The Australian IPF Registry (AIPFR), launched in 2012, recruits IPF patients from across Australia and a broad spectrum of impairment exists within its data set. Using this cohort, we sought to compare the FVC ≥ 80% with other severity criteria in their ability to distinguish differences in death and disease progression as measured by annual FVC decline, between mild and moderate-severe cohorts. Additionally, we investigated factors predicting poorer prognosis for patients with mild physiological impairment, to ascertain whether further characterisation may help select patients who would especially merit early drug intervention.

Methods

Participants

The Australian IPF Registry is a multi-centre, prospective, observational registry of incident and prevalent IPF patients across Australia. Details regarding the Australian IPF Registry data collection, structure and operations have previously been published [16]. The Registry has ethical approval to operate in all States and Territories and this analysis has ethical approval from the Sydney Local Health District ethics committee (protocol No X14–0264). All participants in the Registry were eligible for inclusion in this analysis.

Classification of mild disease

Using data from the Registry, patients were categorised as having mild physiological impairment using four different criteria. The primary analysis focused on FVC ≥ 80% predicted (exploratory analysis for FVC ≥ 90% FVC ≥ 75%, FVC ≥ 70%) [13], as this is the criteria used clinically to restrict anti-fibrotic therapies in many regions. Secondary analysis included: DLco ≥55% (exploratory analysis of DLco ≥50%, DLco ≥40%, DLco ≥30%) [12]; CPI ≤ 40 (exploratory analysis CPI ≤ 30, CPI ≤ 50) [14]; GAP stage 1 [15].

Only patients who had all the necessary information for calculation of all scores were included. The CPI was calculated using the formula: CPI = 91.0 - (0.65 × % predicted DLco) - (0.53 × % predicted FVC) + (0.34 × % predicted FEV_1) [14]. The GAP score was calculated using gender, age and physiology as outlined in Additional file 1: Table S1 [15].

Statistical methods

Data are presented as mean ± standard deviation (SD) and also range, or n (%), as appropriate. The agreement between the different criteria used to define mild impairment was assessed using kappa values. Univariable and multivariable Cox proportional models were performed to investigate the relationships between baseline variables, including disease severity classifications, with survival. All patients who received lung transplantation were censored at the date of transplant for time to event analyses. Survival curves were compared using the Kaplan-Meier method and log rank test.

An unstructured, linear mixed model for changes in FVC % predicted per year was fitted with random intercepts and slopes to compare the disease trajectory for patients with mild compared with moderate-severe physiological impairment, over the entire time of patient follow up in the Registry. Finally, logistic regression assessing a composite end-point of death or disease progression (defined as a relative fall in FVC ≥ 10% and/or DLco ≥ 15% from baseline) at 12 months was performed in patients with mild impairment (FVC ≥ 80%) at baseline, to determine markers associated with poorer short-term prognosis in this group.

Results

Baseline characteristics

Of the 647 patients in the Australian IPF Registry, there were 416 patients who had complete data for severity score measurements at baseline, and so available for inclusion in this study. Their baseline characteristics are displayed in Table 1. Interestingly, though less severe, patients with mild physiological impairment still had significant symptoms as measured by the St George Respiratory Questionnaire (SGRQ) and University of California San Diego shortness of breath Questionnaire (UCSD SOBQ). Comparisons of baseline demographic parameters of patients excluded from this analysis are available in Additional file 2: Table S2. Overall, patients who were excluded were slightly older and had more severe symptoms, similar to patients categorised as severe impairment using FVC ≤ 80% criteria (Table 1).

There were 114 deaths (27.4%) over a median follow up period of 2.09 years (IQR 1.56, 2.78 years) providing

Table 1 Baseline characteristics of patients in the Australian IPF Registry

Variable	n	overall	Mild (FVC ≥ 80%)	Moderate-Severe (FVC < 80%)	P[a]	Min	Max
			216	200			
Age, years	416	70.4 (8.6)	71.6 (7.9)	69.0 (9.1)	0.003	31.5	89.9
Male, n (%)	416	290 (69.7%)	125 (57.9%)	165 (82.5%)	<0.001		
Ever smoker, n (%)	416	308 (74.0%)	160 (74%)	148 (74%)	0.986		
BMI, kg/m^2	412	28.8 (4.8)	28.9 (5.0)	28.6 (4.6)	0.565	15.8	46.4
FVC, L	416	2.6 (0.8)	2.96 (0.79)	2.30 (0.54)	<0.001	0.9	4.8
FVC, % pred	416	81.7 (21.2)	97.3 (16.6)	64.9 (9.8)	<0.001	40.9	219.5
FEV_1/FVC ratio%	416	82.2 (8.4)	80.1 (8.6)	84.4 (7.5)	<0.001	27.0	135.0
DLco, % pred	416	48.5 (16.8)	54.6 (17.4)	41.8 (13.2)	<0.001	9.4%	143.7%
CPI	416	45.1 (14.1)	37.5 (13.2)	53.3 (9.7)	<0.001	54.2	74.5
GAP stage	416				<0.001		
GAP stage 1		192 (46.2%)	152 (70.4%)	40 (20.0%)			
GAP stage 2		186 (44.7%)	64 (29.6%)	122 (61.0%)			
GAP stage 3		38 (9.1%)	0 (0%)	38 (19.0%)			
6MWT distance, m	164	431.0 (119)	433 (115)	430 (122)	0.894	48.0	706.0
Initial SpO_2, %	163	95.5 (3.19)	95.8 (3.4)	95.4 (3.1)	0.482	83.0	100.0
End SpO_2, %	160	86.2 (7.2)	89.0 (7.0)	84.4 (6.8)	<0.001	58.0	99.0
Nadir SpO_2, %	153	85.3 (7.1)	87.9 (7.3)	83.6(6.5)	<0.001	58.0	99.0
SGRQ	383	43.0 (19.7)	38.7 (19.0)	47.6 (44.8)	<0.001	0.0	96.6
UCSD SOBQ	243	40.8 (29.3)	33.7(27.1)	48.6 (29.6)	<0.001	0.0	119.0
Cough severity	347	39.5 (23.5)	36.9 (22.9)	42.3(23.9)	0.034	0.0	100.0
Anti-fibrotic therapy	416	102 (24.5%)	52 (24.1%)	50 (25.0%)	0.826		

[a]comparison between mild and severe physiological impairment

914 patient-years of follow up. 17 (4.1%) patients underwent lung transplantation during the follow up period.

Agreement of proposed criteria for mild IPF

The FVC ≥ 80% categorised almost equal numbers of patients as having mild (*n* = 216, 52%) compared to moderate-severe impairment (*n* = 200, 48%), while a DLco ≥55% classified the least patients as having mild disease (*n* = 131, 32%) (Fig. 1). We also undertook exploratory analysis of other threshold levels and as expected, the change in threshold values had a significant impact on the proportion of patients classified as mild for FVC, DLco and in particular CPI (Additional file 3: Figure S1).

Mild physiological impairment defined by FVC ≥ 80% had modest agreement with GAP stage 1 (k = 0.50) and CPI ≤ 40 (k = 0.48) and only fair agreement with DLco ≥ 55% (k = 0.30). CPI ≤ 40 had the best agreement with other variables including DLco ≥ 55% (k = 0.74) and GAP

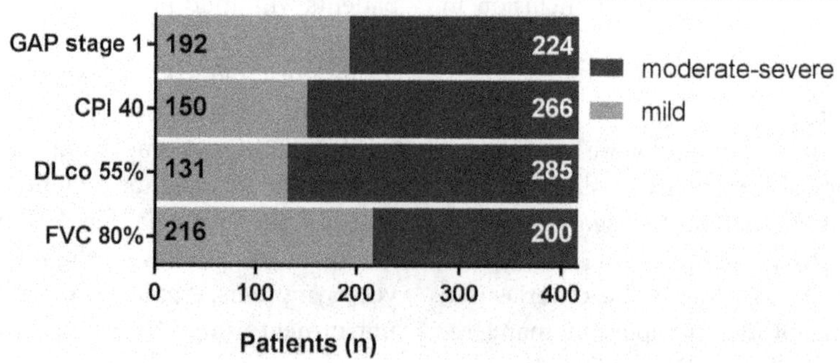

Fig. 1 Classification as mild disease using different mild definitions

stage 1 (k = 0.68). There was good agreement between GAP stage 1 and DLco ≥ 55% (k = 0.61).

Factors predictive of death

As demonstrated in Table 2, on univariable analysis, demographic characteristics (age, gender, BMI, smoking status), physiology, and symptom scores (SGRQ, UCSD SOBQ), except cough severity (measured at baseline on a visual analogue scale), all predicted increased mortality for the entire IPF population.

The presence of mild impairment at baseline (by all proposed criteria) was also predictive of better survival than those patients with moderate-severe disease, on univariable as well as multivariable analysis including age, gender, BMI and smoking status (Table 3). There was a wide separation in the Kaplan-Meier curves for mild versus moderate-severe physiological impairment (Fig. 2).

Disease progression

The disease progression of patients with mild impairment, measured as change in FVC % predicted per year compared to those with moderate-severe impairment are shown in Table 4 and Fig. 3. There was no difference in the annual rate of FVC% predicted decline between the mild and moderate-severe cohorts, regardless of the disease severity classification used, with the predicted annual fall for the entire cohort calculated at 4.4 units (of FVC % predicted)/year. In a exploratory analysis, locally weighted scatterplots of FVC% predicted were constructed for patients with mild and moderate-severe disease and again demonstrated similar disease trajectories in these groups (Additional file 4: Figure S2).

Table 2 Univariable Cox analysis

	n	HR	95% CI		p
Age	416	1.03	1.01	1.05	0.013
male	416	1.96	1.25	3.08	0.003
BMI	412	0.94	0.89	0.98	0.003
Smoking	416	1.93	1.20	3.11	0.007
Physiology					
FVC (L)	416	0.56	0.43	0.74	<0.001
FVC (%pred)[a]	416	0.71	0.64	0.79	<0.001
DLco (%pred)[a]	416	0.56	0.49	0.64	<0.001
6MWD[b]	164	0.82	0.73	0.92	0.001
SpO2 at rest	163	0.88	0.82	0.95	0.001
SpO2 at end	160	0.92	0.88	0.95	<0.001
SpO2 nadir	153	0.92	0.89	0.96	<0.001
CPI	416	1.09	1.07	1.11	<0.001
GAP stage	416	4.48	3.37	5.95	<0.001
Patient reported outcomes					
SGRQ total[c]	383	1.11	1.06	1.15	<0.001
UCSD SOBQ[a]	243	1.23	1.13	1.33	<0.001
Cough severity[a]	347	1.08	0.99	1.17	0.069

BMI body mass index, *FVC* forced vital capacity, *DLco* diffusion capacity for carbon monoxide, *CPI* composite physiological index, *GAP* gender age physiology, *6MWD* 6 min walk distance, *SpO2* peripheral blood oxygen saturation, *SGRQ* St George's Respiratory Questionniare, *UCSD- SOBQ* University of California San Diego shortness of breath questionnaire. [a]For every 10 unit change; [b] for every 50 m change; [c]for every 4 point change

Table 3 Univariable and multivariable Cox analysis for disease severity

	HR	95% CI	p	HR	95% CI	p
	Univariable analysis			Multivariable analysis[a]		
FVC < 80%	3.21	2.17–4.75	<0.001	3.15	2.11–4.71	<0.001
DLco < 55%	6.28	3.28–12.03	<0.001	5.55	2.88–10.70	<0.001
CPI > 40	7.28	3.90–13.57	<0.001	6.60	3.52–12.39	<0.001
GAP stage 1	7.09	4.27–11.76	<0.001	7.44	4.18–13.25	<0.001

[a]Multivariable model includes age, gender, BMI and smoking status and includes 412 of 416 available for univariable model

Factors predicting progression or death at 12 month in the mild disease group

There were 216 patients with FVC ≥ 80% categorised as having mild impairment. Overall, these patients had preserved lung volume with a mean FVC of 97.3% predicted, DLco of 54.6% predicted and were mostly categorised as GAP stage 1 (70.4%) with the remainder as GAP stage 2 (29.6%). Unsurprisingly, they were less symptomatic than those with more severe disease, though they still had significant symptoms. Interestingly, patients with mild impairment were slightly older and more likely to be female (Table 1).

Within the cohort of patients with mild impairment, the prognostic markers which predicted death or progression at 12 months were evaluated using univariable logistic regression. There were 22 patients (10.2%) who died or progressed within 12 months. The only factor that predicted death or progression at 12 months was oxygen desaturation during 6 min walk testing at baseline (OR 0.89, 95% CI 0.81, 0.98; $p = 0.024$ for every 1% change in nadir SpO_2) (Table 5).

Unsurprisingly, within this cohort with mild impairment, other lung function parameters and composite scores were not predictive of death or progression. On a multivariable logistic regression model including age, gender, BMI and smoking status, nadir oxygen saturation during 6MWT remained a significant predictor of poorer outcome (OR 0.89, 95%CI 0.80, 0.98; p = 0.024).

Discussion

In our cohort of IPF patients from the Australian IPF Registry, we demonstrate that a significant proportion of

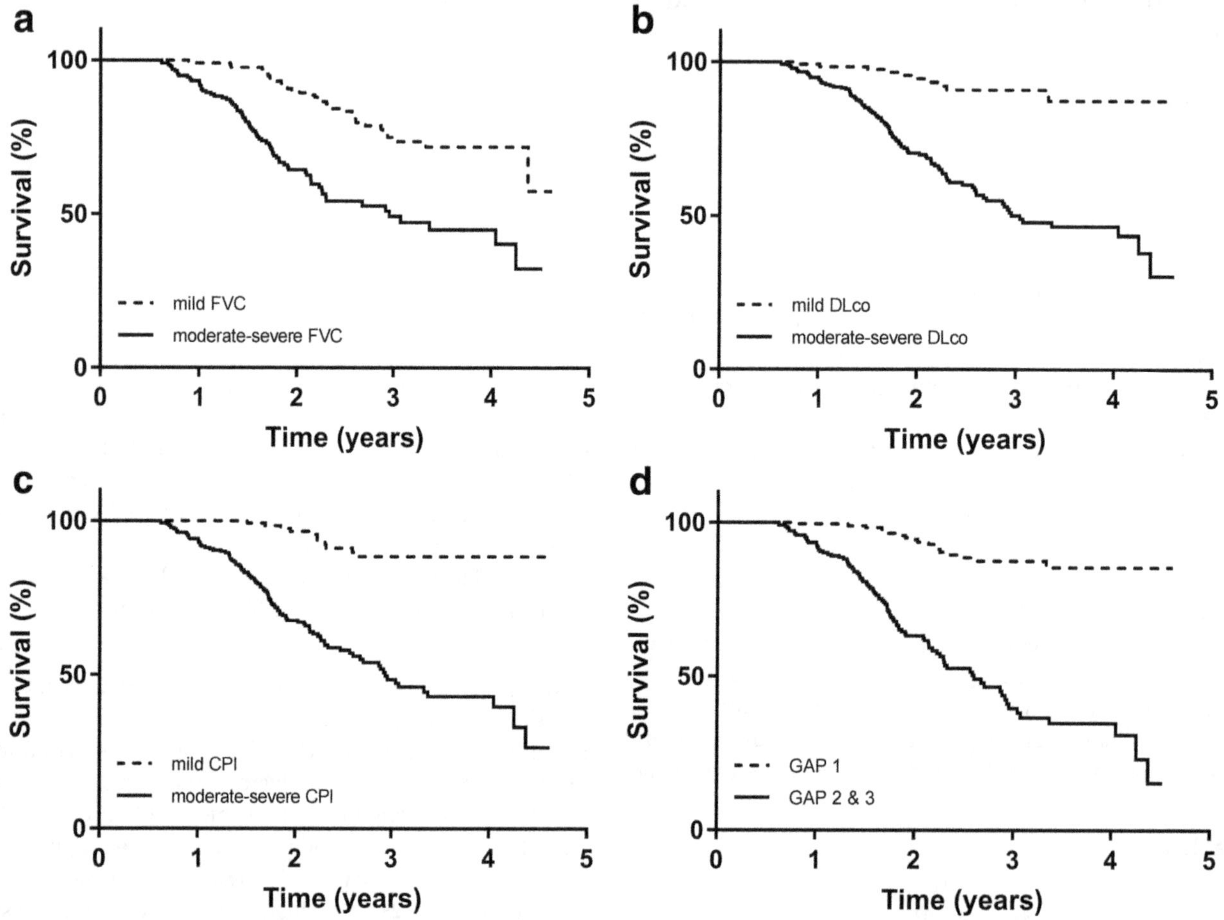

Fig. 2 Kaplan Meier analysis for time to death by disease category. **a**. Kaplan Meier analysis according to FVC 80%. Log rank test $p < 0.001$. **b**. Kaplan Meier analysis according to DLco 55%. Log rank test p < 0.001. **c**. Kaplan Meier analysis according to CPI 40. CPI (composite physiological index). Log rank test p < 0.001. **d**. Kaplan Meier analysis according to GAP stage. GAP (Gender, Age, Physiology). Log rank test p < 0.001

IPF patients have mild physiological impairment; though this proportion varied depending on the criteria and threshold used to define mild impairment. We demonstrate that the agreement for mild impairment using FVC ≥ 80% was modest to fair with other proposed criteria. We also show that patients who are mild have better survival than patients those with moderate-severe physiological impairment. Importantly, we show that patients with mild impairment, regardless of the criteria for categorisation used, have a similar annual rate of

Table 4 Annual FVC % predicted decline by disease category and severity

	mild	95% CI	more severe	95% CI	P[a]
FVC	−4.6%	−5.8;-3.4%	−4.9%	−6.3; −3.5%	0.779
DLco	−4.9%	−6.0;-3.8%	−4.7%	−5.7; −3.7%	0.702
CPI	−5.0%	−6.3; −3.6%	−4.5%	−5.7; −3.3%	0.600
GAP	−5.0%	−6.3; −3.8%	−4.4%	−5.8; −3.0%	0.517

[a]comparison of mild to moderate-severe group

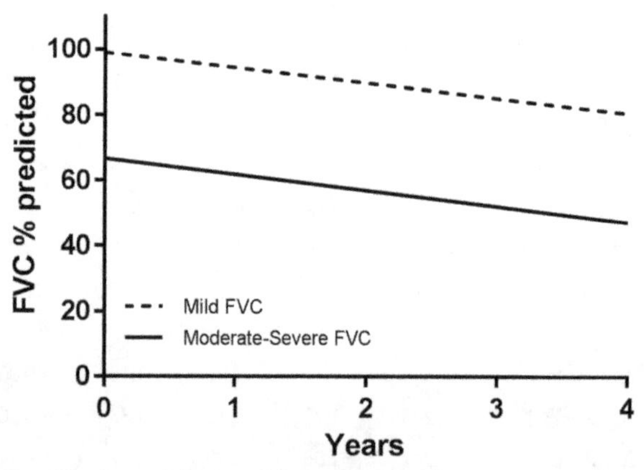

Fig. 3 Decline in FVC % predicted in mild (FVC ≥ 80%) compared with moderate-severe (FVC < 80%) physiological impairment. Graphical representation of annual FVC% decline as calculated by unstructured linear mixed model with random intercept and slopes for mild and moderate-severe disease

Table 5 Logistic regression for death or disease progression at 12 months in patients with FVC ≥ 80%

	n	OR	95% CI		p
Age	216	0.99	0.94	1.05	0.847
male	216	0.86	0.35	2.09	0.739
BMI	212	1.00	0.92	1.10	0.954
Ever smoker	216	0.93	0.34	2.50	0.879
FVC % pred[a]	216	0.81	0.56	1.16	0.241
DLco %pred[a]	216	0.87	0.67	1.14	0.312
CPI[a]	216	1.26	0.86	1.86	0.234
GAP stage	216	1.12	0.43	2.90	0.813
6 MWD[b]	63	0.75	0.54	1.04	0.083
SpO2 at start	63	0.86	0.71	1.03	0.108
SpO2 at end	63	0.89	0.81	0.98	0.021
SpO2 nadir	59	0.89	0.81	0.98	0.024
SGRQ[c]	199	1.02	0.93	1.12	0.688
UCSD SOBQ[a]	126	1.00	0.77	1.28	0.970
Cough severity[a]	177	1.16	0.95	1.41	0.136

BMI body mass index, *FVC* forced vital capacity, *DLco* diffusion capacity for carbon monoxide, *CPI* composite physiological index, *GAP* gender age physiology, *6MWD* 6 min walk distance, *SpO2* peripheral blood oxygen saturation, *SGRQ* St George's Respiratory Questionniare, *UCSD- SOBQ* University of California San Diego shortness of breath questionnaire. [a]For every 10 unit change; [b] for every 50 m change; [c] for every 4 point change

decline in FVC % predicted compared to those with more severe impairment. Finally, we show that in patients with mild impairment, the prognostic marker most predictive of death or progression at 12 months was oxygen desaturation on the 6 min walk test (6MWT).

One important finding of this study was that IPF patients with mild physiological impairment had the same disease trajectory, with comparable annual decline in FVC to those with moderate-severe disease. This mirrors the results found in the post-hoc analysis of pirfenidone [8] and nintedanib trial cohorts [7] whereby patients with mild physiological impairment were shown to have comparable disease progression at 12 months to their more severe counterparts. Unlike the clinical trial cohorts however, Registry patients are real-world, unselected IPF patients with frequent significant co-morbidities. Registry patients also have a wide spectrum of IPF disease severity with 68 patients below the threshold for inclusion in clinical trials (FVC < 50%, n = 9; DLco <30% n = 47, and n = 6 for both), and are managed by respiratory physicians throughout Australia, not limited to tertiary referral centres. The reproducibility of this finding in this heterogeneous cohort strengthens the generalisability of the post-hoc analysis from the large therapeutic clinical trials [7, 8]. It is also important to note that even patients with mild physiological impairment had significant symptoms. Ultimately, these results suggest that patients with preserved physiology are likely to represent an earlier stage of the natural history of IPF, rather than a separate and milder cohort of IPF patients with a specific natural history.

Another important finding of our study was that within the cohort of patients with mild impairment, the degree of oxygen desaturation on the 6MWT was the only significant short-term prognostic marker. Whilst previous studies have demonstrated that the 6MWT distance [17–19] and oxygen desaturation [20, 21] on 6MWT can predict mortality in IPF, this test is often not performed on a regular basis (as demonstrated in this study by the smaller number of patients who have had this test). The desaturation on the 6MWT is likely to represent a complex interplay between, and cumulative impact of, the physiological changes that occur in IPF including pulmonary hypertension, ventilation/perfusion mismatch and diffusion limitation. Our data suggests that in a cohort with relatively preserved lung function, where individual pulmonary function variables provide no additional prognostic value, the performance of the 6MWT is prognostically important.

We also highlight the differences between various proposed criteria for IPF severity, reflecting the need for a standardised approach to disease severity stratification. While we found in our cohort a significant overlap using these various definitions for mild physiological impairment, there were also significant discrepancies. Furthermore, there was only fair concordance between FVC and DLco, with the FVC ≥80% classifying more patients as mild than DLco ≥55%. This likely reflects the effects of the pulmonary function thresholds chosen, and was highlighted by the considerable variability in classification with different thresholds used in the exploratory analysis (see Additional file 3). The better concordance with composite values, as opposed to between single measures such as FVC and DLco, arises from the fact that both these single measures contribute to the calculation of the composite scores. It is interesting to note that the DLco and the composite scores were better at predicting survival suggesting that, while it is commonly used, the FVC threshold may not be the most clinically useful criteria.

Our study has several limitations. Firstly, this was a retrospective analysis of a prospective observational study and all investigations were performed as part of the patients' routine clinical care, resulting in some variability in the investigations performed. In particular, in clinical practice in Australia, there is variability between centres in routinely undertaking a 6MWT, for which we had baseline data for 164 individuals overall, and 63 patients in the groups with FVC ≥ 80%. Despite the limited numbers, we were able to show a significant difference in outcomes, highlighting the strength of this association, a finding that we hope will now affect national clinical practice. Also, while there is a standardised guide for the 6MWT, there is likely to be variation between centres. The potential importance of this association between desaturation on 6MWT and prognosis also highlights the importance of confirming these findings in a larger, prospective cohort with standardised testing.

Conclusion

In summary, accurate clinical staging has important implications in IPF as it can inform initial patient management, prognostication and standardisation of clinical trials and their outcomes. Patients with mild physiological impairment have better overall survival, although their rate of disease progression appears the same as seen in those with moderate-severe impairment, with differences in outcome being attributable to where the patient sits in the natural history of their disease. Given their apparent identical disease trajectory and significant symptoms, this study adds impetus to the view that patients with mild impairment be offered anti-fibrotic therapy early in their disease course. This is particularly so for those with significant desaturation on the 6MWT, as they appear to have the poorest outcomes.

Additional files

Additional file 1: Table S1. GAP stage calculation.

Additional file 2: Table S2. Baseline characteristics of patients excluded from analysis.

Additional file 3: Figure S1. Exploratory analysis of varying thresholds.

Additional file 4: Figure S2. Locally Weighted Scatterplot Smoothing curves for FVC% predicted. a. Mild physiological impairment (FVC ≥ 80%). b. Moderate-severe physiological impairment (FVC < 80%). c. Summary of LOWESS curve means.

Abbreviations

6MWD: 6 min walk distance; 6MWT: 6 min walk test; AIPFR: Australian Idiopathic Pulmonary Fibrosis Registry; ASCEND: Assessment of Pirfenidone to Confirm Efficacy and Safety in Idiopathic Pulmonary Fibrosis; BMI: body mass index; CAPACITY: Clinical Studies Assessing Pirfenidone in idiopathic pulmonary fibrosis: Research of Efficacy and Safety Outcomes; COPD: chronic obstructive pulmonary disease; CPI: composite physiological index; DLco: diffusion capacity for carbon monoxide; FVC: forced vital capacity; GAP: Gender, Age, Physiology; ILD: interstitial lung disease; IPF: idiopathic pulmonary fibrosis; NHS: National Health Service; SD: standard deviation; SGRQ: St George's Respiratory Questionnaire; SpO2: peripheral blood oxygen saturation; TOMORROW: To improve pulmonary fibrosis with BIBF 1120; UCSD SOBQ: University of California San Diego shortness of breath questionnaire

Acknowledgements

The writers thank all the participants and physicians who contribute to the Registry, as well as the Registry secretariat and co-coordinators who work tirelessly to gather and collate information. We also thank Alfred Health Solutions and Alfred Medical Imaging who are integral to the development and maintenance of the web-based radiology database.

Funding

Lung Foundation Australia has established the Australian IPF Registry with the generous support of a philanthropic family and unrestricted educational grants from Foundation partners Roche Products, Pty. Limited and Boehringer Ingelheim and Project partner Bristol-Myers Squibb Australia. This analysis has been funded by support from the National Health and Medical Research Council (APP1066128). All data analysis, interpretation and writing was performed by the authors of the manuscript without input from funding bodies.

Authors' contributions

HJ, TC and IG conceived the study. HJ analysed the data and together with TC, wrote the manuscript. All authors contributed to data collection and read and approved the final manuscript.

Consent for publication

Not applicable. This manuscript does not contain any individual person's data in any form.

Competing interests

The authors declare that they have no competing interests.

Author details

[1]Royal Prince Alfred Hospital, Missenden Road, Camperdown, NSW 2050, Australia. [2]University of Sydney, Camperdown, NSW, Australia. [3]The Alfred Hospital, Melbourne, VIC, Australia. [4]Fiona Stanley Hospital, Murdoch, WA, Australia. [5]Royal Adelaide Hospital, Adelaide, SA, Australia. [6]The Austin Hospital, Heidelberg, VIC, Australia. [7]Prince Charles Hospital, Chermside West, QLD, Australia. [8]Princess Alexandria Hospital, Woolloongabba, QLD, Australia. [9]School of Medicine, Western Sydney University, Parramatta, NSW, Australia. [10]School of Medicine, University of Tasmania, Hobart, TAS, Australia. [11]University of Tasmania, Hobart, TAS, Australia. [12]Royal Brisbane and Women's Hospital, Herston, QLD, Australia. [13]John Hunter Hospital, New Lambton Heights, NSW, Australia. [14]Lung Foundation Australia, Milton, QLD, Australia.

References

1. Raghu G, Collard HR, Egan JJ, Martinez FJ, Behr J, Brown KK, Colby TV, Cordier JF, Flaherty KR, Lasky JA, et al. An official ATS/ERS/JRS/ALAT statement: idiopathic pulmonary fibrosis: evidence-based guidelines for diagnosis and management. Am J Respir Crit Care Med. 2011;183(6):788–824.
2. Hutchinson J, Fogarty A, Hubbard R, McKeever T. Global incidence and mortality of idiopathic pulmonary fibrosis: a systematic review. Eur Respir J. 2015;46(3):795–806.
3. King TE Jr, Bradford WZ, Castro-Bernardini S, Fagan EA, Glaspole I, Glassberg MK, Gorina E, Hopkins PM, Kardatzke D, Lancaster L, et al. A phase 3 trial of pirfenidone in patients with idiopathic pulmonary fibrosis. N Engl J Med. 2014;370(22):2083–92.
4. Richeldi L, du Bois RM, Raghu G, Azuma A, Brown KK, Costabel U, Cottin V, Flaherty KR, Hansell DM, Inoue Y, et al. Efficacy and safety of nintedanib in idiopathic pulmonary fibrosis. N Engl J Med. 2014;370(22):2071–82.
5. Noble PW, Albera C, Bradford WZ, Costabel U, du Bois RM, Fagan EA, Fishman RS, Glaspole I, Glassberg MK, Lancaster L, et al. Pirfenidone for idiopathic pulmonary fibrosis: analysis of pooled data from three multinational phase 3 trials. Eur Respir J. 2016;47(1):243–53.

6. Richeldi L, Cottin V, du Bois RM, Selman M, Kimura T, Bailes Z, Schlenker-Herceg R, Stowasser S, Brown KK. Nintedanib in patients with idiopathic pulmonary fibrosis: combined evidence from the TOMORROW and INPULSIS trials. Respir Med. 2016;113:74–9.
7. Kolb M, Richeldi L, Behr J, Maher TM. Nintedanib in patients with idiopathic pulmonary fibrosis and preserved lung volume. Thorax. 2017;72(4):340–6.
8. Albera C, Costabel U, Fagan EA, Glassberg MK, Gorina E, Lancaster L, Lederer DJ, Nathan SD, Spirig D, Swigris JJ. Efficacy of pirfenidone in patients with idiopathic pulmonary fibrosis with more preserved lung function. Eur Respir J. 2016;48(3):843–51.
9. Kolb M, Collard HR. Staging of idiopathic pulmonary fibrosis: past, present and future. Eur Respir Rev. 2014;23(132):220–4.
10. Sharp C, Adamali HI, Millar AB. A comparison of published multidimensional indices to predict outcome in idiopathic pulmonary fibrosis. ERJ open research. 2017;3:1.
11. King TE Jr, Tooze JA, Schwarz MI, Brown KR, Cherniack RM. Predicting survival in idiopathic pulmonary fibrosis: scoring system and survival model. Am J Respir Crit Care Med. 2001;164(7):1171–81.
12. Mogulkoc N, Brutsche MH, Bishop PW, Greaves SM, Horrocks AW, Egan JJ, Greater Manchester Pulmonary Fibrosis C. Pulmonary function in idiopathic pulmonary fibrosis and referral for lung transplantation. Am J Respir Crit Care Med. 2001;164(1):103–8.
13. Erbes R, Schaberg T, Loddenkemper R. Lung function tests in patients with idiopathic pulmonary fibrosis. Are they helpful for predicting outcome? Chest. 1997;111(1):51–7.
14. Wells AU, Desai SR, Rubens MB, Goh NS, Cramer D, Nicholson AG, Colby TV, du Bois RM, Hansell DM. Idiopathic pulmonary fibrosis: a composite physiologic index derived from disease extent observed by computed tomography. Am J Respir Crit Care Med. 2003;167(7):962–9.
15. Ley B, Ryerson CJ, Vittinghoff E, Ryu JH, Tomassetti S, Lee JS, Poletti V, Buccioli M, Elicker BM, Jones KD, et al. A multidimensional index and staging system for idiopathic pulmonary fibrosis. Ann Intern Med. 2012; 156(10):684–91.
16. Jo HE, Glaspole I, Grainge C, Goh N, Hopkins PM, Moodley Y, Reynolds PN, Chapman S, Walters EH, Zappala C, et al. Baseline characteristics of idiopathic pulmonary fibrosis: analysis from the Australian idiopathic pulmonary fibrosis registry. Eur Respir J. 2017;49:2.
17. Lederer DJ, Arcasoy SM, Wilt JS, D'Ovidio F, Sonett JR, Kawut SM. Six-minute-walk distance predicts waiting list survival in idiopathic pulmonary fibrosis. Am J Respir Crit Care Med. 2006;174(6):659–64.
18. Caminati A, Bianchi A, Cassandro R, Mirenda MR, Harari S. Walking distance on 6-MWT is a prognostic factor in idiopathic pulmonary fibrosis. Respir Med. 2009;103(1):117–23.
19. du Bois RM. 6-minute walk distance as a predictor of outcome in idiopathic pulmonary fibrosis. Eur Respir J. 2014;43(6):1823–4.
20. Flaherty KR, Andrei AC, Murray S, Fraley C, Colby TV, Travis WD, Lama V, Kazerooni EA, Gross BH, Toews GB, et al. Idiopathic pulmonary fibrosis: prognostic value of changes in physiology and six-minute-walk test. Am J Respir Crit Care Med. 2006;174(7):803–9.
21. Hallstrand TS, Boitano LJ, Johnson WC, Spada CA, Hayes JG, Raghu G. The timed walk test as a measure of severity and survival in idiopathic pulmonary fibrosis. Eur Respir J. 2005;25(1):96–103.

3

Effectiveness of nasal highflow in hypercapnic COPD patients is flow and leakage dependent

Jens Bräunlich*†, Friederike Mauersberger† and Hubert Wirtz

Abstract

Background: Nasal Highflow (NHF) delivers a humidified and heated airflow via nasal prongs. Current data provide evidence for efficacy of NHF in patients with hypoxemic respiratory failure. Preliminary data suggest that NHF may decrease hypercapnia in hypercapnic respiratory failure. The aim of this study was to evaluate the mechanism of NHF mediated PCO_2 reduction in patients with chronic obstructive pulmonary disease (COPD).

Methods: In 36 hypercapnic COPD patients ($PCO_2 > 45$ mmHg), hypercapnia was evaluated by capillary gas sampling 1 h after NHF breathing under four conditions A to D with different flow rates and different degrees of leakage (A = 20 L/min, low leakage, two prongs, both inside; B = 40 L/min, low leakage, two prongs, both inside; C = 40 L/min, high leakage, two prongs, one outside and open; D = 40 L/min, high leakage, two prongs, one outside and closed). Under identical conditions, mean airway pressure was measured in the hypopharynx of 10 COPD patients.

Results: Hypercapnia significantly decreased in all patients. In patients with capillary $PCO_2 > 55$ mmHg ($n = 26$), PCO_2 additionally decreased significantly by increased leakage and/or flow rate in comparison to lower leakage/ flow rate conditions (A = 94.2 ± 8.2%; B = 93.5 ± 4.4%; C = 90.5 ± 7.2%; D = 86.8 ± 3.8%). The highest mean airway pressure was observed in patients breathing under condition B (2.3 ± 1.6 mbar; $p < 0.05$).

Conclusions: This study demonstrates effective PCO_2 reduction with NHF therapy in stable hypercapnic COPD patients. This effect does not correlate with an increase in mean airway pressure but with increased leakage and airflow, indicating airway wash out and reduction of functional dead space as important mechanisms of NHF therapy. These results may be useful when considering NHF treatment in hypercapnic COPD patients.

Keywords: COPD, Hypercapnia, Nasal high flow, Type II respiratory failure, Wash-out

Background

Ventilatory support systems have become an important therapeutic mean in patients with chronic respiratory disease. These devices create a gradient between atmospheric pressure and airway pressure, thus establishing a driving pressure during inspiration as well as a variable amount of positive end expiratory airway pressure. Respiratory frequency and a minimum minute volume may be specified. This kind of ventilator support improves alveolar ventilation and consecutively reduces PCO_2 [1]. The aim of non-invasive ventilation support is an improvement of respiratory muscle function by partially relieving respiratory muscle load and, subsequently, the normalization of setpoint values of the sensors of the respiratory system.

A novel development in non-invasive ventilation support is the application of a constant high nasal airflow with 20 to 60 L/min. This technique is known as nasal high flow (NHF) therapy. Patients tolerate flow rates in this order of magnitude when gas is warmed and humidified close to body standard temperature and humidity before entering the nose. In addition, the gas mixture may contain any fraction of oxygen set from 0.21 to 1.0.

* Correspondence: jens.braeunlich@uniklinik-leipzig.de
†Equal contributors
Department of Respiratory Medicine, University of Leipzig, Liebigstrasse 20, 04103 Leipzig, Germany

NHF therapy has become frequently used in the treatment of neonatal patients as an alternative to nasal continuous positive airway pressure (nCPAP) therapy [2]. However, there are increasing data that demonstrate the benefits of NHF therapy also in adult patients. Maggiore et al. [3] were able to show superiority in oxygen delivery and reintubation rate of NHF therapy over Venturi mask oxygen therapy following extubation of patients with acute respiratory failure. In their study, Frat et al. [4] demonstrated that in patients with primary respiratory failure, NHF therapy is equally effective and partially superior to oxygen supply and non-invasive ventilation (NIV) in terms of reduced intubation rates. In the study of Stéphan et al. [5], NHF therapy was shown not to be inferior to NIV in patients who suffered from respiratory failure after cardiothoracic surgery. Furthermore, Hernandez and colleagues documented benefits in patients with low and high risk of postextubation respiratory failure [6, 7]. The results of these studies emphasize the benefits and the safety of NHF therapy in the treatment of acute hypoxemic respiratory failure. However, when compared to conventional NIV, much less experience is available from clinical studies on NHF therapy. In fact, the standard indications of NIV, acute and chronic hypercapnic respiratory failure, have not been investigated yet.

Few studies have investigated the effect of NHF therapy on e.g. hypercapnia in patients with chronic obstructive pulmonary disease (COPD), but the number of patients recruited in these studies is limited [8–13]. In addition, the mechanisms that may lead to a decrease in hypercapnia have not been elucidated so far. Some authors suggest the increase in airway pressure to be responsible for the effects of NHF therapy [14, 15]. However, the increase in airway pressure seems to be rather small. Another possible explanation focuses on the wash out effect within the upper airways [16, 17]. Frizzola et al. [18] investigated the mechanism of NHF therapy in a piglet model of lung injury. In this model, the reduction of PCO_2 during NHF, as opposed to the situation in NIV, did not correlate with tracheal pressure but was more efficient, when leakage of gas from the nose was increased. The authors therefore suggested that wash out of nasopharyngeal dead space by nasally applied high flow improves CO_2 removal in the piglet model. The high flow generated by NHF can pass functional dead space more easily and may therefore economize the work of breathing [19–21]. The aim of this study was therefore to investigate whether the effects of NHF therapy in hypercapnic COPD patients depend on flow rates, airway pressure, and leakage.

Methods

Study design/ outcome parameters

This study had a prospective, unblinded, and single-center design. Outcome parameters were changes in capillary PCO_2, PO_2, and mean airway pressure during various flow rates and leakage conditions.

Patients

For this study, 46 patients were recruited in the department of respiratory medicine of the University hospital Leipzig in 2015. The study was approved (414–14-06102014) and registered (ClinicalTrails NCT02504814) by the ethics committee of the Medical Faculty, University of Leipzig. All patients gave written informed consent to participate in the study. Criteria for inclusion in the study were a diagnosis of COPD (GOLD), $PCO_2 > 45$ mmHg, chronic ventilatory insufficiency with hypercapnia without additional metabolic alterations, > 18 years of age, and a stable stage of disease. Patients with acute ventilatory insufficiency (pH < 7.35), instable disease (e.g. exacerbation, systemic inflammation, pneumonia), incomplete or untapped medical therapy, other lung diseases, inadequate compliance to any kind of treatment, as well as fertile women and patients participating in other trails were excluded.

NHF ventilator

In this study, the TNI20s oxy device (TNI medical AG, Wuerzburg, Germany) was used. The system was equipped with an additional humidifier/heater (Hydrate OMNI™, Hydrate Inc., Midlothian, USA) to ensure the intended higher flow rates because the original humidifier was not able to sufficiently humidify when flow rates were higher than 24 L/min. Flow rates were additionally verified with an electronic flowmeter (TSI 4000 Series®, TSI Inc., Shoreview, USA). With these modifications, the NHF system provided stable flow rates of up to 50 L/min and allowed the admixture of oxygen.

Measuring changes in hypercapnia

Patients were randomly assigned to undergo sequences of treatment conditions. Randomization was computer-generated with a sequence of numbers, and each number was associated with a character (1 = A, 2 = B, 3 = C, 4 = D). Some patients were treated by all conditions. Changes in hypercapnia were measured in 36 COPD patients who had undergone NHF therapy for 1 h. Capillary blood gas samples were taken prior to NHF therapy, 30 min after the beginning, and immediately after completion of one condition at 60 min. The starting PCO_2 prior to NHF therapy was considered as baseline PCO_2. If more than one of the four possible NHF conditions were tested in one patient at 1 day, a treatment-free interval of at least 2 h between the two conditions was assured. Note that if patients were given continuous oxygen insufflations within the scope of their regular therapy, oxygen supply was neither altered nor interrupted during the duration of NHF treatment.

The leakage and flow combinations tested (conditions A – D) were combinations of two different flow rates (20 L/min and 40 L/min) and two degrees of leakage (NHF applied through one or two nostrils; Fig. 1). Note that in condition C, the effective flow rate was 20 L/min with the device set at 40 L/min but with only one of two equal prongs inserted to one nostril.

Blood gas analysis

Blood samples for capillary blood gas analyses were obtained from a hyperemic earlobe after 10 min of treatment with a vasodilatation ointment (Finalgon®, Boehringer Ingelheim Pharma GmbH & Co. KG, Ingelheim am Rhein, Germany). All measurements were performed with constant oxygen supplementation as indicated.

Measuring mean airway pressure in COPD patients

Mean airway pressure was measured in 10 patients with COPD. First, a water-filled thin flexible tube (1 mm in diameter, Original Perfusor®-cable type standard, B. Braun, Melsungen, Germany) was connected to a pressure sensor (GMH3111, Greisinger electronic GmbH, Regenstauf, Germany). The free end was inserted in the nasopharynx under visual control. The electronic pressure sensor was hooked to a computer. A total of 10 breaths were recorded during spontaneous breathing (baseline) and another 10 breaths were recorded during each of the experimental conditions.

Statistics

The sample size of 36 had 85% power, with a type I error rate of 5%, to detect a difference in capillary pCO_2 of 5%. Data were analyzed using single factor ANOVA. If F > F crit, we rejected the null hypothesis. Additionally, we used Student's t-test (Sigma Plot, Systat Software GmbH, Ekrath, Germany) to compare each pair of means (in case of rejecting null hypothesis). A p-value <0.05 was considered as significant.

Results

Demographic data are presented in Table 1. NHF significantly reduced PCO_2 in comparison to baseline in all patients (A: 95.3 ± 8.0%, n = 22; B: 95.6 ± 5.8%, n = 19; C: 94.5 ± 9.9%, n = 20; D: 95.1 ± 8.6%, n = 19). No significant differences were observed between the four experimental conditions with regard to PCO_2 after treatment.

A total of 26 out of 36 patients recruited for PCO_2 measurements had a baseline PCO_2 > 55 mmHg. In this hypercapnic subgroup of COPD patients, PCO_2 was significantly reduced by all conditions (A-D). The reduction of capillary PCO_2 by condition A was more pronounced when the flow rate was increased from 20 to 40 L/min (condition A = > B). The increase of leakage and the reduction of the effective flow rate (by using only one nostril) to 20 L/min (condition C) resulted in an even greater decrease. Yet, the largest reduction of capillary PCO_2 was obtained after increasing the flow rate in a single prong to 40 L/min by occluding the prong that was located outside the nostrils (condition D). Between conditions A and D, there was an additional significant decrease in PCO_2 (Table 2, Fig. 2). There was no significant difference between the capillary PCO_2 values obtained after 30 min and those obtained after 60 min of NHF therapy.

In all measurements, capillary PO_2 did not differ significantly although a trend to lower values was observed under conditions B to D (Fig. 3). PH increased significantly under conditions B, C, and D.

Mean airway pressure was measured in 10 patients (Table 2, Fig. 4). In contrast to the above-mentioned results, mean airway pressure achieved its maximum with condition B (Fig. 4). Significant pressure differences to baseline were only observed with conditions A and B.

Discussion

In this study, we found a leakage and flow dependent decrease of hypercapnia in COPD patients by NHF treatment. These data support the assumption that elimination of CO_2 during NHF therapy is independent of an increase of mean airway pressure.

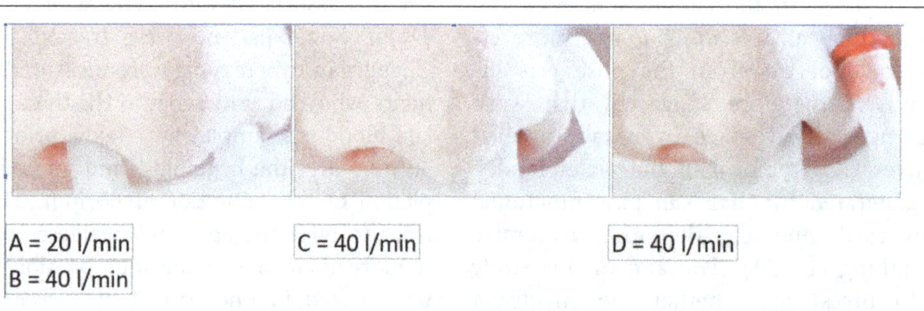

Fig. 1 Experimental conditions. A = 20 L/min, low leakage, two prongs, both inside; B = 40 L/min, low leakage, two prongs, both inside; C = 40 L/min, high leakage, two prongs, one outside and open; D = 40 L/min; high leakage, two prongs, one outside and closed

Table 1 Demographic and clinical data of all patients

Characteristics	Study participants (*n* = 36)
Age (years; mean ± SD)	60.5 ± 14.3
Gender male (n): female (n)	19: 17
Oxygen insufflation (L/min; mean ± SD)	1.9 ± 1.4
FEV1 (% predicted; mean ± SD)	29.9 ± 13.3
FEV1%FVC (predicted; mean ± SD)	54.1 ± 17.5
Rtot (% predicted; mean ± SD)	346.9 ± 153.5
TLC (% predicted; mean ± SD)	111.6 ± 21.3
RV (% predicted; mean ± SD)	210.3 ± 78.3
RV%TLC (% predicted; mean ± SD)	183.4 ± 40.2
pH (mean)	7.4029 ± 0,039
PO_2 (mmHg; mean ± SD)	66.3 ± 18.4
PCO_2 (mmHg; mean ± SD)	58.9 ± 9.8

FEV1 forced expiratory volume in 1 s, *FVC* forced vital capacity, *Rtot* resistance, *RV* residual volume, *TLC* total lung capacity, *SD* standard deviation

NHF therapy is increasingly investigated for use in clinical practice. Its benefits have been demonstrated in the treatment of patients with acute respiratory insufficiency (ARI) due to pulmonary causes and in the prevention of postextubation respiratory failure [3–7]. In addition, smaller reports have suggested the use of NHF therapy in other medical indications [8–11]. Potential NHF applications are still to be defined, and the NHF mechanism of action needs to be further elucidated. In particular, the effects on oxygenation, hypercapnia, and dyspnea need to be characterized [3, 9].

Little is known about the mechanisms that underlie NHF therapy. Previous studies have demonstrated increases in airway pressure [8] but the changes in airway pressure were small. In our study, mean airway pressure increased with NHF therapy, confirming previous results [8, 10]. Increase of flow rates resulted in an increase in airway pressure. It achieved its maximum under the conditions of setting B where gas was supplied through both nostrils (low leakage condition) with the highest flow rate tested (40 L/min). Mean airway pressure appeared to depend on the flow rate since doubling the effective flow rate (A = > B, C = > D) led to increased mean airway pressures in both cases. However, the mean airway pressure also depended on the degree of leakage (B vs. D), in line with the notion that pressure is released through leaking nostrils. Thus, in addition to the confirmation that NHF therapy leads to a flow dependent increase in mean airway pressure, our results indicate that the increase in mean airway pressure also depends on the degree of leakage, or vice versa to the extent to which the upper airways are occluded (nostrils, mouth). In adults, the nostrils are only partially occluded by the prongs, whereas in neonates, the prongs can completely obstruct the nostrils, which leads to a larger increase in mean airway pressure, rendering NHF treatment more similar to nCPAP therapy [2]. This signifies a fundamental difference between the ways in which NHF therapy works in neonates and adults.

If the increase in airway pressure was the principal reason accounting for the clinical effects of NHF therapy in adults, capillary PCO_2 should achieve its minimum when mean airway pressure rises to its maximum, but this is not what was observed in this study. In contrast, in our study, PCO_2 achieved its minimum with condition D, whereas mean airway pressure reached its maximum with condition B. Increased leakage (B = > C) resulted in a greater decrease in PCO_2 that went along with a decrease of mean airway pressure, demonstrating that the reduction in PCO_2 is not due to an increase in mean airway pressure. Rather, it relies on a higher degree of leakage and a concomitant airway wash out. This wash out affects the upper airways, as shown by Möller et al. who demonstrated CO_2 elimination from nasal dead space and reduction of CO_2-rebreathing under NHF therapy [16]. A model study by Bräunlich et al.

Table 2 Changes of mean airway pressure and PCO_2 in patients with baseline PCO_2 > 55 mmHg under different experimental conditions

	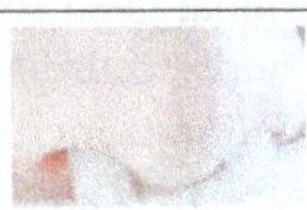	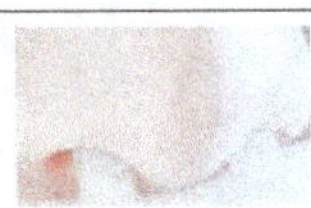	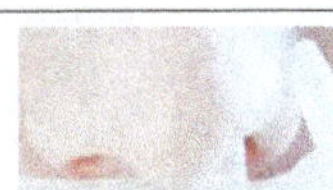	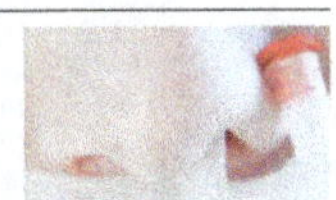
Condition	A	B	C	D
Mechanically gene-rated flow rate (L/min)	20	40	40	40
Effective nasal flow rate (L/min)	20	40	20	40
Mean airway pressure (mbar ± SD)	0.57 ± 0.38 *p* = 0.03	2.3 ± 1.6 *p* = 0.02	1.63 ± 1.4 *p* = 0.08	2.13 ± 1.7 *p* = 0.05
PO_2 (% baseline PO_2 ± SD)	99.2 ± 18.9 *p* = 0.2	93.1 ± 15.7 *p* = 0.18	93.8 ± 17.6 *p* = 0.12	93.5 ± 11.9 *p* = 0.05
PCO_2 (% baseline PCO_2 ± SD)	94.2 ± 8.3 *p* = 0.01	93.5 ± 4.4 *p* = 0.000	90.5 ± 7.2 *p* = 0.005	86.8 ± 3.8 *p* = 0.001

All values are mean ± SD. *SD* standard deviation

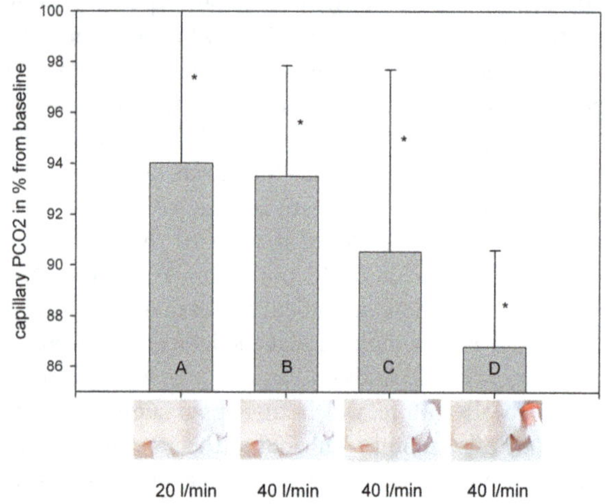

Fig. 2 Percentage decrease in capillary PCO_2 in COPD patients after 1 h of NHF breathing under different experimental conditions. * $= p < 0.05$ vs. baseline; baseline $PCO_2 > 55$ mmHg, **a**: $n = 14$, **b**: $n = 11$, **c**: $n = 9$, **d**: $n = 9$

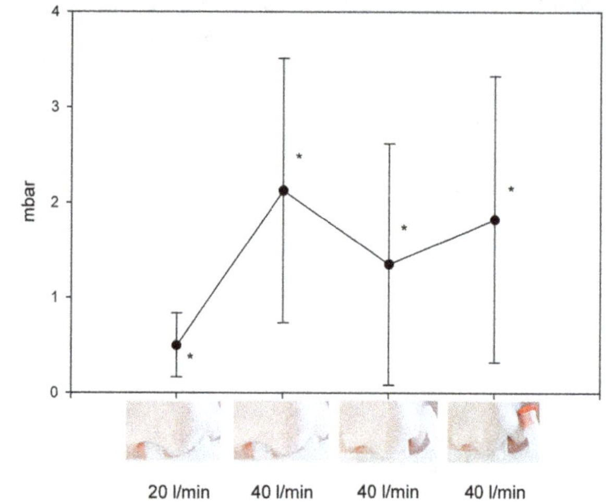

Fig. 4 Changes in mean airway pressure in COPD patients under different experimental conditions. * $= p < 0.05$ vs. baseline; $n = 10$

[17] indicated that CO_2 wash out may extend to the lower airways. Our data confirm previous data obtained by Frizzola et al. who demonstrated that the reduction of PCO_2 with NHF therapy in piglets similarly depends on the degree of leakage [18].

As shown in this study, oxygen saturation tended to slightly decrease when using higher flow rates and constant oxygen supplementation. This observation is not surprising because FIO_2 decreased by applying higher amounts of room air and stable oxygen supplementation. We aimed at integrating this observation into our study because of both insufficient literature data and the hypothesis that reduction in oxygen can lead to a reduction in PCO_2. Interestingly, there was no change in PO_2 under low flow/low leakage of condition A. This study supports the observed necessity to increase rates of supplemented oxygen to keep FIO_2 constant at higher flow rates. The non-significant decrease in oxygen cannot be the reason for decreased PCO_2 levels in this study because of (1) constant oxygen values in different settings and regardless decreasing PCO_2 values (conditions B, C, D) [10], (2) stable PO_2 and decreased PCO_2 values when using 20 L/min (condition A) [8, 10, 12, 21], and (3) documented reduction of respiratory rates despite of PO_2 reduction [8, 10, 22].

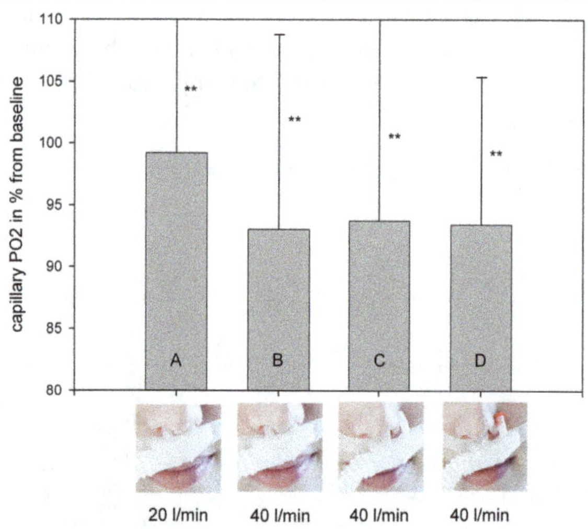

Fig. 3 Percentage decrease of capillary PO_2 in COPD patients after 1 h of NHF breathing under different experimental conditions. ** $= p > 0.05$ vs. baseline; baseline $PCO_2 > 55$ mmHg, **a**: $n = 14$, **b**: $n = 11$, **c**: $n = 9$, **d**: $n = 9$

NHF therapy partially relieves the work of breathing in COPD patients [10, 13, 21]. This is also evidenced from the increase in tidal volume and concomitant decrease in respiratory rate as well as the reduction in minute volume as previously reported [10]. In hypercapnia, respiratory muscle function deteriorates, resulting in reduced tidal volumes and higher respiratory rates. This, in turn, leads to a decrease of alveolar ventilation. Dead space ventilation increases in proportion to overall ventilation. By constantly placing the air/oxygen mixture in the airways, functional dead space is reduced and tidal volume can adjust and, accordingly, declines. If kept constant, alveolar ventilation is increased. Together with the wash out of airways, NHF is able to work as a ventilation support device.

Study limitations

Our study has three limitations. Since experiments were time consuming and some patients tolerated only few measurements, it was not possible to test all four conditions within the clinical setting. Bias cannot entirely be excluded because patients as well as investigators could not be blinded regarding the different experimental conditions. The fact that only COPD patients were tested could limit the generalizability of our findings.

Conclusions

In the present study, we showed that NHF therapy significantly reduces capillary PCO_2 in COPD patients. Higher flow rates and increased leakage of the upper airways appear to increase the effectiveness in reducing PCO_2. At the same time, an increase in airway pressure is not required. Our data indicate that airway wash out is the major mechanism of action in NHF breathing.

Abbreviations

(n) CPAP: (nasal) continuous positive airway pressure; ANOVA: Analysis of variance; ARI: Acute respiratory insufficiency; BGA: Blood gas analysis; COPD: Chronic obstructive pulmonary disease; NHF: Nasal highflow; PCO_2: Partial pressure of CO_2; PO_2: Partial pressure of O_2

Acknowledgements

We thank Sebastian Sewerin for critical revision of the manuscript. We acknowledge support from the German Research Foundation (DFG) and Leipzig University within the program of Open Access Publishing.

Funding

The study was supported by TNI medical AG (Wuerzburg, Germany). TNI medical AG had no influence on the design of the study, collection, analysis, and interpretation of data as well as on the preparation of the manuscript.

Authors' contributions

JB contributed to the literature research, data collection, study design, analysis of data, and manuscript preparation. FM contributed to the literature research, data collection, study design, analysis of data, and manuscript preparation. HW contributed to the literature research, data collection, study design, analysis of data, and revision of the manuscript. All authors read and approved the final manuscript.

Consent for publication

Not applicable.

Competing interests

JB received travel grants and equipment from TNI medical AG (Wuerzburg, Germany). FM declares that he/she has no competing interests. HW received lecture fees from TNI medical AG.

References

1. Dreher M, Storre JH, Schmoor C, Windisch W. High-intensity versus low-intensity non-invasive ventilation in patients with stable hypercapnic COPD: a randomised crossover trial. Thorax. 2010;65:303–8.
2. Manley BJ, Manley BJ, Owen LS, Owen LS, Doyle LW, Doyle LW, et al. High-flow nasal cannulae in very preterm infants after extubation. N Engl J Med. 2013;369:1425–33.
3. Maggiore SM, Idone FA, Vaschetto R, Festa R, Cataldo A, Antonicelli F, et al. Nasal high-flow versus Venturi mask oxygen therapy after Extubation. Effects on oxygenation, comfort, and clinical outcome. Am J Respir Crit Care Med. 2014;190:282–8.
4. Frat J-P, Thille AW, Mercat A, Girault C, Ragot S, Perbet S, et al. Supplementary appendix: high-flow oxygen through nasal cannula in acute hypoxemic respiratory failure. N Engl J Med. 2015;372:2185–96.
5. Stéphan F, Barrucand B, Petit P, Rézaiguia-Delclaux S, Médard A, Delannoy B, et al. High-flow nasal oxygen vs noninvasive positive airway pressure in hypoxemic patients after cardiothoracic surgery. JAMA. 2015;313:2331–9.
6. Hernández G, Vaquero C, González P, Subira C, Frutos-Vivar F, Rialp G, et al. Effect of Postextubation high-flow nasal Cannula vs conventional oxygen therapy on Reintubation in low-risk patients: a randomized clinical trial. JAMA. 2016;315:1354–61.
7. Hernández G, Vaquero C, Colinas L, Cuena R, González P, Canabal A, et al. Effect of Postextubation high-flow nasal Cannula vs noninvasive ventilation on Reintubation and Postextubation respiratory failure in high-risk patients: a randomized clinical trial. JAMA. 2016;316:1565–74.
8. Bräunlich J, Beyer D, Mai D, Hammerschmidt S, Seyfarth H-J, Wirtz H. Effects of nasal high flow on ventilation in volunteers, COPD and idiopathic pulmonary fibrosis patients. Respiration. 2013;85:319–25.
9. Bräunlich J, Seyfarth H-J, Wirtz H. Nasal high-flow versus non-invasive ventilation in stable hypercapnic COPD: a preliminary report. Multidiscip Respir Med. 2015;10:27.
10. Bräunlich J, Köhler M, Wirtz H. Nasal highflow improves ventilation in patients with COPD. COPD. 2016;11:1077–85.
11. Jeong JH, Kim DH, Kim SC, Kang C, Lee SH, Kang T-S, et al. Changes in arterial blood gases after use of high-flow nasal cannula therapy in the ED. Am J Emerg Med Elsevier. 2015;33:1344–9.
12. Fraser JF, Spooner AJ, Dunster KR, Anstey CM, Corley A. Nasal high flow oxygen therapy in patients with COPD reduces respiratory rate and tissue carbon dioxide while increasing tidal and end-expiratory lung volumes: a randomised crossover trial. Thorax. 2016;71:759–61.
13. Pisani L, Fasano L, Corcione N, Comellini V, Musti MA, Brandao M, et al. Change in pulmonary mechanics and the effect on breathing pattern of high flow oxygen therapy in stable hypercapnic COPD. Thorax. 2017; 72:373–5.
14. Groves N, Tobin A. High flow nasal oxygen generates positive airway pressure in adult volunteers. Aust Crit Care. 2007;20:126–31.
15. Parke R, McGuinness S, Eccleston M. Nasal high-flow therapy delivers low level positive airway pressure. Br J Anaesth. 2009;103:886–90.
16. Möller W, Celik G, Feng S, Bartenstein P, Meyer G, Oliver E, et al. Nasal high flow clears anatomical dead space in upper airway models. American Physiological Society. 2015;118:1525–32.
17. Bräunlich J, Goldner F, Wirtz H. Nasal Highflow eliminates CO2 from lower airways. Respir Physiol Neurobiol. 2017;242:86–8.
18. Frizzola M, Miller TL, Rodriguez ME, Zhu Y, Rojas J, Hesek A, et al. High-flow nasal cannula: impact on oxygenation and ventilation in an acute lung injury model. Pediatr Pulmonol. 2011;46:67–74.
19. Delorme M, Bouchard P-A, Simon M, Simard S, Lellouche F. Effects of high-flow nasal Cannula on the work of breathing in patients recovering from acute respiratory failure. Crit Care Med. 2017;
20. Nahum A, Ravenscraft SA, Nakos G, Adams AB, Burke WC, Marini JJ. Effect of catheter flow direction on CO2 removal during tracheal gas insufflation in dogs. J Appl Physiol. 1993;75:1238–46.
21. Biselli PJC, Kirkness JP, Grote L, Fricke K, Schwartz AR, Smith P, et al. Nasal high-flow therapy reduces work of breathing compared with oxygen during sleep in COPD and smoking controls: a prospective observational study. J Appl Physiol. 2017;122:82–8.
22. Roca O, Riera J, Torres F, Masclans JR. High-flow oxygen therapy in acute respiratory failure. Respir Care. 2010;55:408–13.

4

Chronic airflow obstruction in Tanzania

Thomas Zoller[1,2,3,4,5], Elirehema H. Mfinanga[2], Tresphory B. Zumba[2], Peter J. Asilia[2], Edwin M. Mutabazi[2], David Wimmersberger[1,5], Florian Kurth[3,4], Francis Mhimbira[2], Frederick Haraka[1,2,5] and Klaus Reither[1,5,6*]

Abstract

Background: Chronic obstructive pulmonary disease is a global problem and available data from sub-Saharan Africa is very limited.

Methods: A cross-sectional facility-based pilot study among patients and visitors to an urban and a rural primary healthcare facility was conducted in coastal Tanzania. The primary outcome was the prevalence of chronic airflow obstruction.

Results: The final analysis included 598 participants with valid post-bronchodilator spirometry. Applying ATS/ERS spirometric criteria, chronic airflow obstruction was found in $n = 24$ (4%, CI_{95} 2.7–5.9) participants and in $n = 30$ (5%, CI_{95} 3.5–7.1) applying GOLD spirometric criteria. To analyse risk factors for chronic airflow obstruction including those not meeting ATS/ERS or GOLD criteria, FEF_{25-75} and FEV1% predicted was analysed in participants without evidence of pulmonary restriction among those exposed or not exposed to risk factors ($n = 552$). FEV1% predicted, but in particular FEF_{25-75} decreased with increasing symptom severity of shortness of breath as well as limitations in daily activities of participants. Cooking in general and cooking with biomass fuels vs. gas or electricity was associated with significantly lower FEF_{25-75}, but not with lower FEV1% predicted. Participants having refrained from taking a job because of shortness of breath exhibited lower FEF_{25-75} ($p < 0.01$). A history of prior active TB was the most relevant risk factor associated with a decrease in FEF_{25-75} as well as FEV1% predicted.

Conclusion: This study demonstrated a relevant prevalence of chronic airflow obstruction in primary healthcare attendants and healthy visitors of a Tanzanian hospital. Using the baseline data provided, larger and population-based studies are needed to validate these findings. TB may have more impact on development of chronic airway obstruction than smoking in Africa. Due to the influence of age on the GOLD definition of chronic airflow obstruction, studies should report results using both ATS/ERS and GOLD definitions and include age-stratified analysis. Analysis of FEV1 and in particular FEF_{25-75} may yield additional information on risk factors and earlier stages of chronic airflow obstruction.

Keywords: COPD, Airflow obstruction, Tuberculosis, Tanzania

Background

Chronic airflow obstruction (CAO), caused by a chronic inflammation of airways in response to exposure to dusts and fumes is a characteristic feature of chronic obstructive pulmonary disease (COPD). CAO leads to a decline in lung function and to subsequent loss of exercise capacity. Cigarette smoking is the major causative factor for CAO in industrialized countries [1], leading to an overall population prevalence between 5% and 25% in Europe, North America, Latin America and Asia [2–5].

COPD is a disease mainly affecting higher age groups and most studies have so far addressed the population above the age of 40 years. Little is known however on prevalence and risk factors of COPD in developing countries with younger populations, and particularly in sub-Saharan Africa. Recently, the BOLD study investigated prevalences of CAO on a global level and provided data from Latin America and Asia as well as data from

* Correspondence: klaus.reither@swisstph.ch
[1]Swiss Tropical and Public Health Institute, Basel, Switzerland
[5]University of Basel, Basel, Switzerland
Full list of author information is available at the end of the article

two study sites in Africa [2, 3, 6, 7]. Previous studies in sub-Saharan Africa have mostly focussed on risk groups with occupational exposure such as miners [8–11].

Epidemiology and risk factors of COPD in developing countries likely differ from those in the developed world. While cigarette smoking is less common in developing countries, factors like prolonged exposure to biomass fuels from cooking starting from early childhood, cooking indoors in rooms shared for living and sleeping purposes, high TB prevalence and different age structure have relevant influence on COPD epidemiology [12]. At present, it is unclear which effects this life-long exposure to biomass fuels in Africa has for the development of chronic obstructive pulmonary disease. Moreover, there is little data on chronic obstructive pulmonary disease in young African populations.

To gather data on CAO in Tanzania, we examined patients attending primary healthcare facilities as well as persons accompanying patients using a questionnaire and performed pre- and post-bronchodilator spirometry. Tanzanian Lung Health Study (TLHS) aims to provide first estimates on CAO in Tanzania and to explore risk factors as well as medical and social aspects of CAO, providing baseline data for further studies on a larger scale. Moreover, TLHS aims to give additional information on analysis of spirometric outcomes other than the standard definitions of CAO and their diagnostic value to detect earlier stages of small airways disease in an African setting.

Methods

A cross-sectional facility-based study was conducted among attendants, accompanying persons and visitors to the rural Bagamoyo District Hospital (Bagamoyo, Pwani, Tanzania), and the urban Mwananyamala Regional Hospital (Dar es Salaam, Tanzania) between October 2015 and September 2016. Both study centres are located in coastal Tanzania without mining industry or exposure to other region-specific lung hazards. The primary outcome was spirometric evidence of CAO. Secondary outcomes were risk factors and parameters indicating social impact. Participants were eligible for inclusion if they were at least 18 years of age and either attendants of a primary healthcare clinic for any reason other than an acute respiratory problem, persons accompanying patients or visitors to the hospital visiting inpatients. Participants visiting the hospital for other reasons, having medical contraindications against bronchodilator drugs or having any other physical or mental condition limiting the ability to obtain a valid spirometry result were excluded (hospitalisation within <3 months, newly diagnosed heart disease within <3 months, uncontrolled hypertension, resting heart rate > 100/min., uncontrolled diabetes, pregnancy, acute infections or fever, acute pain, smoking during the last 2 h, thoracic or abdominal surgery within <3 months or any other severe physical or mental disease limiting the ability to comply with instructions for spirometry). To allow analysis of outcomes in patients across all relevant age groups, age-stratified sampling was used. Within age-strata, participants were invited randomly using a predefined selection procedure.

A sample size of 600 participants was intended to provide an acceptable prevalence estimate with 2.5% precision for this pilot study assuming a prevalence of 10% of chronic airflow obstruction.

After obtaining informed consent either in writing or by an impartial witness, participants were interviewed by a trained physician or a study nurse to obtain data on lung health and TB history and trained in performing spirometry supported by a video.

After spirometry was performed, patients inhaled 4 times 100 μg of salbutamol under supervision of a nurse using a spacer. Spirometry was repeated after 15 min. Quality criteria for spirometry were applied according to the 2005 ATS/ERS guidelines [13]. Spirometer readings were checked for acceptability and repeatability criteria by the physician performing the test and checked again by a senior pulmonologist. Only spirometer readings meeting all acceptability as well as repeatability criteria (minimum grade A and B) were finally accepted. Spirometry was performed using the NDD EasyONE World Spirometer (Zürich, Switzerland). Spirometric prediction equations of the Global Lung Function Initiative for African Americans were used [14].

Spirometric data was analysed for prevalence of CAO applying the FEV1/FVC < 5th percentile predicted (LLN) method (ATS/ERS spirometric criteria) as well as the GOLD definition with a fixed FEV1/FVC ratio < 0.7. A positive bronchodilator response was defined as an increase of FEV1 and/or FVC >12% and at least 200 ml compared to baseline. To further assess airflow obstruction including earlier stages, the post-bronchodilator forced expiratory flow at 25–75% of forced vital capacity (FEF_{25-75}) [15] and the FEV1% predicted were used. As pulmonary restriction influences FEF_{25-75} and FEV1% predicted, participants with evidence of restriction (FVC < 5th percentile of FVC predicted and FEV1/FVC >0.85, as defined by ATS/ERS criteria [16]) were excluded from this analysis.

Data was analysed using JMP ver. 14. Median FEF_{25-75} and FEV1% predicted values were compared among participants exposed vs. unexposed to risk factors for CAO. Parameters were compared between risk groups using the Mann-Whitney-U-test to compare two and the Kruskal-Wallis-Test to compare multiple groups. X_2 test was used to compare categorical outcomes between groups. Differences were considered significant when p was <0.05.

Results

Study population

A total of 1224 participants either attending or visiting the two health facilities of the study gave informed consent. 195 participants were excluded due to violating exclusion criteria and 32 participants due to incomplete datasets. 399 patients did not produce a post-bronchodilator spirometry meeting ATS/ERS quality criteria despite intensive video-assisted training and were excluded. The study population included 598 participants with valid post-bronchodilator spirometry.

We analysed if the population of participants not able to produce a spirometry according to ATS/ERS quality criteria was different from the study population in the final analysis. Slightly more women were excluded based on this criterion (54.6% vs. 45.3%, $p = 0.05$), but there was no significant difference in terms of age (median 46 vs. 45 years, $p = 0.23$), history of active TB infection ($p = 0.93$), visitors vs. patients ($p = 0.4$), education ($p = 0.46$), reason for seeking medical attention among patients ($p = 0.71$) and smoking status ($p = 0.07$).

Demographic and social characteristics

The median age of the study population was 46 years (IQR 37–57 years) across the different age groups invited for participation, and 72% of patients were at least 40 years old (for details see Table 1). There was an equal gender distribution. The majority of participants (60%) were visitors to the hospital or persons accompanying patients to primary healthcare clinics. The level of education was generally low, with most participants having either no (29%) or only primary school (48%) education. Main occupations were business and trade (29%) as well as farming and agriculture (24%). The leading reasons for seeking medical attention for patients attending primary healthcare clinics were infections/fevers (17%), musculosceletal problems and injuries (15%) and cardiovascular problems (14%). The majority of participants cooked with charcoal (60%) and wood (25%), and only few participants with gas (8%).

CAO prevalence and bronchodilator response

Applying ATS/ERS criteria, CAO was found in $n = 24$ (4.0%, CI_{95} 2.7–5.9) participants and $n = 30$ (5.0%, CI_{95} 3.5–7.1) met GOLD spirometric criteria for CAO. There was an obvious difference in CAO prevalence across age groups using the two definitions. Applying ATS/ERS criteria, prevalence of CAO increased only moderately with age from 3.6% to 5.6% in 4 age groups, whereas prevalence defined by GOLD spirometric criteria was only 1.8% in participants <40 years of age, but 11.3% in participants >60 years of age (for details see Table 2). Overall, $n = 46$ (7.7%, CI_{95} 5.8–10.1) showed a positive bronchodilator response. Most participants meeting either ATS/ERS or GOLD spirometric criteria had either mild or moderate levels of obstruction (see Table 3).

Table 1 Demographic and social characteristics of the study population

		N	% of study population
Age group	18–39	169	28
	40–59	299	50
	60–79	124	21
	> = 80	6	1
Gender	Male	310	52
	Female	288	48
Type of participant	Patient of hospital	242	40
	Visitor to hospital	356	60
Education	No formal education	173	29
	Primary school	289	48
	Secondary school	99	17
	University/college	31	1
Occupation[a]	Business and trade	172	29
	Farming and agriculture	141	24
	Craftsmen	38	6
	Drivers	21	4
Reasons for seeking medical attention (patients)[a]	Infections/fevers	41	17
	Musculosceletal problems	35	15
	Cardiovascular problems	33	14
	Gastrointestinal problems	29	12
	Non-acute respiratory problems	25	10
	Urogenital/ reproductive problems	13	5
Cooking fuel	Charcoal	360	60
	Wood in open stove	137	23
	Wood in open fire	12	2
	Gas	49	8
Smoking status	Never smoker	435	73
	Current or recent smoker	87	15
	Ex-smoker (≥6 months abstinence)	76	13

[a]Only major categories shown

Correlation of symptoms and limitations of daily activities with spirometry

Current definitions of CAO only allow to define presence or absence of obstruction and may not capture

Table 2 Prevalence of chronic airflow obstruction in the study population according to spirometric criteria of ATS/ERS using FEV1/FVC < 5th percentile predicted (LLN) method or the Global Initiative for Chronic Obstructive Lung Disease (GOLD) criteria

Risk factor	Group	n	Meet criteria	%	CI_{95}
CAO (LLN)	All	598	24	4.0	2.7–5.9
	Age groups				
	18–39	169	6	3.6	1.6–7.5
	40–59	299	11	3.7	2.0–6.5
	60–79	124	7	5.6	2.8–11.2
	> = 80	6	0	0	
CAO (GOLD)	All	598	30	5.0	3.5–7.1
	Age groups				
	18–39	169	3	1.8	0.6–5
	40–59	299	13	4.3	2.5–7.3
	60–79	124	14	11.3	6.8–18
	> = 80	6	0	0	

more subtle changes in airflow obstruction; we analysed therefore FEF_{25-75} as well as FEV1% predicted values in participants without evidence of restriction ($n = 552$) in an exploratory analysis and correlated spirometric values with symptoms and limitations in daily life, and with parameters causing social impact. Participants graded the level of respiratory symptoms (shortness of breath, coughing) and social impact (limitation of daily activities or at work, limitation of activities at home) on a scale between 0 (no symptoms) and 3 (severe/frequent symptoms), and for coughing up to 4 (constant symptoms). The results are shown in Fig. 1. Symptom severity increased and indicators for social impact deteriorated with decreasing FEF_{25-75} and FEV1% predicted.

Table 3 Severity of CAO according to spirometric criteria of ATS/ERS using FEV1/FVC < 5th percentile predicted (LLN) method or the Global Initiative for Chronic Obstructive Pulmonary Disease (GOLD) criteria

		n	%	FEV1% of predicted
CAO (LLN)	All	24		
	Very severe	2	8.3	<35%
	Severe	0	0	35–49%
	Moderately severe	3	12.5	50–59%
	Moderate	6	25.0	60–69%
	Mild	13	54.2	≥70%
CAO (GOLD)	All	30		
	Very severe	2	6.7	<30
	Severe	0	0	30–49
	Moderate	15	50.0	50–79
	Mild	13	43.3	≥ 80

Risk factors for airflow obstruction

To identify risk factors promoting airflow obstruction, data from the patient interview was used to classify patients into exposed and non-exposed groups and FEF_{25-75} as well as FEV1% predicted values in patients without restriction were compared. The results are given in Table 4. There was no significant difference in lung function parameters between participants who smoked or were exposed to dusts and fumes at their workplace. Cooking in general and cooking with biomass fuels vs. gas or electricity was associated with significantly lower FEF_{25-75}, but not with lower FEV1% predicted. The biggest and significant differences in both lung function parameters were observed between participants with a history of TB vs. those who reported no history of prior TB ($p < 0.01$). Symptoms of chronic bronchitis were associated with a decrease in both lung function parameters ($p = 0.02$). Participants having refrained from taking a job because of shortness of breath exhibited lower FEF_{25-75} and FEV1% predicted values, but the difference was only significant for FEF_{25-75}.

Discussion

Chronic airflow obstruction is an important cause of morbidity and mortality, and has major impact on the lives of those affected. Data from this pilot study in coastal Tanzania indicate a relevant level of CAO among urban and rural inhabitants. CAO can be found across all age groups and those affected may suffer from limitations in their ability to work and in quality of life.

This study showed that approximately one out of twenty inhabitants of coastal Tanzania has CAO according to both definitions currently used. Whereas the ATS/ERS definition using the LLN method showed only a moderate increase of prevalence with age, the GOLD definition showed a six-fold higher prevalence of CAO in the highest vs. the youngest age group. As the GOLD definition uses a fixed FEV1/FVC ratio of 0.7 as cut-off to define CAO, older age groups are overrepresented as the FEV1/FVC ratio declines physiologically with increasing age [17]. There is a persisting controversy on which classification to use; the LLN method indicating CAO is better suited for research purposes as it controls for ageing of the lung whereas the GOLD spirometric criteria are preferred by many clinicians due to their simplicity. The results from this study however underscore the concerns regarding over-diagnosis of elderly patients using the GOLD definition as well as potential under-diagnosis in younger patients, and demonstrate this effect in an African setting. Future epidemiological studies in Africa should therefore report results using both definitions until a universally accepted method has been developed. Moreover, results should include prevalences stratified by age groups, as exposure to biomass fuel smoke starting from birth or

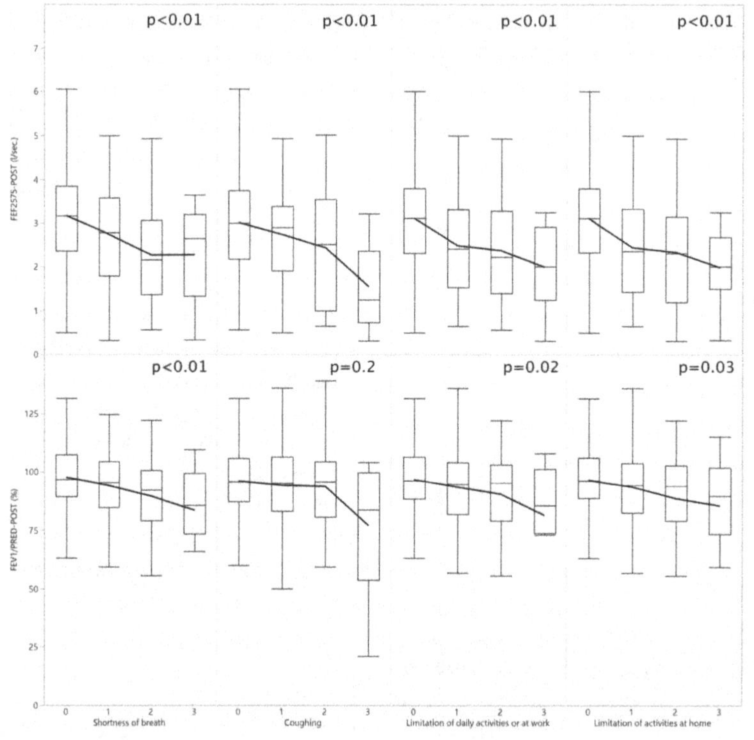

Fig. 1 Chronic airflow obstruction in relation to severity of symptoms: post-bronchodilator median FEF_{25-75} (l/s.) and FEV1 in patients without restriction by symptom severity (0 no symptoms, 3 severe symptoms). Boxplot shows median & interquartile ranges and whiskers denote the furthest point within 1.5× interquartile range. Number of subjects in severity groups (from 0 to 3): shortness of breath $n = 331, 140, 67, 13$; coughing $n = 447, 75, 20, 9$; limitation of daily activities or at work $n = 409, 84, 43, 15$; limitation of activities at home $n = 418, 81, 38, 14$, respectively. Note: the symptom "coughing" was assessed in 4 severity grades. Only one participant graded coughing with severity 4; this participant and was removed from the figure, as no boxplot could be drawn from a single value. The patient had a FEF_{25-75} of 1.99 l/s and a FEV1/PRED of 76.39%

even in utero [12] may lead to an earlier onset and higher prevalence of CAO in young African populations.

Few studies have reported prevalence of CAO in general populations from sub-Saharan Africa not exposed to special risk factors (e.g. gold miners). The reports available so far do not give consistent results across African regions; the prevalences found in this study were lower than in a recent study from Nigeria (5.1%–10% (LLN)) [6], Malawi (14% (GOLD)) [18] or from Uganda (12.4% (LLN), 16.2% (GOLD)) [19], but higher than in Cameroon (2.4% (LLN), 0.5% (GOLD)) [20]. Consistent across all studies, the majority of patients had either mild or moderate severity of obstruction. There is still no sufficient data from large population-level spirometry-based and quality-assured studies in sub-Saharan Africa to give a good CAO prevalence estimate in general or specific to African regions; the data presented in this study add relevant baseline data for planning studies on a larger scale and underscore the importance of reporting data in different age groups.

Risk factors for CAO likely differ from other regions of the world due to different living circumstances, living standards and lifestyle of populations. Smoking [1] and exposure to particulate matter [21] in the air are the predominant risk factors for CAO in industrialized countries. Data from China, Latin America and Turkey show a moderately increased risk of CAO after exposure to smoke from biomass fuels, with a stronger effect for firewood than for charcoal [22]. Following these principles, indoor air pollution is generally assumed to be a major risk factor in Sub-Saharan Africa [23]. Four recent studies however did not demonstrate a clear association between indoor use of biomass fuel with CAO [6, 7, 19, 20]. Chronic airflow obstruction may begin early in life and investigation of first signs may be missed by applying the ATS/ERS or GOLD criteria only – the predominant method of analysis used in studies from Africa. Large population based epidemiological studies have however demonstrated excellent sensitivity for early detection of airway pathology using continuous analysis of FEV1 and in particular FEF_{25-75} [21, 24, 25] as well as FEV1 as a percentage of FVC [21]. In an exploratory approach, we therefore used FEF_{25-75} as well as FEV1% predicted to detect more subtle changes in airway pathology. Analysis of FEF_{25-75} seemed to have a higher sensitivity and better correlation with severity of symptoms and physical limitations than FEV1% predicted. Both parameters indicated

Table 4 Post-bronchodilator FEF_{25-75} (l/s.) and FEV1% predicted in participants without restriction, with risk factors, symptoms and limitations caused by chronic airflow obstruction in participants without evidence of restriction)

	Exposure	N	% of n	Median FEF_{25-75} (IQR), post bronchodilator (L/s.)	Δ FEF_{25-75} (L/s.)	p	Median FEV1% PRED (IQR)	Δ FEV1% PRED	p
Smoking	Current or former smoker	155	28.1	3.1 (2.15–3.76)	0.2	0.4	96.44 (87.39–104.12)	1.23	0.59
	Never smoker	397	71.9	2.9 (2.05–3.65)			95.21 (86.14–106.34)		
Exposure to dusts and fumes at workplace	Exposure	442	80.1	2.97 (2.03–3.7)	0.19	0.78	95.15 (85.94–104.42)	3.74	0.07
	No exposure	110	19.9	2.78 (2.2–3.63)			98.88 (89.31–107.82)		
Cooking	Regular cooking	317	57.4	2.74 (1.93–3.47)	0.43	<0.01	95.19 (85.61–105.79)	0.2	0.12
	No regular cooking	231	41.8	3.16 (2.34–3.99)			95.39 (88.62–105.37)		
Biomass fuels for cooking	Cooking with wood or coal	472	85.5	2.84 (1.96–3.61)	0.53	<0.01	95.15 (85.62–104.93)	1.33	0.39
	Cooking with gas or electricity	47	8.5	3.36 (2.5–3.99)			96.47 (72.93–106.29)		
History of active TB	History of active TB	71	12.9	2.07 (1.5–3.12)	0.95	<0.01	96.2 (87.48–106.34)	6.34	<0.01
	No history of active TB	481	87.1	3.02 (2.23–3.71)			89.86 (77.11–101.86)		
Chronic bronchitis (chronic cough and sputum)	Yes	46	8.3	2.41 (1.44–3.49)	0.58	0.02	90.73 (74.02–103.34)	4.86	0.02
	No	506	91.7	2.99 (2.1–3.67)			95.6 (86.89–105.86)		
Having ever refrained from taking a job because of shortness of breath	Yes	87	15.8	2.43 (1.56–3.28)	0.6	<0.01	95.25 (81.58–103.25)	0.28	0.14
	No	465	84.2	3.02 (2.17–3.71)			95.53 (86.99–105.96)		

differences among participants exposed and unexposed to risk factors for CAO typical for an African setting and indicated their potential significance for causing social impact. We therefore recommend that in larger studies on CAO in Africa, results should be reported both using the standard CAO definitions, but also using analysis of continuous spirometric values such as FEF_{25-75} and FEV1% predicted.

Recent meta-analyses and studies on a global scale were able to demonstrate that active tuberculosis as an infection causing chronic pulmonary inflammation over a prolonged period of time is a major factor contributing to CAO [26–28]. In this study, a history of active TB infection was the most relevant risk factor associated with a lower FEF_{25-75} as well as a lower FEV1% predicted. The observed effect of TB infection is consistent with other recently published studies from local African populations [6, 18, 29] and underscores the significance of TB for development of chronic lung disease in Africa.

This study had limitations. In order to examine CAO in a sufficient number of subjects in each age class in this study, age-stratified sampling was used. The population sample examined consisted of a mixed population composed of hospital visitors and patients. Therefore, particularly the prevalence of CAO should not necessarily be regarded as representative for the general population. An unexpectedly high number of study participants was unable to produce a spirometry meeting ATS/ERS quality criteria despite intensive and standardized pre-spirometry training including a training video two times. In previous studies in developing country settings in Latin America and Africa [6, 19, 30], observed spirometry failure rates were lower except for one study from Malawi with a similar rate of exclusions [7]. Local cultural and religious factors in this community causing people not to expose themselves in a medical examination requiring their participation with maximum muscular force used, together with a generally low level of education probably have contributed to this high failure rate. Main findings in this study, particularly with regard to risk factors for CAO need to be confirmed in larger population-based studies.

Conclusions

In conclusion, this study demonstrated a relevant burden of CAO in a Tanzanian population and showed major differences in prevalence as well as age-specific prevalence between the two standard definitions of CAO used. Although most individuals with evidence of CAO had only mild or moderate obstruction, CAO likely has relevant social and social and economic impact for those affected. TB may have more impact on development of chronic airway obstruction than smoking in Africa. Analysis of FEV1 and FEF_{25-75} in epidemiologic studies on CAO may give important information on risk factors and impact in addition to using standard definitions for CAO alone.

Abbreviations
ATS/ERS: American Thoracic Society/European Respiratory Society; BOLD: Burden of Obstructive Lung Disease Initiative; CAO: Chronic airflow obstruction; COPD: Chronic obstructive pulmonary disease; FEF: Forced exspiratory flow; FEV1: Forced expiratory volume in 1 s; FVC: Forced vital capacity; GOLD: Global Initiative for Chronic Obstructive Lung Disease; LLN: Lower limit of normal; TB: Tuberculosis

Acknowledgements
Not applicable.

Funding
Rudolf Geigy Foundation, Basel, Switzerland.

Authors' contributions
TZ, EHM, DW and KR conceived the study. TBZ, PJA recruited patients and performed spirometry under supervision of TZ, EHM, FM, FH. All authors contributed to and revised the final manuscript. All authors read and approved the final manuscript.

Consent for publication
Not applicable.

Competing interests
All authors declare no competing interest.

Author details
[1]Swiss Tropical and Public Health Institute, Basel, Switzerland. [2]Ifakara Health Institute, Dar es Salaam, Tanzania. [3]Charité - Universitätsmedizin Berlin, corporate member of Freie Universität Berlin, Humboldt-Universität zu Berlin, and Berlin Institute of Health, Berlin, Germany. [4]Department of Infectious Diseases and Respiratory Medicine, Charité – Universitätsmedizin Berlin, Berlin, Germany. [5]University of Basel, Basel, Switzerland. [6]Clinical Research Unit, Schweizerisches Tropen- und Public Health Institut, Socinstr. 57, 4051 Basel, Switzerland.

References
1. Vogelmeier CF, Criner GJ, Martinez FJ, et al. Global Strategy for the Diagnosis, Management, and Prevention of Chronic Obstructive Lung Disease 2017 Report: GOLD Executive Summary. Eur Respir J. 2017;49: 1700214. [https://doi.org/10.1183/13993003.00214-2017].
2. Buist AS, McBurnie MA, Vollmer WM, Gillespie S, Burney P, Mannino DM, et al. International variation in the prevalence of COPD (the BOLD study): a population-based prevalence study. Lancet. 2007;370:741–50.
3. Menezes AMB, Perez-Padilla R, Jardim JRB, Muiño A, Lopez MV, Valdivia G, et al. Chronic obstructive pulmonary disease in five Latin American cities (the PLATINO study): a prevalence study. Lancet Lond Engl. 2005;366:1875–81.
4. Caballero A, Torres-Duque CA, Jaramillo C, Bolívar F, Sanabria F, Osorio P, et al. Prevalence of COPD in five Colombian cities situated at low, medium, and high altitude (PREPOCOL study). CHEST J. 2008;133:343–9.
5. WHO | Causes of COPD [Internet]. WHO. [cited 2017 Apr 3]. Available from: http://www.who.int/respiratory/copd/causes/en/
6. Obaseki DO, Erhabor GE, Gnatiuc L, Adewole OO, Buist SA, Burney PG. Chronic airflow obstruction in a black African population: results of BOLD study, Ile-Ife, Nigeria. COPD J Chronic Obstr Pulm Dis. 2016;13:42–9.
7. Meghji J, Nadeau G, Davis KJ, Wang D, Nyirenda MJ, Gordon SB, et al. Noncommunicable lung disease in sub-Saharan Africa. A community-based cross-sectional study of adults in urban Malawi. Am J Respir Crit Care Med. 2016;194:67–76.
8. Park HH, Girdler-Brown BV, Churchyard GJ, White NW, Ehrlich RI. Incidence of tuberculosis and HIV and progression of silicosis and lung function impairment among former Basotho gold miners. Am J Ind Med. 2009;52:901–8.
9. Ehrlich RI, Myers JE, te Water Naude JM, Thompson ML, Churchyard GJ. Lung function loss in relation to silica dust exposure in south African gold miners. Occup Environ Med. 2011;68:96–101.
10. Hamatui N, Naidoo RN, Kgabi N. Respiratory health effects of occupational exposure to charcoal dust in Namibia. Int J Occup Environ Health. 2016;22:3, 240-48. https://doi.org/10.1080/10773525.2016.1214795.
11. Isara AR, Adam VY, Aigbokhaode AQ, Alenoghena IO. Respiratory symptoms and ventilatory functions among quarry workers in Edo state, Nigeria. Pan Afr Med J. 2016;23:212.
12. Eisner MD, Anthonisen N, Coultas D, Kuenzli N, Perez-Padilla R, Postma D, et al. An official American Thoracic Society public policy statement: novel risk factors and the global burden of chronic obstructive pulmonary disease. Am J Respir Crit Care Med. 2010;182:693–718.
13. Miller MR. Standardisation of spirometry. Eur Respir J. 2005;26:319–38.
14. Quanjer PH, Stanojevic S, Cole TJ, Baur X, Hall GL, Culver BH, et al. Multi-ethnic reference values for spirometry for the 3–95-yr age range: the global lung function 2012 equations. Eur Respir J. 2012;40:1324–43.
15. McNulty W, Usmani OS. Techniques of assessing small airways dysfunction. Eur. Clin Respir J. 2014;1:25898.
16. Pellegrino R. Interpretative strategies for lung function tests. Eur Respir J. 2005;26:948–68.
17. Do not adopt the GOLD definition [Internet]. [cited 2017 Apr 5]. Available from: http://spirxpert.ers-education.org/en/gold-controversy/background/
18. Fullerton DG, Suseno A, Semple S, Kalambo F, Malamba R, White S, et al. Wood smoke exposure, poverty and impaired lung function in Malawian adults. Int J Tuberc Lung Dis. 2011;15:391–8.
19. van Gemert F, Kirenga B, Chavannes N, Kamya M, Luzige S, Musinguzi P, et al. Prevalence of chronic obstructive pulmonary disease and associated risk factors in Uganda (FRESH AIR Uganda): a prospective cross-sectional observational study. Lancet Glob Health. 2015;3:e44–51.
20. Pefura-Yone EW, Kengne AP, Balkissou AD, Magne-Fotso CG, Ngo-Yonga M, Boulleys-Nana JR, et al. Prevalence of obstructive lung disease in an African country using definitions from different international guidelines: a community based cross-sectional survey. BMC Res Notes. 2016;9:124.
21. Downs SH, Schindler C, L-JS L, Keidel D, Bayer-Oglesby L, Brutsche MH, et al. Reduced exposure to PM10 and attenuated age-related decline in lung function. N Engl J Med. 2007;357:2338–47.
22. Kurmi OP, Semple S, Simkhada P, Smith WCS, Ayres JG. COPD and chronic bronchitis risk of indoor air pollution from solid fuel: a systematic review and meta-analysis. Thorax. 2010;65:221–8.
23. Perez-Padilla R, Schilmann A, Riojas-Rodriguez H. Respiratory health effects of indoor air pollution. Int. J. Tuberc. Lung dis. Off. J. Int. Union Tuberc Lung Dis. 2010;14:1079–86.
24. Avol EL, Gauderman WJ, Tan SM, London SJ, Peters JM. Respiratory effects of relocating to areas of differing air pollution levels. Am J Respir Crit Care Med. 2001;164:2067–72.
25. Gauderman WJ, Gilliland GF, Vora H, Avol E, Stram D, McConnell R, et al. Association between air pollution and lung function growth in southern California children: results from a second cohort. Am J Respir Crit Care Med. 2002;166:76–84.
26. Amaral AFS, Coton S, Kato B, Tan WC, Studnicka M, Janson C, et al. Tuberculosis associates with both airflow obstruction and low lung function: BOLD results. Eur Respir J. 2015;46:1104–12.
27. Byrne AL, Marais BJ, Mitnick CD, Lecca L, Marks GB. Tuberculosis and chronic respiratory disease: a systematic review. Int J Infect Dis. 2015;32:138–46.
28. Menezes AMB, Hallal PC, Perez-Padilla R, Jardim JRB, Muino A, Lopez MV, et al. Tuberculosis and airflow obstruction: evidence from the PLATINO study in Latin America. Eur Respir J. 2007;30:1180–5.
29. Manji M, Shayo G, Mamuya S, Mpembeni R, Jusabani A, Mugusi F. Lung functions among patients with pulmonary tuberculosis in Dar es Salaam – a cross-sectional study. BMC Pulm Med. 2016;16:58. https://doi.org/10.1186/s12890-016-0213-5.
30. Idolor LF, De Guia TS, Francisco NA, Roa CC, Ayuyao FG, Tady CZ, et al. Burden of obstructive lung disease in a rural setting in the Philippines: BOLD in a rural Philippines community. Respirology. 2011;16:1111–8.

5

Risk factors for acute respiratory infections in children under five years attending the Bamenda Regional Hospital in Cameroon

Alexis A. Tazinya[1], Gregory E. Halle-Ekane[2*], Lawrence T. Mbuagbaw[1], Martin Abanda[1], Julius Atashili[3] and Marie Therese Obama[4]

Abstract

Background: Acute respiratory infections (ARI) are a leading cause of morbidity and mortality in under-five children worldwide. About 6.6 million children less than 5 years of age die every year in the world; 95% of them in low-income countries and one third of the total deaths is due to ARI. This study aimed at determining the proportion of acute respiratory infections and the associated risk factors in children under 5 years visiting the Bamenda Regional Hospital in Cameroon.

Methods: A cross-sectional analytic study involving 512 children under 5 years was carried out from December 2014 to February 2015. Participants were enrolled by a consecutive convenient sampling method. A structured questionnaire was used to collect clinical, socio-demographic and environmental data. Diagnosis of ARI was based on the revised WHO guidelines for diagnosing and management of childhood pneumonia. The data was analyzed using the statistical software EpiInfo™ version 7.

Results: The proportion of ARIs was 54.7% (280/512), while that of pneumonia was 22.3% (112/512). Risk factors associated with ARI were: HIV infection OR_{adj} 2.76[1.05–7.25], poor maternal education (None or primary only) OR_{adj} 2.80 [1.85–4.35], exposure to wood smoke OR_{adj} 1.85 [1.22–2.78], passive smoking OR_{adj} 3.58 [1.45–8.84] and contact with someone who has cough OR_{adj} 3.37 [2.21–5.14].

Age, gender, immunization status, breastfeeding, nutritional status, fathers' education, parents' age, school attendance and overcrowding were not significantly associated with ARI.

Conclusion: The proportion of ARI is high and is associated with HIV infection, poor maternal education, exposure to wood smoke, passive cigarette smoking, and contact with persons having a cough. Control programs should focus on diagnosis, treatment and prevention of ARIs.

Keywords: Acute, Respiratory infections, Risk factors, Proportion, Under-five

Background

Acute respiratory infections (ARIs) are a major cause of morbidity and mortality worldwide [1, 2]. Each year, about 1.3 million children under 5 years die from acute respiratory infections worldwide [3]. ARI constitute one third of the deaths in under five in low income countries [4]. The World Health Organization (WHO) estimates that respiratory infections account for 6% of the total global burden of disease; this is a higher percentage compared with the burden of diarrheal disease, cancer, human immunodeficiency virus (HIV) infection, ischemic heart disease or malaria [5]. Each year ARIs account for over 12 million hospital admissions in children less than 5 years [6]. In a 16 year study on the causes and circumstances of death in northern Cameroon, 67% of all deaths were in children and a majority 24% (167) of the deaths were caused by ARIs, followed by malaria 21% (152) and diarrheal diseases 19% (133) making ARIs one of the leading public health problems in under-fives in Cameroon [7].

* Correspondence: halle-ekane.edie@ubuea.cm; gregory@yahoo.fr
[2]Department of Surgery and Obstetrics/Gynecology, Faculty of Health Sciences, University of Buea, P.O Box 12, Buea, Cameroon
Full list of author information is available at the end of the article

Despite the burden of acute respiratory infection on morbidity and mortality in children under the age of five in the world, there is limited data to evaluate the problem in Cameroon. The availability of data on the proportionand risk factors of ARIs is vital because, achieving the Sustainable Development Goal on improving health and wellbeing, will depend on the existing efforts to prevent and control ARIs in all WHO regions [1, 8].

There are many socio-cultural, demographic and environmental risk factors that predispose children less than 5 years to acquire Respiratory Tract Infections (RTIs). Even though many of these risk factors are preventable [9], they have not been documented in many regions in Cameroon making it difficult to develop algorithms for the management of this group of patients.

This study therefore aimed at determining the proportion of ARIs and their associated risk factors amongst children under 5 years of age who attend the Bamenda Regional Hospital.

Methods

Study design and setting

This was a hospital-based cross-sectional analytic study carried out in the peak period of the dry season from December 2014 to February 2015. Bamenda is the capital of the North West Region. It is located 366 km north-west of the Cameroonian capital, Yaoundé. It has an estimated population of about 500,000 inhabitants [10] Bamenda like other parts of Cameroon has two seasons in a year. The dry season starts in November and ends by March while the rainy season starts in April and ends in October. The dry season is characterized by cool, dry and very dusty harmattan winds which blow during the peak periods of the dry season (December, January and March), with temperatures ranging between 9°c and 30°c. Many people in Bamenda use wood for cooking and this produces smoke rendering the children vulnerable to its effects.

The Bamenda Regional Hospital (BRH) is the biggest health care facility in the region receiving about 150 patients daily, about one-third being children. The hospital is a second level health facility and serves as a teaching hospital for the Faculty of Health Sciences, of the University of Bamenda. It has an HIV treatment center with over 80 children in care who visit the hospital at least monthly for a refill of their medication. This study was carried out in the pediatric unit of the Regional Hospital which has a capacity of 34 and 15 beds for pediatric patients and neonates respectively. It has a level of occupancy of more than 85% most times of the year [11]. Health care services are provided by a pediatrician, 3 general practitioners and 15 nurses. Children visiting this hospital benefit from the Expanded Program of Immunisation which offers many vaccines for various ages including the influenza vaccine, pneumococcal vaccine and the measles vaccines.

Sample size calculation

The sample size was calculated using the formula for estimating proportions [12]. A pre-study estimate of prevalence of ARI from a systematic review of literature from 12 developing countries was 22% [13] with a precision of 0.036. The calculated sample size w as508. Five hundred and twelve children were included in the study.

Study population and sampling

All children under 5 years who visited the Bamenda Regional Hospital during the study period and whose parents or guardians gave consent were included in the study. Children less than 2 months were excluded from this study because the clinical definitions of ARIs have low sensitivity and specificity in this age group and the clinical presentation is nonspecific. Children whose parents or guardians did not give consent were also excluded from the study.

Study procedure

Approach to participants

Participants were recruited between 8 am and 5 pm from Monday to Saturday from both the out-patient and inpatient departments. The parents or guardians of the child were informed about the study at the outpatient waiting room or in the wards and their written consent sought. Those who gave their consent to the study were met in the pediatrician's consultation room or in the wards and a designed questionnaire was administered by the principal investigator. Findings from the consultation were used and additional information needed was obtained from a complementary history and physical examination.

Data collection

Data was collected using a structured questionnaire on the; demographic, clinical and the socioeconomic variables of the child and the parents or guardians.

Data management

Data was entered, cleaned, and analyzed using the statistical software Epi info version 7.

Case definition for ARI was was based on the Integrated Management of Childhood Illnesses (IMCI) classification for children presenting with cough or difficulty breathing.: Mild ARI (no pneumonia), Moderate ARI (pneumonia) and Severe ARI (severe pneumonia) [14]. Potential risk factors included: age, sex, birth weight, co-infection with HIV (diagnosed using a rapid test- Determine) passive smoking (any child living with someone who smokes at home), attendance at day care, exposure to wood smoke (any child who spends more than 30 min in wood smoke daily), living in the same house with someone have a cough, poor parental education (primary school level or less), malnutrition (Z-scores<2SD), inadequate immunization (if a child was lacking some vaccines for age) and mixed breastfeeding (if the child was not exclusively breastfed for at least 4 months) overcrowding (either ≥6 persons in a house, or ≥3 people using one bed) [5]. The predictor variables were grouped into three categories; socio-demographic, environmental, and clinical factors. The prevalence of ARI in children attending the BRH was calculated as; Number of children 2–59 months diagnosed with ARI during the study period, divided by the total number of children 2–59 months who visited the hospital during the same) multiplied by 100%.

The chi square test was used to evaluate significance of associations between ARI and potential risk factors, which were coded as categorical variables. The odds ratio (OR) of having ARI was calculated for all the assessed risk factors as follows: OR = (a/b)/(c/d) where a = exposed with ARI, c = not exposed with ARI, b = exposed without ARI, d = not exposed without ARI.

Multivariable analysis was performed using a logistic regression model, which included as explanatory variables all risk factors whose *p*-value was lower than 0.20 in univariable analysis.

Results

A total of 620 children visited the hospital during the study period. Forty eight children were under 2 months of age, 36 parents did not give consent either because they presented as emergencies or did not want any delay in the consultation process. Eighteen guardians did not give consent either because they were not sure of child's history or they did not want to enroll the children without their parents consent. Six questionnaires had incomplete information. In total, 512 children participated in the study. A majority (58%) were male and aged between 13 to 59 months (56%), with a median age of 15 months. Children older than 1 year had an average of 2.2 (SD2.4) episodes of ARIs before reaching their first birthday. Those with ARI spent a mean number of 6 (SD4.1) days with symptoms before consulting a health centre or hospital.

The proportion of ARIs in children under 5 years in the BRH was 54.7% (280 children) with a 95% CI of 50.3%–59.0%. Using IMCI guidelines, a total of 166/280 (59%) were mild ARIs (No Pneumonia), 69/280 (25%) were moderate ARI (Pneumonia) and 45/280 (16%) were severe ARI (Severe Pneumonia) as shown in Fig. 1. The ARIs as diagnosed by consultants were: rhinitis 170/280 (60%%), pharyngitis 120 (43%), tonsillitis 54 (19%), acute otitis media 39 (14%), bronchopneumonia 88 (31%) as shown in Fig. 2. One hundred and ninety one (37.3%) of the 512 children had an URTI (rhinitis, pharyngitis, tonsillitis, acute otitis media), 88 (17.2%) had a LRTI (bronchopneumonia) and 35 had both upper and lower RTI.

Of the 280 children who had ARIs, 118 of them were also found to have other co-morbid conditions like: malnutrition 51 (18.2%), malaria 25 (8.9%), diarrheal disease 26 (9.3%), measles-like rash 8(2.9%), and HIV infection 23 (8.2%) as shown in Fig. 3.

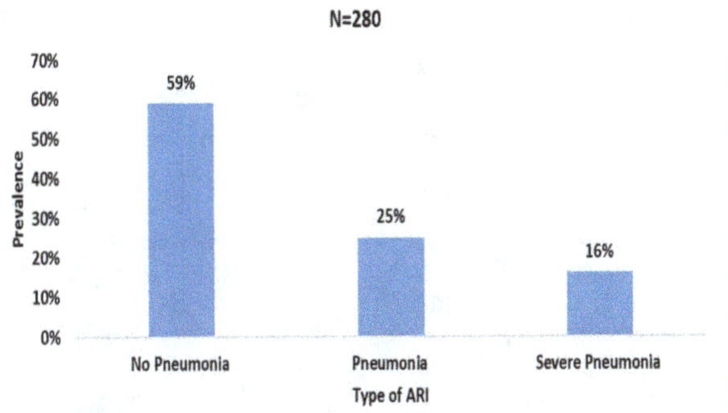

Fig. 1 Proportion of ARI using IMCI definition in children less than 5 years

As shown on Table 1, children aged more than 12 months, males, children with low birth weight, poor paternal education and children with younger fathers (≤30 years), accounted for a higher proportion of ARIs than their comparative groups.. However, the difference was not statistically significant ($p > 0.05$).

Children with poorly educated mothers had significantly higher proportion of ARIs ($P < 0.001$) with an OR of 3.13 (95% CI: 2.11–4.64).

The evaluated clinical risk factors (Table 2) revealed that malnourished children [OR 3.01 (95% CI: 1.66–5.43)] and children infected with HIV [OR 2.88 CI: 1.21–6.83], had a significantly higher proportion ($P < 0.05$) of ARI than well-nourished and HIV negative children.

Children who were inadequately breastfed and inadequately immunized did not have a significantly different proportion of ARIs when compared those who were exclusively breastfed and immunized respectively. ($P > 0.05$).

Environmental factors such as exposure to wood smoke, cigarette smoke, and contact or living with someone who had a cough were found to significantly increase the proportion of ARIs ($P < 0.05$). While the association of school attendance and overcrowding was not significant. (Table 3).

After multivariate analysis, all significant variable remained significant except for the children's nutritional status with a *p*-value of 0.06. Table 4.

Discussion

This study aimed at determining the proportion of ARIs and identifying some related risk factors in children under 5 years attending the Bamenda Regional Hospital. A high proportion of ARI of 54.7% was probably because this study was carried out during the peak of the dry season (December, January and February) which is characterized by dry, cold and dusty harmattan winds. Though high, this result is lower than 69.7% obtained by Sikoilia et al. in Kenya [15] and 70% obtained by Rhamam in Bangladesh

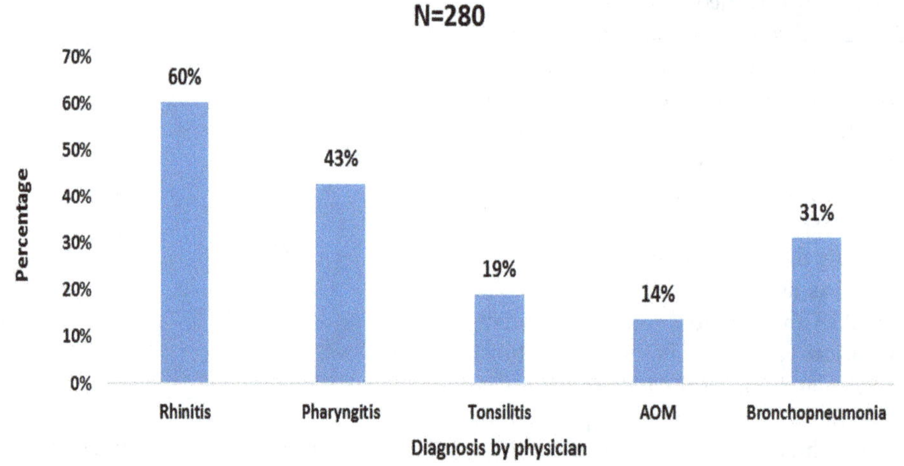

Fig. 2 Proportion of the different types of ARI as diagnosed by physician

[16]. This is probably because participants in this study were found to have a lower average of 3.7 ± 4.5 infections a year, compared to 6–8 episodes obtained in under-five children in Nigeria by Ujunwa et al. [4]. The number of hospital visits for ARI(2.1 ± 2.2) compared to the number episodes of ARIs in our study are similar to findings in a study in India [17] where only 42.5% of mothers regarded ARIs as serious enough to present to the hospital.

On the other hand our study found a higher proportion of ARI compared to the 10–40% in found in other studies [18]. This differences in the proportions of ARI could be as a result of different study populations, different study settings, differences in age groups studied, or because this study used mainly clinical definitions for the cases which is more sensitive than laboratory confirmed cases. A study lasting at least one complete calender year could help get the proportion of infections for a typical year. In order to reduce this high burden of ARI on the population, the ministry of public health in developing countries could include control of ARIs in their community intervention activities.

The proportion of pneumonia in this study was 22.3%, higher than the 19.4% for the Northwest Region of Cameroon as reported in 2004 by Tchatchou [19]. The proportion of a LRTI in our study (17.35%) is very similar to the 17.4% found in the Far North Region in 2011 [20] and higher than the prevalence for the Northwest Region (9.5%) in the same survey. No particular reason was found for this differences.

The proportion of pneumonia alone in this study (22.3%) is higher than the proportion of all LRTI (17.2%) in the same study. This is because the diagnostic criteria of pneumonia according to Integrated Management of Childhood

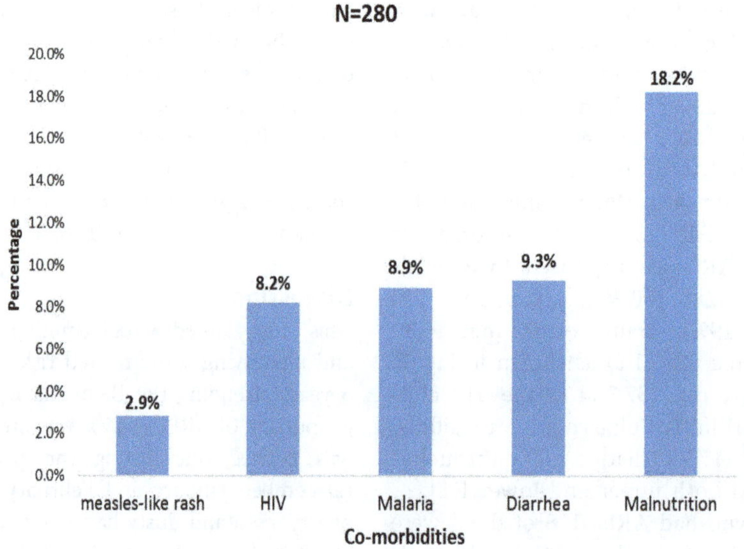

Fig. 3 ARI and co-morbidities

Table 1 Socio-demographic factors associated with ARI in children under 5 years

Factor	Total	ARI	Odds ratios	95% CI	*P*-value
Age(months)					
2–12	225	117(52.00%)	1		
13–59	287	163(56.79%)	1.21	0.85–1.72	0.28
Gender					
Female	218	113(51.83%)	1		
Male	294	167(56.80%)	1.21	0.85–1.72	0.29
Birth weight					
Normal	463	251(54.21%)	1		
Low birth weight < 2.5 kg	19	12(63.16%)	1.45	0.56–3.74	0.45
Overweight ≥4 kg	30	17(58.62%)	1.19	0.55–2.53	0.66
Mothers age (years)					
Age > 20	407	212(52%)	1		
Age ≤ 20	20	11(55%)	1.12	0.45–2.7	0.80
Fathers age(years)					
Age > 30	303	153(50.50%)	1		
Age ≤ 30	108	61(56.48%)	1.27	0.82–1.98	0.28
Mother's level of education					
Secondary + tertiary	316	144(45.57%)	1		
None + primary	183	131(71.58%)	3.13	2.11–4.64	< 0.001
Father's level of education					
Secondary + tertiary	330	173(52.42%)	1		
None + primary	159	97(61.01%)	1.42	0.97–2.09	0.07

Illnesses (IMCI) guidelines is highly sensitive [14] and will include some false positive cases of pneumonia, made up of children with a severe URTI because of the presence of cough, difficulty breathing with or danger signs which are sensitive but not specific to pneumonia alone. The proportion of LRTI of 17.2% in our study is similar to 19% in a study in India [21]. The diagnostic challenges of respiratory illnesses in our setting compels many clinicians to use the IMCI which does not specify the different types of ARIs but uses the term pneumonia to facilitate management in resource poor settings. Community health workers should be trained on the use of IMCI guidelines so that they can recognize ARI early enough and take appropriate actions to prevent its spread and severity.

Of the risk factors identified in our study, malnutrition was found to be significant with an odds ratio of 3.01 (95%

Table 2 Clinical factors associated with ARI

Factor	Total	ARI	Odds ratios	95% CI	*P*-value
Nutritional status					
Malnourished	67	51(76.12%)	3.01	1.66–5.43	< 0.001
Normal	445	229(51.45%)	1		
HIV status					
Positive	30	23(76.67%)	2.88	1.21–6.83	< 0.016
Negative	482	257(53.32%)	1		
Immunization status					
No/ incomplete vaccination	11	4(36.36%)	0.69	0.20–2.39	0.56
Up to date with EPI	501	227(55.29%)	1		
Breastfeeding					
Mixed	74	43(58.11%)	1.17	0.71–1.92	0.54
Exclusive	438	238(54.34%)	1		

Table 3 Environmental and social factors associated with ARI

Factor	Total	ARI	Odds ratios	95% CI	*P*-value
Exposure to wood smoke					
Not exposed	203	82(40.39%)	1		
Exposed	309	198(64.08%)	2.63	1.83–3.79	< 0.001
Cigarette smoke					
Non passive smoker	474	249(52.53%)	1		
Passive smoker	37	31(83.78%)	4.67	1.91–11.40	< 0.001
History of contact[a]					
No contact	313	134(42.81%)	1		
Had contact	199	147(73.87%)	3.78	2.56–5.56	< 0.001
School attendance					
Do not go to school	391	210(53.71)	1		
Go to school	121	70(57.85%)	1.18	0.78–1.79	0.42
Overcrowding					
Not overcrowded	303	167(55.12%)	1		
Overcrowded	209	114(54.55%)	0.97	0.69–1.39	0.90

[a]contact with someone who has a cough

CI: 1.66–5.43). This finding is consistent with a similar study in Nigeria by Ujunwa et al. in 2014 [4] where malnutrition was a significant risk factor with a relative risk of 3.33 (95% CI: 2.65–4.21) and Rahman in Bangladesh who obtained the prevalence of ARI in malnourished children to be 63.1% ($p < 0.001$). After multivariate analysis, the nutrition status was only marginally significant ($p = 0.06$) this could be attributed to statistical methods because the influence of malnutrition on ARIs is well known from many different studies [18, 21–25]. Supplementation of common foods for children and routine education of mothers during vaccination clinics could help address the problem of malnutrition and reduce the impact of ARIs.

Table 4 Multivariate logistic regression analysis of potential risk factors for ARI

Factor	Adjusted Odds ratios	95% CI	*P*-value
Nutritional status			
Normal	1		
Malnourished	1.91	0.97–3.76	0.06
History of contact			
No	1		
Yes	3.37	2.21–5.14	< 0.01
Exposure to wood smoke			
Not exposed	1		
Exposed	1.85	1.22–2.78	< 0.01
HIV status			
Negative	1		
Positive	2.76	1.05–7.25	0.04
Mother's level of education			
Secondary + tertiary	1		
Primary + none	2.80	1.85–4.25	< 0.01
Passive smoking			
No	1		
Yes	3.58	1.45–8.84	< 0.01

The prevalence of HIV infection in Cameroon stood at 5.5% by 2007 with 420,000 new infections in children under 15 years [26]. Children who tested positive for HIV in this study (30) were more likely to have an ARI than those who were negative (OR 2.88 95% CI:1.21–6.83). Although 14 (45%) of the 31 children who tested positive for the HIV rapid test (Alere Determine ™ HIV- 1/2) were exposed children, the association of HIV and ARI is expected because HIV infection is known to weaken the immune system and increase the spectrum of organisms that infect the respiratory system [27]. Children who tested positive for the rapid HIV test had a higher risk and a poorer outcome than the HIV negative children [27, 28]. The presence of the HIV treatment center in the hospital can account for the considerably large number of HIV exposed and infected children. The diagnosis of HIV using rapid test will include exposed noninfected children accounting for a large proportion (8.2) of children diagnosed with HIV.

Children from mothers who had no education or primary education only, had a higher chance of developing an ARI than children from more educated mothers (secondary education and above). This is probably because children spend more time with their mothers, and mothers' educational level will determine the quality of care and many social and environmental factors that the child will be exposed to. Ujunwa et al. also found an association with maternal education but it was significant only for LRTI and not for URTI. Other studies have also found a positive association between poor maternal education and ARI [4, 16–18, 21, 29]. Infant welfare clinics could be used as an area to reinforce maternal health education and care of infants and children.

The odds of developing an ARI after exposure to wood smoke was 2.63 compared to those who were not exposed. WHO reports that children who are exposed to cooking fuels increase the risk of developing pneumonia [1]. A similar association between wood fuel and ARI has also been found to be significant in some studies [15, 18, 21, 24, 30, 31]. The community has to be educated on the dangers of wood smoke especially because it is the main source of cooking fuel in the local communities.

Passive cigarette smoking from this study, was found to be a significant risk factor of ARI increasing the odds by 4.67 (1.91–11.40) compared to children who were not passive smokers. This is a consistent finding with other studies [4, 18, 24, 25] in which the risk of passive smoking increased by about 2 to 4 fold that of non-passive smokers [32]. This association was expected and could be explained by the fact that smoking destroys the natural protective mechanism of the respiratory tract making it easier for pathogens to overcome the first line defense of the respiratory system [33]. Anti smoking campaigns could help sensitise the population on the dangers of tobacco smoke in general and on the health of children in particular.

Coming in contact with someone who had symptoms of respiratory disease significantly increases the risk of a child to develop an ARI. This result only confirms the fact that ARIs are communicable diseases transmitted by droplets from infected persons. This is an association that has been found in other studies like Ariane et al. in the Netherlands [29]. Children should be kept away from people who present with cough so as to prevent them from getting infected.

The age, and gender of a child in this study did not significantly affect the proportions of acute respiratory infections. The meta-analysis by Jackson et al. reported an inconsistency in the effect of age and gender on ARI as 4 of the studies reviewed found a significant association and 3 others studies agree with our finding in that they did not also find a significant association of the age and gender with ARI [30].

The WHO in a report on pneumonia, brings out the importance of low birth weight in the prevalence of ARIs [24]. We did not find any significant association between the birth weight and ARIs in our study. Similarly, Lira et al., in Brazil did not find any significant difference between low birth weight and the prevalence of cough [34]. This is probably because the effect of low birth weight on ARI is more significant in neonates and our study excluded neonates.

Factors like inadequate breastfeeding and poor immunization in our study, are in great contrast with the results from many other studies [4, 18, 21, 23, 29, 30, 32]. Many breastfed children are given water and other liquids foods like corn soup frequently before 4 months of life, classifying them as mixed feeding in this study. Giving clean water and corn soup to children less than 4 months may not increase their risk of infection. Children in Bamenda receive the pneumococcal and *Haemophilus influenza* type b vaccines at 6 weeks, 10 weeks and 14 weeks and at 6 months they receive the miseasles vaccine as required by the EPI calendar. Our study did not find a significant association between vaccination and ARI probably because some of the inadequately vaccinated children according to the definition, might have received some doses of the pneumococcal and *Haemophilus influenza* type b vaccine which are known to reduce morbidity and mortality from ARI [1]. Analyzing nasal swabs could also determing the specific predisposing germs.

Study limitations

The diagnosis of the various ARIs was made based on clinical findings and compared to the gold standards is less sensitive and specific.

This study is a hospital-based study and less than 50% of children with ARIs go to the hospital for medical care so the proportion may not be a true reflection of what is in the community.

A longitudinal study would better illustrate the effects of the potential risk factors than this cross sectional study.

Conclusion

The proportion of ARI in the BRH was 54.7% and that of pneumonia was 22.3%. The risk factors significantly associated with ARI were: infection with HIV, poor maternal education, passive smoking, exposure to wood smoke and contact with person having ARI. Measures taken to abate these conditions will reduce the morbidity and mortality associated with ARI.

Abbreviations

ARI: Acute Respiratory Infection; BRH: Bamenda Regional Hospital; CI: Confidence Interval; EPI: Expanded Program of Immunization; HIV: Human Immunodeficiency Virus; IMCI: Integrated Management of Childhood Illnesses; LRTI: Lower Respiratory Tract Infection; OR: Odds Ratio; RTI: Respiratory Tract Infection; SD: Standard Deviation; URTI: Upper Respiratory Tract Infection; WHO: World Health Organization

Acknowledgements

We are grateful to all the children who took part in the study and their guardians for accepting to participate. We thank the administration of the Bamenda Regional Hospital for permitting us to conduct this study.

Funding
This study was not funded.

Authors' contributions
This work was carried out in collaboration with all authors. Authors AAT, JA, MTO did the study design and wrote the protocol. Authors LTM, GEHE did the literature search, cross-checked the statistical analysis and made important inputs in the drafting of the manuscript. LTM cross-checked the data entry while AAT and MA analysed the data. GEHE is the corresponding author. All authors read and approved the final manuscript.

Consent for publication
Not applicable.

Competing interests
The authors declare that they have no competing interests.

Author details
[1]Department of Internal Medicine and Pediatrics, Faculty of Health Sciences University of Buea, P. O. Box 63, Buea, Cameroon. [2]Department of Surgery and Obstetrics/Gynecology, Faculty of Health Sciences, University of Buea, P.O Box 12, Buea, Cameroon. [3]Department of Public Health and Hygiene, Faculty of Health Sciences, University of Buea, P.O Box 12, Buea, Cameroon. [4]Faculty of Medicine and Biomedical Sciences, University of Yaoundé 1, Yaoundé, Cameroon.

References
1. WHO. Pneumonia, the forgotten killer of children. Geneva 27: UNICEF/WHO; 2006. 10: 92-806-4048-8
2. The UN Inter-agency Group for Child Mortality Estimation . Levels & Trends in Child Mortality: Report 2014. New York: UNICEF; 2014.
3. Organization WH, UNICEF. Ending preventable child deaths from pneumonia and diarrhoea by 2025: the integrated global action plan for pneumonia and diarrhoea (GAPPD). 2013.
4. Ujunwa F, Ezeonu C. Risk factors for acute respiratory tract infections in under-five children in Enugu Southeast Nigeria. Ann Med Health Sci Res. 2014;4(1):95–9.
5. Mizgerd JP. Lung infection–a public health priority. PLoS Med. 2006;3(2):e76.
6. Nair H, Simoes EA, Rudan I, Gessner BD, Azziz-Baumgartner E, Zhang JS, et al. Global and regional burden of hospital admissions for severe acute lower respiratory infections in young children in 2010: a systematic analysis. Lancet (London, England). 2013;381(9875):1380–90.
7. Einterz EM, Bates M. Causes and circumstances of death in a district hospital in northern Cameroon, 1993-2009. Rural Remote Health. 2011;11(3):1623.
8. Griggs D, Stafford-Smith M, Gaffney O, Rockstrom J, Ohman MC, Shyamsundar P, et al. Policy: Sustainable development goals for people and planet. Nature. 2013;495(7441):305–7.
9. Schluger NW, Koppaka R. Lung disease in a global context. A call for public health action. Ann Am Thorac Soc. 2014;11(3):407–16.
10. Council BC. Bamenda City profile 2015 [1st February 2015]. Available from: bamendacity.com/index.php?option=com_content&view= article&id=61&Itemid=339.
11. Suzuki M, Thiem VD, Yanai H, Matsubayashi T, Yoshida LM, Tho LH, et al. Association of environmental tobacco smoking exposure with an increased risk of hospital admissions for pneumonia in children under 5 years of age in Vietnam. Thorax. 2009;64(6):484–9.
12. Wechsler S. Statistics at Square One. Ninth Edition, revised by M. J. Campbell, T. D. V. Swinscow, BMJ Publ. Group, London, 1996. No. of pages: 140. ISBN 0-7279-0916-9. Statistics in Medicine. 1997;16(22):2629-30.
13. Selwyn BJ. The epidemiology of acute respiratory tract infection in young children: comparison of findings from several developing countries. Coordinated Data Group of BOSTID Researchers. Rev Infect Dis. 1990; 12(Suppl 8):S870–88.
14. Patwari AK, Raina N. Integrated Management of Childhood Illness (IMCI): a robust strategy. Indian J Pediatr. 2002;69(1):41–8.
15. Sikolia DN, Mwololo K,HC. The prevalence of acute respiratory infections and the associated risk factors: a study of children under five years of age in Kibera Lindi village, Nairobi, Kenya. J Natl Inst Public Health. 2002;51(1):32-38
16. Rahman MM, Shahidullah M. Risk factors for acute respiratory infections among the slum infants of Dhaka city. Bangladesh Med Res Counc Bull. 2001;27(2):55–62.
17. Debasism B, Ahemed T. Study of knowledge, attitude and practice among mothers towards acute respiratory infection in urban and rural communitiesof burdwan district, West Bengal, India. Rev Progr. 2013; 1(8):1–6.
18. Arifeen S, Black RE, Antelman G, Baqui A, Caulfield L, Becker S. Exclusive breastfeeding reduces acute respiratory infection and diarrhea deaths among infants in Dhaka slums. Pediatrics. 2001;108(4):e67-e.
19. Tchatchou ND. Variations Regionales de la Survenance des Infections Respiratoires Aigues chez les Enfants de Moins de Cinq Ans Au Cameroun: Maters[Dissertation]Yaounde, Universite de Yaounde II; 2011.
20. INS I. Enquête Démographique et de Santé et à Indicateurs Multiples du Cameroun 2011. Calverton, MD: International I. 2012;423.
21. Mathew JL, Patwari AK, Gupta P, Shah D, Gera T, Gogia S, et al. Acute respiratory infection and pneumonia in India: a systematic review of literature for advocacy and action: UNICEF-PHFI series on newborn and child health, India. Indian Pediatr. 2011;48(3):191–218.
22. Mtango FD, Neuvians D, Korte R. Magnitude, presentation, management and outcome of acute respiratory infections in children under the age of five in hospitals and rural health centres in Tanzania. Trop Med Parasitol. 1989;40(2):97-102.
23. Bellos A, Mulholland K, O'Brien KL, Qazi SA, Gayer M, Checchi F. The burden of acute respiratory infections in crisis-affected populations: a systematic review. Confl Health. 2010;4:3.
24. WHO. Programme for the control of acute respiratory infections. Acute respiratory infections in children: case management in small hospitals in developing countries A manual for doctors and other senior health workers. Geneva: World Health Organization; 1990.
25. Rahman M, Rahman A. Prevalence of acute respiratory tract infection and its risk factors in under five children. Age. 1997;23(2):47-50
26. Mbanya D. Current status of HIV/AIDS in Cameroon: how effective are control strategies? Int J Environ Res Public Health. 2008;5(5):378–83.
27. Zar HJ. Pneumonia in HIV-infected and HIV-uninfected children in developing countries: epidemiology, clinical features, and management. Curr Opin Pulm Med. 2004;10(3):176–82.
28. Madhi SA, Petersen K, Madhi A, Khoosal M, Klugman KP. Increased disease burden and antibiotic resistance of bacteria causing severe community-acquired lower respiratory tract infections in human immunodeficiency virus type 1-infected children. Clin Infect Dis. 2000;31(1):170–6.
29. Macedo SE, Menezes AM, Albernaz E, Post P, Knorst M. Risk factors for acute respiratory disease hospitalization in children under one year of age. Rev Saude Publica. 2007;41(3):351–8.
30. Jackson S, Mathews KH, Pulanic D, Falconer R, Rudan I, Campbell H, et al. Risk factors for severe acute lower respiratory infections in children: a systematic review and meta-analysis. Croat Med J. 2013;54(2):110–21.
31. Morris K, Morganlander M, Coulehan JL, Gahagen S, Arena VC. WOod-burning stoves and lower respiratory tract infection in american indian children. Am J Dis Children. 1990;144(1):105–8.
32. Arcavi L, Benowitz NL. CIgarette smoking and infection. Arch Intern Med. 2004;164(20):2206–16.
33. Valencia-Gattas M, Conner GE, Fregien NL. Gefitinib, an EGFR tyrosine kinase inhibitor, prevents smoke-mediated ciliated airway epithelial cell loss and promotes their recovery. PLoS One. 2016;11(8):e0160216.
34. Lira PI, Ashworth A, Morris SS. Low birth weight and morbidity from diarrhea and respiratory infection in northeast Brazil. J Pediatr. 1996;128(4):497–504.

Prevalence and characteristics of COPD among pneumoconiosis patients at an occupational disease prevention institute

Yating Peng[1,2,3†], Xin Li[4†], Shan Cai[1,2,3], Yan Chen[1,2,3], Weirong Dai[4], Wenfeng Liu[4], Zijing Zhou[1,2,3], Jiaxi Duan[1,2,3] and Ping Chen[1,2,3*]

Abstract

Background: Pneumoconiosis may play an important role in the development of chronic obstructive pulmonary disease (COPD), and the complication of COPD may impose a heavy burden of illness.

Methods: The study was conducted in Hunan Province in China from December 1, 2015, to December 1, 2016. Consecutive underground male pneumoconiosis patients employed for at least 1 year were recruited from the Hunan Occupational Disease Prevention Institute. Patient information, respiratory symptoms and clinical data were collected using a structured questionnaire. The diagnosis of COPD were assessed using the Global Initiative for Chronic Obstructive Lung Disease (GOLD) criteria. Logistic regression analyses were conducted to examine the clinical and demographic risk factors of COPD among pneumoconiosis patients.

Results: The prevalence of COPD in our sample of pneumoconiosis patients was 18.65% (119/638). In pneumoconiosis patients with and without smoking history, the prevalence of COPD was 19.32 and 16.77%. Compared with non-COPD patients, those with COPD are older in age, have longer exposure time, have lower body mass index (BMI), have a higher smoking index and have worse pulmonary function (all $p < 0.05$). For the five respiratory symptoms (cough, sputum, wheeze, dyspnea, and chest tightness), only the presence of wheeze and the severity scores for wheeze or dyspnea showed significant differences between the COPD and non-COPD groups ($p < 0.01$). Multivariate logistic regression analysis revealed that advanced pneumoconiosis category, older age and the presence of wheeze symptoms were significant risk factors for the development of COPD among pneumoconiosis patients.

Conclusion: Pneumoconiosis patients are at a high risk of COPD, and pneumoconiosis patients with COPD may suffer more severe respiratory symptoms, such as wheeze and dyspnea, than patients without COPD. Advanced pneumoconiosis category, older age and the presence of wheeze symptoms are associated with an increased risk of COPD in pneumoconiosis. We proposed that a routine assessment of lung function is necessary for timely and adequate clinical management.

Keywords: Pneumoconiosis, COPD, Prevalence, Risk factors

* Correspondence: pingchen0731@csu.edu.cn
†Equal contributors
[1]Department of Respiratory Medicine, The Second Xiangya Hospital, Central South University, Changsha, Hunan 410011, China
[2]Research Unit of Respiratory Diseases, Central South University, Changsha, Hunan 410011, China
Full list of author information is available at the end of the article

Background

Coal or silicosis dust exposure are risks for a range of chronic respiratory diseases, including coal workers' pneumoconiosis (CWP), silicosis, diffuse dust-related fibrosis, and COPD. Pneumoconiosis is one of the most common occupational diseases, and it is associated with the inhalation of mineral or organic dust [1] and poor personal protection [2]. The destruction of the pulmonary parenchyma and the upper airway is progressive and irreversible throughout the disease, and there is no effective therapy for the disease according to current guidelines [3]. China is one of the world's leading countries in the number of cases of pneumoconiosis, and the prevalence has remained very high in recent decades. A total of 23,152 new cases of pneumoconiosis were diagnosed in 2013, accounting for 87.72% of all reported occupational diseases in China [4].

COPD is characterized by partial reversible airflow limitation, and it is predicted to be ranked as the third most frequent cause of death in 2020 [5]. In addition to cigarette smoking, genetic factors, longstanding asthma, outdoor air pollution, secondhand smoke exposure, biomass smoke and occupational exposures are also recognized as risk factors for COPD [6–8]. In China, COPD was associated with high exposure to dust or gas/fume with no evidence of effect modification by smoking and the overall population attributable fraction for COPD due to occupational exposure was reported as 10.4% [9]. Moreover, pneumoconiosis was found to be a factor of severity in acute exacerbation of COPD (AECOPD) [10]. Patients admitted for AECOPD complicated with CWP had longer hospitalization times, a higher cost of hospitalization, and higher rates of infective microorganisms in respiratory secretions and/ or blood cultures compared to patients without pneumoconiosis [10]. This study aimed to assess the prevalence and risk factors for developing COPD and to compare the clinical difference between pneumoconiosis patients with and without COPD.

Methods

Study objectives and design

The Strengthening the reporting of observational studies in epidemiology (STROBE) checklist was followed with respect to the study design as much as possible [11]. Pneumoconiosis patients who worked underground for at least 1 year were consecutively recruited in the Hunan Occupational Disease Prevention Institute from Dec 2015 to Dec 2016. Detailed questionnaires and comprehensive clinical examinations were conducted for the participants. The study was approved by the ethics review board of the Hunan Occupational Disease Prevention Institute, and written informed consent was obtained from each participant.

Subjects with identified cases of acute pulmonary infection or pneumothorax, pulmonary tuberculosis/intrapulmonary infection, emphysema, chronic bronchitis, asthma, bronchiectasis or pulmonary interstitial fibrosis were excluded from the study. Subjects who were unable to cooperate with lung function tests were also excluded from the study.

Data collection

Upon participants' follow-up visits to the institute, medical records were reviewed from the database, and complete check-up procedures were performed for eligible participants. Basic medical information and questionnaires for COPD were collected, and pulmonary function tests were conducted. The interviewer-administered questionnaire (Appendix i) comprised specific questions related to possible risk factors. This information included age, height, weight, smoking status, duration of employment in different professions and workplaces, exposure duration time, past medical history, family history, exposure to silicosis or coal dust, and whether or not air drills were engaged. Cigarette smoking history was collected as the smoking index (SI = pack per day * smoking year) and classified into four types: heavy (≥20 pack-years), moderate (≥10, <19 pack-years), mild (<10 pack-years) and never cigarette smokers. BMI status was classified into below normal (< 18.5 kg/m^2), normal (18.5~ 23.9 kg/m^2), overweight (24.0~ 27.9 kg/m^2), and obesity (≥28 kg/m^2). The diagnosis of radiography pneumoconiosis was performed according to the China National Diagnostic Criteria [12], which is the same as that of the 1980 International Labour Organization (ILO) in the judgment of opacity profusion. The pneumoconiosis patients were classified into category I, category II, and category III according to the size, profusion, and distribution range of the opacity of the chest X-ray [13]. Pulmonary function was measured using a spirometer MasterScreen™ pulmonary function test (PFT) system (Germany), and spirometric measurements met the standards of the American Thoracic Society and the European Respiratory Society [14]. A portable diffusion carbon monoxide detector was used to measure carbon monoxide diffusion capacity. The diagnosis of COPD was performed according to the update 2015 GOLD guideline [15]. The criterion for the confirmation of a diagnosis of COPD was made through clinical manifestations, risk factors, and a post-bronchodilator forced expiratory volume in the first second/forced vital capacity (FEV_1/FVC) ratio of < 0.7 on PFT. The level of GOLD spirometric was as follows: $FEV_1\% \geq 80\%$ predicted was designated mild airflow limitation; $50\% \leq FEV_1 < 80\%$ predicted was designated moderate airflow limitation; $30\% \leq FEV_1 < 50\%$ predicted was designated severe airflow limitation; and $FEV_1 < 30\%$ predicted was designated very severe airflow limitation.

Respiratory symptoms (cough, sputum, wheeze, dyspnea and chest tightness), as well as the COPD Assessment Test (CAT) [16] and the COPD clinical questionnaire (CCQ) [17], were completed individually. The questions regarding respiratory symptoms are listed as follows: "Do you usually have a cough in the absence of a cold and cough most days, at least three times per week each year? Yes/No"; "Do you have sputum most days, at least three times per week each year? Yes/No"; "Did you have chest wheezing in the past 12 months? Yes/No"; "Do you have shortness of breath when walking faster on flat ground or on a slight slope or walk slower than others your age on flat ground due to shortness of breath? Yes/No"; and "Do you have chest tightness most days, especially after force? Yes/No". Positive respiratory symptoms were determined when the answer was "Yes". At the same time, quantitative data on the severity of symptoms were evaluated on a scale from 0 to 5 (severity scale: 0 = Not at all, 1 = Just a little, 2 = Somewhat, 3 = Moderately, 4 = Quite a lot, 5 = Very much).

Statistical analysis

Statistical analysis was performed using the Statistical Package for Social Sciences 17.0 (SPSS Inc.®, Chicago, IL, USA) software. The continuous variables had a skewed distribution and were expressed as medians (interquartile ranges). Chi-square test analysis was conducted to compare the frequencies between two groups and among four groups. Comparisons of continuous and rank variables were determined by using the Mann-Whitney U test. Correlations between pulmonary functions and scale scores were analyzed using Spearman correlation analysis. Univariate and multivariate logistic regression analysis was used to determine the risk factors of COPD, and the enter method was used to build the statistical model in the univariate regression analysis. ORs with 95% CI are presented. A p-value was used to characterize statistically significant results.

Results

A total of 650 male pneumoconiosis patients were recruited during the study period. A total of 12 pneumoconiosis patients were excluded because of their inability to cooperate with lung function tests. Finally, 638 eligible radiography pneumoconiosis patients were included in our study (Fig. 1). The mean age of these 638 subjects was 50.75 years (range 28–80 years), and the mean exposure time was 17.70 years (range 1–38 years).

According to the GOLD guideline, 119 patients (18.65%) had COPD. The prevalence of COPD was 12.32, 22.37, 45.00 and 47.06% in the patients with age of 41–50, 51–60, 61–70 and 71–80 years, respectively. The prevalence of COPD was 41.67, 18.97, 15.26 and 18.18% in the patients with BMI below normal, normal, overweight, and obesity. The prevalence of COPD was 8.24, 13.64 and 46.75% in the patients with category I, category II, category III. The prevalence of COPD was 12.72, 17.54, 27.42 and 11.76% in the patients with exposure time of 0–10, 11–20, 21–30, and 31–40 years, respectively. The prevalence of COPD was 20.42% in patients with silicosis exposure, 18.15% in patients with coal exposure. The prevalence of COPD was 21.89% in patients with air drill and 15.00% in patients without air drill. The prevalence of COPD was 19.32 and 16.77% in patients with and without smoking history and was 23.21%, 7.5%, 17.35% in the patients with heavy, moderate, mild smoking history (Table 1).

Compared with non-COPD group, the combined COPD group have significantly higher pneumoconiosis category ($p = 0.00$), older age ($p = 0.00$), longer exposure time ($p = 0.01$), lower BMI ($p = 0.01$), higher SI ($p = 0.02$) and more air drill type ($p = 0.03$). In addition, those with COPD had significantly severe airflow limitation, lower levels of Pre-FEV_1, Pre-FVC, FEV_1/FVC, DLCO and DLCO% compared with non-COPD patients (p all<0.00). The severity scores in wheeze, dyspnea, CAT, and CCQ were significantly

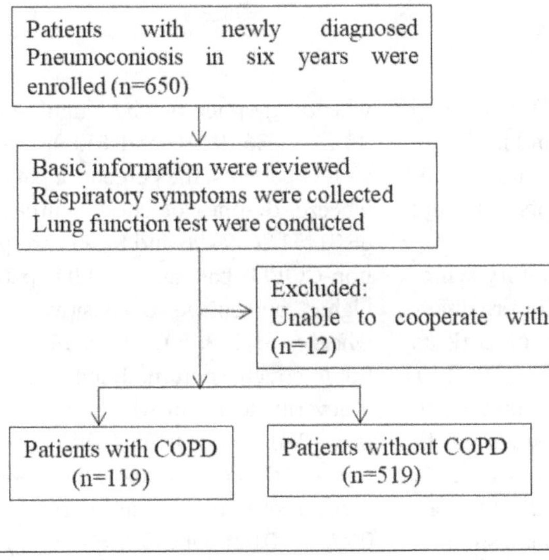

Fig. 1 Study flow diagram

Table 1 Demographic characteristics of the pneumoconiosis patients and prevalence of COPD

Total ($n = 638$)		Subjects		Prevalence of COPD	
		No.	%	No.	%
Age,years	21–30	2	0.31%	0	0%
	31–40	10	1.57%	0	0%
	41–50	341	53.45%	42	12.32%
	51–60	228	35.74%	51	22.37%
	61–70	40	6.27%	18	45.00%
	71–80	17	2.66%	8	47.06%
BMI	Below normal	24	3.76%	10	41.67%
	Normal	369	57.84%	70	18.97%
	Overweight	190	29.78%	29	15.26%
	Obesity	55	8.62%	10	18.18%
Category	I	352	55.17%	29	8.24%
	II	132	20.69%	18	13.64%
	III	154	24.14%	72	46.75%
Exposure time, years	0–10	173	27.12%	22	12.72%
	11–20	228	35.74%	40	17.54%
	21–30	186	29.15%	51	27.42%
	31–40	51	7.99%	6	11.76%
Exposure type	Silicosis dust	142	22.26%	29	20.42%
	Coal dust	496	77.74%	90	18.15%
Air drill type	No	300	47.02%	45	15.00%
	Yes	338	52.98%	74	21.89%
Smoking history	Never	167	26.18%	28	16.77%
	Mild	98	15.36%	17	17.35%
	Moderate	80	12.54%	6	7.5%
	Heavy	293	45.92%	68	23.21%
Education	Below primary school	8	1.25%	1	12.5%
	Primary school	197	30.88%	43	21.83%
	Middle school	423	66.30%	73	17.26%
	High school	6	0.94%	2	33.33%
	Some college	4	0.63%	0	0%

higher in the COPD group than in the non-COPD group (p all<0.00). No significant differences were found in the severity scores of cough, sputum and chest tightness symptoms and degree of education between patients with and without COPD ($p > 0.05$) (Table 2).

The distribution and severity scores of respiratory symptoms between patients with and without COPD were different. In non-COPD patients, the percentages of patients with 0, 1, 2, 3, 4, and 5 positive symptoms were 1.93, 2.70, 12.14, 12.91, 48.36, and 21.97%, respectively. However, in combined COPD patients, the percentage of patients with 0, 1, 2, 3, 4, and 5 positive symptoms was 0, 8.4, 10.92, 12.61, 35.29, and 40.34%, respectively (Fig. 2). In non-COPD patients, the percent of patients have cough, sputum, wheeze, dyspnea or chest tightness symptoms were 85.36, 82.47, 27.36, 92.10 and 81.89%, respectively. In combined COPD patients, the percent of patients have cough, sputum, wheeze, dyspnea or chest tightness symptoms were 89.08, 85.71, 51.26, 94.96 and 82.35%, respectively. Compared with non-COPD patients, COPD patients have significantly higher percentage of positive respiratory symptoms in wheeze (61/119, 50.83% vs 142/519, 27.36%, $p = 0.00$), but not in cough, sputum, dyspnea and chest tightness (Fig. 3).

Severity scores of wheeze were correlated with pre-FEV_1 ($r = -0.41$ $p = 0.00$), FEV_1/FVC ($r = -0.28$, $p = 0.00$), DLCO ($r = -0.16$, $p = 0.08$) and DLCO% ($r = -0.22$, $p = 0.02$). Severity scores of dyspnea correlated with pre-FEV_1 ($r = -0.22$, $p = 0.02$), DLCO ($r = -0.29$, $p = 0.00$) and DLCO% (r

Table 2 Comparison of clinical characteristics between pneumoconiosis patients with and without COPD

Characteristics	Non-COPD (n = 519)		COPD (n = 119)		P Value
	N	%	N	%	
Pneumoconiosis category					
I	323	62.24	29	24.37	0.00 a,**
II	114	21.97	18	15.13	
III	82	15.80	72	60.50	
Exposure type					
Silicosis	113	21.77	29	24.37	0.54 a
Coal	406	78.23	90	75.63	
Engaged in Air drill					
Yes	264	50.87	74	62.18	0.03 a,*
No	255	49.13	45	37.82	
Age,y	49.00(46.00,53.00)		53.00(48.00,60.00)		0.00 b,**
BMI, kg/m^2	23.14(21.30,25.22)		22.32(20.10,24.37)		0.01 b,**
Exposure time, y	15.00 (10.00,25.00)		20.00(13.00,25.00)		0.01 b,*
Smoking index	12.50(0.00,27.00)		20.00(1.25,32.00)		0.02 b,*
Education	2.00(1.00,2.00)		2.00(1.00,2.00)		0.25
Category	1.00(1.00,2.00)		3.00(2.00,3.00)		0.00 b,**
Pulmonary function					
Airflow limitation	0.00(0.00,0.00)		2.00(2.00,3.00)		0.00 b,**
Pre-FEV$_1$	89.70(81.40,98.60)		57.90(41.60,70.60)		0.00 b,**
Pre-FVC	91.30(83.30,99.40)		76.80(65.40,87.20)		0.00 b,**
FEV$_1$/FVC	80.56(75.94,84.55)		62.19(51.84,65.63)		0.00 b,**
DLCO	8.29(7.13,9.44)		6.86(5.42,7.99)		0.00 b,**
DLCO%	91.90(79.20,104.50)		76.40(60.60,88.50)		0.00 b,**
Severity scores					
Cough	1.00(1.00,3.00)		2.00(1.00,3.00)		0.37
Sputum	1.00(1.00,3.00)		2.00(1.00,3.00)		0.39
Wheeze	0.00(0.00,0.00)		0.00(0.00,1.00)		0.00 b,**
Dyspnea	2.00(2.00,2.00)		2.00(2.00,2.00)		0.00 b,**
Chest tightness	2.00(1.00,3.00)		2.00(1.00,3.00)		0.29
CAT	10.00(7.00,14.00)		13.00(8.00,17.00)		0.00 b,**
CCQ	21.00(16.00,26.00)		25.00(21.00,29.00)		0.00 b,**

Note: Airflow limitation are presented as average rating, 1 = mild, 2 = moderate, 3 = severe, 4 = very severe
*p<0.05, **p<0.01
[a]Chi-square test
[b]Mann-Whitney U test

= − 0.23, p = 0.01). Severity scores of cough correlated with pre-FEV$_1$ (r = − 0.24, p = 0.01). Severity scores of sputum correlated with pre-FEV$_1$ (r = − 0.21, p = 0.02). Meanwhile, Severity scores of CAT were correlated with pre-FEV$_1$ (r = − 0.35, p = 0.00) and FEV$_1$/FVC (r = − 0.27, p = 0.00), and CCQ were correlated with pre-FEV$_1$ (r = − 0.39, p = 0.00) and FEV$_1$/FVC (r = − 0.37, p = 0.00). We did not find any associations between chest tightness scores and pulmonary function index (Table 3).

The factors associated with the presence of COPD were analyzed using logistic regression. The factors associated with the presence of COPD were analyzed using logistic regression. In the whole population, in the univariate logistic regression model, pneumoconiosis category (OR, 3.29 [95% CI, 2.49–4.35] per unit higher category; p = 0.00), the presence of wheeze symptoms (OR, 2.84 [95% CI, 1.74–4.60]; p = 0.00), and age (OR, 2.31 [95% CI, 1.68–3.19] per unit older age; p = 0.00) were independent determinants of COPD; In the multivariate logistic regression model, the following factors were independent determinants of COPD: pneumoconiosis category III compared with category II (OR, 10.92 (6.20,19.24) [95% CI, 6.21–19.26]; p = 0.00), pneumoconiosis category II compared with category I (OR, 4.39 [95% CI, 2.29–8.41]; p = 0.00), the presence of wheeze symptoms (OR, 2.94 [95% CI, 1.79–4.83]; p = 0.00), age (OR, 0.90 [95% CI, 0.87–0.93] per 1-year-older age; p = 0.00) and reduction in BMI (OR, 1.09 [95% CI, 1.00–1.18] per 1 m^2/kg reduced BMI; p = 0.04) (Table 4).

However, in pneumoconiosis patients with smoking history, we also found pneumoconiosis category, old age, the presence of wheeze or sputum symptoms were significant risk of COPD in the univariate analysis. Neither type of smoking history or smoking index was a risk of COPD in pneumoconiosis patients with smoking history in the univariate or multivariate analysis (Table 5). In pneumoconiosis patients without smoking history, in the multivariate logistic regression model, pneumoconiosis category III compared with category II (OR, 10.96 [95% CI, 3.50–34.25]; p = 0.00), pneumoconiosis category II compared with category I (OR, 10.00 [95% CI, 1.67–60.13]; p = 0.01), age (OR, 0.92 [95% CI, 0.86–0.99] per 1-year-older age; p = 0.02) were independent determinants of COPD; in the univariate logistic regression model, only pneumoconiosis category (OR, 3.34 [95% CI, 1.88–5.93] per unit higher category; p = 0.00) is independent determinants of COPD (Table 6).

Discussion

In the current study, we found that the prevalence of COPD was 18.65% in pneumoconiosis. The prevalence of COPD in pneumoconiosis in our study was higher than in the average population [18–21]. A large-population, spirometry-based, cross-sectional survey of COPD prevalence in China in 2007 showed that the overall prevalence of COPD was 12.4% in men and 5.1% in women [18]. Another retrospective study showed that the overall prevalence rate of COPD among Chinese population aged over 40 years in 2013 was 7.3%, and reached as high as 15.5% in the elderly aged over 80 years [19]. In England, population-based study showed the prevalence of spirometrically-defined COPD between 2002 and 2004 was 10% [20]. Whereas it was reported that the prevalence of chronic bronchitis is 18.1% in former coal

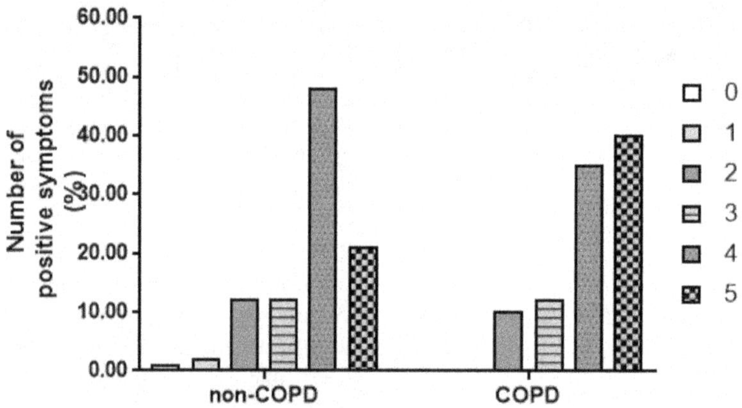

Fig. 2 Percent of patients with a certain number of positive respiratory symptoms in pneumoconiosis patients without COPD and with COPD

miners in Ukrainian [20]. And plenty studies demonstrated that the presence of COPD was significantly associated with occupational exposures [9, 20, 22], it was estimated that 10–15% of the total burden of COPD is associated with workplace exposures to dusts, noxious gases/vapors, and fumes [22–25].

We also found that this high prevalence was mainly associated with older age and advanced pneumoconiosis category. Age is often listed as a risk factor for COPD. It is unclear whether healthy aging leads one to be sensitive to COPD or if age reflects the sum of cumulative dust exposures. Nevertheless, the prevalence of COPD increased steeply with age groups and is appreciably high in those over 40 years of age in our study. In addition to age, those with a high pneumoconiosis severity also showed an overwhelming risk of developing COPD, with the highest prevalence among those in pneumoconiosis category III. Pneumoconiosis category is determined by radiographic changes in lung, and the radiographic abnormalities are closely associated with pulmonary function and prognosis in workers exposed to occupational dust [26, 27]. In predominantly active coal miners, decrements in FEV_1, FVC, and FEV_1/FVC ratios were greater with the increasing profusion of small opacities [27]. It is worth mentioning that radiographic small opacities may be less prominent as emphysema progresses, and moreover, emphysema due to coal mine dust may occur in the absence of radiographic evidence of CWP [26, 28].

Although we found a significant difference in the distribution of COPD in groups with different exposure times and in the average exposure times between the combined COPD and non-COPD group, the exposure time did not significantly contribute to the risk of COPD in the logistic analysis. These results are similar to those of other studies demonstrating that the duration of silica exposure had no independent effects on lung function [29]. The particularly small population of patients exposed for 31–40 years (51 cases) may also influence the results. Patients less susceptible to developing COPD

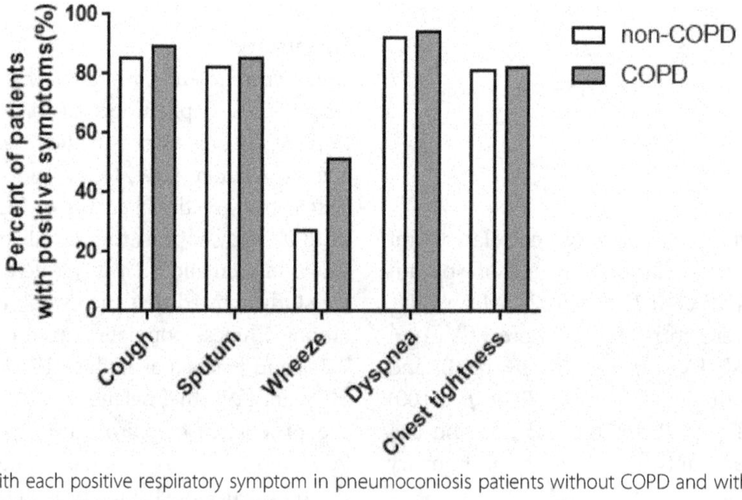

Fig. 3 Percent of patients with each positive respiratory symptom in pneumoconiosis patients without COPD and with COPD

Table 3 Correlation between pulmonary functions and scale scores in pneumoconiosis patients with the complication of COPD

	Pre-FEV$_1$	FEV$_1$/FVC	DLCO	DLCO%
Cough	−0.24(0.01)**	− 0.18(0.06)	− 0.10(0.29)	−0.11(0.22)
Sputum	−0.21(0.02)*	− 0.13(0.16)	− 0.00(0.99)	− 0.04(0.67)
Wheezing	− 0.41(0.00)**	− 0.28(0.00)**	− 0.16(0.08)	− 0.22(0.02)*
Dyspnea	− 0.22(0.02)*	− 0.13(0.16)	− 0.29(0.00)**	− 0.23(0.01)*
Chest tightness	− 0.13(0.17)	− 0.08(0.42)	−0.02(0.83)	− 0.02(0.80)
CAT	−0.35(0.00)**	− 0.27(0.00)**	−0.16(0.08)	− 0.16(0.08)
CCQ	−0.39(0.00)**	− 0.37(0.00)**	−0.14(0.14)	− 0.15(0.10)

Spearman correlation
*p<0.05, **p<0.01

due to occupational exposure may be those exposed for a rather long period of time (longer than 31 years). In the patients exposed for 31–40 years, we didn't find any association with the risk of COPD regards to age, pneumoconiosis category, BMI, SI, respiratory symptoms, exposure type or air drill type in the multivariate analysis. In our study, 26.96% of the patients had been suffering from occupational dusts for less than 10 years, and the prevalence of COPD in these patients still reached up to 12.72%. For these "short time" exposed patients, we found only pneumoconiosis category were associated with COPD in the univariate analysis.

In our observations, 73.82% of those with pneumoconiosis were smokers and 26.18% were never-smokers. Pneumoconiosis without smoking history still have a rather high prevalence of COPD and there were no significant difference in COPD prevalence between patients with and without smoking history (91/471, 19.32% vs 28/167, 16.77%, $p = 0.47$). It is well known that dust exposure is associated with both emphysema and airflow obstruction in non-smoking subjects. In Sweden, prevalence of COPD among never-smokers was 3.0–7.7% depending on definition and occupational exposure to gas, dust or fumes was significantly associated with COPD in never-smokers [30]. In one hospital-based cross-sectional study in Turkey, the prevalence of emphysema in non-smoking subjects with

Table 4 OR with 95% CI for the development of COPD in pneumoconiosis patients according to multiple logistic regression analysis

Variable	Univariate analysis		Multivariate analysis	
	OR(95%CI)	*P* value	OR(95%CI)	*P* value
Age	2.31(1.68,3.19)	0.00**	0.90(0.87,0.93)	0.00**
BMI	0.83(0.60,1.17)	0.29	1.09(1.00,1.18)	0.043*
Smoking	1.01(0.91,1.32)	0.32	0.99(0.98,1.01)	0.30
Exposure time	1.18(0.91,1.54)	0.21	0.99(0.96,1.02)	0.44
Air drill type	1.46(0.90,2.37)	0.12	1.38(0.84,2.26)	0.21
Exposure type	1.13(0.61,2.07)	0.70	1.29(0.68,2.45)	0.43
Category	3.29(2.49,4.35)	0.00**	10.92(6.20,19.24)	0.00**
			4.39(2.29,8.41)	0.00**
Cough	1.73(0.42,7.12)	0.45	1.76(0.42,7.38)	0.44
Sputum	0.51(0.14,1.82)	0.30	0.50(0.14,1.79)	0.29
Wheezing	2.84(1.74,4.60)	0.00**	2.94(1.79,4.83)	0.00**
Dyspnea	1.08(0.37,3.13)	0.89	1.12(0.38,3.34)	0.83
Chest tightness	0.98(0.51,1.90)	0.96	0.93(0.48,1.82)	0.83

In univariate analysis model:
Age (1 = 21–30,2 = 31–40,3 = 41–50,4 = 51–60,5 = 61–70,6 = 71–80)
BMI (1 = Below normal, 2 = Normal, 3 = Overweight, 4 = Obesity)
Smoking (1 = Never smokers, 2 = Mild smokers, 3 = Moderate smokers, 4 = Heavy smokers)
Exposure time (1 = 0–10, 2 = 11–20, 3 = 21–30, 4 = 31–40)
Air drill type (1 = No, 2 = Yes)
Exposure type (1 = Silicosis, 2 = Coal)
Category (1 = I, 2 = II, 3 = III)
Cough: 1 = No, 2 = Yes, Sputum: 1 = No, 2 = Yes, Wheezing: 1 = No, 2 = Yes, Dyspnea: 1 = No, 2 = Yes,
Chest tightness:1 = No, 2 = Yes
In multivariate analysis, age, BMI, exposure time and SI were taken as covariate
OR odd ratio, *CI* confidence interval
*p<0.05, **p<0.01

Table 5 OR with 95% CI for the development of COPD in pneumoconiosis patients with smoking history according to multiple logistic regression analysis

Variable	Univariate analysis		Multivariate analysis	
	OR(95%CI)	*P* value	OR(95%CI)	*P* value
Age	2.55(1.73,3.75)	0.00**	0.89(0.86,0.93)	0.00**
BMI	0.76(0.52,1.12)	0.16	1.09(1.00,1.20)	0.06
Smoking	1.01(0.77,1.56)	0.63	1.00(0.98,1.01)	0.50
Exposure time	1.07(0.78,1.45)	0.68	1.00(0.97,1.03)	0.98
Air drill type	1.51(0.86,2.66)	0.15	1.44(0.81,2.56)	0.22
Exposure type	1.08(0.52,2.25)	0.84	1.22(0.57,2.60)	0.61
Category	3.40(2.43,4.76)	0.00**	11.85(5.97,23.49)	0.00**
			3.92(1.90,8.07)	0.00**
Cough	4.29(0.81,22.65)	0.09	4.16(0.76,22.93)	0.10
Sputum	0.21(0.05,0.95)	0.04*	0.21(0.05,1.00)	0.06
Wheezing	3.00(1.70,5.31)	0.00**	3.10(1.72,5.56)	0.00**
Dyspnea	0.75(0.22,2.53)	0.64	0.75(0.22,2.55)	0.64
Chest tightness	0.94(0.43,2.05)	0.87	0.91(0.41,2.00)	0.81

In univariate analysis model:
Smoking (1 = Mild smokers, 2 = Moderate smokers, 3 = Heavy smokers)
OR odd ratio, *CI* confidence interval
*p<0.05, **p<0.01

Table 6 OR with 95% CI for the development of COPD in pneumoconiosis patients without smoking history according to multiple logistic regression analysis

Variable	Univariate analysis		Multivariate analysis	
	OR(95%CI)	*P* value	OR(95%CI)	*P* value
Age	1.83(0.99,3.37)	0.05	0.92(0.86,0.99)	0.02*
BMI	1.05(0.52,2.12)	0.90	1.08(0.90,1.29)	0.41
Exposure time	1.64(0.92,2.91)	0.09	0.94(0.88,1.00)	0.05
Air drill type	1.23(0.47,3.23)	0.67	1.02(0.38,2.78)	0.97
Exposure type	1.35(0.40,4.60)	0.63	1.29(0.35,4.77)	0.70
Category	3.34(1.88,5.93)	0.00**	10.96(3.50,34.25)	0.00**
			10.00(1.67,60.13)	0.01**
Cough	0.00(0.00–0.00)	1.00	0.00(0.00–0.00)	1.00
Sputum	0.00(0.00–0.00)	1.00	0.00(0.00–0.00)	1.00
Wheezing	2.40(0.91,6.30)	0.08	2.49(0.90,6.92)	0.08
Dyspnea	5.04(0.38,66.58)	0.22	8.81(0.61,128.08)	0.11
Chest tightness	0.93(0.23,3.76)	0.92	0.79(0.19,3.31)	0.75

OR odd ratio, *CI* confidence interval
*$p<0.05$, **$p<0.01$

CWP was 15% [31]. Another autopsied study on coal miners in the United States showed that the average prevalence of emphysema in non-smoking miners was 30% [32]. In a review of occupational exposure and COPD, the population attributable risk (PAR) for COPD attributable to work was estimated to be 40% in never-smokers and 15% in the overall population [33]. Longitudinal studies have shown that exposure to coal dust has a rapidly decreasing effect on FEV_1, independent of cigarette smoking [34]. And the progressive massive fibrosis grade and emphysema index at CT were found to be the best independent determinants of FEV_1,FEV_1/FVC, and TLC in silicosis. Neither duration of silica exposure nor cigarette consumption had an independent influence on the lung function or clinical parameters, with the exception that cigarette consumption affected DLCO [29]. Because smoking is recognized as an undisputed risk factors risk factor of COPD, we stratified the smoking factor according to smoking history. However, in pneumoconiosis patients with smoking history, neither smoking index nor smoking history type were significant risk of COPD. Advanced category of pneumoconiosis, old age and the presence of wheeze symptoms were the determinant factor of development of COPD in the pneumoconiosis patients. However, the relative small population of patients without smoking history and a healthy smoker effect biasing our results.

Within the COPD group, there were close correlations between lung ventilation function and scores for wheeze, dyspnea, cough, sputum, CAT, CCQ, as well as close correlations between diffusing functions and scores for dyspnea and wheeze. This finding is consistent with the literature report showing that obstructive pulmonary function injury was associated with reported symptoms of dyspnea and wheeze [26]. Pneumoconiosis and COPD may share the same symptoms like cough, sputum, wheezing, dyspnea and chest tightness. However, only the presence of wheeze symptoms and the severity of wheeze and dyspnea were significantly higher in the combined COPD group than in the non-COPD group. This finding reminds us that an inquiry of respiratory symptoms is not enough in the early detection of COPD among patients with pneumoconiosis; instead, pulmonary ventilation function is important in the early screening of COPD [35].

Thus far, there is no curative treatment for pneumoconiosis. It is especially important to delay the onset and slow down the progression. According to current guidelines on the management of COPD, active screening of lung function and smoking cessation [36] is recommended. Prevention measures are critical to decreasing front-line exposures and optimally managing these combined COPD patients among coal or silica-exposed workers. Governments, enterprises, physicians should take effective measures against this situation.

There are some limitations in our study. First, our study is only an institution-based study. In epidemiologic research, population-based studies are necessary for the elimination of the "healthy smokers effect" and the "healthy worker effect". Second, mineral dust-exposed workers without radiological pneumoconiosis also have exposure-related declines in FEV_1 and a high prevalence of chronic bronchitis [37, 38]. Therefore, underlying chronic bronchitis cannot be ignored in workers with or without radiological pneumoconiosis, and occupational irritant-induced subclinical lung damage is also worthy of attention. Third, our study did not include female workers because of the extremely low population of female workers in the factories we investigated. Finally, a large population of the patients at the institute are covered by health insurance, which means that there is an unrecognized population of pneumoconiosis patients who are uninsured and probably have a higher prevalence of COPD.

Conclusions

In summary, we observed that the prevalence COPD is rather high, and advanced pneumoconiosis category, older age were associated with the risk of developing COPD in pneumoconiosis patients. This finding indicates that clinicians must remain vigilant for such COPD-susceptible groups when developing screening protocols for COPD, which will help bring down its prevalence and improve the prognosis. Further prospective cohort studies are needed to confirm these results.

Acknowledgements
The authors thank all miner workers who participated in this study.

Funding
This project carried out with the support of the Explore and Innovative Projects of doctoral students in Central South University (2015zzts118), the National Key Clinical Specialist Construction Projects ((2012)No. 650) and National Natural Science Foundation of China (81370143,81170036).

Authors' contributions
PC generated the hypothesis, directed the implementation. YP and XL contribute to data collection, statistical analyses and wrote the manuscript. ZZ, SC, YC, WD, WL, JD supervised the field activities and and edited the manuscript. All authors read and approved the final manuscript.

Consent for publication
Not applicable.

Competing interests
The authors declare that they have no competing interests.

Author details
[1]Department of Respiratory Medicine, The Second Xiangya Hospital, Central South University, Changsha, Hunan 410011, China. [2]Research Unit of Respiratory Diseases, Central South University, Changsha, Hunan 410011, China. [3]Diagnosis and Treatment Center of Respiratory Disease, Central South University, Changsha, Hunan 410011, China. [4]Hunan Institute of Occupational Disease Prevention, Hunan Provincial Center for Disease Control and Prevention, 410011 Changsha, People's Republic of China.

References
1. Cohen RAC. Is the increasing prevalence and severity of coal workers pneumoconiosis in the United States due to increasing silica exposure? J Occup Environ Med. 2010;67(10):649–50.
2. Weston A. Work-related lung diseases. IARC Sci Publ. 2011;163:387–405.
3. McCunney RJ, Morfeld P, Payne S. What component of coal causes coal workers' pneumoconiosis? J Occup Environ Med. 2009;51(4):462–71.
4. Ministry of Health of China. National occupational diseases report for 2013. (2014). Availableat:http://www.nhfpc.gov.cn/jkj/s5899t/201406/ed8ed220d0b74010bcb6dcd8e340f4fb.shtml. Accessed June 2014.
5. Postma DS, Bush A, van den Berge M. Risk factors and early origins of chronic obstructive pulmonary disease. Lancet. 2015;385(9971):899–909.
6. Eisner MD, Anthonisen N, Coultas D, et al. An official American Thoracic Society public policy statement: novel risk factors and the global burden of chronic obstructive pulmonary disease. Am J Resp Crit Care. 2010;182(5):693–718.
7. Yang Y, Mao J, Ye Z, et al. Risk factors of chronic obstructive pulmonary disease among adults in Chinese mainland: a systematic review and meta-analysis[J]. Respir Med. 2017;131:158–65.
8. Salvi SS, Barnes PJ. Chronic obstructive pulmonary disease in non-smokers[J]. Lancet. 2009;374(9691):733–43.
9. Lam KBH, Yin P, Jiang CQ, et al. Past dust and GAS/FUME exposure and COPD in Chinese: the Guangzhou biobank cohort study[J]. Respir Med. 2012;106(10):1421–8.
10. Ornek T, Atalay F, Erboy F, et al. Is pneumoconiosis a factor of severity in acute exacerbation of chronic obstructive pulmonary disease[J]. Clin Ter. 2013;164(6):e473–7.
11. Von Elm E, Altman DG, Egger M, et al. The strengthening the reporting of observational studies in epidemiology (STROBE) statement: guidelines for reporting observational studies. Int J Surg. 2014;12(12):1495–9.
12. Xia Y, Liu J, Shi T, et al. Prevalence of pneumoconiosis in Hubei, China from 2008 to 2013. Inter J Env Res Pub Heal. 2014;11(9):8612–21.
13. ILO. Guidelines for the use of ILO International classification of radiographs of pneumoconiosis. Geneva: International Labour Office 2002 (Occupational Safety and Health Series, No 22 (rev 2000); 2000.
14. Miller MR, Hankinson JA, Brusasco V, Burgos F, et al. Standardisation of spirometry. Eur Respir J. 2005;26(2):319–4.
15. Global strategy for the diagnosis, management, and prevention of chronic obstructive pulmonary disease updated 2015. (http://goldcopd.org/).
16. Gupta N, Pinto LM, Morogan A, et al. The COPD assessment test: a systematic review[J]. Eur Respir J. 2014;44(4):873–84.
17. Zhou Z, Zhou A, Zhao Y, et al. Evaluating the clinical COPD questionnaire: a systematic review[J]. Respirology. 2017;22(2):251–62.
18. Zhong N, Wang C, Yao W, et al. Prevalence of chronic obstructive pulmonary disease in China: a large, population-based survey[J]. Am J Respir Crit Care Med. 2007;176(8):753–60.
19. Zhou M. A subnational analysis for mortality and prevalence of chronic obstructive pulmonary disease in China 1990-2013: findings from global burden of disease study (GBD) 2013[J]. 2016.
20. Melville AM, Pless-Mulloli T, Afolabi OA, et al. COPD prevalence and its association with occupational exposures in a general population[J]. Eur Respir J. 2010;36(3):488–93.
21. Graber JM, Cohen RA, Basanets A, et al. Results from a Ukrainian-US collaborative study: prevalence and predictors of respiratory symptoms among Ukrainian coal miners. Am J Ind Med. 2012;55(12): 1099–109.
22. Sadhra S, Kurmi OP, Sadhra SS, et al. Occupational COPD and job exposure matrices: a systematic review and meta-analysis. Int J Chronic Obstr. 2017;12:725.
23. Omland Ø, Würtz ET, Aasen TB, et al. Occupational chronic obstructive pulmonary disease: a systematic literature review. Scand J Work Environ Health. 2014;40:19–35.
24. Torén K, Järvholm B. Effect of occupational exposure to vapors, gases, dusts, and fumes on COPD mortality risk among Swedish construction workers: a longitudinal cohort study. Chest. 2014;145(5):992–7.
25. Vinnikov D, Semizhon S, Rybina T, et al. Occupation and chronic obstructive pulmonary disease in Minsk tractor plant workers[J]. Am J Ind Med. 2017; 60(12):1049–55.
26. Hnizdo E, Vallyathan V. Chronic obstructive pulmonary disease due to occupational exposure to silica dust: a review of epidemiological and pathological evidence. Occup Environ Med. 2003;60(4):237–43.
27. Blackley DJ, Laney AS, Halldin CN, et al. Profusion of opacities in simple coal worker's pneumoconiosis is associated with reduced lung function. Chest. 2015;148(5):1293–9.
28. Go LHT, Krefft SD, Cohen RA, et al. Lung disease and coal mining: what pulmonologists need to know. Curr Opin Pulm Med. 2016;22(2):170–8.
29. Ooi GC, Tsang KWT, Cheung TF, et al. Silicosis in 76 men: qualitative and quantitative CT evaluation—clinical-radiologic correlation study. Radiology. 2003;228(3):816–25.
30. Hagstad S, Backman H, Bjerg A, et al. Prevalence and risk factors of COPD among never-smokers in two areas of Sweden–occupational exposure to gas, dust or fumes is an important risk factor[J]. Respir Med. 2015;109(11): 1439–45.
31. Altnsoy B, Öz İl, Erboy F, et al. Emphysema and Airflow Obstruction in Non-Smoking Coal Miners with Pneumoconiosis. Med Sci Monit. 2016;22:4887.
32. Kuempel ED, Wheeler MW, Smith RJ, et al. Contributions of dust exposure and cigarette smoking to emphysema severity in coal miners in the United States. Am J Resp Crit Care. 2009;180(3):257–64.
33. Blanc PD. Occupation and COPD: a brief review. J Asthma. 2012;49(1):2–4.
34. Wang ML, Wu ZE, Du QG, et al. Rapid decline in forced expiratory volume in 1 second (FEV1) and the development of bronchitic symptoms among new Chinese coal miners. J Occup Environ Med. 2007;49(10):1143–8.
35. Nishimura K, Mitsuma S, Kobayashi A, et al. COPD and disease-specific health status in a working population. Resp Res. 2013;14(1):61.
36. Chen J, Chen Y, Chen P, et al. Effectiveness of individual counseling for smoking cessation in smokers with chronic obstructive pulmonary disease and asymptomatic smokers[J]. Exp Ther Med. 2014;7(3):716–20.
37. De Zotti R. Chronic obstructive pulmonary disease (COPD) and occupational exposure to mineral dust. G Ital Med Lav Ergon. 2002;24(2):144–6.
38. Cohen RAC, Patel A, Green FHY. Lung disease caused by exposure to coal mine and silica dust. Semin Respir Crit Care Med. 2008;29(6):651–61.

7

Test-retest repeatability of child's respiratory symptoms and perceived indoor air quality – comparing self- and parent-administered questionnaires

Jussi Lampi[1,2*], Sari Ung-Lanki[1], Päivi Santalahti[3] and Juha Pekkanen[1,4]

Abstract

Background: Questionnaires can be used to assess perceived indoor air quality and symptoms in schools. Questionnaires for primary school aged children have traditionally been parent-administered, but self-administered questionnaires would be easier to administer and may yield as good, if not better, information. Our aim was to compare the repeatability of self- and parent-administered indoor air questionnaires designed for primary school aged pupils.

Methods: Indoor air questionnaire with questions on child's symptoms and perceived indoor air quality in schools was sent to parents of pupils aged 7–12 years in two schools and again after two weeks. Slightly modified version of the questionnaire was administered to pupils aged 9–12 years in another two schools and repeated after a week. 351 (52%) parents and 319 pupils (86%) answered both the first and the second questionnaire. Test-retest repeatability was assessed with intra-class correlation (ICC) and Cohen's kappa coefficients (k).

Results: Test-retest repeatability was generally between 0.4–0.7 (ICC; k) in both self- and parent-administered questionnaire. In majority of the questions on symptoms and perceived indoor air quality test-retest repeatability was at the same level or slightly better in self-administered compared to parent-administered questionnaire. Agreement of self- and parent administered questionnaires was generally < 0.4 (ICC; k) in reported symptoms and 0.4–0.6 (ICC; k) in perceived indoor air quality.

Conclusions: Children aged 9–12 years can give as, or even more, repeatable information about their respiratory symptoms and perceived indoor air quality than their parents. Therefore, it may be possible to use self-administered questionnaires in future studies also with children.

Keywords: Repeatability, Symptoms, Indoor air questionnaire

Background

Indoor air quality problems can be caused by inadequate ventilation, unpleasant room temperature, dampness and moisture damages [1], gaseous indoor air pollutants and particulate matter [2]. At group level, for instance at work places or schools, indoor air quality problems can be assessed with indoor air questionnaires. These questionnaires typically contain questions about perceived symptoms and indoor air quality [3, 4]. However, questionnaires alone cannot verify the source or presence of indoor air problems [3]. Questionnaires can, however, point to the cause of the problem, for instance high room temperature or problems in ventilation, and therefore can be used as an aid in the problem management accompanied by adequate building and structural inspections. Indoor air questionnaires used today are validated with adult workers, but not with children [4] and are intended to be parent-administered when for example used among pupils in schools.

Questionnaires concerning child respiratory symptoms have traditionally relied on parent-report. These

* Correspondence: jussi.lampi@thl.fi
[1]Department of Health Security, Environmental Health, National Institute for Health and Welfare, P.O. Box 95, FI-70701 Kuopio, Finland
[2]Social and Health, City of Kuopio, Kuopio, Finland
Full list of author information is available at the end of the article

questionnaires have been shown to have fairly good repeatability e.g. [5–7]. However, in children's health related quality of life questionnaires (HRQL) self-report has been increasingly used [8]. Furthermore, it has been suggested that children aged 6–11 years have basic understanding about concepts of health and have also capacity to associate health to environmental factors [9]. Questionnaires are easier to administer to pupils in schools than to their parents, which often leads to better response rates.

To our knowledge, repeatability of perceived symptoms and indoor air quality collected with self-administered questionnaires from primary school aged children has not been studied earlier. We therefore assessed the test- retest repeatability of two types of questionnaires, self- and parent-administered, on reported symptoms and perceived indoor air quality among primary school children and their parents. If it would be possible to collect reliable and repeatable information about perceived symptoms and environmental quality from the children themselves, self-administered questionnaires could be more widely used in epidemiologic studies also in younger children.

Methods

Study population and data collection

Present study is part of a larger study on indoor air, which was conducted in ten primary schools (age 7–12 years) in five municipalities in Finland between March 17 and April 4, 2014. All 71 regional environmental health units in Finland were approached via e-mail, asking for willingness to participate in the study and for suggestions on schools with current indoor air problems and control schools without indoor air problems. Of twelve suggestions received, five case-control school pairs were included in this study. More detailed criteria for selection of the schools are descripted previously [10]. A parent-administered questionnaire on indoor air quality was sent to all parents of the pupils in the ten schools. The research plan was approved by the Institutional Review Board (IRB) of National Institute for Health and Welfare (THL) (IRB 00007085, FWA 00014588). The study participation was voluntary and parents of the pupils were able to deny participation in advance.

Test-retest repeatability of parent-administered questionnaire was studied with a two week interval in two schools (case and control) and 351 parents (52%) returned both questionnaires. Test-retest repeatability of self-administered questionnaire was studied only among 3rd to 6th graders (age 9–12 years) with a one week interval in another two schools (case and control) and 319 pupils (86%) answered both the first and the second questionnaire. In the schools, which repeatability of self-report was tested, we had data at the baseline also from a parent -administered questionnaire, which made it possible to study also agreement between the self- and parent-administered questionnaires. However, these questionnaires were not administered exactly at the same time, as the interval between questionnaires was about 2 weeks.

Questionnaire

Parent-administered indoor air questionnaire for primary school pupils (7–12 years) was developed to study the prevalence of self-reported symptoms and perceived indoor air quality at school. The questionnaire included two sections on symptoms in the last four weeks, categorized as respiratory symptoms (8 items) and other symptoms (17 items). All items had four response options (no; yes, sometimes; yes, every week; yes, almost every day). Every item was followed by the question "if yes, does the symptom get worse at school" with response options "no", "yes" and "don't know". Symptoms were selected based on previous indoor air questionnaires used in Finland (National institute for Health and Welfare and Finnish Institute of Occupational Health) and Sweden (MM-40). The questionnaire included also questions about perceived indoor air quality at school in the last four weeks (14 items). All items had five response options (never; yes, sometimes; yes, every week; yes, almost every day; don't know). Prevalence of asthma in the study population was determined with the question "Do your child have had following diseases in the past 12 months? Asthma?" with response options "no" and "yes". The parents were instructed to fill in the questions on symptoms together with the child, and 89% of them reported doing so for some or most of the symptoms.

Self-administered indoor air questionnaire was slightly modified version from parent-administered questionnaire. The questionnaire included respiratory symptoms (5 items) and other symptoms (7 items) in the last two weeks. All items had three response options (no; yes, sometimes; yes, almost every day) and every item was followed by the question "Does the symptom get worse at school" with response options "no/no symptom", "yes" and "don't know". The questionnaire included also questions about perceived indoor air quality and other environmental characteristics at school in the last two weeks (7 items). All items had four response options (no; yes, sometimes; yes, almost every day; don't know). Prevalence of asthma in the study population was determined with the question "Do you have asthma?" with response options "no", "yes" and "don't know". Asked symptoms and environmental characteristics in schools used in both parent- and self-administered questionnaire are show in Figs. 1 and 2.

Statistical analysis

Intra-class correlation (ICC) and Cohen's kappa coefficients (k) and percentages of total, negative and positive agreement [11] were used to assess test-retest repeatability of self- and parent- administered questionnaire and agreement between self- and parent-administered questionnaires. As

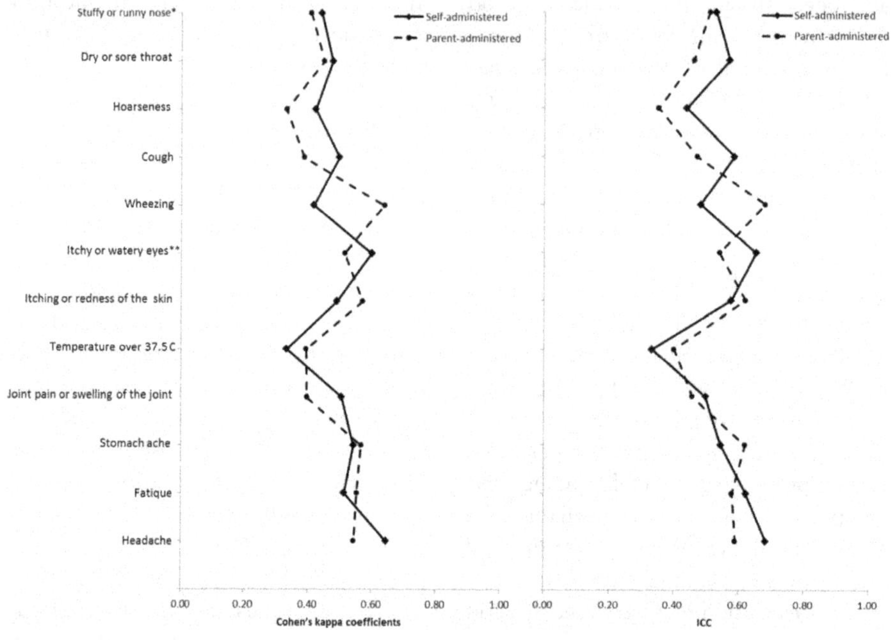

Fig. 1 Test-retest repeatability of reported symptoms from self- and parent-administered questionnaires in primary school age children assessed with Cohen's kappa coefficients and intra-class correlation (ICC). *Asked with two questions in parent administered questionnaire: stuffy nose (0.51 ICC; 0.41 k) and runny nose (0.38 ICC; 0.36 k). ** Asked with two questions in parent administered questionnaire: itchy eyes (0.54 ICC; 0.52 k) and watery eyes (0.41 ICC; 0.40 k)

the response categories in self- and parent-administered questionnaire varied, the parent-administered answers were categorized to 3 classes ("no", "yes, sometimes" or "yes, every week" and "yes almost every day") for these analyses, so that the number of categories would be the same. To calculate Cohen's kappa coefficients and percentages of total, negative and positive agreement, responses were dichotomized to "no" or "yes" (includes all of the different "yes" answer options). All of the analyses were done with SPSS.

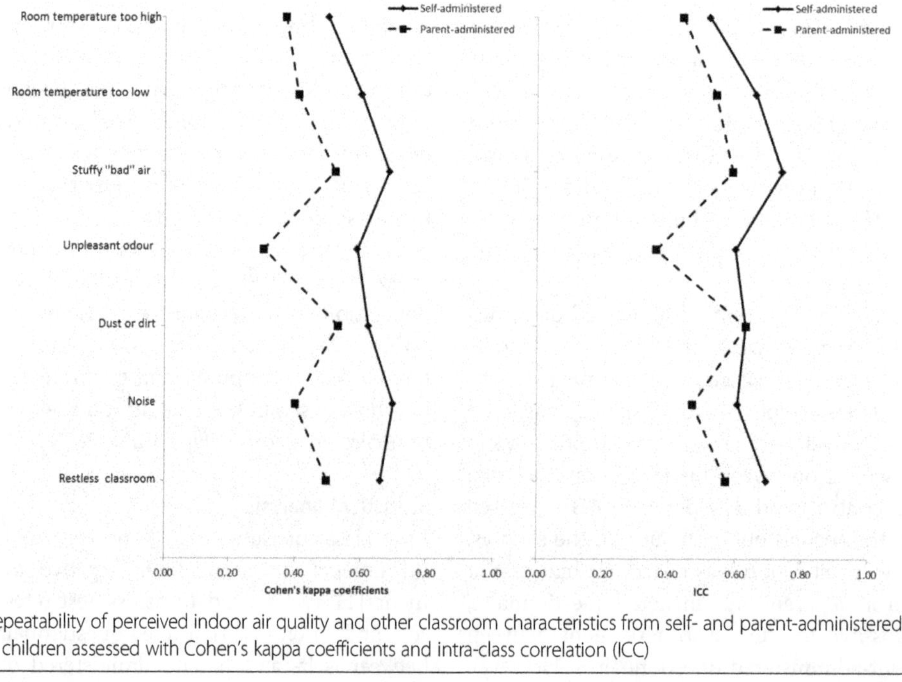

Fig. 2 Test-retest repeatability of perceived indoor air quality and other classroom characteristics from self- and parent-administered questionnaires in primary school age children assessed with Cohen's kappa coefficients and intra-class correlation (ICC)

Results

Test-retest repeatability of parent-administered questionnaire was assessed with 351 pupils aged 7–12 years and from these pupils 49% were boys and 51% girls. Similarly, test-retest repeatability of self-administered questionnaire was assessed with 319 pupils aged 9–12 years and from these pupils 44% were boys and 56% girls. Prevalence of the symptoms, perceived indoor air quality and missing information in these two populations are show in Additional file 1: Table S1 and S2. Prevalence of missing information in symptoms and perceived indoor air quality was low, generally around 1 %, and highest percentage of missing information observed was 2.7% (wheezing in self-administered questionnaire). Highest prevalence of don't know answers was 13.5% in self-administered questionnaire (dust and dirt) and 7.5% (unpleasant odor) in parent-administered questionnaire, but generally lower in both self- and parent- administered questionnaires. Missing information and don't know answers were excluded from further analysis.

Repeatability of the self-administered questionnaire

Test-retest repeatability of questions on symptoms and perceived indoor air quality in schools from self-administered questionnaires were generally within 0.4–0.7 (ICC, k) (Figs. 1 and 2). Only question with repeatability below 0.4 was temperature over 37.5 C in past 2 weeks (0.33 ICC; k). For sensitivity analysis, we stratified the analysis by pupil's grade in schools, but no major differences in test-retest repeatability in self-administered questionnaire for symptoms and perceived indoor air quality between the younger or older pupils were observed (data not shown). Percentages of observed total agreement and proportions of negative and positive agreement of question from self-administered questionnaire are shown in Additional file 1: Table S3.

Repeatability of the parent-administered questionnaire

Test-retest repeatability of reported symptoms and perceived indoor air quality in schools from parent-administered questionnaires were generally at the same level or slightly lower than in self-administered questionnaire and generally was within 0.4–0.7 (ICC, k) in parent-administered questionnaire also (Figs. 1 and 2). The questions with test-retest repeatability below 0.4 were runny nose (0.38 ICC; 0.36 k), hoarseness (0.35 ICC; 0.33 k), and cough (0.47 ICC; 0.39 k). Only symptom where test-retest repeatability was distinctly higher in parent-administered questionnaire was wheezing (0.68 vs. 0.48 ICC; 0.64 vs. 0.42 k). Percentages of observed total agreement and proportions of negative and positive agreement of question from parent-administered questionnaire are shown in Additional file 1: Table S4.

Agreement between the self- and parent administered questionnaires

Agreement between self- and parent administered questionnaires at baseline was generally within 0.2–0.4 (ICC; k) in all reported symptoms expect headache (0.51 ICC; 0.45 k) (Fig. 3). Compared to reported symptoms, agreement between parent- and self-administered questionnaires in perceived indoor air quality was higher, as the intraclass correlation was between 0.47–0.60 and Cohen's kappa coefficient between 0.38–0.58 (Fig. 4). Percentages of observed total agreement and proportions of negative and positive agreement of question between self- and parent administered questionnaires are shown in Additional file 1: Table S5.

Asthma

Prevalence of asthma was 8.8% in both self-administered questionnaires and Cohen's kappa coefficient between self-administered questionnaires was 0.98. In first self-administered questionnaire prevalence of don't know answers was 7.6% and missing information was 0.6%. In second self-administered questionnaire prevalence of don't know answers was 8.8% and missing information was 0.6%.

Prevalence of asthma was 9.3% in the first parent-administered questionnaire and 8.6% in the second parent-administered questionnaire. Cohen's kappa coefficient between parent-administered questionnaires was 0.87 in reported asthma. In first parent-administered

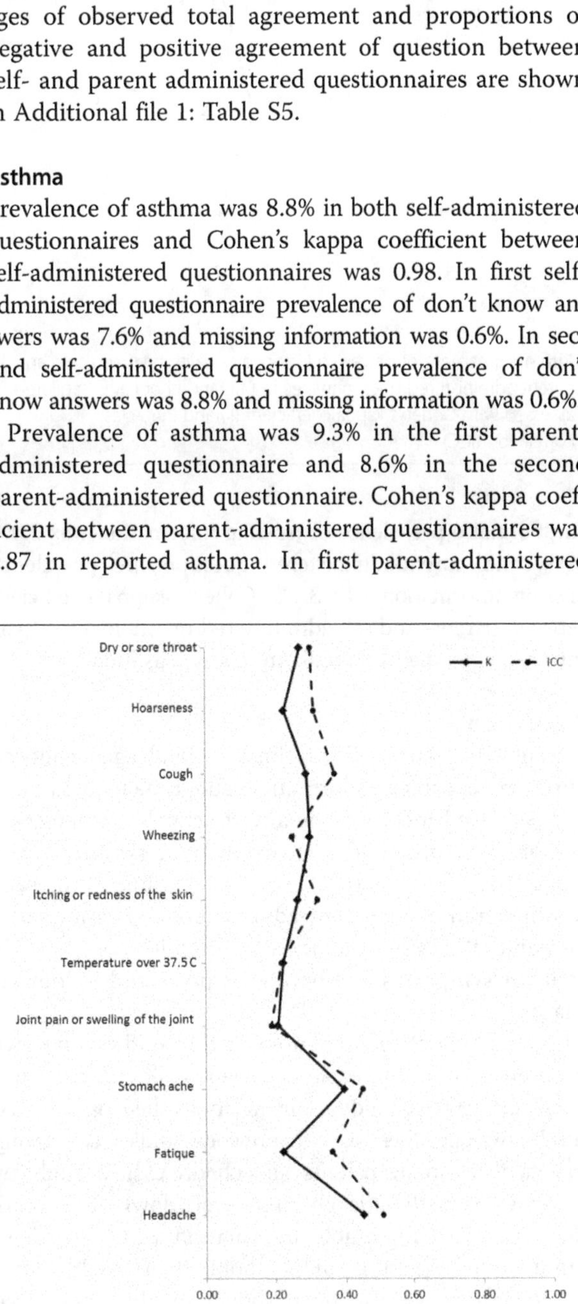

Fig. 3 Agreement of reported symptoms between self- and parent administered questionnaires in primary school aged children assessed with Cohen's kappa coefficient (k) and intra-class correlation (ICC)

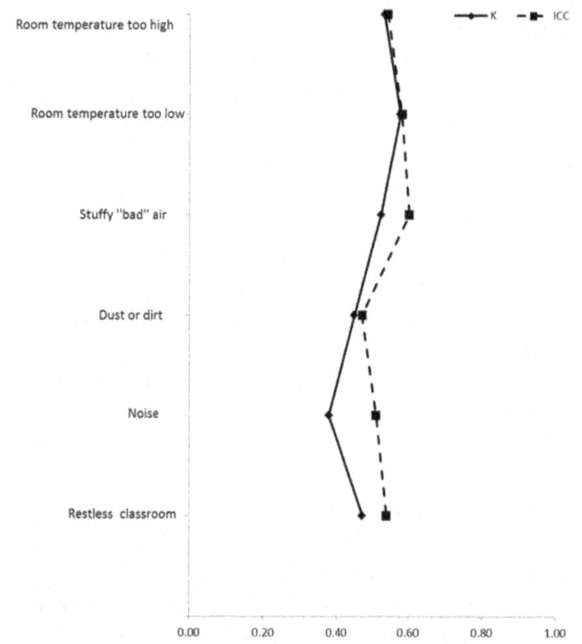

Fig. 4 Agreement of perceived indoor air quality between self- and parent administered questionnaires in primary school aged children assessed with Cohen's kappa coefficient (k) and intra-class correlation (ICC)

questionnaire prevalence of missing information was 2.3%. In second parent-administered questionnaire prevalence missing information was 3.4%. Cohen's kappa coefficient between parent- and self-administered questionnaires (parent-child agreement) was 0.87 in reported asthma.

Discussion

Present study shows that primary school aged children can give repeatable information about their symptoms and perceived indoor air quality at schools. In perceived indoor air quality and with majority of symptoms the repeatability was at the same level or higher in self-administered than parent-administered questionnaire. Agreement between the parent and child was generally poor for symptoms, but better for perceived indoor air quality.

Primary school aged children in this study could give as, or even more, repeatable information about their symptoms and perceived indoor air quality as their parents. To our knowledge, there are no previous studies comparing repeatability among parents and children. In a study by Olson et al. asthmatic children even down to 7 years old could give repeatable information with interview-administered questionnaires about their health [12]. Adolescents have also been shown to give repeatable information about their respiratory symptoms with self-administered questionnaires [13, 14]. Furthermore, it has been reported that children aged 11 years can give repeatable information about their physical and social environment at home and in neighborhood [15]. In our study, only in questions about temperature over 37.5 C and wheezing the test-retest repeatability was distinctly lower in self-administered than in parent-administered questionnaire. Wheezing is a difficult concept even for parents to understand [16, 17], therefore it is not surprising that repeatability of self-reported wheeze was poor in children. Thus, questions should be quite descriptive or should be visualized to be more understandably for children [9]. However, based on this and previous studies, children aged 9–12 years appear to be able to give repeatable information about their symptoms and perceived indoor air quality.

In this study parent-child agreement on symptoms was low, which is in line with previous studies [18–20]. It is possible that this is partly explained by characteristics of the child or the parent, which may lead to under- or over reporting of symptoms. It has been shown that mothers self-reported health is strongly associated with how she reports on the health of the child [21]. Parent's lifestyle factors (e.g. smoking) may also affect their reporting on child's symptoms [22]. Furthermore, psychosocial factors are known to affect environmental complaints and perceived symptoms [23]. However, agreement on perceived indoor air quality was better than for symptoms in the present study.

The validity of the information given by the children cannot be assessed with the present results and study design. Previous studies have suggested that in child perception of asthma symptoms are associated with objective measurements of the lung function and the correlation between symptoms and lung function may be better or at the same level than parent's perception of the symptoms [24, 25] but dependent on age of the child [26]. In this study, child-parent agreement on asthma was excellent which is in line with previous studies [18, 20, 27]. This gives some suggestive indication also for validity of the questionnaire.

The test-retest repeatability of reported symptoms and perceived indoor air quality in both self- and parent-administered questionnaire was generally 0.4–0.7 (ICC, k) in this study. This level of repeatability is generally considered to be acceptable for this type of questionnaires. However, when test-retest repeatability is assessed by using kappa values, the dependence of kappa values on marginal prevalence's (i.e. amount of change in agreement) should be acknowledged. The dependence results directly from definition of kappa [28].

The few limitations of the study should be acknowledged. The self-administered questionnaire was slightly different from the parent-administered questionnaire. There were fewer questions, questions had one less response category, and the time period used was different (2 weeks in self-reported vs. 4 weeks in parent-reported questionnaire). Furthermore, the time interval in which the test-retest was performed was not the same (1 week in self-reported vs. 2 weeks in parent-reported questionnaire). These factors can affect differences between test-retest repeatability of self- and parent-administered questionnaires and agreement between self- and parent- reported symptoms. It should also be noted that the repeatability of self and parent-administered questionnaires were tested in different schools, since otherwise the children would have had to take part in filling of four questionnaires in total, two self-administered and two parent-administered, as parent-administered questionnaires were instructed to be filled in together with the child. Furthermore, the agreement of the reported symptoms between self- and parent administered questionnaire can be partly affected by the fact that questionnaires were not administered exactly at the same time.

Conclusion

Children aged 9–12 years can give as, or even more, repeatable information about their symptoms and perceived indoor air quality than their parents. Therefore, in future it may be possible to use self-administered questionnaires in epidemiologic studies on perceived indoor air quality and symptoms also among primary school age children. If indoor air questionnaires could be administered to pupils during school day, this could lead to better response rates and even more reliable results.

Abbreviations

ICC: intra-class correlation; K: Cohen's kappa coefficients

Acknowledgements

Not applicable.

Funding

This work was partly funded by a grant from the Ministry of Social Affairs and Health, Finland.

Authors' contributions

JL wrote the manuscript, performed the statistical analysis, made substantial contributions to the data interpretation and to the planning of the manuscript. JP and SU-L designed the study, made substantial contributions to the writing and planning of the manuscript, data interpretation and statistical analysis. PS made contributions to the writing of the manuscript, data interpretation and to the planning of the manuscript. All the authors have critically revised and approved the final version of the manuscript.

Consent for publication

Not applicable.

Competing interests

The authors declare that they have no competing interests.

Author details

[1]Department of Health Security, Environmental Health, National Institute for Health and Welfare, P.O. Box 95, FI-70701 Kuopio, Finland. [2]Social and Health, City of Kuopio, Kuopio, Finland. [3]Department of Health, Mental Health Unit, National Institute for Health and Welfare, Helsinki, Finland. [4]Department of Public Health, University of Helsinki, Helsinki, Finland.

References

1. WHO Guidelines. For indoor air quality: dampness and Mould. Geneva: World health Organization; 2009.
2. Bernstein JA, Alexis N, Bacchus H, Bernstein IL, Fritz P, Horner E, Li N, Mason S, Nel A, Oullette J, Reijula K, Reponen T, Seltzer J, Smith A, Tarlo SM. The health effects of non-industrial indoor air pollution. J Allergy Clin Immunol. 2008;121(3):585–91.
3. Reijula K, Sundman-Digert C. Assessment of indoor air problems at work with a questionnaire. Occup Environ Med. 2004;61(1):33–8.
4. Andersson K. Epidemiological approach to indoor air problems. Indoor Air. Supplement: 4 Pages: 32–39 Published: 1998.
5. Strippoli MP, Silverman M, Michel G, Kuehni CE. A parent-completed respiratory questionnaire for 1-year-old children: repeatability. Arch Dis Child. 2007;92(10): 861–5.
6. Faniran AO, Peat JK, Woolcock AJ. Measuring persistent cough in children in epidemiological studies: development of a questionnaire and assessment of prevalence in two countries. Chest. 1999;115(2):434–9.
7. Brunekreef B, Groot B, Rijcken B, Hoek G, Steenbekkers A, de Boer A. Reproducibility of childhood respiratory symptom questions. Eur Respir J. 1992;5(8):930–5.
8. Upton P, Lawford J, Eiser C. Parent-child agreement across child health-related quality of life instruments: a review of the literature. Qual Life Res. 2008;17(6):895–913.
9. Bevans KB, Riley AW, Moon J, Forrest CB. Conceptual and methodological advances in child-reported outcomes measurement. Expert Rev Pharmacoecon Outcomes Res. 2010;10(4):385–96.
10. Ung-Lanki S, Lampi J, Pekkanen J. Analyzing symptom data in indoor air questionnaires for primary schools. Indoor Air. 2017 Sep;27(5):900–8.
11. Cicchetti DV, Feinstein AR. High agreement but low kappa: II. Resolving the paradoxes. J Clin Epidemiol. 1990;43(6):551–8.
12. Olson LM, Radecki L, Frintner MP, Weiss KB, Korfmacher J, Siegel RM. At what age can children report dependably on their asthma health status? Pediatrics. 2007;119(1):e93–102.
13. Shaw RA, Crane J, Pearce N, Burgess CD, Bremner P, Woodman K, Beasley R. Comparison of a video questionnaire with the IUATLD written questionnaire for measuring asthma prevalence. Clin Exp Allergy. 1992;22(5):561–8.
14. Braun-Fahrländer C, Gassner M, Grize L, Minder CE, Varonier HS, Vuille JC, Wüthrich B, Sennhauser FH. Comparison of responses to an asthma symptom questionnaire (ISAAC core questions) completed by adolescents and their parents. SCARPOL-Team Swiss Study on Childhood Allergy and Respir Symptoms with respect to Air Pollut Pediatr Pulmonol. 1998;25(3):159–66.
15. Hume C, Ball K, Salmon J. Development and Reliability of a self-report questionnaire to examine children's perceptions of the physical activity environment at home and in the neighbourhood. Int J Behav Nutr Phys Act. 2006;3:16.
16. Cane RS, Ranganathan SC, McKenzie SA. What do parents of wheezy children understand by "wheeze"? Arch Dis Child. 2000;82(4):327–32.
17. Cane RS, McKenzie SA. Parents' interpretations of children's respiratory symptoms on video. Arch Dis Child. 2001;84(1):31–4.
18. Sweeting H, West P. Health at age 11: reports from schoolchildren and their parents. Arch Dis Child. 1998;78(5):427–34.
19. Hoek G, Wypij D, Brunekreef B. Self-reporting versus parental reporting of acute respiratory symptoms of children and their relation to pulmonary function and air pollution. Int J Epidemiol. 1999;28(2):293–9.

20. Wong TW, Yu TS, Liu JL, Wong SL. Agreement on responses to respiratory illnesses questionnaire. Arch Dis Child. 1998;78(4):379–80.
21. Waters E, Doyle J, Wolfe R, Wright M, Wake M, Salmon L. Influence of parental gender and self-reported health and illness on parent-reported child health. Pediatrics. 2000;106(6):1422–8.
22. Dales RE, White J, Bhumgara C, McMullen E. Parental reporting of childrens' coughing is biased. Eur J Epidemiol. 1997;13(5):541–5.
23. Lahtinen M, Sundman-Digert C, Reijula K. Psychosocial work environment and indoor air problems: a questionnaire as a means of problem diagnosis. Occup Environ Med. 2004;61(2):143–9.
24. Yu TS, Wong TW. Can school children provide valid answers about their respiratory health experiences in questionnaires? Implications for epidemiological studies. Pediatr Pulmonol. 2004;37(1):37–42.
25. Lara M, Duan N, Sherbourne C, Lewis MA, Landon C, Halfon N, Brook RH. Differences between child and parent reports of symptoms among Latino children with asthma. Pediatrics. 1998;102(6):E68.
26. Guyatt GH, Juniper EF, Griffith LE, Feeny DH, Ferrie PJ. Children and adult perceptions of childhood asthma. Pediatrics. 1997;99(2):165–8.
27. Andersen A, Krølner R, Holstein BE, Due P, Hansen EH. Medicine use among 11- and 13-year-olds: agreement between parents' reports and children's self-reports. Ann Pharmacother. 2007;41(4):581–6.
28. Vach W. The dependence of Cohen's kappa on the prevalence does not matter. J Clin Epidemiol. 2005;58(7):655–61.

8

Long-term progression-free survival in an advanced lung adenocarcinoma patient harboring EZR-ROS1 rearrangement

Liang Dong[†], Jingwen Xia[†], Jing Zhang, Yuanyuan Zhang, Ning Zhu, Peng Zhang, Youzhi Zhang, Xiujuan Zhang and Shengqing Li[*]

Abstract

Background: Crizotinib is recommended as first-line therapy in ROS1-driven lung adenocarcinoma. However, the optimal first-line therapy for this subgroup of lung cancer is controversial according to the available clinical data.

Case presentation: Here, we describe a 57-year-old man who was diagnosed with stage IIIB lung adenocarcinoma and EGFR/KRAS/ALK-negative tumors. The patient received six cycles of pemetrexed plus cisplatin as first-line therapy and then pemetrexed as maintenance treatment, with a progression-free survival (PFS) of 42 months. The patient relapsed and underwent re-biopsy. EZR-ROS1 fusion mutation was detected by next-generation sequencing (NGS). The patient was prescribed crizotinib as second-line therapy and achieved a PFS of 6 months. After disease progression, lorlatinib was administered as third-line therapy, with a favorable response.

Conclusions: Prolonged PFS in patients receiving pemetrexed chemotherapy might be related to the EZR-ROS1 fusion mutation. Lorlatinib is an optimal choice in patients showing crizotinib resistance.

Keywords: Lung adenocarcinoma, ROS1 rearrangement, Pemetrexed, Crizotinib, Lorlatinib

Background

Prolonging the overall survival (OS) of advanced lung cancer patients remains a challenge. The advent of targeted therapeutic approaches led to the classification of NSCLC into subgroups according to factors such as histology and the molecular makeup of the tumor. C-ros oncogene 1 (ROS1) rearrangements are detected in approximately 1–2% of patients with NSCLC [1, 2]. ROS1 is a receptor tyrosine kinase (RTK) related to the anaplastic lymphomakinase/lymphocyte-specific protein tyrosine kinase (ALK/LTK) and insulin receptor (INSR) RTK families [3, 4]. Preclinical and clinical data support the efficacy of tyrosine kinase inhibitors (TKIs) against these receptors, such as crizotinib (first generation) [5, 6], ceritinib (second generation) [7], and lorlatinib (third generation) [8, 9], in ROS1-positive NSCLC patients. However, a case series study reported prolonged PFS with pemetrexed as first-line and maintenance therapy in patients with ROS1-driven lung adenocarcinoma [10], indicating that patients in this subgroup may be optimal candidates for pemetrexed chemotherapy.

We herein report a case of advanced lung adenocarcinoma with EZR-ROS1 rearrangement treated by first-line pemetrexed/cisplatin and then pemetrexed mono-drug for maintenance therapy. After progression, crizotinib was used as second-line treatment, and lorlatinib as third-line treatment. The patient showed an excellent response and achieved long-term progression-free survival (PFS).

Case presentation

A 57-year-old man with a 20-pack-year smoking history presented to the hospital in March 2013 with a persistent cough for 2 months and a palpable right cervical mass for 4 days. Enhanced computed tomography (CT)

* Correspondence: shengqingli@hotmail.com
[†]Equal contributors
Department of Pulmonary and Critical Care Medicine, Huashan Hospital, Fudan University, #12, Urumqi middle Road, Shanghai 200040, China

showed a 9 × 11 mm nodule in the lower lobe of the left lung and multiple enlarged lymph nodes (Fig. 1a). The serum levels of carcinoembryonic antigen (CEA) were 21.86 μg/L (Fig. 1, lower panel). A cervical lymph node biopsy confirmed the diagnosis of lung adenocarcinoma. The biopsy sample was genotyped negative for EGFR and KRAS mutations using an amplification refractory mutation system (ARMS)-polymerase chain reaction (PCR) method and negative for ALK rearrangement by fluorescent in situ hybridization (FISH). At that time, ROS1 rearrangement was not detected because of the lack of a detection method and no targeted drug available in clinical practice. The patient's clinical stage was determined as cT1aN3M0 (stage IIIB). Accordingly, he received first-line chemotherapy with six cycles of pemetrexed (500 mg/m^2) and cisplatin (75 mg/m^2), achieving a partial response (Fig. 1b). Maintenance therapy consisted of nine cycles of pemetrexed (500 mg/m^2) every month (Fig. 1c). Assessment of CEA levels and a lung CT scan were performed every 2–3 months during the follow-up period. In March 2016, the patient showed a marked increase in serum CEA levels from 1.78 μg/L to 10.21 μg/L, and a CT scan showed pulmonary disease progression with an enlarged 31 × 15 mm nodule (Fig. 1d). The patient was treated with four cycles of pemetrexed (500 mg/m^2) and cisplatin (75 mg/m^2) at a local hospital. At last, the pemetrexed-based regimen for this patient resulted in a PFS of 42 months.

The patient was referred to our hospital because of disease progression. Following admission, a positron emission tomography (PET)/CT scan revealed a 32 × 17 mm nodule in the left lower lobe with intense uptake of 18F–fluorodeoxyglucose and multiple hypermetabolic lymph nodes (Figs. 1e and 2a). To understand the

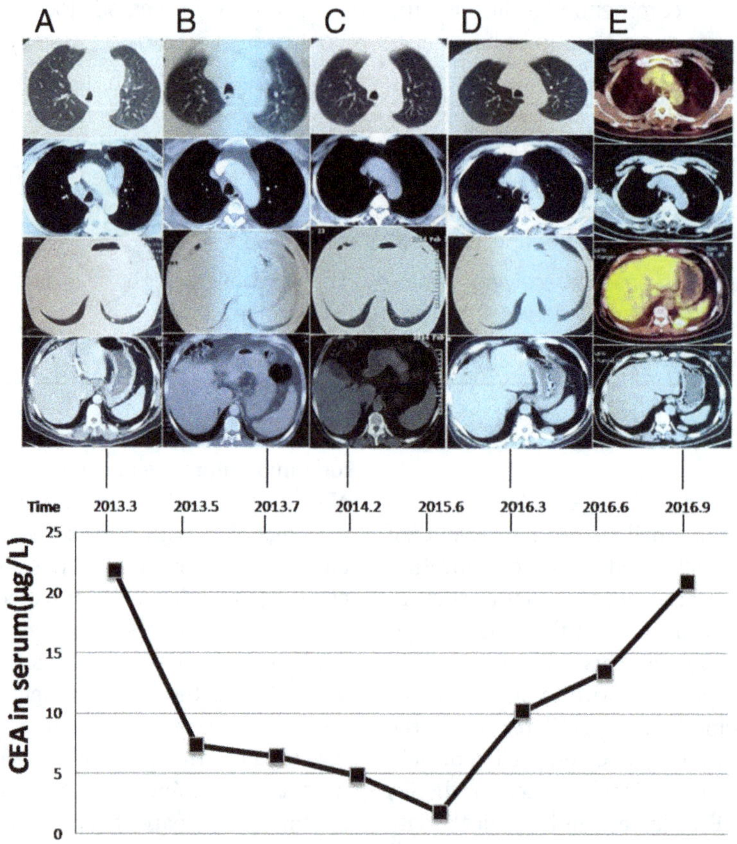

Fig. 1 Follow-up schematic diagram between March 2013 and September 2016. The top panel shows a series of CT scans (columns **a**–**d**) and a PET/CT scan (column **e**) at different time points as indicated. The upper two rows of images of the lung window and mediastinal window depict the changes of enlarged mediastinal lymph nodes, which shrunk after six cycles of pemetrexed plus cisplatin chemotherapy and nine cycles of pemetrexed maintenance (columns **a**–**c**). They remained stable after four cycles of pemetrexed plus cisplatin chemotherapy (columns **d**–**e**). The lower two rows of images of the lung window and mediastinal window depict the changes of the primary lesion as a 9 × 11 mm nodule (column **a**) in the left lung lower lobe. The lesion decreased in size after six cycles of pemetrexed plus cisplatin chemotherapy and nine cycles of pemetrexed maintenance (columns **a**–**c**), but relapsed with an enlarged 31 × 15 mm nodule in March 2016 (column **d**). Four cycles of pemetrexed plus cisplatin chemotherapy were unsuccessful in controlling the lesion, and a growing nodule of 32 × 17 mm was detected (column **e**). The bottom panel depicts the follow-up changes of serum CEA levels, which markedly decreased after chemotherapy, but increased in March 2016 after disease progression. CT, computed tomography; PET, positron emission tomography; CEA, carcinoembryonic antigen

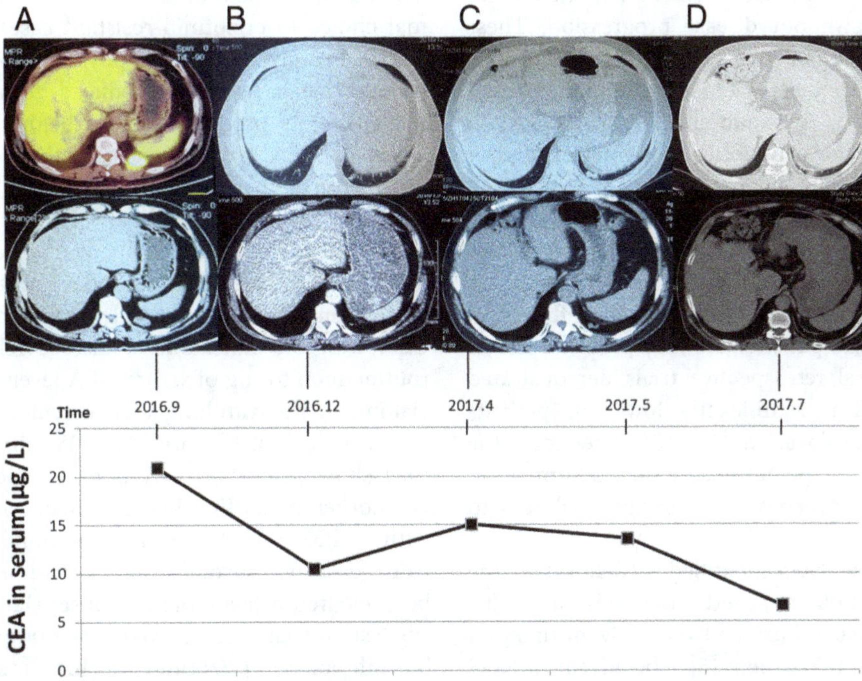

Fig. 2 Follow-up schematic diagram between September 2016 and July 2017. The top panel shows a PET/CT scan (column **a**) and a series of CT scans of the lung window and mediastinal window (columns **b**–**d**) of the primary lesion, which decreased in size after crizotinib treatment targeting the EZR-ROS1 fusion protein (columns **a** and **b**). However, relapse was detected in April 2017 (column **c**), which was controlled with lorlatinib until now (column **d**). The bottom panel depicts the follow-up changes of serum CEA levels, which markedly decreased after crizotinib treatment, and increased in April 2017 after disease progression, showing a decreasing trend after lorlatinib treatment. CT, computed tomography; PET, positron emission tomography; CEA, carcinoembryonic antigen

histological and molecular evolution of cancer tissues, a secondary biopsy was performed by endobronchial ultrasonography with a guide sheath (EBUS-GS), which confirmed the diagnosis of adenocarcinoma by immunohistochemical staining. Target-capture sequencing on an Illumina platform was performed in a laboratory certified by the College of American Pathologists using a next-generation sequencing (NGS) method across a 123 gene panel. Tumor samples showed activating mutations in EZR-ROS1, as well as the concomitant alterations NQO1(P187S), TYMS (− 6 bp non-frame shift deletion), UGT1A1(G71R), XRCC1(Q339R), CYP2D6(P34S), DPYD (I543V), and MTHFR (A222V). The tumor was therefore identified as ROS1-driven lung cancer, and the patient was immediately started on second-line therapy with crizotinib (250 mg/twice daily), which targets ROS1 rearrangements. Within 3 months of crizotinib treatment, the patient had achieved excellent radiological partial remission (Fig. 2b) according to the Response Evaluation Criteria in Solid Tumors version 1.1 (RECIST*v*1.1). In April 2017, serum CEA levels were increased, and a lung CT scan showed an enlarged nodule (Fig. 2c). The PFS on crizotinib was determined as 6 months. Lorlatinib, a third-generation macrocyclic ALK/ROS1-TKI (100 mg/once daily), was used as third-line therapy after obtaining consent from the patient. After 3 months, the patient achieved a favorable response (Fig. 2d), which was maintained at the time of publication.

Written informed consent was obtained from the patient for the publication of this case report.

Discussion and conclusions

Crizotinib is approved by the US Food and Drug Administration (FDA) for the first-line treatment of NSCLC patients with ROS1 rearrangements with a median PFS of at least 19.2 months [6, 11]. Pemetrexed-based regimens are recommended as first-line and maintenance therapy for advanced lung adenocarcinoma, particularly in patients without driven mutations [12–14]. However, pemetrexed shows superior efficacy as first-line and maintenance chemotherapy in NSCLC cases with ROS1 rearrangements. Pemetrexed showed beneficial results as first-line and maintenance therapy in four metastatic NSCLC patients with ROS1 translocations, with a PFS period of > 47 months in one patient [10]. This was considerably longer than the median PFS of 19.2 months reported for crizotinib as first-line therapy [6]. Similar results were obtained in the present case with EZR-ROS1 translocation. This patient received a pemetrexed-based regimen as front-line and maintenance therapy for 42 months overall without disease progression. These findings suggest that patients with ROS1-driven lung cancer are optimal candidates for first-line pemetrexed-based chemotherapy. A randomized control trial is needed to validate the superiority of pemetrexed over crizotinib as a first-line regimen.

The molecular mechanism underlying the prolonged PFS in ROS1-driven lung cancer treated with pemetrexed remains unknown. Low thymidylate synthase (TS) expression is positively related to the efficacy of pemetrexed in NSCLC patients and may predict a longer PFS [15, 16]. Several retrospective trials demonstrated that TS expression is significantly lower in patients harboring ROS1 translocation [17, 18]. Therefore, the favorable outcomes of pemetrexed-based treatment in ROS1-driven lung cancer could be partly attributed to low TS expression.

In the present case, NGS identified EZR-ROS1 as the oncogenic driver mutation, and crizotinib, a multi-targeted TKI, showed robust and clinically meaningful efficacy endpoints in this patient [6]. The advent of NGS revolutionized the molecular mutational spectrum of lung cancer by increasing the feasibility and range of DNA sequencing from whole genome sequencing to targeted panels, allowing the identification of targetable mutations and predicting the emergence of drug resistance [19]. NGS is capable of detecting low frequency mutations, and can screen the mutational status of different critical samples such as biopsies, cytological samples, and circulating plasma DNA, offering innovative diagnostic opportunities [20, 21]. NGS represents a highly attractive system to identify mutations and thus improve the outcome of lung cancer patients before the start of treatment [22]. An important challenge for lung cancer treatment is the spatial and temporal tumor heterogeneity, as well as clonal selection or evolution in NSCLC tumors [23, 24]. Despite the success of targeted treatment for EGFR-mutant NSCLC, the outcomes are limited by the development of TKI resistance. To dynamically monitor the histological and molecular evolution of lung cancer, secondary biopsy after each relapse combined with NGS would benefit the individualized selection of treatment regimens.

Lorlatinib is a third-generation macrocyclic ALK/ROS1 TKI with a novel chemical scaffold that shows potent antineoplastic activity against all known mutations resistant to first- and second-generation inhibitors [25–27]. The safety and efficacy of lorlatinib for ALK/ROS1-driven lung cancers were demonstrated in a phase I/II clinical trial. A recent case report described a patient who responded to lorlatinib for 8 months after becoming refractory to crizotinib [28]. The same phenomenon was observed in the present case. Therefore, we believe that lorlatinib may be the optimal choice in crizotinib-resistant cases.

CEA is a glycosylphosphatidylinositol-anchored glycoprotein that is normally produced during fetal development, and its production stops before birth [29]. High levels of CEA strongly suggest the presence of lung cancer rather than benign lung disease [30]. A rapid increase in the serum levels of CEA provides prognostic and predictive information about recurrence and mortality in NSCLC patients independent of treatment [31]. In the present case, the markedly increased serum levels of CEA were an indication of disease relapse. Therefore, routine monitoring of serum CEA levels could be beneficial in patients with lung adenocarcinoma.

In conclusion, the present ROS1-driven lung cancer case showed a positive response to pemetrexed-based chemotherapy as first-line and maintenance treatment, with a PFS of 42 months. Crizotinib and lorlatinib were used as second- and third-line therapies and both elicited a favorable response. Data from this case suggested that pemetrexed-based regimens may not be inferior to crizotinib as first-line treatment for ROS1-driven lung cancers, and lorlatinib may be an alternative treatment choice in crizotinib-resistant disease. Secondary biopsy after each relapse combined with NGS would help to dynamically monitor the histological and molecular evolution of lung cancer and may benefit the individualized selection of treatment regimens. CEA serum levels may be useful for monitoring relapse in lung adenocarcinoma.

Abbreviations

ALK/LTK: Anaplastic lymphomakinase/lymphocyte-specific protein tyrosine kinase; ARMS: Amplification refractory mutation system; CEA: Carcinoembryonic antigen; CT: Computed tomography; EBUS-GS: Endobronchial ultrasonography with a guide sheath; FDA: Food and Drug Administration; FISH: Fluorescent in situ hybridization; INSR: Insulin receptor; NGS: Next-generation sequencing; OS: Overall survival; PCR: Polymerase chain reaction; PET: Positron emission tomography; PFS: Progression-free survival; ROS1: C-ros oncogene 1; TKIs: Tyrosine kinase inhibitors; TS: Thymidylate synthase

Acknowledgments

The authors would like to thank Dr. Corina Marx and Francis Donnelly for providing assistance with English language editing.

Funding

No source of funding.

Authors' contributions

LD prepared the initial manuscript. JWX edited and submitted the manuscript. SQL drafted the article and gave final approval of the version to be published. JZ, YYZ, NZ, PZ, YZZ, and XJZ were involved in the diagnosis and treatment of the patient. All authors have read and approved the final manuscript.

Consent for publication

Written informed consent was obtained from the permitted assigns for publication of this case report and any accompanying images. A copy of the written consent is available for review by the editor of this journal.

Competing interests

The authors declare that they have no competing interests.

References

1. Cai W, Li X, Su C, Fan L, Zheng L, Fei K, Zhou C, Manegold C, Schmid-Bindert G. ROS1 fusions in Chinese patients with non-small-cell lung cancer. Ann Oncol. 2013;24(7):1822–7.
2. Bergethon K, Shaw AT, Ou SH, Katayama R, Lovly CM, McDonald NT, Massion PP, Siwak-Tapp C, Gonzalez A, Fang R, et al. ROS1 rearrangements define a unique molecular class of lung cancers. J Clin Oncol. 2012;30(8): 863–70.
3. Acquaviva J, Wong R, Charest A. The multifaceted roles of the receptor tyrosine kinase ROS in development and cancer. Biochim Biophys Acta. 2009;1795(1):37–52.
4. Robinson DR, Wu YM, Lin SF. The protein tyrosine kinase family of the human genome. Oncogene. 2000;19(49):5548–57.
5. Mazieres J, Zalcman G, Crino L, Biondani P, Barlesi F, Filleron T, Dingemans AM, Lena H, Monnet I, Rothschild SI, et al. Crizotinib therapy for advanced lung adenocarcinoma and a ROS1 rearrangement: results from the EUROS1 cohort. J Clin Oncol. 2015;33(9):992–9.
6. Shaw AT, Ou SH, Bang YJ, Camidge DR, Solomon BJ, Salgia R, Riely GJ, Varella-Garcia M, Shapiro GI, Costa DB, et al. Crizotinib in ROS1-rearranged non-small-cell lung cancer. N Engl J Med. 2014;371(21):1963–71.
7. Lim SM, Kim HR, Lee JS, Lee KH, Lee YG, Min YJ, Cho EK, Lee SS, Kim BS, Choi MY, et al. Open-label, multicenter, phase II study of Ceritinib in patients with non-small-cell lung cancer harboring ROS1 rearrangement. J Clin Oncol. 2017;35(23):2613–8.
8. Basit S, Ashraf Z, Lee K, Latif M. First macrocyclic 3rd-generation ALK inhibitor for treatment of ALK/ROS1 cancer: clinical and designing strategy update of lorlatinib. Eur J Med Chem. 2017;134:348–56.
9. Johnson TW, Richardson PF, Bailey S, Brooun A, Burke BJ, Collins MR, Cui JJ, Deal JG, Deng YL, Dinh D, et al. Discovery of (10R)-7-amino-12-fluoro-2,10,16-trimethyl-15-oxo-10,15,16,17- tetrahydro-2H-8,4-(metheno)pyrazolo[4,3-h][2,5,11]-benzoxadiazacyclotetradecine-3-carbonitrile (PF-06463922), a macrocyclic inhibitor of anaplastic lymphoma kinase (ALK) and c-ROS oncogene 1 (ROS1) with preclinical brain exposure and broad-spectrum potency against ALK-resistant mutations. J Med Chem. 2014;57(11):4720–44.
10. Riess JW, Padda SK, Bangs CD, Das M, Neal JW, Adrouny AR, Cherry A, Wakelee HA. A case series of lengthy progression-free survival with pemetrexed-containing therapy in metastatic non–small-cell lung cancer patients harboring ROS1 gene rearrangements. Clin Lung Cancer. 2013;14(5):592–5.
11. Kazandjian D, Blumenthal GM, Luo L, He K, Fran I, Lemery S, Pazdur R. Benefit-risk summary of Crizotinib for the treatment of patients with ROS1 alteration-positive, metastatic non-small cell lung cancer. Oncologist. 2016;21(8):974–80.
12. Paz-Ares L, de Marinis F, Dediu M, Thomas M, Pujol JL, Bidoli P, Molinier O, Sahoo TP, Laack E, Reck M, et al. Maintenance therapy with pemetrexed plus best supportive care versus placebo plus best supportive care after induction therapy with pemetrexed plus cisplatin for advanced non-squamous non-small-cell lung cancer (PARAMOUNT): a double-blind, phase 3, randomised controlled trial. Lancet Oncol. 2012;13(3):247–55.
13. Scagliotti GV, Parikh P, von Pawel J, Biesma B, Vansteenkiste J, Manegold C, Serwatowski P, Gatzemeier U, Digumarti R, Zukin M, et al. Phase III study comparing cisplatin plus gemcitabine with cisplatin plus pemetrexed in chemotherapy-naive patients with advanced-stage non-small-cell lung cancer. J Clin Oncol. 2008;26(21):3543–51.
14. Ettinger DS, Wood DE, Aisner DL, Akerley W, Bauman J, Chirieac LR, D'Amico TA, DeCamp MM, Dilling TJ, Dobelbower M, et al. Non-small cell lung cancer, version 5.2017, NCCN clinical practice guidelines in oncology. J Natl Compr Cancer Netw. 2017;15(4):504–35.
15. Sun JM, Ahn JS, Jung SH, Sun J, Ha SY, Han J, Park K, Ahn MJ. Pemetrexed plus Cisplatin versus Gemcitabine plus Cisplatin according to Thymidylate Synthase expression in Nonsquamous non-small-cell lung cancer: a biomarker-stratified randomized phase II trial. J Clin Oncol. 2015;33(22):2450–6.
16. Nicolson MC, Fennell DA, Ferry D, O'Byrne K, Shah R, Potter V, Skailes G, Upadhyay S, Taylor P, André V, et al. Thymidylate Synthase expression and outcome of patients receiving Pemetrexed for advanced Nonsquamous non–small-cell lung cancer in a prospective blinded assessment phase II clinical trial. J Thorac Oncol. 2013;8(7):930–9.
17. Song Z, Su H, Zhang Y. Patients with ROS1 rearrangement-positive non-small-cell lung cancer benefit from pemetrexed-based chemotherapy. Cancer Med. 2016;5(10):2688–93.
18. Zhang L, Jiang T, Zhao C, Li W, Li X, Zhao S, Liu X, Jia Y, Yang H, Ren S, et al. Efficacy of crizotinib and pemetrexed-based chemotherapy in Chinese NSCLC patients with ROS1 rearrangement. Oncotarget. 2016;7(46):75145–54.
19. Ahmad A, Gadgeel SM. Lung cancer and personalized medicine: novel therapies and clinical management. Preface. Adv Exp Med Biol. 2016;890:v–vi.
20. Mehrad M, Roy S, Bittar HT, Dacic S. Next-Generation Sequencing Approach to Non-Small Cell Lung Carcinoma Yields More Actionable Alterations. Arch Pathol Lab Med. 2017. https://doi.org/10.5858/arpa.2017-0046-OA. [Epub ahead of print]
21. Illei PB, Belchis D, Tseng LH, Nguyen D, De Marchi F, Haley L, Riel S, Beierl K, Zheng G, Brahmer JR, et al. Clinical mutational profiling of 1006 lung cancers by next generation sequencing. Oncotarget. 2017;8(57):96684–96.
22. Drilon A, Wang L, Arcila ME, Balasubramanian S, Greenbowe JR, Ross JS, Stephens P, Lipson D, Miller VA, Kris MG, et al. Broad, hybrid capture-based next-generation sequencing identifies actionable genomic alterations in lung Adenocarcinomas otherwise negative for such alterations by other genomic testing approaches. Clin Cancer Res. 2015;21(16):3631–9.
23. Burrell RA, McGranahan N, Bartek J, Swanton C. The causes and consequences of genetic heterogeneity in cancer evolution. Nature. 2013; 501(7467):338–45.
24. de Bruin EC, McGranahan N, Mitter R, Salm M, Wedge DC, Yates L, Jamal-Hanjani M, Shafi S, Murugaesu N, Rowan AJ, et al. Spatial and temporal diversity in genomic instability processes defines lung cancer evolution. Science. 2014;346(6206):251–6.
25. Tucker ER, Danielson LS, Innocenti P, Chesler L. Tackling Crizotinib resistance: the pathway from drug discovery to the pediatric clinic. Cancer Res. 2015;75(14):2770–4.
26. Infarinato NR, Park JH, Krytska K, Ryles HT, Sano R, Szigety KM, Li Y, Zou HY, Lee NV, Smeal T, et al. The ALK/ROS1 inhibitor PF-06463922 overcomes primary resistance to Crizotinib in ALK-driven Neuroblastoma. Cancer Discov. 2016;6(1):96–107.
27. Zou HY, Friboulet L, Kodack DP, Engstrom LD, Li Q, West M, Tang RW, Wang H, Tsaparikos K, Wang J, et al. PF-06463922, an ALK/ROS1 inhibitor, overcomes resistance to first and second generation ALK inhibitors in preclinical models. Cancer Cell. 2015;28(1):70–81.
28. Shaw AT, Friboulet L, Leshchiner I, Gainor JF, Bergqvist S, Brooun A, Burke BJ, Deng YL, Liu W, Dardaei L, et al. Resensitization to Crizotinib by the Lorlatinib ALK resistance mutation L1198F. N Engl J Med. 2016;374(1):54–61.
29. Thomas SN, Zhu F, Schnaar RL, Alves CS, Konstantopoulos K. Carcinoembryonic antigen and CD44 variant isoforms cooperate to mediate colon carcinoma cell adhesion to E- and L-selectin in shear flow. J Biol Chem. 2008;283(23):15647–55.
30. Okamura K, Takayama K, Izumi M, Harada T, Furuyama K, Nakanishi Y. Diagnostic value of CEA and CYFRA 21-1 tumor markers in primary lung cancer. Lung Cancer. 2013;80(1):45–9.
31. Grunnet M, Sorensen JB. Carcinoembryonic antigen (CEA) as tumor marker in lung cancer. Lung Cancer. 2012;76(2):138–43.

9

Successful eradication of newly acquired MRSA in six of seven patients with cystic fibrosis applying a short-term local and systemic antibiotic scheme

Alexander Kiefer[1*], Christian Bogdan[2] and Volker O. Melichar[1]

Abstract

Background: In individuals with cystic fibrosis (CF), colonization with methicillin-resistant *Staphylococcus aureus* (MRSA) was reported to be associated with a deterioration of pulmonary disease as reflected by an accelerated decline in lung function. Thus, an early eradication of MRSA could be beneficial in these patients. Here, we report on an intensified MRSA eradication protocol.

Methods: Since 2012 a protocol for the eradication of newly acquired MRSA has been used in our CF Clinic, combining oral rifampicin and fusidic acid, inhaled vancomycin, nasal mupirocin, local antiseptic treatment and hygienic directives all of which are applied for only 7 days during an inpatient hospital stay.

Results: Since 2012 seven patients (3 male, 4 female; age range 4 to 30 years) newly acquired MRSA. In 6 of the 7 patients (86%) successful eradication of MRSA was achieved upon first treatment using the protocol described above. In one patient a second course of treatment was performed which, however, also failed to eliminate the colonizing MRSA.

Conclusions: Our protocol led to an eradication rate of 86%. The impact of each individual component of the protocol remains to be determined.

Keywords: Cystic fibrosis, Methicillin- resistant *Staphylococcus aureus* (MRSA), Eradication

Background

The prevalence of methicillin-resistant *Staphylococcus aureus* (MRSA) colonization in patients with cystic fibrosis (CF) has increased over the past years. The carrier rate significantly varies between regions, ranging from 3,4% in some CF populations in the United Kingdom [1] as high as 30% in the United States [2–5]. The chronic colonization with MRSA seems to be associated with a worsening of the pulmonary disease, with an accelerated decline in lung function and/or a prolonged recovery period after clinical exacerbations [1–3, 6, 7]. Several protocols for an early eradication of MRSA have been reported to prevent negative consequences that might result from chronic MRSA colonization [1, 2, 8]. To the best of our knowledge, studies systematically comparing these protocols are lacking in the literature, as recently also highlighted by a Cochrane review [1, 9, 10]. The aim of this retrospective study was to evaluate the efficacy of our protocol which consists of oral rifampicin and fusidic acid, inhaled vancomycin, nasal mupirocin, and hygienic directives over 7 days. This protocol has been used in our CF center since 2012.

Methods

In 2012 we established a standardized eradication protocol for newly colonized patients with CF. This protocol consists of oral rifampicin (7.5–10 mg/kg, maximum 300 mg twice daily) and oral fusidic acid (15 mg/kg maximum 500 mg three times daily). The combination of these two antibiotics seems to be effective against MRSA in CF patients [1, 8, 11]. In addition, an inhalation therapy with vancomycin (4 mg/kg, maximum

* Correspondence: alexander.kiefer@uk-erlangen.de
[1]Department of Pediatrics and Adolescent Medicine, Clinic for Cystic Fibrosis, Universitätsklinikum Erlangen, Loschgestraße 15, 91054 Erlangen, Germany
Full list of author information is available at the end of the article

250 mg, dissolved in 4 ml sodium chloride 0,9% twice daily) is applied. None of the MRSA strains isolated from the CF patients was resistant to the above-mentioned antibiotics. Supplementary hygienic measurements including the application of mupirocin ointment and the use of disinfectants were performed as stated in Table 1. All these measures were performed under in-patient hospital conditions and contact precautions over 7 days; the inhalation therapy was supervised by a trained physiotherapist. Before starting the treatment, every family member and the pets living in the same household were also tested for MRSA. These test remained negative in each of our patients.

Since 2012 seven patients (3 male, 4 female) were newly colonized with MRSA and all were treated according to the above-mentioned protocol. The age of the patients ranged from 4 to 30 years, with a median age of 15 years. Prior to the start of the treatment each patient or its parents or legal guardian, if the patient was under 18 years old, gave oral informed consent to undergo this therapy scheme. None of the patients who were offered eradication refused to undergo the treatment, and all patients completed the treatment. New colonization with MRSA was defined by one positive culture for MRSA using either sputum analysis or an oropharyngeal swab. The cultures were performed as part of our routine monitoring, which in our CF center is carried out at least every 3 months. One patient acquired MRSA again 9 months after the first successful eradication and therefore underwent eradication for a second time. The age of the patients ranged from 4 to 30 years, with a median age of 15 years. The MRSA was either detected in sputum cultures (4 patients) or in deep oropharyngeal swabs (3 patients). Clinical data of the patients such as age, sex, and FEV1 determined at the time of MRSA detection are summarized in Table 2.

Bacterial cultures of sputum and/or of oropharyngeal swabs were obtained on day 4, 5 and 6 after the eradication attempt. If all the tests remained negative for MRSA, a successful eradication was assumed. The patients were then followed up every 3 months. In addition to the microbiological analyses a lung function test was performed if the patient was able to do it. The entire lung function tests were executed in a MasterScreenTM Body plethysmograph (Jaeger) by a specially trained nurse.

Table 1 Local measures

- Hand sanitation (Alcohol-based: Desderman ®, Sterillium®) as often as possible and reasonable
- Application of mupirocin into the nasal atrium: three times daily
- Disinfecting full body wash including the hair using antiseptic solutions (octenidin, polihexanide): once daily
- Rinse of the oropharynx with antiseptic: chlorhexidine, hexetidine or octenidin: three times daily
- Replacement of toothbrush or soaking in chlorhexidine: after use
- Change of underwear, clothes and bedding and disinfecting laundering: once daily
- Disinfection of all surfaces in the room with glucoprotamin 0,5%: once daily

Results

Successful eradication was achieved in 6 of 7 patients (86%). In one patient the first eradication attempt was unsuccessful and was repeated using the same protocol, which, however, also failed. In another patient MRSA was detected again after 9 months, but was again successfully eradicated. As the MRSA isolates were not subjected to molecular typing, we cannot tell whether the patient had a recurrent colonization with the same MRSA strain or whether he acquired a new MRSA strain.

Due to the retrospective design of our study, the follow-up period of the patients varied between 7 and 38 months (median 16 months) (see Table 3 for more details).

One of the patients (number 6) that successfully underwent the MRSA eradication protocol, was too young to perform a standard lung function test. In the other patients the rate of change in FEV1% predicted varied between a decline of 8.49 per year (patient with a co-colonization with *Burkholderia cepacia*) and an improvement of 0.86 points. The absolute change in FEV1% predicted between the time of initial MRSA detection and the end of the follow up period is shown in Fig. 1. The details of changes in FEV1% predicted per year are shown in Table 3.

Discussion

The impact of a chronic colonization with MRSA in individuals with cystic fibrosis is still a matter of debate. Some studies documented a worsening of pulmonary disease and accelerated loss of lung function in CF patients colonized with MRSA [1–3, 6, 7]. On the other hand, some studies suggest that acquisition of MRSA is not associated with an accelerated loss of lung function [12]. Although a positive effect on pulmonary disease and lung function parameters is not proven yet, there are other issues that have to be considered. Because of the contact precautions, which are necessary for patients with chronic MRSA colonization, they are often unable to receive important therapeutic measures which are part of the routine treatment for CF patients in Germany: In particular the outpatient physiotherapy, which is performed once a week by a specially trained physiotherapist and the rehabilitations are frequently withheld from the patients. This might be different in other countries, but in our opinion this is an important reason to eradicate MRSA. Several CF centers therefore

Table 2 Clinical data of the patients (at the time of the first MRSA detection)

Patient no.	Genotype	FEV1% predicted	bacterial colonization (other than MRSA)
Patient 1	F508del/2721del11	76,4%	*Pseudomonas aeruginosa*
Patient 2	F508del/F508del	31,3%	*Pseudomonas aeruginosa*
Patient 3	F508del/Arg334Trp	72,0%	MSSA[a]
Patient 4	F508del/F508del	80,1%	none
Patient 5	F508del/del17	51,5%	MSSA, *Burkholderia cepacia*
Patient 6	F508del/F508del	Not possible	none
Patient 7	F508del/F508del	76,3%	MSSA, *Pseudomonas aeruginosa*

[a]MSSA, methicillin-susceptible *Staphylococcus aureus*

aim at an early eradication of MRSA immediately after its first detection. The protocols used for the eradication attempts are difficult to compare as they differ in terms of the type, administration route and duration of antibiotic therapy. The success rate of eradication observed with our protocol (86%) compares well to other published schemes, in which the success rates ranged from 55% (Solis et al.) [13] to 94% (Macfarlane et al.) [8]. However, the published studies are not directly comparable, as there are many differences especially with respect to the applied antibiotics, the duration of the therapy, and the follow-up period (see Table 4 for more details). A notable advantage of our eradication protocol is its short duration of 7 days. This might not only lead to a better compliance of the patients, but should also have a positive impact with respect to side effects and the development of antibiotic resistance. The fact that the eradication scheme was performed in an inpatient hospital setting is likely to be an important factor for the high success rate, because adherence to the therapy and especially the implementation of the local measures will be higher under direct supervision than at home. In our opinion eradication according to this protocol at home would lead to a significantly lower success rate. However, as there was no control group who underwent the eradication protocol at home, this remains to be formally demonstrated. In Germany, the inpatient hospital stays are covered by the health insurances. Therefore, we have to admit that this protocol may not be feasible in other countries. Our protocol consists of three parts (local measures, oral rifampicin and fusidic acid and inhaled vancomycin). Unfortunately, we are unable to make a statement on the impact of each individual measurement on the overall success of our protocol. In particular the value of the inhaled vancomycin remains unclear. However, treatment periods longer than 7 days are probably not more successful, as we observed comparable clearance rates. In summary our protocol was well tolerated an accepted by the patients and provided an effective way to eradicate MRSA. The fact that none of the patients who have been offered the eradication procedure refused to undergo the treatment or interrupted the protocol emphasizes the compliance of the patients and the acceptance of the procedure.

Major limitations of our study are the low number of cases and the retrospective design. In addition, we used different specimens (sputum and/or deep oropharyngeal swab) to detect MRSA. This was necessary because some patients were unable to produce sputum. Previous publications suggested that cultures of oropharyngeal swabs are not reliable to predict the presence of bacterial pathogens in the lower airways of cystic fibrosis patients [14, 15]. However, given the fact that we collected three independent specimens for culture after MRSA eradication and that the patients remained negative for a median period of 16 months, we believe that the risk of a

Table 3 Rate of change in FEV1% predicted and time of follow up

Patient no	Change in FEV1% predicted per year	Time of follow up (months)
1	- 0.82	59
2	−1.26	57
3	+ 0.86	28
5	- 8.49	24
7	−0.7	17

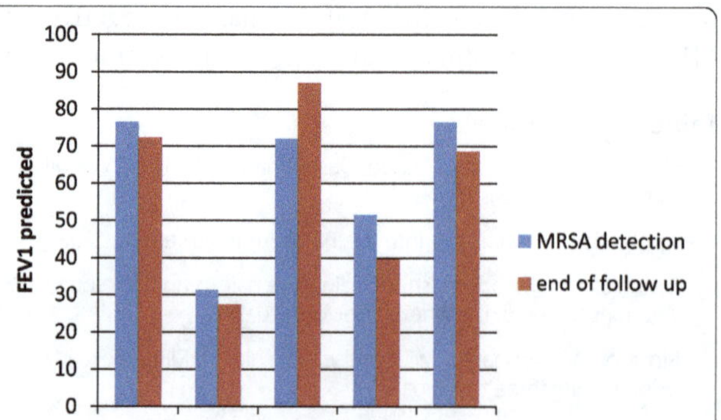

Fig. 1 FEV1% predicted in patients who underwent successful eradication of MRSA. In patient 4 MRSA was not eradicated; patient 6 was too young to perform lung function test

Table 4 Overview on studies that evaluated different antibiotic protocols for the eradication of MRSA after its first detection

Author	Patients treated	Age of patients (years)	Treatment protocol	Eradication success (%)
Solis et al. [13]	12	median 9.8 (0,6–17)	5 days topic/inhaled vancomycin	58
Macfarlane et al. [8]	17	mean 12.3 (1.8–16.5)	1. oral rifampicin and fusidic acid over 5 days	47%
			2. If still positive: oral rifampicin and fusidic acid over additional 5 days	71%
			3. If still positive: intravenous teicoplanin	94%
Hall et al. [1]	29	mean 30 (17–62)	either single or dual oral antibiotic therapy, until negative sputum, minimum 2 weeks, maximum 8 weeks	single therapy 50% dual therapy 85%
Kappler et al. [17]	37	mean 15.3 (0.6–36.9)	3 weeks dual intravenous + 6 weeks dual oral antibiotics + inhaled vancomycin if still positive 6 weeks inhaled vancomycin	84
Muhlebach et al. *Treatment* [16]	22	mean 12.3 (SD 6.6)	2 weeks dual oral antibiotics (rifampicin and trimethoprim/sulfamethoxazole or rifampicin an minocycline)	82
Muhlebach et al. *Observational control* [16]	19	mean 10.5 (SD 5.5)	none	26
this study	7	Median 15 (4–30)	Oral rifampicin and fusidic acid + inhaled vancomycin over 7 days	86

false negative result is minimal. Moreover, the heterogeneity of the patients with respect to age, sex and coinfection or co-colonization with other bacteria such as *Pseudomonas aeruginosa* and *Burkholderia cepacia* made it impossible to demonstrate a positive clinical effect of MRSA eradication in our patients. Furthermore, we were unable to compare our results to a control group of patients that were not offered eradication. A recent publication showed a spontaneous elimination of MRSA of only 26% of the affected patients [16]. In our opinion this emphasizes the importance of MRSA eradication, which, in our opinion will be beneficial for the patients in the long run.

As mentioned above and confirmed recently by the Cochrane Collaboration [9, 10], a comparison of all published eradication schemes is not possible. Further and prospective studies comparing several eradication protocols for MRSA would be useful.

Conclusion

Our short term antibiotic protocol led to the eradication of newly acquired MRSA at a rate of 86%, which compares well to other published schemes. The impact of each individual component of the protocol remains to be determined.

Abbreviations

CF: Cystic fibrosis; FEV1: Forced expiratory volume in one second; MRSA: Methicillin-resistant *Staphylococcus aureus*; MSSA: Methicillin-susceptible *Staphylococcus aureus*

Acknowledgements

We would like to thank our physiotherapist team for the teaching and supervision of vancomycin inhalation and Mrs. Ines Yawa for performing the lung function test.

Funding

Not applicable

Authors' contributions

AK analyzed the data and wrote the manuscript; CB revised the manuscript critically for important intellectual content; VM conceived and designed the eradication scheme; CB and VM edited the manuscript; all authors reviewed and approved the manuscript.

Consent of publication

Not applicable

Competing interests

The authors declare that they have no competing interests.

Author details

[1]Department of Pediatrics and Adolescent Medicine, Clinic for Cystic Fibrosis, Universitätsklinikum Erlangen, Loschgestraße 15, 91054 Erlangen, Germany. [2]Microbiology Institute – Clinical Microbiology, Immunology and Hygiene, Universitätsklinikum Erlangen, Friedrich-Alexander-Universität (FAU) Erlangen-Nürnberg, Wasserturmstraße 3/5, 91054 Erlangen, Germany.

References

1. Hall H, Gadhok R, Alshafi K, Bilton D, Simmonds NJ. Eradication of respiratory tract MRSA at a large adult cystic fibrosis centre. Respir Med. 2015;109(3):357–63. https://doi.org/10.1016/j.rmed.2015.01.013.
2. Chmiel JF, Aksamit TR, Chotirmall SH, Dasenbrook EC, Elborn JS, LiPuma JJ, et al. Antibiotic management of lung infections in cystic fibrosis. I. The microbiome, methicillin-resistant Staphylococcus Aureus, gram-negative bacteria, and multiple infections. Ann Am Thorac Soc. 2014;11(7):1120–9. https://doi.org/10.1513/AnnalsATS.201402-050AS.
3. Dasenbrook EC. Update on methicillin-resistant Staphylococcus Aureus in cystic fibrosis. Curr Opin Pulm Med. 2011;17(6):437–41. https://doi.org/10.1097/MCP.0b013e32834b95ed.

4. Harik NS, Com G, Tang X, Melguizo Castro M, Stemper ME, Carroll JL. Clinical characteristics and epidemiology of methicillin-resistant Staphylococcus Aureus (MRSA) in children with cystic fibrosis from a center with a high MRSA prevalence. Am J Infect Control. 2016;44(4):409–15. https://doi.org/10.1016/j.ajic.2015.10.015.
5. Salsgiver EL, Fink AK, Knapp EA, LiPuma JJ, Olivier KN, Marshall BC, et al. Changing epidemiology of the respiratory bacteriology of patients with cystic fibrosis. Chest. 2016;149(2):390–400. https://doi.org/10.1378/chest.15-0676.
6. Dasenbrook EC, Merlo CA, Diener-West M, Lechtzin N, Boyle MP. Persistent methicillin-resistant Staphylococcus Aureus and rate of FEV1 decline in cystic fibrosis. Am J Respir Crit Care Med. 2008;178(8):814–21. https://doi.org/10.1164/rccm.200802-327OC.
7. Ren CL, Morgan WJ, Konstan MW, Schechter MS, Wagener JS, Fisher KA, et al. Presence of methicillin resistant Staphylococcus Aureus in respiratory cultures from cystic fibrosis patients is associated with lower lung function. Pediatr Pulmonol. 2007;42(6):513–8.
8. Macfarlane M, Leavy A, McCaughan J, Fair R, Reid AJ. Successful decolonization of methicillin-resistant Staphylococcus Aureus in paediatric patients with cystic fibrosis (CF) using a three-step protocol. J Hosp Infect. 2007;65(3):231–6.
9. Lo DK, Hurley MN, Muhlebach MS, Smyth AR. Interventions for the eradication of meticillin-resistant Staphylococcus Aureus (MRSA) in people with cystic fibrosis. Cochrane Database Syst Rev. 2015;2:CD009650. https://doi.org/10.1002/14651858.CD009650.pub3.
10. Goss CH, Muhlebach MS. Review: Staphylococcus Aureus and MRSA in cystic fibrosis. J Cyst Fibros. 2011;10(5):298–306. https://doi.org/10.1016/j.jcf.2011.06.002.
11. Garske LA, Kidd TJ, Gan R, Bunting JP, Franks CA, Coulter C, et al. Rifampicin and sodium fusidate reduces the frequency of methicillin-resistant Staphylococcus Aureus (MRSA) isolation in adults with cystic fibrosis and chronic MRSA infection. J Hosp Infect. 2004;56:208–14.
12. Sawicki GS, Rasouliyan L, Pasta DJ, Regelmann WE, Wagener JS, Waltz DA, et al. The impact of incident methicillin resistant Staphylococcus Aureus detection on pulmonary function in cystic fibrosis. Pediatr Pulmonol. 2008;43(11):1117–23. https://doi.org/10.1002/ppul.20914.
13. Solis A, Brown D, Hughes J, Van Saene HK, Heaf DP. Methicillin-resistant Staphylococcus Aureus in children with cystic fibrosis: an eradication protocol. Pediatr Pulmonol. 2003;36(3):189–95.
14. Kabra SK, Alok A, Kapil A, Aggarwal G, Kabra M, Lodha R, et al. Can throat swab after physiotherapy replace sputum for identification of microbial pathogens in children with cystic fibrosis? Indian J Pediatr. 2004;71(1):21–3.
15. Ramsey BW, Wentz KR, Smith AL, Richardson M, Williams-Warren J, Hedges DL, et al. Predictive value of oropharyngeal cultures for identifying lower airway bacteria in cystic fibrosis patients. Am Rev Respir Dis. 1991;144(2):331–7.
16. Muhlebach MS, Beckett V, Popowitch E, Miller MB, Baines A, Mayer-Hamblett M, et al. Microbiological efficacy of early MRSA treatment in cystic fibrosis in a randomised controlled trial. Thorax. 2017;72(4):318–26. https://doi.org/10.1136/thoraxjnl-2016-208949.
17. Kappler M, Nagel F, Feilcke M, Kroner C, Pawlita I, Naehrig S, et al. Eradication of methicillin resistant Staphylococcus Aureus detected for the first time in cystic fibrosis: a single center observational study. Pediatr Pulmonol. 2016; https://doi.org/10.1002/ppul.23519.

10

The prevalence, burden and risk factors associated with chronic obstructive pulmonary disease in Commonwealth of Independent States (Ukraine, Kazakhstan and Azerbaijan)

Damilya Nugmanova[1], Yuriy Feshchenko[2], Liudmyla Iashyna[2], Olga Gyrina[3], Kateryna Malynovska[4], Eljan Mammadbayov[5], Irada Akhundova[5], Nadezhda Nurkina[1], Luqman Tariq[6], Janina Makarova[7,8*] and Averyan Vasylyev[4]

Abstract

Background: In the Commonwealth of Independent States (CIS) countries the epidemiology of chronic obstructive pulmonary disease (COPD) is poorly characterized. The objective of this analysis is to present the prevalence, burden and risk factors associated with COPD in three CIS countries as part of the CORE study (Chronic Obstructive Respiratory Diseases), the rationale and design of which have been described elsewhere.

Methods: A total of 2842 adults (≥18 years) were recruited (964 in Ukraine, Kiev, 945 in Kazakhstan, Almaty and 933 in Azerbaijan, Baku) between 2013 and 2015 during household visits. Two-step cluster randomization was used for the sampling strategy. All respondents were interviewed about respiratory symptoms, smoking status and medical history, and underwent spirometry with bronchodilator. COPD was defined as (i) "previously diagnosed" when the respondent reported that he/she had previously been diagnosed with COPD by a doctor, (ii) "diagnosed by spirometry" using the GOLD criteria (2011) based on spirometry conducted during the study ($FEV_1/FVC < 0.70$), and (iii) "firstly diagnosed by spirometry", when the patient had received the COPD diagnosis for the first time based on the spirometry results obtained in this study.

Results: The prevalence of "previously diagnosed" COPD was 10.4, 13.8 and 4.3 per 1000, and the prevalence of COPD "diagnosed by spirometry" was 31.9, 66.7 and 37.5 per 1000 in Ukraine, Kazakhstan, and Azerbaijan, respectively. Almost all respondents with COPD were diagnosed for the first time during this study. A statistically significant relationship was shown between smoking and COPD in Kazakhstan (odds ratio, OR: 3.75) and Azerbaijan (OR: 2.80); BMI in Ukraine (OR: 2.10); tuberculosis in Ukraine (OR: 32.3); and dusty work in Kazakhstan (OR: 2.30). Co-morbidities like cardiovascular diseases and a history of pneumonia occurred significantly ($p < 0.05$) more frequently in the COPD population compared to the non-COPD population across all participating countries. For hypertension, this was the case in Ukraine and Azerbaijan.

(Continued on next page)

* Correspondence: yana.j.makarova@gsk.com
[7]GlaxoSmithKline, Moscow, Russia
[8]GSK Russia Business Park "Krylatsky Hills", 17, Krylatskaya Street, Building 3 ("Air"), 121614 Moscow, Russia
Full list of author information is available at the end of the article

(Continued from previous page)

Conclusion: In CIS countries (Ukraine, Kazakhstan and Azerbaijan), the prevalence of COPD "diagnosed by spirometry" was significantly higher than the prevalence of previously diagnosed COPD. Compared to many other countries, the prevalence of COPD seems to be relatively low in CIS countries. Factors such as limited funding from the government; lack of COPD knowledge and the attitude within the population, and of primary care physicians; as well as low access to high-quality spirometry may play a role in this under-diagnosis of COPD. The information provided in this paper will be helpful for healthcare policy makers in CIS countries to instruct COPD management and prevention strategies and to allocate healthcare resources accordingly.

Keywords: Chronic obstructive pulmonary disease (COPD), Prevalence, Risk factors, Ukraine, Kazakhstan, Azerbaijan

Background

Chronic obstructive pulmonary disease (COPD) is a chronic respiratory disease with high worldwide prevalence, which is increasing, particularly in developing countries [1, 2]; moreover, it is associated with a high social burden. It was estimated in 2010, that over 230 million people living in urban areas (prevalence of 13.6%), and more than 153.7 million people living in rural areas (prevalence of 9.7%), are affected by COPD [2]. By 2010 COPD had become the third leading cause of death worldwide [3], and the majority of COPD-related deaths occurred in low– and middle-income countries [2].

COPD is characterized by chronic diffuse irreversible airflow obstruction involving mainly small airways. This condition is a growing cause of morbidity, disability, and mortality in both developed and developing countries that can be related to environmental exposures, smoking and respiratory infectious diseases [4]. Although the importance of early diagnosis is undisputed, patients with COPD often consult a physician at the late stages of the disease [5]. According to the European Respiratory Society (ERS), only 25% of cases are diagnosed at the early stages [6].

Previously published studies evaluating the prevalence of COPD have provided a range of estimates across different countries. The prevalence of previously diagnosed COPD (when diagnosis was made in the past and reported by a respondent) ranged from 18 per 1000 (Sweden) to 222 per 1000 (Russia); and the prevalence of COPD diagnosed by spirometry ranged from 37 per 1000 (United Arab Emirates) to 240 per 1000 (The Netherlands). In the multinational BOLD study the overall prevalence of COPD diagnosed by spirometry using a standardized approach was 193 per 1000 [7]. COPD prevalence estimates from across the globe are summarized in Table 1.

More than half of those with chronic respiratory diseases live in low and middle income countries, including some Commonwealth of Independent States (CIS) countries [8], where there are no population-based epidemiology studies conducted to evaluate the prevalence of these diseases. The CORE study (Chronic Obstructive REspiratory diseases in CIS countries) has been conducted to bridge this gap. The aim of the study was to evaluate the country-specific point prevalence of COPD, bronchial asthma and allergic rhinitis in selected CIS countries in order to obtain a clear "epidemiological picture" of the disease. The rationale and design of the CORE study (including the key steps of the recruitment phase, inclusion and exclusion criteria, study population, demographic characteristics, employment status, education and marital status of participants and the questionnaires used in the study) have been described previously [9]. In this manuscript, data obtained on the prevalence and burden of COPD will be presented. In addition, the potential relationship between the presence of COPD and its risk factors will be assessed.

Methods

Study area and population

The CORE study is a multi-national, cross-sectional population-based epidemiological study conducted across major cities in Ukraine, Kazakhstan and Azerbaijan (Kiev, Almaty and Baku, respectively) from the first half of 2013 until the end of 2015. The study enrolled subjects who were ≥18 years old, had lived in the selected city for ≥10 years and provided written informed consent to participate in the study.

Subjects for whom spirometry could not be performed, and subjects who were not able to answer the study questionnaires (American Thoracic Society (ATS) Respiratory Symptoms Questionnaire, COPD Assessment Test (CAT™), Alcohol Intake, Tobacco Smoking Questions) or had any contraindication for spirometry or hypersensitivity to bronchodilator (Salbutamol) were excluded from the study. Contraindications for spirometry were established based on the judgment of the investigator and defined according to Cooper BG, 2011 [10] including absolute (myocardial infarction, ascending aortic aneurysm, pulmonary embolism, angina) or relative (thoracic/abdominal surgery; brain, eye, ear, nose or throat surgery; pneumothorax, haemoptysis, acute diarrhea, severe hypertension, confused/demented patients; patient discomfort, or infection control issue) contraindications.

Table 1 Reported prevalence of COPD across different regions

Source and study location	Survey period	Estimated prevalence per 1000 (95% CI)		
		Previously diagnosed[a]	Diagnosed by spirometry[b]	Firstly diagnosed by spirometry[c]
Menezes AM et al. Montevideo, Uruguay (PLATINO study) [20]	2002	ND	197 (172–222)	ND
Menezes AM et al. Mexico City, Mexico (PLATINO study) [20]	2002	ND	78 (59–97)	ND
Doney B et al. USA [19]	2004–2011	ND	42 (40–43)	ND
Buist AS et al.12 sites across Europe, Asia, USA, Canada, South Africa and Australia (BOLD study) [7]	2005–2007	ND	193 (ND)	ND
Bárbara C et al. Lisbon, Portugal [28]	2006–2007	ND	142 (111–181)	ND
Danielsson P et al. Uppsala, Sweden (BOLD study) [34]	2006–2007	ND	162 (CI: ND)	ND
Minas M et al. Greece [15]	2006–2007	57 (CI: ND)	184 (CI: ND)	127 (CI: ND)
Soriano JB et al. Spain [16]	2007	ND	45 (24–66)	ND
Vanfleteren LE et al. Maastricht, Netherlands [23]	2007–2009	88 (CI: ND)	240 (CI: ND)	ND
Carlsson AC et al. Stockholm, Sweden [21]	2007–2011	18 (CI: ND)	ND	ND
Yoo KH et al. South Korea [17]	2008	ND	134 (CI: ND)	ND
Sousa CA et al. São Paulo, Brazil [25]	2008–2009	42 (31–54)	ND	ND
Al Zaabi A et al. Abu Dhabi, United Arab Emirates [22]	2009–2010	ND	37 (20–53)	ND
Lâm HT et al. Northern Vietnam [18]	2009–2010	ND	71 (CI: ND)	ND
Chuchalin AG et al. Russia (GARD Study) [26]	2010–2011	222 (212–232)	218 (195–245)	ND
Van Gemert F et al. Uganda [27]	2012	ND	162 (CI: ND)	ND
Tageldin MA et al. Middle East and North Africa (BREATHE study) [35]	2012	36 (35–37)	ND	ND

COPD – chronic obstructive pulmonary disease; *95% CI* – 95% confidence interval; *ND* – not determined
[a]Defined as: when diagnosis was made in the past and reported by a respondent
[b]Defined as: diagnosed and confirmed by spirometry conducted during the course of the study
[c]Defined as: diagnosed for the first time based on spirometry

Case definition and severity

Diagnosis of COPD was established based on the study questionnaire and/or spirometry conducted without bronchodilator (pre-dose) and with bronchodilator (post-dose: 15–20 min after administration of 200–400 mcg Salbutamol (GlaxoSmithKline). Consequently, FEV_1 (forced expiratory volume in one second) and FVC (forced vital capacity) were estimated during the spirometry using a standardized approach defined by Miller MR et al., 2005 [11]. Spirometry quality and results were regularly reviewed by members of the Study Executive Committee.

COPD was identified through three definitions:

1. Previously diagnosed: When self-reported by the respondent while completing the study questionnaire. Respondents were asked to answer the following question to identify "previously diagnosed COPD":

Has a doctor ever told you that you have chronic obstructive pulmonary disease (COPD)?

If YES, please, indicate number of exacerbations during the last year.

2. Diagnosed by spirometry: confirmed by spirometry results based on the GOLD (Global Initiative for Chronic Obstructive Lung Disease) guideline (2011) ($FEV_1/FVC < 0.70$). Spirometry was conducted as part of the study (Table 2).
3. Firstly diagnosed by spirometry: when the respondent was diagnosed with COPD for the first time based on spirometry outcomes.

As shown in Table 2, severity of COPD was investigated based on the GOLD guidelines (2011) [5] while using four categories for severity based on spirometry results only.

Data collected

The data were collected from participants during household visits. Two-step cluster randomization (first step, administrative district; second step, street) was used for the sampling strategy. Districts and streets for household visits were selected by the Study Executive Committee. The interviewers visited households sequentially, starting with the first apartment of the first house in the selected street, and continuing in ascending order. At every household the interviewers assessed the eligibility of all inhabitants. Participants who provided their consent and were eligible to participate in the study provided their socio-demographic information and medical history, underwent weight/height measurement and spirometry with bronchodilator and completed the study questionnaires, as described previously [9].

Table 2 COPD diagnosis and severity based on spirometry outcomes (GOLD 20115)

Diagnosis	Post-dose parameters
No disease	$FEV_1/FVC \geq 0.70$
COPD GOLD stage:	
Stage I: Mild	$FEV_1/FVC < 0.70$ $FEV_1 \geq 80\%$ predicted
Stage II Moderate:	$FEV_1/FVC < 0.70$ $50\% \leq FEV_1 < 80\%$ predicted
Stage III: Severe	$FEV_1/FVC < 0.70$ $30\% \leq FEV_1 < 50\%$ predicted
Stage IV: Very Severe	$FEV_1/FVC < 0.70$ $FEV_1 < 30\%$ predicted or $FEV_1 < 50\%$ predicted plus chronic respiratory failure

FEV_1 forced expiratory volume in one second; *FVC* forced vital capacity; respiratory failure: arterial partial pressure of oxygen (PaO_2) less than 8.0 kPa (60 mmHg) with or without arterial partial pressure of CO_2 ($PaCO_2$) greater than 6.7 kPa (50 mmHg) while breathing air at sea level

Socio-demographic data were collected to describe the characteristics of the overall study population, including gender, age and ethnicity distribution, body mass index (BMI), smoking status and alcohol intake. COPD prevalence data were collected using the case definition described above and the impact of age, gender and severity were assessed. Additionally, the type and frequency of co-morbidities and any potential association between COPD and its related risk factors (i.e. smoking, BMI, alcohol intake, tuberculosis, dusty work, open fire cooking) were investigated.

The COPD Assessment Test (CAT™) and the modified Medical Research Council (mMRC) Dyspnoea Scale were used to assess additional characteristics of COPD in this study. All respondents answered the CAT™ and were assessed by the mMRC Dyspnoea Scale at the interview. The CAT™ is a validated short questionnaire for measurement of the impact of COPD on a patient's health status [12]. It comprises eight items, each with a scoring range of 0–5. The total CAT™ score is derived based on the sum of responses given to the eight items with a range of 0–40. The mMRC Dyspnoea Scale was used as a simple grading system to assess the level of dyspnoea/shortness of breath in five categories from 0 to 4: 0 - Responder is not affected by shortness of breath, except when engaging in strenuous exercise; 1 - Responder has shortness of breath when walking briskly on flat ground or slightly uphill; 2 - Responder walks more slowly on flat surfaces than other people his/her age because of shortness of breath, or he/she has to stop to catch his/her breath when walking at his/her own pace on flat ground; 3 - Responder has to stop to catch his/her breath after walking around 100 m or after walking for a few minutes on flat ground; 4 - Responder's shortness of breath prevents him/her from leaving home or he/she has shortness of breath when dressing or undressing.

Statistical analysis

The point prevalence of COPD, (overall and separate stages/categories), is defined as the number of COPD individuals divided by total number of subjects included in the study, and is expressed as a number per 1000 for each country. Prevalence was calculated in the subject population with valid data. 95% confidence intervals (CI) were calculated for each frequency using the Clopper-Pearson method [13]. Odds ratios (OR) and 95% CI were calculated to estimate the statistical significance (p‹0.05) of associations between risk factors and COPD. Statistical analysis was performed using IBM SPSS Statistics software (IBM Corp., USA) version 21.0 and R software version 3.1.2 (R Core Team, Austria).

Results

Study sample and demographics

A total of 2842 adult subjects were included in the CORE study (964 in Ukraine, 945 in Kazakhstan and 933 in Azerbaijan). The majority of study population were women across the three countries: 58.2% in Ukraine; 63.2% in Kazakhstan and 58.3% in Azerbaijan. The mean age was slightly above 40 years old in all participating countries. As expected, the majority of participants were Caucasian in Ukraine (99.7%) and Azerbaijan (100%), and almost two-thirds of participants in Kazakhstan were Asian (62.8%). The mean BMI was at the boundary of overweight in Ukraine, (25.0 (5.1) kg/m^2), and in Kazakhstan, (25.7 (5.1) kg/m^2), while it was slightly higher in Azerbaijan (26.4 (5.3) kg/m^2). Approximately one-third of participants were either current or past smokers (33.7% in Ukraine, 40.2% in Kazakhstan, 26.0% in Azerbaijan). Heavy alcohol consumption was reported by 53.4% of respondents in Ukraine, 44.8% in Kazakhstan and 22.7% in Azerbaijan. See Table 3.

Prevalence of COPD

Subjects who fulfilled the definitions used in this study for COPD are shown in Table 4. Prevalence of previously diagnosed COPD was 10.4 (95% CI 5.0–19.1) per 1000 in Ukraine, 13.8 (95% CI 7.3–23.4) per 1000 in Kazakhstan, and 4.3 (95% CI 1.2–11.0) per 1000 in Azerbaijan. The estimated prevalence of COPD diagnosed by spirometry was higher among all participating countries compared to previously diagnosed COPD estimates: 31.9 (95% CI 21.7–45.3) per 1000 in Ukraine, 66.7 (95% CI 51.6–84.5) per 1000 in Kazakhstan, and 37.5 (95% CI 26.3–51.8) per 1000 in Azerbaijan. Almost all participating subjects were firstly diagnosed for COPD by spirometry. See Fig. 1.

A similar picture was obtained for the prevalence of COPD among respondents ≥40 years old (Fig. 2). The estimated prevalence of COPD diagnosed by spirometry was: 47.3 (95% CI 29.9–70.8) per 1000 in Ukraine, 114.1 (95% CI 87.3–145.6) per 1000 in Kazakhstan, and 60.1 (95% CI 40.3–85.7) per 1000 in Azerbaijan; compared to the prevalence of previously diagnosed COPD which was 14.7 (95% CI 5.9–30.1) per 1000 in Ukraine, 26.5 (95% CI 14.2–44.9) per 1000 in Kazakhstan, and 8.6 (95% CI 2.3–21.9) per 1000 in Azerbaijan.

GOLD stage classification (2011) [5] was used for COPD severity (airflow limitation) estimation. COPD patients identified in this study were distributed between stages I ($FEV_1/FVC < 0.70$, $FEV_1 \geq 80\%$ normal) and II ($FEV_1/FVC < 0.70$, FEV_1 50–79% normal). In all three participating countries, more patients were found in stage II (18.1 (95% CI 10.6–28.8) per 1000 in Ukraine; 48.7 (95% CI 35.9–64.4) per 1000 in Kazakhstan and 21.4 (95% CI 13.1–32.9) per 1000 in Azerbaijan) (Fig. 3).

A higher prevalence of previously diagnosed COPD was observed in the age group ≥65 years old compared to the younger age groups in Kazakhstan and Azerbaijan: 73.5 (95% CI 24.3–163.3) and 38.5 (95% CI 4.7–132.1) per 1000 respectively. However, in Ukraine, the highest prevalence was observed in the 40–64 years old age group: 14.8 (95% CI 5.4–31.9) per 1000 (Fig. 4). A higher prevalence of COPD diagnosed by spirometry was observed in the population aged ≥65 years old compared to younger age groups in Ukraine, Kazakhstan and Azerbaijan: 153.8 (95% CI 76.3–264.8), 264.7 (95% CI 165.0–385.7) and 192.3 (95% CI 96.3–325.4) per 1000 respectively.

In all three participating countries, COPD was more common in men. This applied to both previously diagnosed COPD and COPD confirmed based on spirometry. The prevalence of previously diagnosed COPD was 14.9 (95% CI 5.5–32.2) per 1000 in men vs 7.2 (95% CI 2.0–18.3) per 1000 in women in Ukraine; 17.2 (95% CI 6.4–37.2) per 1000 in men vs 11.7 (95% CI 4.7–24.0) per 1000 in women in Kazakhstan and 10.3 (95% CI 2.8–26.1) per 1000 in men vs 0.0 (95% CI 0.0–6.8) in women in Azerbaijan. The prevalence of COPD diagnosed by spirometry was 45.6 (95% CI 27.2–71.1) per 1000 in men vs 22.1 (95% CI 11.4–38.2) per 1000 in women in Ukraine; 120.7 (95% CI 88.4–159.6) per 1000 in men vs 35.2 (95% CI 21.9–53.3) per 1000 in women in Kazakhstan and 54.0 (95% CI 33.7–81.3) per 1000 in men vs 25.7 (95% CI 14.1–42.8) per 1000 in women in Azerbaijan (Figs. 5 and 6).

The ethnicity-specific prevalence of COPD was estimated only in Kazakhstan, because most Ukrainians and Azerbaijanians were Caucasians. Generally, in Kazakhstan, the prevalence of COPD in Caucasians was slightly higher than in Asians, both for previously diagnosed COPD (17.2 (95% CI 6.3–37.1) per 1000 in Caucasians vs 11.8 (95% CI 4.8–24.2) per 1000 in Asians), and for COPD diagnosed by spirometry (68.8 (95% CI 44.6–100.6) per 1000 in Caucasians vs 64.1 (95% CI 45.7–86.9) per 1000 in Asians).

Risk factors associated with COPD

The relationship between the presence of COPD and smoking status (current/past smoker), alcohol intake (severe alcohol intake), BMI (BMI ≥ 25 kg/m^2), tuberculosis (ever diagnosed), dusty work, and open fire cooking was investigated and statistical significance was found between COPD and smoking in Kazakhstan (OR 3.756 (CI 2.156–6.543) $p < 0.001$) and Azerbaijan (OR 2.808 (CI 1.423–5.542) $p = 0.002$). Tuberculosis was a significant risk factor associated with COPD in Ukraine (OR 32.393 (CI 4.403–238.330) $p < 0.001$). Dusty work might increase the appearance of COPD in Kazakhstan (OR 2.306 (CI 1.328–4.002) $p = 0.002$)

Table 3 Demographic characteristics of respondents

		Ukraine	Kazakhstan	Azerbaijan
Gender	Male	403 (41.8%)	348 (36.8%)	389 (41.7%)
	Female	561 (58.2%)	597 (63.2%)	544 (58.3%)
	Total	964	945	933
Ethnicity	Asian	3 (0.3%)	593 (62.8%)	0
	Black	0	1 (0.1%)	0
	Caucasian	961 (99.7%)	349 (36.9%)	933 (100.0%)
	Other	0	2 (0.2%)	0
	Total	964	945	933
Age, years	Mean (SD)	40.7 (15.1)	42.5 (15.3)	40.7 (14.8)
	18–39 years old	482 (50.1%)	454 (48.0%)	467 (50.1%)
	40–64 years old	408 (42.4%)	423 (44.8%)	414 (44.4%)
	≥ 65 years old	72 (7.5%)	68 (7.2%)	52 (5.6%)
BMI, kg/m^2	Mean (SD)	25.0 (5.1)	25.7 (5.1)	26.4 (5.3)
Overweight/obesity (BMI ≥ 25 kg/m^2)	Overall population	437 (45.4%)	449 (47.6%)	511 (54.9%)
	Males	210 (52.1%)	165 (47.6%)	212 (54.5%)
	Females	227 (40.5%)	284 (47.6%)	299 (55.3%)
Smoking	Never smoked	629 (65.2%)	564 (59.7%)	690 (74,.0%)
	Current/past smoker	325 (33.7%)	380 (40.2%)	243 (26.0%)
Alcohol intake	Standard drinks[a], mean (SD)	2.63 (4.15)	2.99 (7.54)	1.40 (2.82)
	Not at all	77 (8.0%)	240 (26.3%)	536 (57.4%)
	Moderate[b]	371 (38.6%)	263 (28.9%)	185 (19.8%)
	Heavy[b]	514 (53.4%)	408 (44.8%)	212 (22.7%)

BMI – body mass index; *SD* – standard deviation
[a]One drink was defined as 12 fluid ounces of regular beer (5% alcohol), 5 fluid ounces of wine (12% alcohol), or 1.5 fluid ounces of 80 proof (40% alcohol) distilled spirits. One drink contains 0.6 fluid ounces of alcohol
[b]Moderate alcohol consumption was defined as the consumption of up to 1 drink per day for women and up to 2 drinks per day for men. Heavy (or high-risk) drinking was defined as the consumption of more than 3 drinks on any day or more than 7 per week for women and more than 4 drinks on any day or more than 14 per week for men

COPD assessment test and the modified Medical Research Council dyspnoea scale

The CAT™ and mMRC dyspnoea scale were assessed in respondents with COPD diagnosed by spirometry (COPD population) and those without COPD (non-COPD population). As seen in Table 5, the total CAT™ score and intensity of dyspnoea/shortness of breath by mMRC were significantly higher among respondents with COPD than in the non-COPD population in all countries. In all non-COPD respondents and COPD respondents in Kazakhstan, the median CAT™ score did not exceed 5 points, which corresponds to the upper limit of normal in healthy non-smokers, and in the COPD population of Ukraine and Azerbaijan the median CAT™ score

Table 4 Number of respondents with COPD previously diagnosed and diagnosed by spirometry during the study

	Ukraine ($n = 939$)	Kazakhstan ($n = 945$)	Azerbaijan ($n = 933$)
Previously diagnosed COPD	$N = 10$ (1.0%)	$N = 13$ (1.4%)	$N = 4$ (0.4%)
Diagnosed by spirometry	$N = 30$ (3.2%)	$N = 63$ (6.7%)	$N = 35$ (3.8%)
Firstly diagnosed by spirometry	$N = 27$ (2.9%)	$N = 58$ (6.1%)	$N = 33$ (3.5%)
COPD severity by GOLD stage[a]:			
I (Mild)	13 (1.4%)	26 (2.8%)	13 (1.4%)
II (Moderate)	17 (1.8%)	37 (3.9%)	22 (2.4%)

GOLD Stage I (Mild): $FEV_1/FVC < 0.70$ and $FEV1 \geq 80\%$ predicted
GOLD Stage II (Moderate): $FEV_1/FVC < 0.70$ and $50\% \leq FEV_1 < 80\%$ predicted
[a]There were no respondents diagnosed with COPD III or IV GOLD stages

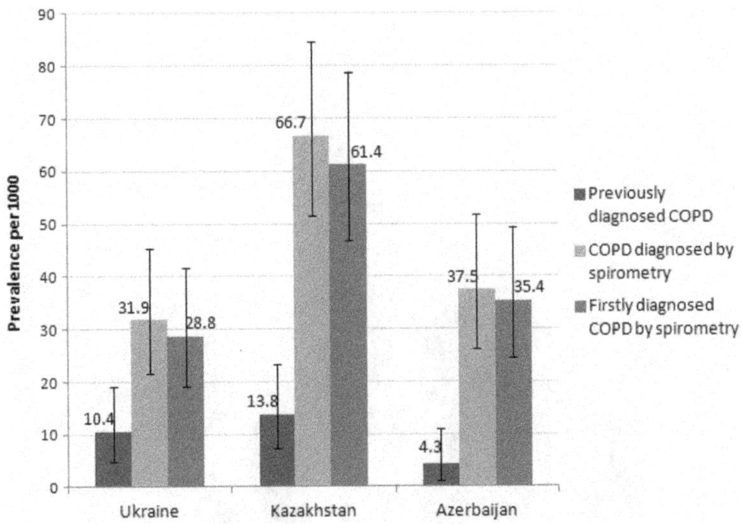

Fig. 1 Point prevalence of COPD in the whole population. The prevalence was calculated per 1000 persons and expressed with 95% confidence intervals, for three COPD definitions: *previously diagnosed COPD* (when self-reported by the respondent while completing the study questionnaire); *COPD diagnosed by spirometry* (confirmed by spirometry results based on GOLD Guidelines (2011), i.e. $FEV_1/FVC < 0.70$), and *firstly diagnosed COPD by spirometry* (when the respondent was diagnosed with COPD for the first time based on spirometry outcomes)

corresponds to a low (< 10) impact of COPD on health status [12]. According to the mMRC dyspnoea scale, 70–80% respondents without COPD and only half of COPD respondents had no dyspnoea (grade 0).

Co-morbidities

While completing the study questionnaire the respondents were asked to report the presence of other chronic medical conditions except for respiratory diseases. Co-morbidities were reported by 44.2% of respondents in Ukraine, 23.5% respondents in Kazakhstan and 54.6% respondents in Azerbaijan. The respondents with COPD diagnosed by spirometry (COPD population) were compared to the rest of the respondents (non-COPD population) by the rate of co-morbidities. In all participating countries, the number of subjects that reported suffering from a chronic health condition was higher in the COPD population compared to

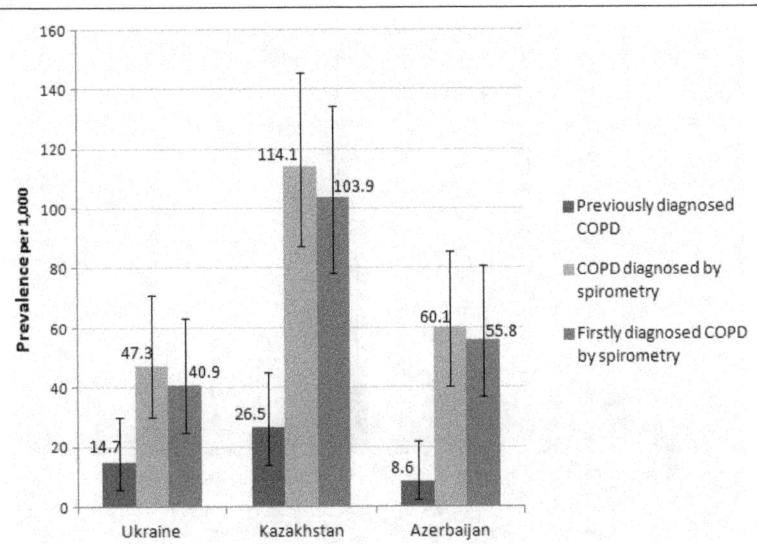

Fig. 2 Point prevalence of COPD among respondents ≥40 years old. The prevalence was calculated per 1000 persons and expressed with 95% confidence intervals, for three COPD definitions: *previously diagnosed COPD* (when self-reported by the respondent while completing the study questionnaire); *COPD diagnosed by spirometry* (confirmed by spirometry results based on the GOLD guideline (2011), i.e. $FEV_1/FVC < 0.70$), and *firstly diagnosed COPD by spirometry* (when the respondent was diagnosed with COPD for the first time based on spirometry outcomes)

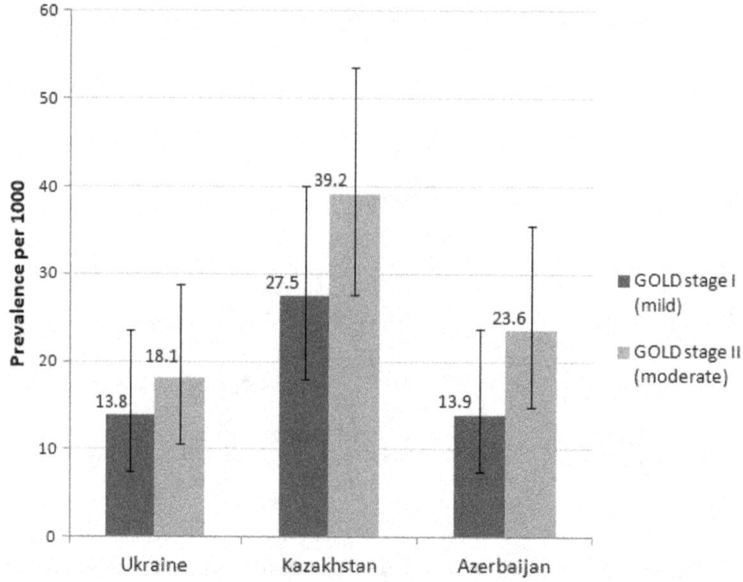

Fig. 3 Point prevalence of COPD (diagnosed by spirometry) by GOLD stage. The prevalence of various GOLD stages of COPD was calculated per 1000 persons and expressed with 95% confidence intervals, for *COPD diagnosed by spirometry* (confirmed by spirometry results based on GOLD Guidelines (2011), i.e. FEV1/FVC < 0.70). There were no respondents diagnosed with COPD III or IV GOLD stages in this study

the non-COPD population: 57% vs 43% in Ukraine, 51% vs 27% in Kazakhstan, and 74% vs 54% in Azerbaijan, respectively (Table 6).

A history of pneumonia was significantly more frequent in the COPD population than in the non-COPD population in all investigated countries (36.7% vs 19.4%, $p = 0.024$ in Ukraine, 31.7% vs 14.9%, $p = 0.001$ in Kazakhstan and 17.1% vs 5.9%, $p = 0.019$ in Azerbaijan). The same results were obtained for a previous cardiovascular disease (26.7% vs 6.0%, $p < 0.001$ in Ukraine, 22.2% vs 7.8%, $p = 0.001$ in Kazakhstan and 22.9% vs 3.5%, p˂0.001 in Azerbaijan in COPD and non-COPD populations respectively). Additionally, hypertension occurred significantly more often in the COPD population

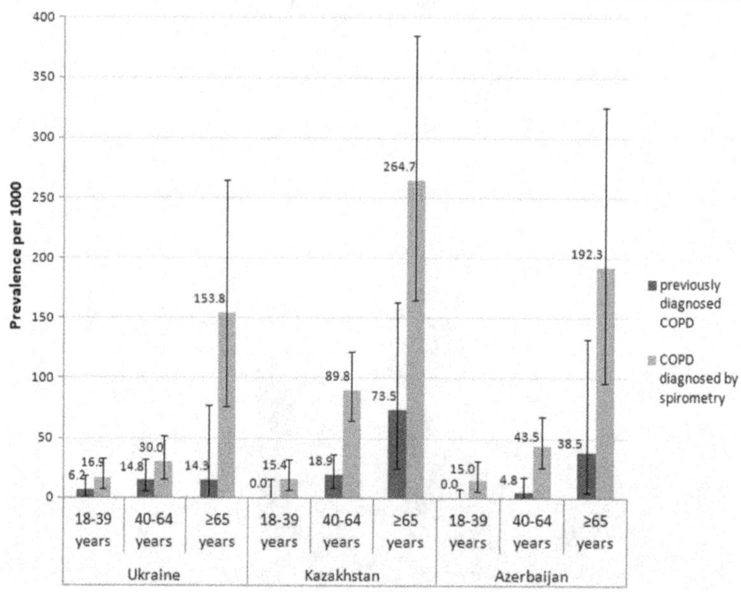

Fig. 4 Point prevalence of COPD stratified by age. The prevalence of COPD was calculated per 1000 persons and expressed with 95% confidence intervals in three age groups: 18–39, 40–64, and ≥65 years old, for *previously diagnosed COPD* (when self-reported by the respondent while completing the study questionnaire) and *COPD diagnosed by spirometry* (confirmed by spirometry results based on GOLD Guidelines (2011), i.e. $FEV_1/FVC < 0.70$)

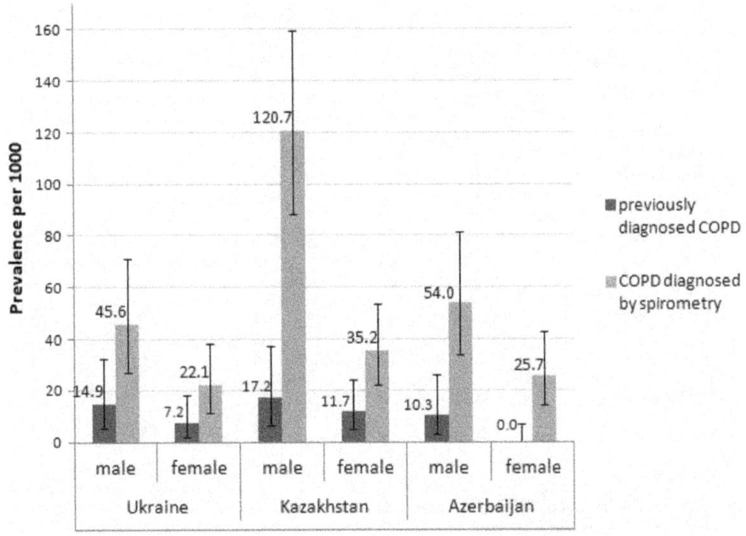

Fig. 5 Point prevalence of COPD stratified by gender. The prevalence of COPD was calculated per 1000 persons and expressed with 95% confidence intervals, among men and women, for *previously diagnosed COPD* (when self-reported by the respondent while completing the study questionnaire) and *COPD diagnosed by spirometry* (confirmed by spirometry results based on GOLD Guidelines (2011), i.e. $FEV_1/FVC < 0.70$)

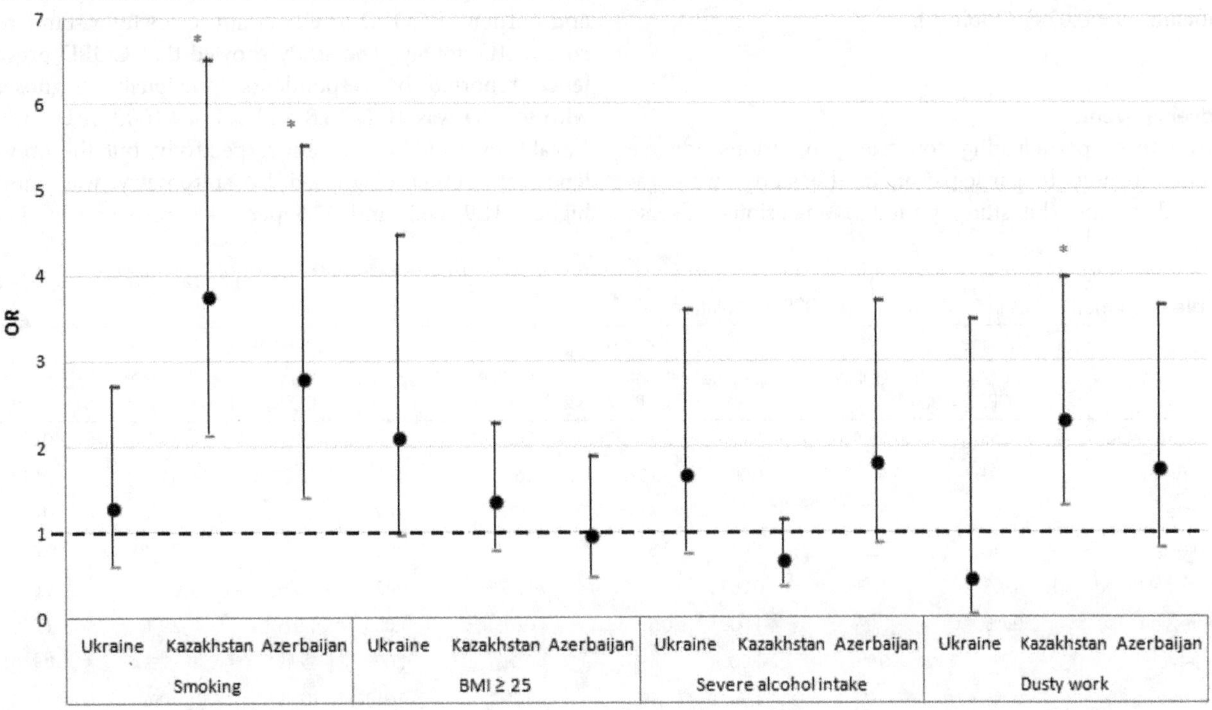

Fig. 6 Association between risk factors and COPD diagnosed by spirometry. Odds ratios [OR] and 95% confidence intervals for OR are presented for each potential risk factor. Asterisk (*) denotes as statistically significant association between risk factor and COPD diagnosed by spirometry ($p < 0.05$). For tuberculosis in anamnesis, a significant association was found in Ukraine, but not included in the figure due to the high OR value: 32.393 (CI 4.403–238.330)

Table 5 CAT™ and mMRC Dyspnoea Scale in COPD and non-COPD population

	Ukraine		Kazakhstan		Azerbaijan	
	Non-COPD	COPD	Non-COPD	COPD	Non-COPD	COPD
CAT™ total score						
median [25–75-percentiles]	2 [0–6]	6 [2–13]	2 [0–5]	4 [2–9]	3 [0–8]	8 [2–14]
p-value[a]	0.003		< 0.001		0.004	
mMRC grade, %						
Grade 0	79.4%	50.0%	70.0%	49.2%	75.2%	45.7%
Grade 1	16.1%	43.3%	25.5%	36.5%	22.2%	34.3%
Grade 2	2.4%	6.7%	3.7%	6.3%	1.7%	11.4%
Grade 3	0.9%	0.0%	0.6%	6.3%	0.4%	8.6%
Grade 4	0.4%	0.0%	0.0%	0.0%	0.0%	0.0%
Missing[b]	0.8%	0.0%	0.2%	1.6%	0.0%	0.0%
p-value[a]	< 0.001		< 0.001		< 0.001	

[a]two-sided Mann-Whitney U test for a comparison between COPD and non-COPD populations
[b]Respondents with 'missing' are not included in calculating *p*-values
COPD population: respondents with COPD diagnosed by spirometry (post-dose $FEV_1/FVC < 0.70$)
Non-COPD population: respondents without COPD diagnosed by spirometry (post-dose $FEV_1/FVC \geq 0.70$)

compared to the non-COPD population in Ukraine (40.0% vs 14.0%, $p = 0.001$) and Azerbaijan (34.3% vs 16.8%, $p = 0.012$). In Kazakhstan, hypertension was also more frequently observed in the COPD population (36.5%) compared to the non-COPD population (25.5%) but the difference was not shown to be significant ($p = 0.074$) (Table 6).

Adverse events

In all three participating countries, no serious adverse events (related to participation in the study) were recorded during the study period. Non-serious adverse events were not collected, as there was no investigational drug administration in this study.

Discussion

The CORE study is, to our knowledge, the first epidemiological study conducted to evaluate the prevalence and burden of COPD in CIS countries using a standardized methodology. The study showed that COPD prevalence reported by respondents 'previously diagnosed' with COPD was 10.4, 13.8 and 4.3 per 1000 in Ukraine, Kazakhstan, and Azerbaijan, respectively, but the prevalence of COPD diagnosed by spirometry was much higher, 31.9, 66.7 and 37.5 per 1000 respectively. This

Table 6 Co-morbidities in COPD and non-COPD population

	Ukraine			Kazakhstan			Azerbaijan		
	Non-COPD*N* = 909	COPD*N* = 30	*p*-value[a]	Non-COPD*N* = 882	COPD*N* = 63	*p*-value[a]	Non-COPD*N* = 898	COPD*N* = 35	*p*-value[a]
Any co-morbidity	42.5%	56.7%	0.136	26.9%	50.8%	< 0.001	53.8%	74.3%	0.023
Hypertension	14.0%	40.0%	0.001	25.5%	36.5%	0.074	16.8%	34.3%	0.012
Diabetes	3.4%	6.7%	0.621	3.4%	7.9%	0.078	5.2%	8.6%	0.428
Cardiovascular disease	6.0%	26.7%	<0.001	7.8%	22.2%	0.001	3.5%	22.9%	<0.001
Abnormal blood lipids	4.9%	13.3%	0.062	11.7%	15.9%	0.421	1.3%	0.0%	1.000
Depression	0.7%	0.0%	1.000	0.6%	0.0%	1.000	1.9%	2.9%	1.000
Anxiety	0.2%	0.0%	1.000	0.6%	0.0%	1.000	2.6%	5.7%	0.240
Osteoporosis	0.7%	0.0%	1.000	1.6%	3.2%	0.618	0.6%	0.0%	1.000
Tuberculosis	0.2%	6.7%	0.006	2.3%	0.0%	0.391	1.4%	2.9%	1.000
Pneumonia	19.4%	36.7%	0.024	14.9%	31.7%	0.001	5.9%	17.1%	0.019

[a]two-sided Pearson Chi-Square test for a comparison between COPD and non-COPD populations
COPD population: respondents with COPD diagnosed by spirometry (post-dose $FEV_1/FVC < 0.70$)
Non-COPD population: respondents without COPD diagnosed by spirometry (post-dose $FEV_1/FVC \geq 0.70$)

can be explained by under diagnosis of the disease in CIS countries. Therefore, the majority of respondents with COPD were diagnosed for the first time in this study. As highlighted by Pasko (2002), COPD is often under-reported which could explain why official data on COPD prevalence are up to 10-fold lower than actual population data [14]. The prevalence of COPD observed in Kazakhstan was high compared to Ukraine and Azerbaijan; one possible explanation for this may be the relatively poor ecological conditions in Almaty. This city is surrounded by high mountains (3000–5000 m) and experiences little wind, whereas the climate in Kiev and Baku is windy and there is a river or sea. However, this assumption needs further investigation.

A statistically significant relationship was shown between smoking and COPD in Kazakhstan and Azerbaijan; tuberculosis and COPD in Ukraine; and dusty work and COPD in Kazakhstan. Co-morbidities were significantly more frequent in the COPD population compared to the non-COPD population.

In all countries studied, the frequency of COPD diagnosed by spirometry had a tendency to increase with age (peak prevalence occurred at the age of 65 years and older). This trend has been observed in many studies [15–17] and can be explained by greater exposure to risk factors and physiological decrease in lung function with age. In epidemiological studies, high prevalence of COPD in the elderly has been reported widely, in age groups > 50 years [18], 55–70 years [19], ≥ 60 years [20], 75–84 years [21], ≥ 70 years [22].

In all three countries, COPD was more prevalent in men (both diagnosed by spirometry and previously diagnosed), in line with numerous other studies [7, 15]. This fact can probably be explained by different susceptibility associated with gender or by increased exposure to risk factors in men (smoking, occupational hazards, etc.). A low rate of previously reported COPD compared to spirometry findings was also noted in other studies [15, 23]. This could indicate a significant underestimation of COPD prevalence in these countries, probably related to late visits to doctors (because of limited accessibility to primary medical care or non-specific and/or mild symptoms at early stages of disease) and lack of population screening. It should be noted that not all participants with previously diagnosed COPD underwent spirometry (especially in Kazakhstan and Azerbaijan), so the real prevalence of spirometry changes relevant to COPD may be substantially higher.

Ethnicity-related differences were assessed in Kazakhstan only and revealed a higher prevalence of COPD (both diagnosed by spirometry and previously diagnosed by a physician) in Caucasians compared to Asians, together with more prominent symptoms and spirometry changes. Other studies have mentioned that genetic factors are probably involved in the decreased COPD risk observed in Asian [24].

Comparison with published literature

The prevalence of previously diagnosed COPD shown in the present study is low compared to estimates provided by previous studies (42 in Brazil [25], 57 in Greece [15], 88 in The Netherlands [23] and 222 in Russia [26] per 1000). Sweden was the only country where the reported prevalence was comparable to the present study (18 per 1000) [21]. This can possibly be explained by peculiarities of the healthcare systems. In the CIS countries, a big issue is the lack of COPD knowledge and the attitude to this disease within the population (people do not take a "simple" cough or dyspnea seriously and therefore do not visit a doctor). Another major problem may be related to low access to primary care services; in all the countries that took part in this study primary care is underfinanced and underdeveloped. Under-reporting of COPD may reflect the lack of COPD knowledge not only among patients, but also among healthcare workers, especially general practitioners and internists, who are the primary contact between the healthcare system and the population. For example, in Kazakhstan as early as 10–15 years ago, COPD was considered an "exotic" disease; a COPD diagnosis would be given in specialized institutions, not by primary care physicians. Nowadays COPD is much more well known. However, some public health problems may still exist; for example, patients receive medications for COPD treatment free of cost which may force health authorities to regulate the number of COPD patients registered in primary and specialty care. The forth reason for COPD under-reporting may be related to low availability of spirometry and its low quality in primary care hospitals. From a public health perspective, another important issue is that all respiratory diseases are collected in one statistical pool; there is no separate registration of COPD, asthma, allergic rhinitis and other non-infectious respiratory diseases in the CIS countries.

The COPD prevalence estimates based on spirometry reported in this study were similar to the data published in previous studies (45 in Spain [16], 42 in USA [19] and 37 in United Arab Emirates [22] per 1000). Some other studies reported higher estimates (240 (The Netherlands) [23], 218 (Russia) [26], 197 (Uruguay) [20], 184 (Greece) [15], 162 (Uganda) [27], 162 (Sweden) [21], 142 (Portugal) [28], 134 (Korea) [17], 78 (Mexico) [20] and 71 (Vietnam) [18] per 1000). The variability in prevalence estimates could reflect true differences or be due to the different methodologies used in different studies. Study design aspects such as differences in the rigor of case ascertainment (for example, different diagnostic criteria) or the over-representation of a high-risk sub-population in the study (such as another age range of participants or percentage of smokers) or even differences in healthcare systems (the availability of medical care) could have led to variations in estimates. However, different nations or regions may have a truly increased or decreased burden of the disease as a result of true biological phenomena. It should be noted that in the Russian study (GARD) spirometry was performed only for participants with suspected COPD, so the prevalence may be overstated; in addition, a significantly higher prevalence of previously diagnosed COPD in the Russian study is probably due to different diagnostic criteria. One study estimated the prevalence of COPD firstly diagnosed by spirometry [15]. In line with our study, most cases of COPD diagnosed by spirometry were firstly diagnosed, and prevalence of firstly diagnosed COPD was higher than for the previously diagnosed COPD confirming the observation that COPD is often under-reported.

COPD characteristics

The majority of respondents with COPD diagnosed by spirometry in this study had mild/moderate COPD; there were no respondents with GOLD stages III or IV. The median CAT™ score did not exceed 10 points, which corresponds to a low impact of COPD on health status. Almost half of respondents with COPD did not have dyspnoea/shortness of breath by mMRC scale. At the same time, clear statistically significant differences for CAT™ and mMRC scale were obtained between COPD and non-COPD respondents that additionally confirm the validity of these instruments for evaluation of COPD in research studies and routine use.

Co-morbidities

As for co-morbid conditions, in Ukraine the participants more often reported unburdened anamnesis, than in Kazakhstan and especially in Azerbaijan. A high rate of arterial hypertension was observed, followed by other cardiovascular diseases, diabetes mellitus and blood lipid abnormalities. In other studies, cardiovascular diseases were also the most common co-morbidities [29] and were recorded more frequently than in this study.

As expected, the most significant correlation was found between COPD and cardiovascular diseases. The rate of hypertension was also higher among respondents with COPD compared to the non-COPD population (although this difference was only statistically significant in Ukraine and Azerbaijan). It is well established, that COPD is a precursor to cardiovascular disease development and/or its aggravation [30, 31]. The association between a history of pneumonia and COPD confirms available data. Pneumonia and COPD can aggravate each other. One study indicated that previous exacerbations of pneumonia are significantly associated with a higher rate of COPD exacerbation [32]. Another study confirmed that COPD increases mortality in patients with pneumonia [33].

Strengths and limitations

This study has several strengths. It is a multi-national, cross-sectional, population-based study with a large sample size using consistent methodology across all countries, providing a standardized measure of prevalence in the CIS countries. In addition, the case definition of COPD used is based on both (i) self-reported diagnosis and (ii) diagnosis confirmed by spirometry. Furthermore, severity of COPD has been assessed based on the validated international GOLD guidelines. As it is the first time such an epidemiological study has been conducted in CIS countries, this study could facilitate increased recognition of COPD in CIS countries and allow preparation of educational interventions to optimize management of patients with COPD. Whereas many previously published studies on COPD concern patients only over 40 years of age, this study evaluates COPD prevalence in the overall adult population.

We acknowledge that the current study has several limitations. The method of district and street sampling may not ensure completely random selection of streets and participants. The relatively small number of COPD patients limits the analysis of risk factors associated with COPD and can limit the power for specific types of within-city analysis, such as detailed subgroup analyses. The subjectivity of the diagnostic criteria based on symptoms can lead to over or under diagnosis. Spirometry was the only objective diagnostic measure in the present study and its results were reviewed centrally, but difficulties encountered when conducting spirometry can affect the results of this procedure. Additionally, the physiological decrease in lung function in the elderly may influence the estimation of COPD prevalence stratified by age, taking into account that fixed ratio FEV_1/FVC was used as the diagnostic criteria for COPD in this study.

The city population may not be representative of each country in general, because risk factors and healthcare provision (including the availability of medical care) may vary widely across the country. In particular, the results may only reflect the situation in urban areas and not represent the whole country, since rural areas could have different levels of healthcare provision and accessibility to medical care and different living and working conditions for the people who live in these areas. Finally, some data are missing due to a lack of relevant information from participants, as a lot of study data were collected from respondents' interview.

Conclusion

In conclusion, in Ukraine, Kazakhstan and Azerbaijan the prevalence of COPD diagnosed by spirometry is significantly higher than the prevalence self-reported by respondents and/or based on anamnesis, demonstrating that COPD is under-reported in these countries. Compared to other countries, the COPD prevalence estimates in these CIS countries were relatively low. Factors such as limited funding from the government, lack of COPD knowledge, attitude within the population and of primary care physicians, and low access to high-quality spirometry may play a role in the under-reporting of COPD in these countries. A higher rate of COPD prevalence was observed in Kazakhstan (Almaty) compared to Ukraine (Kiev) and Azerbaijan (Baku) likely due to poor ecological conditions, but this assumption needs further investigation. The information provided in this paper will be helpful for healthcare policy makers in CIS countries to instruct COPD disease management and prevention strategies and allocate healthcare resources accordingly.

Abbreviations
ATS: American Thoracic Society; BMI: Body mass index; CAT™: COPD Assessment Test; CI: Confidence interval; CIS: Commonwealth of Independent States; COPD: Chronic Obstructive Pulmonary Disease; ERS: European Respiratory Society; FEV_1: Forced Expiratory Volume in one second; FVC: Forced Vital Capacity; GARD: Global Alliance against Chronic Respiratory Diseases; GOLD: Global Initiative for Chronic Obstructive Lung Disease; GSK: GlaxoSmithKline; mMRC: Modified Medical Research Council; OR: Odds Ratio; $PaCO_2$: Arterial partial pressure of carbon dioxide; PaO_2: Arterial partial pressure of oxygen; SD: Standard Deviation

Acknowledgments
National Institute of Phthisiology and Pulmonology F.G. Yanovsky National Academy of Medical Sciences of Ukraine (NIPP), Kiev, Ukraine and Semey State Medical University, Almaty, Kazakhstan provided advisory support to the study. Editorial support in the form of draft outline, editorial suggestions to draft versions of this paper, collating author comments, assembling tables and figures, referencing, and copyediting was provided by Julia She at Synergy Research Group and was funded by GSK.
We thank all investigators for their contribution to the study, allowing the first clinical epidemiology research to happen with a high level of integrity, and the contract research organization, Synergy Research Group, which was funded by GSK, and oversaw the study organization and conduct.

Funding
Funding for this study was provided by GSK (GSK Study Number RES116757, GSK study acronym: CORE).

Authors' contributions
All listed authors meet the criteria for authorship set forth by the International Committee for Medical Journal Editors. YF, LI, DN, AV provided support in the study concept and protocol development. DN, YF, LI, OG, KM, EM, IA, NN, LT, JM, AV were actively involved in the study design, acquisition of data, analysis and interpretation of the study data. Authors participated in critical revisions of the manuscript and have approved the article for publication. The authors contributed to the manuscript review, applying their clinical, epidemiology, and study design expertise and take responsibility for the integrity of the data and the accuracy of the data analysis. All authors read and approved the final manuscript.

Ethics approval and consent to participate
The study was reviewed and approved by an Independent Ethics Committee in Kazakhstan (Central Commission for Ethics at the Ministry of Health of the Republic of Kazakhstan) and by Local Ethics Committees in Kazakhstan, Azerbaijan and Ukraine (Ethics Committee at Semey State Medical University, Almaty, Kazakhstan; Ethics Committee at Scientific Research Institute of Lung Diseases in Baku, Azerbaijan; Commission for Ethics at National Institute of Phthisiology and Pulmonology F.G. Yanovsky of NAMS, Kiev, Ukraine; Commission for Ethics at Center for Primary Health Care #2 of Shevchenko District, Kiev, Ukraine), according to the local legal requirements. Written informed consent was obtained from each participant before any procedures or data collection related to the study.

Consent for publication
Not applicable.

Competing interests
The study was sponsored by GlaxoSmithKline (GSK) marketing a number of treatments for COPD, Allergic Rhinitis, and Asthma.
DN, YF, LI, OG, EM, IA, NN report grants from GSK, during the conduct of the study; personal fees from GSK, outside the submitted work.
KM and JM are employees of GSK. AV and LT are GSK employees and shareholders.

Author details
[1]Semey State Medical University, Almaty, Kazakhstan. [2]National Institute of Phthisiology and Pulmonology F.G. Yanovsky of NAMS, Kiev, Ukraine. [3]National Medical University n.a. O.O. Bogomoletz, Kiev, Ukraine. [4]GlaxoSmithKline, Kiev, Ukraine. [5]Scientific Research Institute of Lung Diseases, Baku, Azerbaijan. [6]GlaxoSmithKline, Dubai, UAE. [7]GlaxoSmithKline, Moscow, Russia. [8]GSK Russia Business Park "Krylatsky Hills", 17, Krylatskaya Street, Building 3 ("Air"), 121614 Moscow, Russia.

References
1. Raherison C, Girodet PO. Epidemiology of COPD. Eur Respir Rev. 2009; 18(114):213–21. https://doi.org/10.1183/09059180.00003609.
2. Adeloye D, Chua S, Lee C, Basquill C, Papana A, Theodoratou E, et al. Global Health epidemiology reference group (GHERG). Global and regional estimates of COPD prevalence: systematic review and meta-analysis. J Glob Health. 2015;5(2):020415. https://doi.org/10.7189/jogh.05-020415/.
3. Lozano R, Naghavi M, Foreman K, Lim S, Shibuya K, Aboyans V, et al. Global and regional mortality from 235 causes of death for 20 age groups in 1990 and 2010: a systematic analysis for the global burden of disease study 2010. Lancet. 2012;380(9859):2095–128. https://doi.org/10.1016/S0140-6736(12)61728-0. Erratum in: Lancet. 2013;381(9867):628.
4. Ignatiev VA, Titov OH, Gultyaeva OI. Chronic obstructive pulmonary disease: epidemiology and economic damage. Bulletin of St. Petersburg University. 2007; Issue 4: 37–46.
5. Global Strategy for the Diagnosis, Management and Prevention of COPD [Revised 2011], Global Initiative for Chronic Obstructive Lung Disease. Accessed from: http://www.goldcopd.org April 2011 (GOLD 2011).
6. Xu W, Collet JP, Shapiro S, Lin Y, Yang T, Wang C, et al. Negative impacts of unreported COPD exacerbations on health-related quality of life at one year. Eur Respir J. 2009;6.
7. Buist AS, McBurnie MA, Vollmer WM, Gillespie S, Burney P, Mannino DM, et al; BOLD Collaborative Research Group. International variation in the prevalence of COPD (the BOLD Study): a population-based prevalence study. Lancet. 2007;370(9589):741–50. Erratum in: Lancet. 2012;380(9844):806.
8. Bousquet J, Khaltaev N. Global surveillance, prevention and control of Chronic Respiratory Diseases. A comprehensive approach. www.who.int/gard/publications/GARD%20Book%202007.pdf. Date last updated: 2007.
9. Feshchenko Y, Iashyna L, Nugmanova D, Gyrina O, Polyanskaya M, Markov A, et al. Chronic obstructive pulmonary disease, bronchial asthma and allergic rhinitis in the adult population within the commonwealth of independent states: rationale and design of the CORE study. BMC Pulm Med. 2017;17:131.

10. Cooper BG. An update on contraindications for lung function testing. Thorax. 2011;66(8):714–23. https://doi.org/10.1136/thx.2010.139881.
11. Miller MR, Hankinson J, Brusasco V, Burgos F, Casaburi R, Coates A, et al. Standardisation of spirometry. Series "ATS/ERS task force: standardisation of lung function testing". Edited by V. Brusasco, R. Crapo and G. Viegi. Number 2 in this series. Eur Respir J. 2005;26:319–38.
12. Jones PW, Tabberer M, Chen WH. Creating scenarios of the impact of COPD and their relationship to COPD assessment test (CAT™) scores. BMC Pulm Med. 2011;11:42. https://doi.org/10.1186/1471-2466-11-42.
13. Clopper C, Pearson ES. The use of confidence or fiducial limits illustrated in the case of the binomial. Biometrika. 1934;26:404–13.
14. Pasko EN. Asthma. Following the standards of diagnosis and treatment. Medicus Amicus. 2002, #2.
15. Minas M, Hatzoglou C, Karetsi E, Papaioannou AI, Tanou K, Tsaroucha R, et al. COPD prevalence and the differences between newly and previously diagnosed COPD patients in a spirometry program. Prim Care Respir J. 2010; 19(4):363–70.
16. Soriano JB, Ancochea J, Miravitlles M, García-Río F, Duran-Tauleria E, Muñoz L, et al. Recent trends in COPD prevalence in Spain: a repeated cross-sectional survey 1997-2007. Eur Respir J. 2010;36(4):758–65.
17. Yoo KH, Kim YS, Sheen SS, Park JH, Hwang YI, Kim SH, et al. Prevalence of chronic obstructive pulmonary disease in Korea: the fourth Korean National Health and nutrition examination survey, 2008. Respirology. 2011;16(4):659–65.
18. Lâm HT, Ekerljung L, Tuòng NV, Rönmark E, Larsson K, Lundbäck B. Prevalence of COPD by disease severity in men and women in northern Vietnam. COPD. 2014;11(5):575–81.
19. Doney B, Hnizdo E, Syamlal G, Kullman G, Burchfiel C, Martin CJ, et al. Prevalence of chronic obstructive pulmonary disease among US working adults aged 40 to 70 years. National Health Interview Survey data 2004 to 2011. J Occup Environ Med. 2014;56(10):1088–93.
20. Menezes AM, Perez-Padilla R, Jardim JR, Muiño A, Lopez MV, Valdivia G, et al. PLATINO team. Chronic obstructive pulmonary disease in five Latin American cities (the PLATINO study): a prevalence study. Lancet. 2005; 366(9500):1875–81.
21. Carlsson AC, Wändell P, Ösby U, Zarrinkoub R, Wettermark B, Ljunggren G. High prevalence of diagnosis of diabetes, depression, anxiety, hypertension, asthma and COPD in the total population of Stockholm, Sweden - a challenge for public health. BMC Public Health. 2013;13:670.
22. Al Zaabi A, Asad F, Abdou J, Al Musaabi H, Al Saiari MB, Buhussien AS, et al. Prevalence of COPD in Abu Dhabi, United Arab Emirates. Respir Med. 2011; 105(4):566–70.
23. Vanfleteren LE, Franssen FM, Wesseling G, Wouters EF. The prevalence of chronic obstructive pulmonary disease in Maastricht, the Netherlands. Respir Med. 2012;106(6):871–4.
24. Tran HN, Siu S, Iribarren C, Udaltsova N, Klatsky AL. Ethnicity and risk of hospitalization for asthma and chronic obstructive pulmonary disease. Ann Epidemiol. 2011;21(8):615–22.
25. Sousa CA, César CL, Barros MB, Carandina L, Goldbaum M, Pereira JC. Prevalence of chronic obstructive pulmonary disease and risk factors in São Paulo, Brazil, 2008-2009. Rev Saude Publica. 2011;45(5):887–96.
26. Chuchalin AG, Khaltaev N, Antonov NS, Galkin DV, Manakov LG, Antonini P, et al. Chronic respiratory diseases and risk factors in 12 regions of the Russian Federation. Int J Chron Obstruct Pulmon Dis. 2014;9:963–74.
27. Van Gemert F, Kirenga B, Chavannes N, Kamya M, Luzige S, Musinguzi P, et al. Prevalence of chronic obstructive pulmonary disease and associated risk factors in Uganda (FRESH AIR Uganda): a prospective cross-sectional observational study. Lancet Glob Health. 2015;3(1):e44–51.
28. Bárbara C, Rodrigues F, Dias H, Cardoso J, Almeida J, Matos MJ, et al. Chronic obstructive pulmonary disease prevalence in Lisbon, Portugal: the burden of obstructive lung disease study. Rev Port Pneumol. 2013; 19(3):96–105.
29. Dal Negro RW, Bonadiman L, Turco P. Prevalence of different comorbidities in COPD patients by gender and GOLD stage. Multidiscip Respir Med. 2015; 10(1):24.
30. Calverley PM, Scott S. Is airway inflammation in chronic obstructive pulmonary disease (COPD) a risk factor for cardiovascular events? COPD. 2006;3(4):233–42.
31. Caram LM, Ferrari R, Naves CR, Coelho LS, Vale SA, Tanni SE, et al. Risk factors for cardiovascular disease in patients with COPD: mild-to-moderate COPD versus severe-to-very severe COPD. J Bras Pneumol. 2016;42(3):179–84.
32. Hwang YI, Lee SH, Yoo JH, Jung BH, Yoo KH, Na MJ, et al. History of pneumonia is a strong risk factor for chronic obstructive pulmonary disease (COPD) exacerbation in South Korea: the epidemiologic review and prospective observation of COPD and health in Korea (EPOCH) study. J Thorac Dis. 2015;7(12):2203–13.
33. Restrepo MI, Mortensen EM, Pugh JA, Anzueto A. COPD is associated with increased mortality in patients with community-acquired pneumonia. Eur Respir J. 2006;28:346–51.
34. Danielsson P, Ólafsdóttir IS, Benediktsdóttir B, Gíslason T, Janson C. The prevalence of chronic obstructive pulmonary disease in Uppsala, Sweden—the burden of obstructive lung disease (BOLD) study: cross-sectional population-based study. Clin Respir J. 2012;6(2):120–7.
35. Tageldin MA, Nafti S, Khan JA, Nejjari C, Beji M, Mahboub B, et al. BREATHE study group. Distribution of COPD-related symptoms in the Middle East and North Africa: results of the BREATHE study. Respir Med. 2012;106(Suppl 2): S25–32.

11

Secondary pulmonary alveolar proteinosis

Dongmei Zhang[1,5], Xinlun Tian[1*], Ruie Feng[2], Xiaobei Guo[1], Peng Wang[3], Yusen Situ[4], Yi Xiao[1] and Kai-Feng Xu[1]

Abstract

Background: Secondary pulmonary alveolar proteinosis (sPAP) is an extremely rare disease. The clinical features of sPAP patients remain to be summarizeds.

Methods: Patients pathologically diagnosed with PAP and with negative results for anti-granulocyte macrophage colony stimulating factor (GM-CSF) autoantibodies from Peking Union Medical College Hospital between January 2000 and July 2016 were retrospectively studied. The PubMed database was also searched for literature to collect published cases.

Results: In our center, nine patients were diagnosed as sPAP with a median age of 37 years. Hematological disorders, including myelodysplastic syndrome (MDS), chronic myelogenous leukemia (CML), and pulmonary tuberculosis (TB) infection were the underlying diseases. Cases secondary to MDS had very poor prognosis as all of them survived less than 2 years after their diagnosis, while those secondary to TB had favorable prognosis. Only 33.3% of cases showed interlobular septal thickening in our sPAP group. Through literature review, 164 sPAP cases were collected. The age at diagnosis was 45.0 ± 14.8 years old and the gender radio was 1.20:1 (M:F). 61.9% of cases were diagnosed by bronchoscopy. MDS and CML were common underlying diseases in 34.1% and 15.2% of patients, respectively. Patients with sPAP secondary to hematological diseases had a short survival time and half of them died within 14.95 months after diagnosis.

Conclusions: MDS and TB infection were the most frequent underlying causes of sPAP in this single-center research in China, with cases secondary to MDS having a poor survival rate. sPAP was more likely to be secondary to hematological disorders, especially MDS and CML and had a fairly poor prognosis in published cases. sPAP should be suspected in PAP patients whose CT scan presents only ground-glass opacities without interlobular septal thickening.

Keywords: Secondary pulmonary alveolar proteinosis (sPAP), Anti-granulocyte macrophage colony stimulating factor autoantibodies (GM-CSF-Ab), Myelodysplastic syndrome (MDS), Tuberculosis (TB)

Background

Pulmonary alveolar proteinosis (PAP), a rare disease with an estimated prevalence of 3.7 to 6.2 cases per million persons [1, 2], is characterized by the accumulation of lipoprotein material in alveoli and terminal respiratory airways [3]. Current knowledge about PAP is based on case studies and individual case reports, and as such, the prevalence of PAP may vary due to differences in medical systems and facilities in different countries. According to the pathogenesis, PAP can be classified in three ways: congenital PAP, secondary PAP (sPAP) and autoimmune PAP (or acquired PAP, or idiopathic PAP) [4]. sPAP mainly develops as a result of hematological diseases, the use of immunosuppression drugs, dust inhalation and certain chronic infections with impaired alveolar macrophage function. Autoimmune PAP, which accounts for over 90% of PAP cases, is an

* Correspondence: xinlun_t@sina.com
[1]Department of Respiratory Medicine, Peking Union Medical College Hospital, Chinese Academy of Medical Sciences & Peking Union Medical College, Beijing, China
Full list of author information is available at the end of the article

autoimmune disease with autoantibodies targeting granulocyte macrophage colony stimulating factor (GM-CSF) [5].

According to previous reports, sPAP is different from autoimmune PAP in aspects besides the pathogenesis. For example, sPAP has different features on high-resolution computed tomography (HRCT) compared to autoimmune PAP [6] and sPAP has a much poorer prognosis compared with autoimmune PAP [7]. Knowledge of the clinical characteristics of sPAP are still limited as the majority of current literature is in the form of case reports, the largest series being a report by Ishii H which included 40 Japanese patients [7]. As we do not know whether the prevalence of sPAP in China has any differences compared to other countries, we retrospectively collected sPAP patients hospitalized from 2000 to 2016 in our hospital, listed their clinical features and symptoms, and we also reviewed all published cases in literature to learn more about the characteristics of sPAP around the world.

Methods

Study design and participants

This is a case study of patients who were diagnosed with PAP in Peking Union Medical College Hospital (PUMCH) between Jan. 1st, 2000 and July 1st, 2016. Medical files were retroactively collected on Feb. 2017. The study was approved by the Ethical Committee of PUMCH (S-K-215), and universal informed consent forms were signed when each subject was admitted to our hospital. The patients or their kin have given written informed consent to publish these case details. Patients had a clinical diagnosis of PAP, which was further confirmed pathologically by testing for amorphous periodic Acid-Schiff (PAS)-positive granules, found either in milky broncho-alveolar lavage fluid (BALF) or in alveolar structures of lung biopsy tissues. Patients under 18 years old were excluded. Serum GM-CSF autoantibodies were evaluated using an enzyme-linked immunosorbent assay, as previously described [8–10]. Patients with positive serum GM-CSF autoantibodies (> 5 μg/mL) were also excluded.

Methods of data analysis

The patients' quantitative characteristics such as age at diagnosis were summarized by median and range. The qualitative characteristics such as general appearance, imaging features and other organ complications were presented as a frequency distribution or percentage. Authors had no access to information that could identify individual participants during or after data collection.

Results

Demographic characteristics

In total, among 157 hospitalized PAP cases, 9 patients were diagnosed with sPAP. Their clinical characteristics are summarized in Table 1. In these 9 patients, 3 were female and 6 were male, and they ranged in age from 20 to 56 years (median age 37 years). At the time of administration, 5 (5/9) of the cases complained of fever and cough, followed by weakness (4/9), weight loss (3/9), and dyspnea or exertional dyspnea (3/9). Diagnostic procedures included BALF (3/9), CT guided biopsy (2/9), open lung biopsy (2/9), transbronchial lung biopsy (TBLB) plus BALF (1/9), and video-assisted thoracic surgery (VATS) (1/9).

Primary diseases

The primary diseases of these 9 sPAP cases were variable, as 5 cases arose from hematologic disorders (4 myelodysplastic syndrome (MDS) and 1 chronic myelogenous leukemia (CML)) and 4 cases from tuberculosis (TB). *Mycobacterium chelonei* infection was detected in one patient with underlying MDS using a subcutaneous nodule biopsy, and another patient was affected by hospital-acquired pneumonia with obscure pathogens, and neither of their sputum nor BALF cultures tested positive.

CT features

As shown in Table 1, all of our cases presented bilateral ground-glass opacities (GGO) on their CT scans. Among them, GGO with a diffuse pattern was the most frequent pattern, presenting in 5 (5/9) patients, while a patchy geographic pattern and crazy paving pattern each presented in 2 (2/9) patients respectively. Small scattered nodules were found in both TB (2/4) and MDS patients (2/4). The patient infected with *M. chelonei* showed enlarged mediastinal lymph nodes. Interlobular septal thickening, which was thought to be a typical feature of PAP, could only be recognized in three (3/9) of our sPAP patients.

Pulmonary function tests

At the time of diagnosis, 8 patients underwent arterial blood gas tests and the mean arterial partial oxygen pressure (PaO_2) was 62.2 mmHg (34.1, 97.4 mmHg) in room air. In 7 patients who performed pulmonary function tests during administration, 6 had normal forced vital capacity (FVC) and forced expiratory volume in the first 1 s (FEV_1). All 5 cases evaluated for diffusing function showed a remarkable reduction in diffusing capacity for carbon monoxide (DL_{CO}) with a mean of 43.1% (22.1%, 58.9%) of the normal predicted value.

Table 1 Characteristics of Patients with secondary pulmonary alveolar proteinosis in Peking Union Medical College Hospital

	Gender	Age	Smoking	Clinical Symptoms	Diagnostic Procedure	Primary Disease	PaO_2 mmHg
1	Male	38	Current	Weight loss, weakness, night sweats	BALF	MDS-MLD	64.1
2	Female	26	Never	Fever, productive cough	CT guided percutaneous lung biopsy	TB	94.5
3	Male	20	Current	Exertional dyspnea, dry cough	Surgical biopsy	CML	97.4
4	Male	26	Never	Weakness, fever	BALF+TBLB	MDS-SLD	NA
5	Male	37	Never	Dyspnea, dry cough	BALF	MDS-U	48
6	Male	33	Never	Fever, weight loss, weakness	Surgical biopsy	MDS-EB	34.6
7	Male	56	Never	Fever, dry cough	VATS	TB	84.1
8	Female	54	Never	Weight loss,weakness, fever	CT guided percutaneous lung biopsy	TB	39
9	Female	51	Never	Dyspnea, productive cough	BALF	TB	35.6
	CT Scan Features				Comorbidity/Complication	Treatment	Outcomes
1	diffused bilateral GGO				None	WLL, Danazol, Retinoic acid,	Die
2	bilateral GGO patchy geographic pattern, interlobular septal thickening,small scattered nodules				Hepatitis	INH, RIF, EMB, Levofloxacin	Recovery
3	bilateral GGO patchy geographic pattern, bilateral cysts				None	Hydroxyurea	NA
4	diffused bilateral GGO, small nodules				Type B viral hepatitis	Prednisone	Die
5	bilateral GGO with a crazy paving pattern,enlarged mediastinal lymph nodes				*Mycobacterium chelonei*infection	Antibiotics, traditional medicine	Die
6	diffused bilateral GGO, interlobular septal thickening,small scattered nodules				Hospital acquired pneumonia	Danazol, Retinoic acid, WLL	Die
7	bilateral GGO with a crazy paving pattern, interlobular septal thickening				None	INH, RIF, EMB,Clarithromycin, Oxifloxacin	Improved
8	diffused bilateral GGO, small scattered nodules				None	INH, RIF, EMB,Rifapentine	Stable
9	diffused bilateral GGO, septal thickening				Thrombopenia, Sjogren's syndrome	INH, RIF, EMB,Levofloxacin, WLL	Improved

BALF **broncho-alverolar lavage fluid,** ***CML*** **chronic myelogenousleukemia;*****EMB*** **ethambutol,** ***GGO*** **ground-glass opacities,** ***INH*** **isonicotinic acid hydrazide,** ***MDS*** **myelodysplastic syndrome(SLD:single lineage dysplasia; MLD: multilineage dysplasia; EB: excess blasts; U: unclassifiable),** ***NA*** **not available,** ***RIF*** **rifampicine,** ***TB*** **tuberculosis,** ***TBLB*** **transbronchial lung biopsy,** ***VATS*** **via video-assisted thoracic surgery,** ***WLL*** **whole lung lavage**

Treatment and prognosis

The median follow-up duration was 4.7 years in these patients. All 4 patients with underlying MDS died within 2 years after diagnosis, and whole lung lavage (WLL) was performed in 2 of them, but symptoms only improved temporarily. Both the symptoms and the CT scans improved in 3 of the 4 patients with TB after anti-TB therapy, and the remaining patient with TB remains stable throughout 8 years of follow-up. Unfortunately, the patient with CML could not be followed-up on. The patient with *M.chelonei* complications (patient 5) had his condition worsen rapidly even with antibiotic administration based on drug sensitivity tests and died 3 months after diagnosis.

Literature reviews

Texts were searched for using the terms "pulmonary alveolar lipoproteinosis [Title/abstract]" or "pulmonary alveolar proteinosis [Title/abstract]" in the PubMed database. Cases published only in abstract without full-text were excluded. For cases with a history of dust inhalation, only those that tested negative for GM-CSF autoantibodies were included as dust exposure was not a specified factor of sPAP [11].

Using the above search strategy, 1291 articles on PAP were identified. These articles were carefully reviewed to remove reviews, abstracts, commitments, animal researches, relevant pathophysiological studies or pharmaceutical researches, articles about congenital PAP, and articles about autoimmune PAP. We also removed those diagnosed by autopsy post-mortem and pediatric patients less than 18 years old. In the end, 155 cases of sPAP with underlying diseases were found (Additional file 1: Figure S1). In Table 2, we summarized the available characteristics of the 164 cases in total (including our 9 cases).

The patients were diagnosed at an age of 45.0 ± 14.8. The male to female ratio was 1.20:1. Bronchoscopy, including BALF and/or TBLB, was the most frequent method used to diagnose sPAP, with 61.9% of cases diagnosed in this manner. Other procedures used included VATS and open lung biopsy, with 17.7% and 18.9% of cases being diagnosed in those manners respectively. Approximately 70% of cases were secondary to hematological diseases, such as MDS (34.1%), CML (15.2%) and AML (acute myelogenous leukemia) (5.5%).

Underlying infectious diseases, mainly due to TB, non-TB mycobacteria, human immunodeficiency virus, and *Aspergillosis*, consisted of 7.9% of all cases. Autoimmune diseases including Behcet's disease, vasculitis, Sjogren's syndrome, and dermatomyositis accounted for 6.7% of the underlying causes. 10.4% of sPAP patients were secondary to lung or kidney transplantation. The other rare underlying diseases were non-hematological tumors and dust inhalation. As shown in Fig. 1, the median survival in 92 cases secondary to hematological diseases was only 14.95 months, which was significantly shorter than sPAP secondary to other causes ($p < 0.001$).

Table 2 Summary of characteristics of 159 secondary pulmonary alveolar proteinosis cases

sPAP	164	Underlying disease	
Age in years	45.0 ± 14.8	Myelodysplastic syndrome	56 (34.1)
Sex ratio (Male: Female)	1.20:1	Chronic myeloid leukemia	25 (15.2)
Clinical symptoms	99	Acute myeloid leukemia	9 (5.5)
Asymptomatic	11 (11.1)	Acute lymphoid leukemia	5 (3.0)
Dyspnea with effort	53 (53.5)	Lymphoma	6 (3.7)
Cough	32 (32.3)	Myelofibrosis	3 (1.8)
fever	38 (38.3)	Other hematological disorders	9 (5.5)
Diagnostic procedure		Infection diseases	13 (7.9)
Bronchoscopy	101 (61.6)	Autoimmune diseases	11 (6.7)
CT guided biopsy	3 (1.8)	Post transplantation	17 (10.4)
VATS	29 (17.7)	non-hematological tumors	5 (3.0)
Surgery lung biopsy	31 (18.9)	Dust inhalation	5 (3.0)

Data is present by number (percentage, %)
VATS via video-assisted thoracic surgery

Discussion

Since sPAP is a rare disease, less than 200 cases have been reported throughout the world, with most of them in form of case reports. H. Ishii [7] summarized the characteristics of 40 Japanese sPAP patients, which was the largest retrospective observational study about sPAP that we found. To the best of our knowledge, our study is the largest series of sPAP from a single center in China. We present some interesting findings. Firstly, TB is also a frequent underlying disease of sPAP in China, and fortunately, after effective anti-TB therapy, sPAP can be improved concurrently. Furthermore, hematologic disorders, especially MDS, are the predominant primary disease of sPAP, and these patients have a terrible prognosis with the majority dying within 2 years after diagnosis. Complications from other infections may accelerate the advancement of the disease.

In our center, 5.73% of PAP cases were determined to be sPAP, which is slightly lower than the percentage of sPAP (8.3% to 10%) in the Japanese case series [6, 7]. Both our study and existing literature illustrates that hematologic disorders are the most frequent underlying disease of sPAP. The study including 31 cases of sPAP with MDS found that sPAP is an important risk factor predicting adverse outcome of MDS with a 2-year survival of 46.2% [12]. In our cases, all of the 4 patients with MDS as the

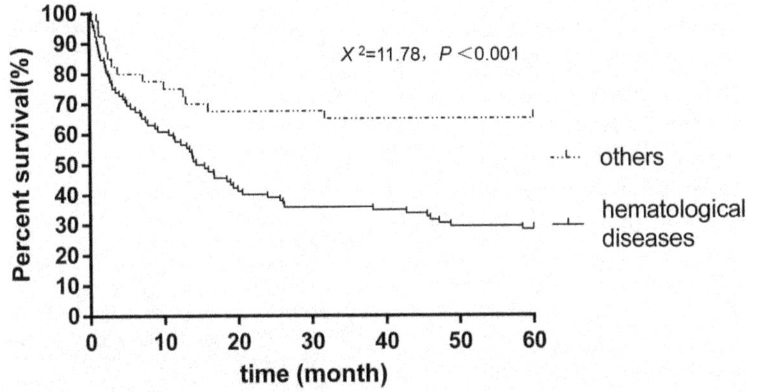

Fig. 1 Survival probability of secondary pulmonary alveolar proteinosis cases. In our 9 cases and 155 cases from literatures, 132 cases had the survival information. In 92 cases secondary to hematological diseases, the median survival was 14.95 months as 66 (71.3%) died within 5 years. In 40 cases secondary to other causes, the median survival was to months and 14 (35%) died within 5 years. Log-rank (Mantel-Cox) test $X^2 = 11.78$, $P < 0.001$

underlying disease died within 2 years. The pathomechanism of sPAP secondary to hematological diseases remains unknown. Mutations in GATA2 may be associated with sPAP [13, 14] since an autosomal dominant familial MDS and AML carried a heritable GATA2 mutation [15] and approximately one third of GATA2 mutation carriers also complicated sPAP [16]. It is speculated that a GATA2 deficiency leads to the alteration of alveolar cellular immunity because these patients had neither GM-CSF receptor mutations nor anti-GM-CSF autoantibodies. In the mice model, T-bet–over expressing T cells act to initiate the pathogenesis of sPAP [17]. Treatment of sPAP should focus on curing the underlying diseases. Bone marrow transplantation or cord blood transplantation can cure sPAP in these patients, but at the cost of an increased risk of infection and mortality [12, 18].

Some infectious diseases such as TB can cause sPAP, possibly due to microorganisms impairing the function of macrophages. The heavy burden of TB in China makes it a significant underlying disease in our cases. In this circumstance, treating the underlying infection(s) can ameliorate sPAP, as shown in our cases, 3 cases improved and 1 case remained stable after anti-TB therapy. However, autoimmune PAP might cause complications with infections including TB, *Nocardia*, and *Aspergillus*. An anti-GM-CSF autoantibody test is effective to distinguish these two situations since it is negative in the former while positive in the later. Besides antibiotics, GM-CSF replacement is ineffective to the former but of benefit to the latter.

In our study, only 33.3% of cases show interlobular septal thickening, which is regarded as a typical feature in the CT scan of autoimmune PAP patients [19]. Additionally, only 22.2% of them present GGO with patchy geographic pattern, which is more common in autoimmune PAP [6]. As a result, sPAP should be suspected in PAP patients whose CT scans only present GGO without interlobular septal thickening or in the absence of a geographic pattern. More detailed evaluation about infectious and hematologic diseases should be performed. Moreover, qualification of anti-GM-CSF-Ab is valuable for the differentiation of autoimmune or secondary PAP.

Several limitations must be stressed with regards to this study. First, since PAP is a rare disease, the value of this study is limited by its small sample size. Our study was also limited in scope in that the underlying disease in our sPAP cases only included hematological diseases and infections, without covering dust inhalation, autoimmune disease or tumors. Secondly, as a retrospective study, some patient characteristics and information are not comprehensive, such as arterial blood gas and lung function. Furthermore, because our hospital is the largest rare disease treatment center in China, patients admitted are usually more complex and serious cases, and as such, we cannot avoid selection bias. Meanwhile, occupational diseases were restrictively diagnosed and treated in designated hospitals in China, so PAP secondary to occupational exposure is difficult to diagnose in our hospital. It is also difficult to compare the result of a single Chinese center with those all over the world. Thus, we conducted a comprehensive review of all the available cases published in available literature to minimize selection bias. Finally, in the review, we did not account for other factors that may affect the variation of sPAP, such as the geographical features of the patients.

Conclusions

In summary, this study found that MDS and TB infection were the most frequent underlying causes of sPAP in this single center research in China and cases that secondary to MDS had a poor survival rate. However, after taking all the published cases into consideration, hematological disorders, especially MDS and CML, are the major primary disease in 68.9% of cases. sPAP was often middle age onset, but it had a fairly poor prognosis when the underlying diseases were hematologic disorders. The diagnosis of sPAP should be considered in PAP patients whose CT scan only presents GGO without interlobular septal thickening.

Abbreviations

AML: Acute myelogenous leukemia; BALF: Bronchoalveolar lavage fluid; CML: Chronic myelogenous leukemia; CT: Computed tomography; DL_{CO}: Diffusing capacity for carbon monoxide; FEV_1: Forced expiratory volume in the first 1 second; FVC: Forced vital capacity; GGO: Ground-glass opacities; GM-CSF-Ab: Granulocyte macrophage colony stimulating factor autoantibodies; HRCT: High-resolution computed tomography; MDS: Myelodysplastic syndrome; PAP: Pulmonary alveolar proteinosis; PAS: Periodic Acid-Schiff; PUMCH: Peking Union Medical College Hospital; sPAP: Secondary pulmonary alveolar proteinosis; TB: Tuberculosis; TBLB: Transbronchial lung biopsy; VATS: Video-assisted thoracic surgery; WLL: Whole lung lavage.

Acknowledgements

The authors would like to thank Tao Liu, Yongjian Liu, Juhong Shi, Chi Shao, and Xiaoming Huang for their efforts in performing and aiding the clinical diagnosis and following of sPAP patients.

Funding

This work was supported by "State Key Project, Clinical Cohort Study of Rare Diseases. Rare Lung Disease Research Group in China" (2016YFC0901502) and The Capital of the Public Health Program: Study on the Evaluation of Diagnosis and Treatment on Seven Treatable Rare Diseases (Z151100003915126)

Authors' contributions

DZ and XT conception, design, obtaining consent, and drafting manuscript; RF reviewed all the pathologicalslides of all the patients, PW detected pathogenic microbes of all the patients. XG collection of data; YS design and drafting manuscript; YX and KFX data analysis and interpretation. All authors read and approved the final manuscript.

Consent for publication

The patients or their kin have given written informed consent to publication.

Competing interests

The authors declare that they have no competing interests.

Author details

[1]Department of Respiratory Medicine, Peking Union Medical College Hospital, Chinese Academy of Medical Sciences & Peking Union Medical College, Beijing, China. [2]Department of Pathology, Peking Union Medical College Hospital, Chinese Academy of Medical Sciences & Peking Union Medical College, Beijing, China. [3]Laboratory Department, Peking Union Medical College Hospital, Chinese Academy of Medical Sciences & Peking Union Medical College, Beijing, China. [4]Department of Biochemistry, Faculty of Medicine and Dentistry, University of Alberta, Edmonton, Canada. [5]Present address: Department of Respiratory and Critical Care Medicine, Beijing Institute of Respiratory Medicine and Beijing Chaoyang Hospital, Capital Medical University, Beijing, China.

References

1. Ben-Dov I, Kishinevski Y, Roznman J, Soliman A, Bishara H, Zelligson E, et al. Pulmonary alveolar proteinosis in Israel: ethnic clustering. Isr Med Assoc J. 1999;1:75–8. PMID:10731299
2. Inoue Y, Trapnell BC, Tazawa R, et al. Characteristics of a large cohort of patients with autoimmune pulmonary alveolar proteinosis in Japan. Am J Respir Crit Care Med. 2008;177(7):752–62. https://doi.org/10.1164/rccm.200708-1271OC. PMID:18202348
3. Rosen SH, Castleman B, Liebow AA. Pulmonary alveolar proteinosis. N Engl J Med. 1958;258:1123–42. https://doi.org/10.1056/NEJM195806052582301. PMID:13552931
4. Trapnell BC, Whitsett JA, Nakata K. Pulmonary alveolar proteinosis. N Engl J Med. 2003;349:2527–39. https://doi.org/10.1056/NEJMra023226. PMID: 14695413
5. Borie R, Danel C, Debray MP, et al. Pulmonary alveolar proteinosis. Eur Respir Rev. 2011;20(120):98–107. https://doi.org/10.1183/09059180.00001311. PMID:21632797
6. Ishii H, Trapnell BC, Tazawa R, Inoue Y, Akira M, Kogure Y, et al. Comparative study of high-resolution CT findings between autoimmune and secondary pulmonary alveolar proteinosis. Chest. 2009;136:1348–55. https://doi.org/10.1378/chest.09-0097. PMID:19892674
7. Ishii H, Tazawa R, Kaneko C, Saraya T, Inoue Y, Hamano E, et al. Clinical features of secondary pulmonary alveolar proteinosis: pre-mortem cases in Japan. Eur Respir J. 2011;37:465–8. https://doi.org/10.1183/09031936.00092910. PMID:21282812
8. Xu KF, Chen Y, Guo ZJ, Zhu YJ. Autoantibody against granulocyte-macrophage colony-stimulating factor and other serum markers in pulmonary alveolar proteinosis. Zhonghua Jie He He Hu Xi Za Zhi. 2004;27:824–8. PMID:15730782
9. Uchida K, Nakata K, Trapnell BC, Terakawa T, Hamano E, Mikami A, et al. High-affinity autoantibodies specifically eliminate granulocyte-macrophage colony-stimulating factor activity in the lungs of patients with idiopathic pulmonary alveolar proteinosis. Blood. 2004;103:1089–98. https://doi.org/10.1182/blood-2003-05-1565. PMID:14512323
10. Li Y, Tian X, Gui Y, Ma A, Li X, Zeng N, Zhang P, Li G, Xu K. Serum markers in patients with idiopathic pulmonary alveolar proteinosis. Zhonghua Jie He He Hu Xi Za Zhi. 2014;37(7):497–501. PMID:25262689
11. Costabel U, Nakata K. Pulmonary alveolar proteinosis associated with dust inhalation: not secondary but autoimmune. Am J Respir Crit Care Med. 2010;181:427–8. https://doi.org/10.1164/rccm.200912-1800ED. PMID:20185750
12. Ishii H, Seymour JF, Tazawa R, Inoue Y, Uchida N, Nishida A, et al. Secondary pulmonary alveolar proteinosis complicating myelodysplastic syndrome results in worsening of prognosis: a retrospective cohort study in Japan. BMC Pulm Med. 2014;14:37. https://doi.org/10.1186/1471-2466-14-37. PMID: 24597668
13. Ballerie A, Nimubona S, Meunier C, et al. Association of pulmonary alveolar proteinosis and fibrosis: patient with GATA2 deficiency. Eur Respir J. 2016;48(5):1510–4. https://doi.org/10.1183/13993003.00252-2016. PMID:27799394
14. Griese M, Zarbock R, Costabel U, Hildebrandt J, Theegarten D, Albert M, et al. GATA2 deficiency in children and adults with severe pulmonary alveolar proteinosis and hematologic disorders. BMC Pulm Med. 2015;15:87. https://doi.org/10.1186/s12890-015-0083-2. PMID: 26264606
15. Hahn CN, Chong CE, Carmichael CL, Wilkins EJ, Brautigan PJ, Li XC, et al. Heritable GATA2 mutations associated with familial myelodysplastic syndrome and acute myeloid leukemia. Nat Genet. 2011;43:1012–7. https://doi.org/10.1038/ng.913. PMID:21892162
16. Chaulagain CP, Pilichowska M, Brinckerhoff L, Tabba M, Erban JK. Secondary pulmonary alveolar proteinosis in hematologic malignancies. Hematol Oncol Stem Cell Ther. 2014;7:127–35. https://doi.org/10.1016/j.hemonc.2014.09.003. PMID:25300566

17. Iriguchi S, Kikuchi N, Kaneko S, et al. T-cell-restricted T-bet overexpression induces aberrant hematopoiesis of myeloid cells and impairs function of macrophages in the lung. Blood. 2015;125(2):370–82. https://doi.org/10.1182/blood-2014-05-575225. PMID: 25349175
18. Tabata S, Shimoji S, Murase K, Takiuchi Y, Inoue D, Kimura T, et al. Successful allogeneic bone marrow transplantation for myelodysplastic syndrome complicated by severe pulmonary alveolar proteinosis. Int J Hematol. 2009; 90:407–12. https://doi.org/10.1007/s12185-009-0404-4. PMID:19693450
19. Mehrian P, Homayounfar N, Karimi MA, Jafarzadeh H. Features of idiopathic pulmonary alveolar proteinosis in high resolution computed tomography. Pol J Radiol. 2014;79:65–9. https://doi.org/10.12659/PJR.890218. PMID:24707326

12

Emphysematous change with scleroderma-associated interstitial lung disease: the potential contribution of vasculopathy?

Hideaki Yamakawa[1,6*], Tamiko Takemura[2], Tae Iwasawa[3], Yumie Yamanaka[1,6], Satoshi Ikeda[1], Akimasa Sekine[1], Hideya Kitamura[1,6], Tomohisa Baba[1], Shinichiro Iso[4], Koji Okudela[5], Kazuyoshi Kuwano[6] and Takashi Ogura[1]

Abstract

Background: Pulmonary emphysema combined with systemic sclerosis (SSc)-associated interstitial lung disease (ILD) occurs more often in smokers but also in never-smokers. This study aimed to describe a new finding characterized by peculiar emphysematous change with SSc-associated ILD (SSc-ILD).

Methods: We conducted a retrospective review of 21 consecutive patients with SSc-ILD diagnosed by surgical lung biopsy and focused on the radio-pathological correlation of the emphysematous change.

Results: Pathological pulmonary emphysema (p-PE) with SSc-ILD was the predominant complication in 16 patients (76.2%) with/without a smoking history, of whom 62.5% were never-smokers. A low attenuation area (LAA) within interstitial abnormality on high-resolution computed tomography (HRCT) was present in 31.3%. Diffusing capacity of the lung for carbon monoxide (D_{LCO}) was lower, disease extent on HRCT higher, and intimal/medial thickening in muscular pulmonary arteries more common in the patients with p-PE with SSc-ILD. However, forced vital capacity (FVC) was well preserved regardless of whether p-PE was observed. Most SSc-ILD patients had pulmonary microvasculature changes in arterioles (90.5%), venules (85.7%), and interlobular veins (81.0%).

Conclusions: Pulmonary emphysematous changes (LAA within interstitial abnormalities on HRCT and destruction of fibrously thickened alveolar walls) are specific and novel radio-pathological features of SSc-ILD. Peripheral vasculopathy may help to destroy the fibrously thickened alveolar walls, resulting in emphysematous change in SSc-ILD.

Keywords: Systemic sclerosis, Emphysematous change, Vasculopathy

Background

Interstitial lung disease (ILD) is common in patients with systemic sclerosis (SSc), and a minority of patients evolve to end-stage respiratory insufficiency [1]. Ground-glass opacity, reticular intralobular interstitial thickening, and traction bronchiectasis are the most common findings on high-resolution computed tomography (HRCT) [2, 3]. The HRCT features of ILD in patients with SSc closely resemble those in patients with idiopathic nonspecific interstitial pneumonia (NSIP) [3]. In terms of pathological findings, NSIP is increasingly regarded as the more prevalent histologic pattern in patients with SSc-associated ILD (SSc-ILD) and in those with other connective tissue diseases (CTD) [4–8].

We previously reported that SSc-related autoantibody-positive ILD, but not CTD, is a different disease entity from that of SSc or mixed CTD associated with ILD [9]. In that report, pathological pulmonary emphysema (p-PE) with ILD was observed more frequently (56%) in the patients with SSc or mixed CTD associated with ILD. Interestingly, a high proportion (64.3%) of these patients were never-smokers [9], and another recent report found that pulmonary emphysema combined with SSc-ILD was also present in some never-smokers [10]. In contrast, Overbeek et al. attached importance to the correlation between vasculopathy and ILD in the patients with SSc [11].

* Correspondence: hide1144@jikei.ac.jp
[1]Department of Respiratory Medicine, Kanagawa Cardiovascular and Respiratory Center, 6-16-1 Tomioka-higashi, Kanazawa-ku, Yokohama 236-0051, Japan
[6]Department of Respiratory Medicine, Tokyo Jikei University Hospital, Tokyo, Japan
Full list of author information is available at the end of the article

Detailed radiological and pathological features of pulmonary emphysema combined with SSc-ILD have not yet been described. Therefore, this study aimed to clarify the clinico-radio-pathological characteristics of SSc-ILD, focusing on pulmonary emphysema and vasculopathy.

Methods

This retrospective cohort study was approved by the institutional review board of Kanagawa Cardiovascular and Respiratory Center (no. 28–11). Because of the retrospective nature of the study, the review board waived the need for written informed consent from the patients.

The study population consisted of patients who had been diagnosed as having SSc-ILD, which was proven by surgical lung biopsy, at Kanagawa Cardiovascular and Respiratory Center between March 1997 and April 2016. The patients fulfilled the criteria for SSc of the American College of Rheumatology/European League Against Rheumatism classification [12]. One patient with SSc-rheumatoid arthritis overlap was excluded from this study, whereas 3 patients who developed manifestations of SSc during their follow-up period (0.42–2.17 years) were included. Baseline clinical measurements, radiological finding of HRCT, and right ventricular systolic pressure of echocardiography as indicator of pulmonary hypertension were obtained within 3 months of the histological diagnosis of ILD by surgical lung biopsy. The definition of chronic kidney disease were not a GFR below 60 mL/min/1.73m^2 for three months or more or a GFR 60 mL/min/1.73m^2 with kidney damage (i.e. marked of high levels of albumin in urine) [13]. Two radiologists (T. I. and S. I.) reviewed the HRCT scans for consensus of the diagnosis of ILD without knowledge of the patients' clinical data. Patients were classified as presenting a HRCT pattern either "suggestive or consistent with NSIP" or "suggestive of usual interstitial pneumonia (UIP)" [14, 15]. The HRCT scans were analyzed for the following characteristics: honeycombing, ground-glass opacity, consolidation, reticulation, emphysema, cyst, traction bronchiectasis, bronchial wall thickening, mosaic attenuation, pulmonary artery dilation, enlarged mediastinal lymph nodes, micro-nodules, pleural thickening or effusion, and volume loss. These features were selected on the basis of previous studies [9, 16]. Moreover, low attenuation areas (LAA) within the interstitial abnormalities were also evaluated. This term was defined as low attenuation within an area such as a reticular shadow or traction bronchiectasis/bronchiolectasis, and the LAA itself had an apparent wall thickness of not more than 1 mm. Any disagreements between the two radiologists after the first assessment were resolved by discussion. The extent (%) of pulmonary abnormalities on HRCT was calculated with computer-aided 3D quantitative analysis [9, 17]. We also categorized the study patients by the easily applied disease staging of Goh's criteria: 1) limited disease or 2) extensive disease [18]. The surgical lung biopsy slides were reviewed by two pulmonary pathologists (K. O. and T. T.) who were blinded to the patients' clinical and radiologic information. Histologic patterns were classified according to the current classification of idiopathic interstitial pneumonia [15]. The pathological features of lung parenchyma, airway, and pleural lesions were semi-quantitatively graded as 0 (absent), 1 (mild), 2 (moderate), or 3 (severe) [9, 19–21]. Pathological emphysema was defined as grade based on the number of alveolar pores due to alveolar wall destruction and the degree of enlarged alveolar lumina [22]. "Cicatricial emphysema," defined as permanent enlargement of air spaces distal to terminal bronchioles caused by severe fibrosis (e.g. idiopathic pulmonary fibrosis), was excluded from the definition of emphysema [23]. Pulmonary vasculopathies, which include 1) muscular pulmonary arteries (from 200 to 300 μm in diameter) by the Heath-Edwards scoring system [24], 2) cellular and/or fibrotic intimal thickening and muscularisation in the interlobular veins and venules, and 3) changes such as medial hypertrophy and/or intimal thickening in the arterioles along the alveolar ducts (< 100 μm in diameter), were also evaluated based on previous reports [11, 25]. Any disagreements between the two pathologists were discussed until consensus was reached.

Data analysis

Categorical baseline characteristics are summarized by frequency and percentage, and continuous characteristic are reported as mean ± SD. To detect differences between groups, the Wilcoxon test, Fisher's exact test, or Mann-Whitney U test was used as appropriate. We considered $P < 0.05$ to represent statistical significance. All data were analyzed with SPSS version 22.0 (IBM Japan, Tokyo, Japan).

Results

Patient characteristics

Clinical characteristics of the 21 patients with SSc-ILD are summarized in Table 1. The proportion of patients who had smoke was 38.1%, and 3 patients (14.3%) had Sjögren syndrome. The median follow-up period was 2.44 years, and only 2 patients (9.5%) died during this period.

p-PE was observed in 16 patients (76.2%) of the patients with SSc-ILD. We classified the patients into two groups according to the existence or non-existence of p-PE with SSc-ILD. The proportion of never-smokers in the patients with p-PE with SSc-ILD was 62.5%. Smoking history for patients with each group was not significantly different. The diffusing capacity of the lung for carbon monoxide (D_{LCO}) was significantly lower ($P = 0.0163$) and the disease extent on HRCT was significantly greater ($P = 0.013$) in the patients with p-PE with SSc-ILD. However, forced vital capacity (FVC) was well

Table 1 Patient characteristics at surgical lung biopsy between the existence and non-existence of pathological emphysema with SSc-associated ILD

Characteristics	All subjects	Existence of pathological pulmonary emphysema		*P* value
		Yes (p-PE with SSc-ILD)	No	
No. of patients	21	16	5	
Female N (%)	18 (85.7)	14 (87.5)	4 (80.0)	> 0.999
Age, mean ± SD	60.3 ± 10.5	60.5 ± 10.5	59.8 ± 11.7	0.679
Never smoker N (%)	13 (61.9)	10 (62.5)	3 (60.0)	> 0.999
Sjögren's syndrome N (%)	3 (14.3)	2 (12.5)	1 (20.0)	> 0.999
Digital ulcers N (%)	4 (19.0)	3 (18.8)	1 (20.0)	> 0.999
Hypertension N (%)	4 (19.0)	3 (18.8)	1 (20.0)	> 0.999
Chronic kidney disease N(%)	1 (4.8)	1 (6.3)	0 (0.0)	> 0.999
KL-6, U/mL	1350.5 ± 1042.8	1517.1 ± 1102.8	684.0 ± 255.1	0.089
SP-D, ng/mL	223.84 ± 132.42	214.86 ± 139.17	259.75 ± 109.89	0.395
Pulmonary function tests				
FEV_1/FVC ratio, %	81.17 ± 5.95	80.67 ± 6.70	82.78 ± 2.02	0.741
FVC, % predicted	92.79 ± 16.76	90.52 ± 17.00	100.04 ± 15.33	0.215
D_{LCO}, % predicted	69.85 ± 20.56	65.02 ± 20.11	87.98 ± 9.68	0.0163*
FVC/D_{LCO}, ratio	1.41 ± 0.37	1.46 ± 0.39	1.22 ± 0.14	0.253
Disease extent on HRCT, %	24.93 ± 10.78	28.13 ± 10.56	15.35 ± 2.94	0.013*
RVSP on echocardiography (available N)	18	15	3	
RVSP, mmHg	33.3 ± 11.8	34.8 ± 12.5	26.2 ± 0.7	0.279
RVSP (< 35/ 35- < 50/ ≥50)	11/ 4/ 3	8/ 4/ 3	3/ 0/ 0	0.730
Staging				
Limited disease N (%)	13 (61.9)	8 (50.0)	5 (100.0)	0.114
Extensive disease N (%)	7 (33.3)	7 (43.7)	0 (0.0)	
Unknown N (%)	1 (8.3)	1 (6.3)	0 (0.0)	
Medication (during follow-up)				
PAH-specific drug therapy use[a]	2 (9.5)	1 (6.3)	1 (20.0)	0.429
Ca channel blocker or ACE inhibitor	5 (23.8)	4 (25.0)	1 (20.0)	> 0.999
Steroid use	10 (47.6)	9 (56.3)	1 (20.0)	0.311
Cyclophosphamide use	4 (19.0)	4 (25.0)	0 (0.0)	0.532
Cyclosporine, tacrolimus or azathioprine use	5 (23.8)	4 (25.0)	1 (20.0)	> 0.999
Pirfenidone or nintedanib use	3 (14.3)	3 (18.8)	0 (0.0)	0.549
Deaths N (%) (during follow-up)	2 (9.5)	2 (12.5)	0 (0.0)	
Median follow-up years (range)	2.44 (0.21–16.06)	2.23 (0.21–16.06)	5.07 (0.81–12.5)	

Data are presented as mean ± SD, unless otherwise stated. *SSc* systemic sclerosis, *ILD* interstitial lung disease, *p-PE* pathological pulmonary emphysema, *KL-6* Krebs von den Lungen-6, *SP-D* surfactant protein-D, FEV_1 forced expiratory volume in 1 s, *FVC* forced vital capacity, D_{LCO} diffusing capacity of the lung for carbon monoxide, *HRCT* high-resolution computed tomography, *RVSP* right ventricular systolic pressure, *PAH* pulmonary arterial hypertension. [a]PAH-specific drugs include only beraprost sodium ($N = 2$). *P value less than 0.05

preserved in the patients regardless of whether p-PE was observed. The radiological and pathological characteristics of the patients are summarized in Tables 2, 3. The major HRCT pattern was NSIP in 19 patients (90.5%). The frequency of diffuse distribution of reticulation was more common in the patients with p-PE with SSc-ILD than in those without p-PE ($P = 0.009$). The association of vasculopathy with SSc-ILD patients are summarized in Table 4. LAA within the interstitial abnormalities was seen only in patients with p-PE with SSc-ILD (31.3%) (Figs. 1a, 2a, 3a, 4a). Fibrotic NSIP was the major histologic pattern seen in the SSc-ILD patients (85.7%). Of the SSc-ILD patients with p-PE, 12 (75.0%) had grade 1 emphysema, and 4 (25.0%) had grade 2 emphysema (Figs. 1b, 2b, 3b, 4b). Notably, emphysematous change in the SSc-ILD patients seemed to occur in the fibrotic

Table 2 Comparison of HRCT findings in patients with SSc-associated ILD

Characteristics	All subjects	Existence of pathological pulmonary emphysema		*P* value
		Yes (p-PE with SSc-ILD)	No	
HRCT pattern N (%)				
Suggestive of UIP	2 (9.5)	2 (12.5)	0 (0.0)	> 0.999
Suggestive or consistent with NSIP	19 (90.5)	14 (87.5)	5 (100.0)	
HRCT findings N (%)				
GGO	21 (100.0)	16 (100.0)	5 (100.0)	N/A
Consolidation	2 (9.5)	1 (6.3)	1 (20.0)	0.429
Reticulation	21 (100.0)	16 (100.0)	5 (100.0)	N/A
Honeycombing	1 (4.8)	1 (6.3)	0 (0.0)	> 0.999
Traction bronchiectasis	20 (95.2)	16 (100.0)	4 (80.0)	0.238
Bronchial wall thickening	10 (47.6)	7 (43.8)	3 (60.0)	0.635
Micro-nodules	3 (14.3)	3 (18.7)	0 (0.0)	0.549
Emphysema (LAA around no fibrotic appearance)	4 (19.0)	3 (18.7)	1 (20.0)	> 0.999
LAA within interstitial abnormalities	5 (23.8)	5 (31.3)	0 (0.0)	0.278
Cyst (non-honeycombing, emphysema)	5 (23.8)	4 (25.0)	1 (20.0)	> 0.999
Mosaic attenuation (air trapping)	7 (33.3)	4 (25.0)	3 (60.0)	0.280
Enlarged mediastinal lymph node	4 (19.0)	3 (18.7)	1 (20.0)	> 0.999
Pleural thickening or effusion	3 (14.3)	3 (18.7)	0 (0.0)	0.549
Pulmonary artery dilatation	6 (28.6)	5 (31.3)	1 (20.0)	> 0.999
Volume loss	17 (81.0)	14 (87.5)	3 (60.0)	0.228

Data are presented as mean ± SD, unless otherwise stated. *SSc* systemic sclerosis, *ILD* interstitial lung disease, *p-PE* pathological pulmonary emphysema, *HRCT* high-resolution computed tomography, *UIP* usual interstitial pneumonia, *NSIP* nonspecific interstitial pneumonia, *GGO* ground glass opacity

Table 3 Comparison of pathological findings (grade 0/1/2/3) in patients with SSc-associated ILD

Characteristics	All subjects	Existence of pathological pulmonary emphysema		*P* value
		Yes (p-PE with SSc-ILD)	No	
Lung parenchyma lesion				
Cellular infiltration	0/9/9/3	0/8/5/3	0/1/4/0	0.589
Lymphoid follicle with germinal center	12/7/1/1	10/5/0/1	2/2/1/0	0.349
Fibrosis	0/2/14/5	0/1/12/3	0/1/2/2	0.728
Honeycombing	15/5/1/0	12/3/1/0	3/2/0/0	0.601
Fibroblastic foci	4/16/1/0	3/12/1/0	1/4/0/0	0.781
Organizing pneumonia (intra-alveolar polyp)	11/8/2/0	8/7/1/0	3/1/1/0	0.927
Atelectasis (collapse)	0/11/5/5	0/10/4/2	0/1/1/3	0.046*
Cyst formation	14/5/2/0	11/3/2/0	3/2/0/0	0.882
Emphysema	5/12/4/0	0/12/4/0	5/0/0/0	< 0.001*
Pulmonary vascular change				
Muscular pulmonary artery	8/7/6/0	4/7/5/0	4/0/1/0	0.105
< none; grade 0/positive = grade 1–3>	8/13	4/12	4/1	0.047*
Arteriole <positive>	19 (90.5)	15 (93.8)	4 (80.0)	0.311
Venule <positive>	18 (85.7)	14 (87.5)	4 (80.0)	> 0.999
Interlobular vein <positive>	17 (81.0)	14 (87.5)	3 (60.0)	0.228

Data are presented as mean ± SD, unless otherwise stated. *SSc* systemic sclerosis, *ILD* interstitial lung disease, *p-PE* pathological pulmonary emphysema, *UIP* usual interstitial pneumonia, *NSIP* nonspecific interstitial pneumonia, *DIP* desquamative interstitial pneumonia. *P value less than 0.05

Table 4 Characteristics of the 21 patients with SSc-associated ILD

Patient	Sex	HRCT findings		Pathological findings		Pulmonary vascular change			
		Disease extent, %	LAA within the interstitial abnormalities	Classification	Emphysema, (grading score)	Muscular type, (grading score)	Arteriole	Venule	Interlobular vein
1	Female	41.37	+	fNSIP	2	1	+	+	+
2	Female	38.24	None	fNSIP	2	1	+	+	+
3	Female	42.37	+	fNSIP	1	2	+	+	+
4	Female	17.54	+	fNSIP	1	1	+	+	+
5	Female	13.65	None	Unclassifiable	1	1	+	+	+
6	Female	33.2	None	fNSIP	1	0	+	+	+
7	Female	13.47	None	fNSIP	1	0	+	+	−
8	Male	25.77	+	fNSIP	2	0	+	−	+
9	Female	18.86	None	fNSIP	1	0	+	+	+
10	Male	29.37	None	fNSIP	1	1	−	+	+
11	Female	N/A	None	fNSIP	1	2	+	+	+
12	Female	42.31	+	fNSIP	2	1	+	−	+
13	Female	16.7	None	fNSIP	1	1	+	+	−
14	Female	23.1	None	fNSIP	1	2	+	+	+
15	Female	36.22	None	Unclassifiable	1	2	+	+	+
16	Female	29.78	None	fNSIP	1	2	+	+	+
17	Female	19.58	None	fNSIP	0	0	+	+	+
18	Female	12.03	None	fNSIP	0	0	−	+	−
19	Male	13.3	None	fNSIP	0	2	+	−	+
20	Female	15.27	None	Unclassifiable	0	0	+	+	+
21	Female	16.55	None	fNSIP	0	0	+	+	−

SSc systemic sclerosis, *ILD* interstitial lung disease, *HRCT* high-resolution computed tomography, *LAA* low attenuation area, *fNSIP* fibrotic nonspecific interstitial pneumonia, *N/A* not applicable

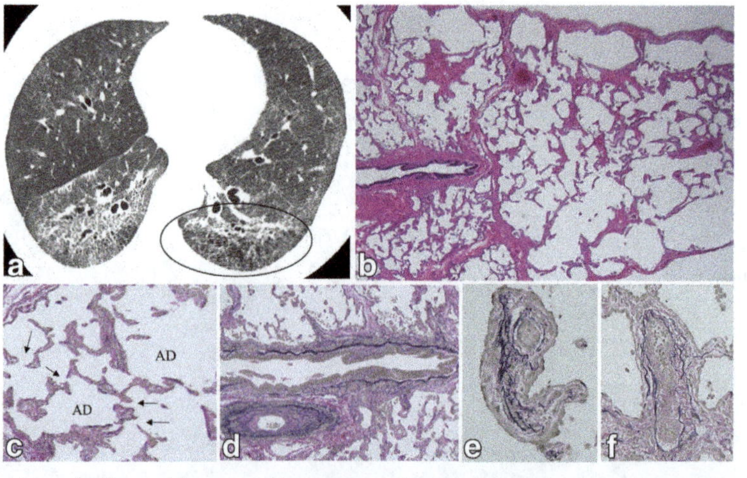

Fig. 1 HRCT and surgical lung biopsy of a 45-year-old never-smoking woman. **a** Computed tomography scan shows traction bronchiectasis, reticulation predominantly in the peribronchovascular zone, and a low attenuation area (circle) in the subpleural area of both lower lungs. **b** Pathologic specimen (H & E staining, × 40) shows fibrotic nonspecific interstitial pneumonia with emphysematous change (grade 2). **c** At high-power magnification, emphysematous change occurs at the fibrously thickened alveolar walls showing an increase in pores (arrows) (Elastica van Gieson staining, × 100); AD: alveolar duct. **d** Muscular pulmonary artery shows intimal thickening (grade 1) (Elastica van Gieson staining, × 80). **e** Pulmonary arteriole lying along the alveolar ducts shows intimal thickening and muscularisation (Elastica van Gieson staining, × 200). **f** A venule shows intimal thickening and muscularisation (Elastica van Gieson staining, × 200)

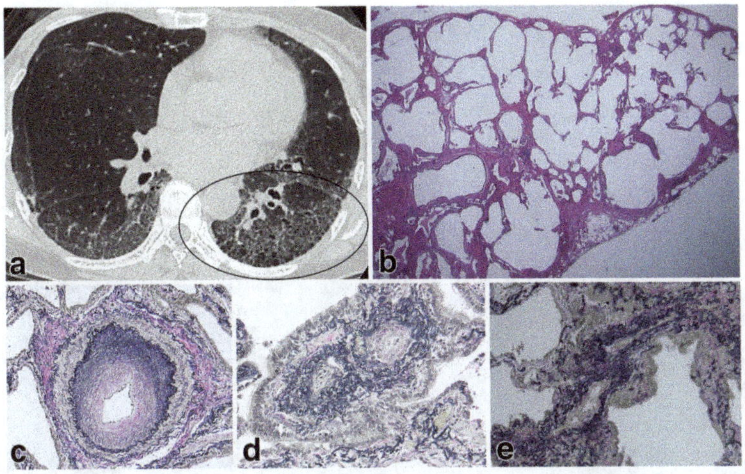

Fig. 2 HRCT and surgical lung biopsy of a 70-year-old never-smoking woman. **a** Computed tomography shows reticulation and a low attenuation area within a ground glass opacity and reticulation (circle). **b** Pathologic specimen (H & E staining, × 40) shows fibrotic nonspecific interstitial pneumonia with emphysematous change (grade 1). **c** Vascular intimal and medial thickening of a muscular pulmonary artery (grade 2) (Elastica van Gieson staining, × 100). **d** Intimal fibrosis of alveolar interstitial vessels (arteriole) and **e**) (venule) (Elastica van Gieson staining, × 200)

alveolar walls and mainly presented as the destruction of fibrous thickened alveolar walls (Fig. 1c).

Although the severity of changes in muscular pulmonary arteries in the patients with p-PE with SSc-ILD was not significantly different from that in the patients without p-PE ($P = 0.105$), its incidence was significantly higher ($P = 0.047$) in the patients with p-PE. Histological analysis found that 61.9% of the muscular pulmonary arteries were of Heath-Edwards grade 1–2 (Figs. 1d, 2c, 4c). Heath-Edwards grading of muscular pulmonary arteries of more than grade 2 (e.g. plexiform lesions) was not detected in our subjects. The incidences of changes in other pulmonary microvasculature were as follows: 90.5% showing arteriolar changes of intimal fibrosis and musculisation (Figs. 1e, 2d, 3c, 4d), 85.7% showing venular intimal thickening (Fig. 1f, 2e, 3d, 4e), and 81.0% showing intimal thickening of the interlobular veins (Fig. 4e). Most of the patients with SSc-ILD had arteriolar and venous-venular changes in their pulmonary microvasculature whether pathological emphysema coexist or not.

Discussion

We investigated characteristic radiological and pathological features of 21 patients with SSc-ILD. This study presented that pulmonary emphysematous changes (LAA within interstitial abnormalities on HRCT and

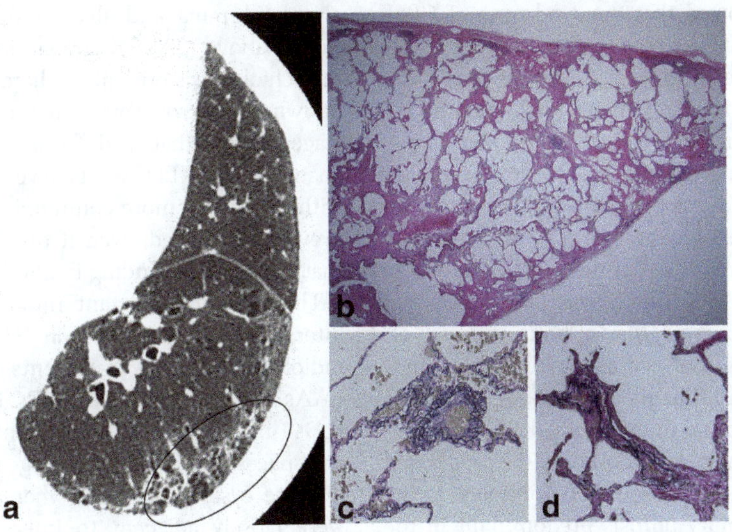

Fig. 3 HRCT and surgical lung biopsy of 66-year-old ex-smoking man. **a** Computed tomography shows reticulation and a low attenuation area within the interstitial abnormalities (circle). **b** Pathologic specimen (H & E staining, × 40) shows fibrotic nonspecific interstitial pneumonia with emphysematous change (grade 2). **c** Intimal fibrosis of alveolar interstitial vessels (arteriole) and **d** (venule) (Elastica van Gieson staining × 200)

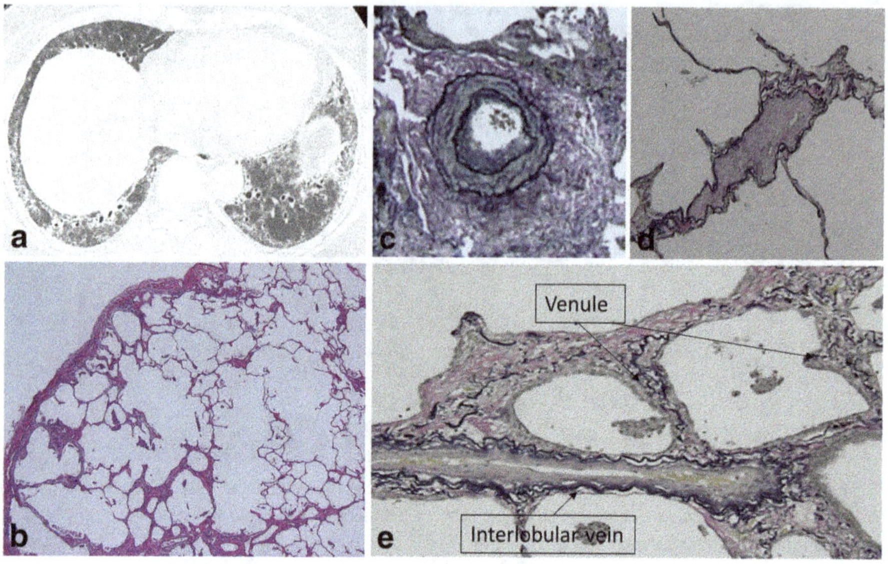

Fig. 4 HRCT and surgical lung biopsy of 58-year-old never-smoking woman. **a** Computed tomography scan shows traction bronchiectasis, reticulation, and ground-glass opacity predominantly in the peribronchovascular zone of both lower lungs. **b** Pathologic specimen (H & E staining, × 40) shows fibrotic nonspecific interstitial pneumonia with emphysematous change (grade 2). **c** Muscular pulmonary artery shows medial hypertrophy (grade 1) (Elastica van Gieson staining, × 100). **d** Pulmonary venule lying along the alveolar ducts shows no apparent intimal thickening (Elastica van Gieson staining, × 200). **e** Venule and interlobular vein show intimal thickening (Elastica van Gieson staining, × 200)

destruction of fibrously thickened alveolar walls) are specific and novel radio-pathological features of SSc-ILD. We provided two important findings. First, among patients with SSc-ILD, the complication of p-PE was frequently present in patients regardless of whether they had ever smoked. Surprisingly, 62.5% of the patients with p-PE with SSc-ILD were never-smokers. Historically, the syndrome of combined pulmonary fibrosis and emphysema (CPFE) has been individualized within the spectrum of smoking-induced chronic lung disease [26]. Later, Cottin et al. reported that the syndrome of CPFE warrants recognition as a novel distinct pulmonary manifestation within the spectrum of lung diseases associated with CTD, especially in patients with rheumatoid arthritis and SSc, whether current- or ex-smokers; however, 11.8% of their patients with CTD complicated by CPFE never smoked. [27] Antoniou et al. recently reported a prevalence of emphysema in patients with SSc-ILD of 12%; emphysema was present more often in current or former smokers, but it was also present in 7.5% of the never-smokers [10]. In both reports, although emphysema was analyzed as a radiological finding, the patients with CPFE had a lower D_{LCO}, preserved FVC, which were also found in our study, and wider disease extent. However, their definition of CPFE was based on the presence of both emphysema predominant in the upper lobes and pulmonary fibrosis predominant in the lower lung zones [10, 27]. Because the emphysema in our study was analyzed pathologically, it is unclear whether these disease entities were evaluated from the same viewpoint in the previous studies. Our analysis emphasizes that the emphysematous change occurring with SSc-ILD is different from the usual form of smoking-related emphysema, which presents as destructive holes in the center of the secondary lobules and is generally well demarcated from the adjacent parenchyma and which also centers around the respiratory bronchioles and alveolar ducts [28]. In contrast, the emphysematous change in SSc-ILD mainly presents as destruction of fibrously thickened alveolar walls, resulting in abnormal dilatation of the alveolar lumina and alveolar ducts. Obviously, as mentioned above [23], "cicatricial emphysema" together with bronchiolectasis presents a characteristic gross appearance known as microscopic honeycombing that reflects end-stage fibrosis that is different from the emphysematous change in SSc-ILD. We believe that the presence of p-PE with SSc-ILD is more commonly seen in SSc patients than previously realized, even if they have never smoked, and that this is a new finding in SSc-ILD.

The second important finding was that LAA within interstitial abnormalities on HRCT might be a specific radiological finding in patients with SSc-ILD. Although LAAs are also shown on HRCT in a variety of fibrotic ILDs (in the extreme, honeycombing is composed of cystic spaces) [29], this finding refers to the fusing of discrete cysts with walls, whereas LAAs in our analysis were closely adjacent to interstitial abnormalities, and the LAAs themselves did not have an apparent wall thickness of more than 1 mm. This radiological finding was only seen in some of the patients with p-PE with

SSc-ILD, and therefore, it might correlate with the pathological emphysema of SSc-ILD, though all our hypotheses were not corroborated.

In the vast majority of people, smoking is the cause of emphysema [30]. A previous radiological analysis showed that pulmonary microvascular blood flow is reduced in mild chronic obstructive pulmonary disease (COPD) [31]. In the aspects of the pathological analysis, pulmonary vascular changes in COPD or CPFE are characterized by a thickening of the vessel wall that begins early in the process of emphysematous change [25]. Thickening of the intima is the first structural change and is followed by an increase in smooth muscle cells and infiltration of the vessel wall by inflammatory cells [32]. In contrast, pulmonary vascular abnormalities are common in SSc patients, and the pulmonary hypertensive vascular changes manifest as concentric intimal thickening by fibromyxoid tissue and medial hypertrophy leading to thickened and stenotic pulmonary arterioles [33]. Most SSc patients with or without pulmonary artery hypertension (PAH) have intimal fibrosis and medial hypertrophy of the pulmonary arteries with an external diameter between 101 and 200 μm, which lie beside bronchioles [34]. Overbeek et al. reported that PAH in SSc patients is characterized by intimal fibrosis in the small vessels (arterioles, venules, and interlobular veins) [11]. Because changes were seen in 61.9% of the muscular pulmonary arteries in our patients with SSc-ILD, and in 90.5% of the arterioles and 85.7% of the venules in the microvasculature, these findings could be caused by reduced pulmonary microvascular blood flow, which might be one factor contributing to the emphysematous changes occurring in ILD.

Our study has several limitations. First, it was a single-institution, retrospective study with a small sample size. Second, there was selection bias because only the patients who could undergo surgical lung biopsy were included. Additionally, only two patients received PAH-specific drug therapy during the follow-up period, and most patients could not be evaluated for PAH by right heart catheterization. Therefore, more severe cases might present different radiological and pathological findings. Third, although this study reveals characteristic radio-pathological features in SSc-ILD, a comparable analysis was not performed for other etiologies of ILD (e.g. CTD-ILD). Fourth, although previous research showed that increased matrix metalloproteinases expression may play a role in accelerating the process of destruction as emphysema [35], immunohistochemical analysis could not be performed in our analysis and would be an issue in the future. Fifth, we used several types of HRCT scanning with the times. Therefore, imaging protocol may lead to a little different interpretation of radiological finding.

Conclusions

Emphysematous changes, i.e. LAA within the interstitial abnormalities on HRCT and destruction of the fibrously thickened alveolar walls, are specific and novel radio-pathological features of SSc-ILD. Histopathological analysis suggested that peripheral vasculopathy may participate in the destruction of the fibrously thickened alveolar walls, resulting in the emphysematous changes seen in patients with SSc-ILD. Our results might help to provide more information for patients who do not fulfil the diagnosis of SSc (such as patients classified as having interstitial pneumonia with autoimmune features [36]) and suffer from a specific CTD diagnosis from the pulmonology viewpoint. Further studies are needed to clarify the quantitative loss of alveolar septa in the peripheral vascular bed that occurs with the emphysematous changes of SSc-ILD.

Abbreviations

COPD: Chronic obstructive pulmonary disease; CPFE: Combined pulmonary emphysema with fibrosis; CTD: Connective tissue disease; D_{LCO}: Diffusing capacity of the lung for carbon monoxide; FVC: Forced vital capacity; HRCT: High-resolution computed tomography; ILD: Interstitial lung disease; LAA: Low attenuation area; MCTD: Mixed connective tissue disease; NSIP: Nonspecific interstitial pneumonia; PAH: Pulmonary artery hypertension; PMBF: Pulmonary microvascular blood flow; p-PE: Pathological pulmonary emphysema; SSc: Systemic sclerosis

Acknowledgments

We offer our sincerest thanks to Yosuke Sasaki of Satista Co., Ltd. for his advice on statistical analysis. The authors would like to thank Rise Japan LLC for the professional English language review.

Funding

Not applicable.

Authors' contributions

HY was the primary author of the manuscript, had full access to all of the data in the study, and takes responsibility for the integrity of the data and the accuracy of the data analysis. TT, AS, HK, TB, and TO contributed to the study design; YY, SaI, AS, HK, TB, and TO contributed to collecting samples and carrying out experiments; AS, TI, and KK contributed to data analysis; TT, SaI, ShI, KO, and TO contributed to data interpretation; TT, TI, KO, and TO contributed to writing the manuscript. All authors read and approved the final version of the manuscript.

Consent for publication

Not applicable.

Competing interests

The authors declare that they have no competing interests.

Author details

[1]Department of Respiratory Medicine, Kanagawa Cardiovascular and Respiratory Center, 6-16-1 Tomioka-higashi, Kanazawa-ku, Yokohama

236-0051, Japan. [2]Department of Pathology, Japanese Red Cross Medical Center, Tokyo, Japan. [3]Department of Radiology, Kanagawa Cardiovascular and Respiratory Center, Yokohama, Japan. [4]Department of Radiology, Yokohama Rousai Hospital for Labour Welfare Corporation, Yokohama, Japan. [5]Department of Pathobiology, Yokohama City University Graduate School of Medicine, Yokohama, Japan. [6]Department of Respiratory Medicine, Tokyo Jikei University Hospital, Tokyo, Japan.

References

1. Bussone G, Mouthon L. Interstitial lung disease in systemic sclerosis. Autoimmun Rev. 2011;10:248–55.
2. Goldin JG, Lynch DA, Strollo DC, Suh RD, Schraufnagel DE, Clements PJ, et al. High-resolution CT scan findings in patients with symptomatic scleroderma-related interstitial lung disease. Chest. 2008;134:358–67.
3. Desai SR, Veeraraghavan S, Hansell DM, Nikolakopolou A, Goh NS, Nicholson AG, et al. CT features of lung disease in patients with systemic sclerosis: comparison with idiopathic pulmonary fibrosis and nonspecific interstitial pneumonia. Radiology. 2004;232:560–7.
4. Fujita J, Yoshinouchi T, Ohtsuki Y, Tokuda M, Yang Y, Yamadori I, et al. Non-specific interstitial pneumonia as pulmonary involvement of systemic sclerosis. Ann Rheum Dis. 2001;60:281–3.
5. Kim DS, Yoo B, Lee JS, Kim EK, Lim CM, lee SD, et al. the major histopathologic pattern of pulmonary fibrosis in scleroderma is nonspecific interstitial pneumonia. Sarcoidosis Vasc Diffuse Lung Dis. 2002;19:121–7.
6. Bouros D, Wells AU, Nicholson AG, Colby TV, Polychronopoulos V, Pantelidis P, et al. Histopathologic subsets of fibrosing alveolitis in patients with systemic sclerosis and their relationship to outcome. Am J Respir Crit Care Med. 2002;165:1581–6.
7. Katzenstein AL, Fiorelli RF. Nonspecific interstitial pneumonia/fibrosis. Histologic features and clinical significance Am J Surg Pathol. 1994;18:136–47.
8. Nicholson AG, Colby TV, wells AU. Histopathological approach to patterns of interstitial pneumonia in patient with connective tissue disorders. Sarcoidosis Vasc Diffuse Lung Dis. 2002;19:10–7.
9. Yamakawa H, Hagiwara E, Kitamura H, Yamanaka Y, Ikeda S, Sekine A, et al. Clinical features of idiopathic interstitial pneumonia with systemic sclerosis-related autoantibody in comparison with interstitial pneumonia with systemic sclerosis. PLoS One. 2016;11:e0161908.
10. Antoniou KM, Margaritopoulos GA, Goh NS, Karagiannis K, Desai SR, Nicholson AG, et al. Combined pulmonary fibrosis and emphysema in scleroderma-related lung disease has a major confounding effect on lung physiology and screening for pulmonary hypertension. Arthritis Rheumatol. 2016;68:1004–12.
11. Overbeek MJ, Vonk MC, Boonstra a, Voskuyl AE, Vonk-Noordegraaf a, smit EF, et al. pulmonary arterial hypertension in limited cutaneous systemic sclerosis: a distinctive vasculopathy. Eur Respir J. 2009;34:371–9.
12. van den Hoogen F, Khanna D, Fransen J, Johnson SR, Baron M, Tyndall A, et al. 2013 classification criteria for systemic sclerosis: an American College of Rheumatology/European league against rheumatism collaborative initiative. Arthritis Rheum. 2013;65:2737–47.
13. Lopez-Giacoman S, Madero M. Biomarkers in chronic kidney disease, from kidney function to kidney damage. World J Nephrol. 2015;4:57–73.
14. American Thoracic Society. European Respiratory Society. American Thoracic Society/European Respiratory Society international multidisciplinary consensus classification of the idiopathic interstitial pneumonias. This joint statement of the American Thoracic Society (ATS), and the European Respiratory Society (ERS) was adopted by the ATS board of directors, June 2001 and by the ERS executive committee, June 2001. Am J Respir Crit Care Med. 2002;166:426.
15. Travis WD, Costabel U, Hansell DM, King TE Jr, Lynch DA, Nicholson AG, et al. ATS/ERS Committee on idiopathic interstitial pneumonias. An official American Thoracic Society/European Respiratory Society statement: update of the international multidisciplinary classification of the idiopathic interstitial pneumonias. Am J Respir Crit Care Med. 2013;188:733–48.
16. Hansell DM, Bankier AA, MacMahon H, McLoud TC, Müller NL, Remy J. Fleischner society: glossary of terms for thoracic imaging. Radiology. 2008; 246:697–722.
17. Iwasawa T, Kato S, Ogura T, Kusakawa Y, Iso S, Baba T, et al. Low-normal lung volume correlates with pulmonary hypertension in fibrotic idiopathic interstitial pneumonia: computer-aided 3D quantitative analysis of chest CT. AJR Am J Roentgenol. 2014;203:W166–73.
18. Goh NS, Desai SR, Veeraraghavan S, Hansell DM, Copley SJ, Maher TM, et al. Interstitial lung disease in systemic sclerosis: a simple staging system. Am J Respir Crit Care Med. 2008;177:1248–54.
19. Song JW, Do KH, Kim MY, Jang SJ, Colby TV, Kim DS. Pathologic and radiologic differences between idiopathic and collagen vascular disease-related usual interstitial pneumonia. Chest. 2009;136:23–30.
20. Enomoto Y, Takemura T, Hagiwara E, Iwasawa T, Okudela K, Yanagawa N, et al. Features of usual interstitial pneumonia in patients with primary Sjögren's syndrome compared with idiopathic pulmonary fibrosis. Respir Investig. 2014;52:227–35.
21. Flaherty KR, Colby TV, Travis WD, Toews GB, Mumford J, Murray S, et al. Fibroblastic foci in usual interstitial pneumonia: idiopathic versus collagen vascular disease. Am J Respir Crit Care Med. 2003;167:1410–5.
22. Wright JL. The importance of ultramicroscopic emphysema in cigarette smoke-induced lung disease. Lung. 2001;179:71–81.
23. Corrin, B, Nicholson AG: Pathology of the lungs. 3rd ed. Philadelphia, Elsevier, 2011,pp 91–134.
24. Heath D, Edwards JE. The pathology of hypertensive pulmonary vascular disease; a description of six grades of structural changes in the pulmonary arteries with special reference to congenital cardiac septal defects. Circulation. 1958;18:533–47.
25. Awano N, Inomata M, Ikushima S, Yamada D, Hotta M, Tsukuda S, et al. Histological analysis of vasculopathy associated with pulmonary hypertension in combined pulmonary fibrosis and emphysema: comparison with idiopathic pulmonary fibrosis and emphysema alone. Histopathology. 2017;70:896–905.
26. Cottin V, Nunes H, Brillet PY, Delaval P, Devouassoux G, Tillie-Leblond I, et al. Groupe d'Etude et de Recherche sur les maladies Orphelines Pulmonaires (GERM O P): combined pulmonary fibrosis and emphysema: a distinct underrecognised entity. Eur Respir J. 2005;26:586–93.
27. Cottin V, Nunes H, Mouthon L, Gamondes D, Lazor R, Hachulla E, et al. Groupe d'Etudes et de Recherche sur les maladies "Orphelines" Pulmonaires: combined pulmonary fibrosis and emphysema syndrome in connective tissue disease. Arthritis Rheum. 2011;63:295–304.
28. Wright JL, Tazelaar HD, Churg A. Fibrosis with emphysema. Histopathology. 2011;58:517–24.
29. Raoof S, Bondalapati P, Vydyula R, Ryu JH, Gupta N, Raoof S, et al. cystic lung diseases: algorithmic approach. Chest. 2016;150:945–65.
30. Wilson JS, Galvin JR. Normal diffusing capacity in patients with PiZ alpha(1)-antitrypsin deficiency, severe airflow obstruction, and significant radiographic emphysema. Chest. 2000;118:867–71.
31. Hueper K, Vogel-Claussen J, Parikh MA, Austin JH, Bluemke DA, Carr J, et al. pulmonary microvascular blood flow in mild chronic obstructive pulmonary disease and emphysema. The MESA COPD study. Am J Respir Crit Care Med. 2015;192:570–80.
32. Seimetz M, Parajuli N, Pichl A, Veit F, Kwapiszewska G, Weisel FC, et al. Inducible NOS inhibition reverses tobacco-smoke-induced emphysema and pulmonary hypertension in mice. Cell. 2011;147:293–305.
33. Vivero M, Padera RF. Histopathology of lung disease in the connective tissue diseases. Rheum Dis Clin N Am. 2015;41:197–211.
34. Yousem SA. The pulmonary pathologic manifestations of the CREST syndrome. Hum Pathol. 1990;21:467–74.
35. Cardoso WV, Sekhon HS, Hyde DM, Thurlbeck WM. Collagen and elastin in human pulmonary emphysema. Am Rev Respir Dis. 1993;147:975–81.
36. Fischer A, Antoniou KM, Brown KK, Cadranel J, Corte TJ, du bois RM, et al. "ERS/ATS task force on undifferentiated forms of CTD-ILD". An official European Respiratory Society/American Thoracic Society research statement: interstitial pneumonia with autoimmune features. Eur Respir J. 2015;46:976–87.

13

Implementation of a successful eradication protocol for *Burkholderia Cepacia* complex in cystic fibrosis patients

Bryan A. Garcia[1], Jacque L. Carden[1], Dana L. Goodwin[1], Tim A. Smith[1], Amit Gaggar[1,2], Kevin Leon[1,2], Veena B. Antony[1,2], Steven M. Rowe[1,2] and George M. Solomon[1,2*]

Abstract

Background: Infection with *Burkholderia cepacia complex* (*Bcc*) results in a heterogeneous clinical course ranging from asymptomatic colonization of the airways to fulminant respiratory failure in patients with cystic fibrosis (CF). Early eradication of *Pseudomonas aeruginosa* improves clinical outcomes. The efficacy and clinical outcomes following implementation of an eradication protocol for *Bcc* are less well understood.

Methods: We developed and implemented a single center *Bcc* eradication protocol that included an intensive combination of intravenous, inhaled, and oral antibiotic therapies based on in vitro sensitivities. We conducted a retrospective cohort analysis of clinical outcomes compared to patients with chronic *Bcc* infection.

Results: Six patients were identified as having a newly acquired *Bcc* colonization and were placed on the eradication protocol. Sequential sputum samples after completion of the protocol demonstrated sustained clearance of *Bcc* in all patients. Lung function and nutritional status remained stable in the year following eradication.

Conclusion: Clearance of *Bcc* from sputum cultures using a standardized protocol was successful at one year and was associated with clinical stability.

Keywords: *Burkholderia cepacia, Burkholderia Cepacia complex (BCC)*, Cystic fibrosis, Infection eradication

Background

Cystic Fibrosis (CF) is characterized by development of viscous airway mucus which provides a fertile media for opportunistic respiratory pathogens [1]. Chronic respiratory infection with recurrent exacerbations and inflammation results in progressive bronchiectasis and ultimately respiratory failure [2, 3]. Aggressive management of chronic respiratory infections is crucial to prevent lung function decline. *Pseudomonas aeruginosa* is a common respiratory pathogen in the CF airway and chronic colonization is associated with impaired lung function for these patients [4, 5]. Early eradication upon initial positive sputum culture with *P. aeruginosa* has been shown to stabilize lung function and improve clinical outcomes with successful eradication ranging from 62 to 93% although the long-term clinical benefit may be uncertain [6–8].

Though less prevalent than *P. aeruginosa*, CF patients may acquire other respiratory pathogens including species of the *Burkholderia cepacia* complex *(Bcc)* [9]. *Bcc* represents a group of genetically related bacteria associated with a heterogeneous clinical course ranging from asymptomatic colonization to fulminant respiratory failure [10, 11]. Chronic colonization with *Bcc* is associated with antibiotic resistance, increased risk of respiratory failure, and worsened mortality [10, 12]. Although *Bcc* eradication has been previously described, implementation of a protocolized approach toward *Bcc* eradication has not been fully studied [13, 14].

* Correspondence: msolomon@uab.edu
[1]Department of Medicine, Division of Allergy, Pulmonary and Critical Care Medicine, 1900 University Blvd, THT 422, Birmingham, AL 35294, USA
[2]Gregory Fleming James Cystic Fibrosis Research Center, Birmingham, AL, USA

Methods

Patient identification and data collection-

We obtained institutional review board approval to conduct a retrospective chart review of CF patients infected with *Bcc* at our center. Beginning January 2012 through June 2015, patients were placed on the eradication protocol if they were found to have a sputum culture positive for *Bcc,* which had not been isolated from sputum during the two prior years. Patients who were known to have chronic airway colonization by *Bcc* were treated with guideline-based standard of care [15]. Lung function (forced expiratory volume in one second, FEV_1% predicted), nutritional status (Body mass index, BMI), and serial sputum cultures were obtained during clinic appointments that generally occurred at 3-month intervals, per CF guidelines. The genomovar of *Bcc* strains isolated was confirmed at the *B. cepacia* Research Laboratory and Repository at the University of Michigan. Successful eradication of *Bcc* was defined as clearance of *Bcc* following the induction stage of therapy with maintenance of at least three additional negative respiratory cultures at 3-month intervals during the 12-month follow-up.

Treatment protocol

Patients included in the eradication group following sputum culture isolation of newly acquired *Bcc* were placed on the eradication protocol (Table 1). Antibiotic selection was based on identifying an aggressive combination of inhaled and intravenous therapies with broad coverage to obtain maximal in-vivo treatment synergy as multiple patient strains demonstrated pan-resistance based on in-vitro antibiotic sensitivity testing. Tobramycin was included for empiric coverage of *P. aeruginosa* given the high rate of co-infection in this population. The rationale for antibiotic selection is included in Table 1.

Statistical analysis

Statistical analysis was performed using GraphPad Prism version 6.0c (GraphPad Software, Inc., San Diego, CA). Continuous variables were described using means with standard deviations, or medians with ranges as sample sizes were small, and were analyzed using Mann-Whitney *t*-test or Two-way ANOVA testing as data were non-parametric. Change in lung function and nutritional status was compared between groups using Two-way ANOVA; Fisher's post hoc test was used when ANOVA was significant. All statistical tests were two-sided and *P*-values < 0.05 were considered statistically significant.

Results

Patient cohort

From January 2012 to June 2015, 14 adult patients were found to have *Bcc* isolated in sputum cultures. Seven of these patients were found to have a newly acquired *Bcc* colonization (no isolation of *Bcc* from sputum in the two preceding years), of which six were placed on eradication protocol. The remaining patient was not included in analysis due to a new acquisition of *P. aeruginosa* during the maintenance phase of the *Bcc* eradication, requiring transition to a *PsA* eradication protocol. Seven additional patients were defined as having chronic colonization with *Bcc* based on prior positive cultures for *Bcc*; these patients were treated based on guidelines for pulmonary exacerbation and were considered as contemporaneous controls. Of these seven control patients, two patients were not included due to inadequate clinic follow up. A third patient with *Bcc* colonization was not included due to identification of only one CF causing mutation despite genetic sequencing. These patients were excluded from further analysis. This control group thus consists of patients with chronic *Bcc* infection and act as case controls for patients with acute infection.

Outcome following bcc *Eradication*

Demographic data for the two groups including age, gender, *CFTR* genotype, baseline lung function, nutritional status, pancreatic functional status, and microbiology culture results at baseline were collected via chart review (Table 2). All patients in both groups were maintained on thrice weekly oral azithromycin therapy for anti-inflammatory effect. In addition, all patients placed

Table 1 *Burkholderia* Eradication Protocol

	Medication	Dosing	Frequency	Route	Bacteria Targeted
Induction Period (21 Days):	Tobramycin	6 mg/kg (per kinetics)	Daily	IV	*PsA, Bcc*
	Ceftazidime	2 g	Every 8 h	IV	*PsA, Bcc*
	Trimethoprim/Sulfamethoxazole	800/160 mg	Twice Daily	Oral	*Bcc*
	Tobramycin inhaled[a]	300 mg	Twice Daily	Nebulized	*PsA, Bcc*
	Azithromycin	250 mg	Daily	Oral	Anti-inflammatory
Consolidation Period (2 months):	Trimethoprim/Sulfamethoxazole	800/160 mg	Twice daily	Oral	*Bcc*
	Tobramycin inhaled[a]	300 mg	Twice daily	Nebulized	*PsA, Bcc*
	Azithromycin	250 mg	Daily	Oral	Anti-inflammatory

[a]Alternative- TIP (tobramycin dry powder for inhalation, 4 caps (28 mg/cap)) every 12 h

Table 2 Baseline characteristics

Group	Gender	Age	Genotype (n)	Pancreatic Insufficient (%)	CFRD (%)	Bcc Species Isolated (*n*)	Additional Pathogens (*n*)	FEV_1% Predicted	BMI
Eradication (*n* = 6)	50% F	23.3 (20–27)	dF508/dF508 [6]	(100%)	83%	B. multivorans [4] B. gladioli [2] *B. cepacia* [1]	PsA [6] MRSA [3] Steno [2] Aspergillus [2]	65.5 (30–96%)	20.2 (15.6–26.9)
Usual Care (*n* = 4)	50% F	28.2 (21–47)	dF508/dF508 [1] 405 3AtoC/V317A Q98X [1] dF508/Q98X [1] dF508/G542X [1]	(75%)	75%	B. multivorans [1] B. cepacia [2] B. arboris [1]	PsA [3] MRSA [4]	55.7 (31–98%)	20.3 (18.9–22)

Abbreviations: F=Female, *CFRD*- CF Related Diabetes, *MRSA*- Methicillin Resistant *Staphylococcus aureus*, *PsA*- Pseudomonas aeruginosa, Steno-*Stenotrophomonas maltophilia*

on *Bcc* eradication were previously colonized with *PsA* and were maintained on every-other-month inhaled tobramycin. Three of the four control patients were also previously maintained on inhaled tobramycin for chronic *PsA* infection.

At baseline there was no significant difference between the group means of the eradication and control groups for FEV_1% predicted (65.5 ± 24.5% vs. 59.7 ± 28.2%, respectively, $p = 0.67$) or BMI (20.2 ± 3.8 vs. 20.3 ± 1.2, respectively, $p = 0.94$). Among patients in the eradication group, 100% of the patients remained free of *Bcc* at the end of the study compared to 25% in the control group. During the one-year follow up period the eradication group experienced a mean number of exacerbation of 1.66 ± 0.42 versus 3.25 ± 1.0 by the control group ($p = 0.166$). The mean time to first exacerbation was 230 days (± 24.55) in the eradication group versus 88 ± 27.6 in the control group ($p = 0.009$). The change from baseline between the eradication and control groups was compared and at three months the groups had a significant difference in change of FEV_1% predicted (10.8 ± 10.7% vs. -6.0 ± 8.8%, $p = 0.01$) (Fig. 1). No significant difference in change of FEV_1% predicted was identified between the eradication and control groups at 6 (1.3 ± 13.0% vs. -7.5 ± 7.5%) or 12 months (– 2.6 ± 15.1% vs. -10.2 ± 11.1%). With regards to nutritional status, no significant difference was identified in change in BMI from baseline between the eradication and control groups at three (0.68 ± 0.71 vs. 0.3 ± 0.64 kg/m^2), six (0.56 ± 1.1 vs. -0.95 ± 1.6 kg/m^2), or 12 months (1.8 ± 2.0 vs. 1.3 ± 0.5 kg/m^2).

We also report absolute FEV_1% and BMI in the eradication group by individual. Among these patients, no significant difference was seen in mean (± standard deviation) FEV_1% predicted at three (76.5 ± 15.0), six (67 ± 20.9), and 12 months (63 ± 24.1) following eradication compared to either baseline (65.6 ± 24.4) or the average of the year prior to *Bcc* acquisition (74.3 ± 15.6). Similarly, no significant difference was seen in BMI at three (20.9 ± 4.1), six (20.8 ± 3.6), and 12 months (22.1 ± 4.4) compared to baseline (20.2 ± 3.8) or the average of the year prior to *Bcc* acquisition (20.4 ± 3.1) (Fig. 2).

Discussion

We describe the implementation of a *Bcc* eradication protocol for CF patients with a newly acquired *Bcc* colonization using an aggressive treatment regimen with a high success rate, suggesting its potential for benefit in

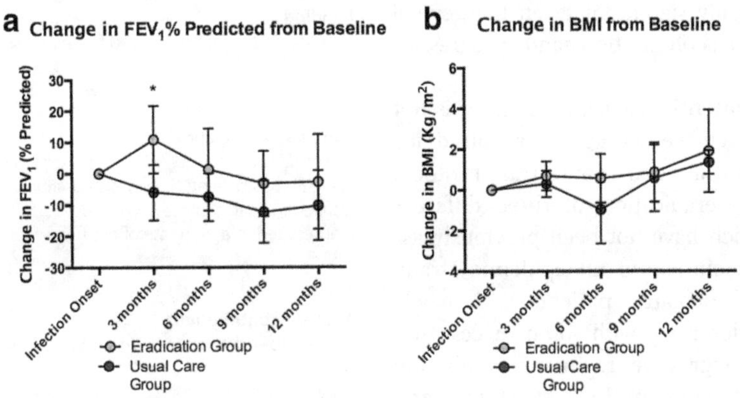

Fig. 1 **a**. Change in mean lung function (FEV_1% predicted) from baseline over time during the course of the cohort study for patients in the eradication group compared to patients treated with standard of care. *$p = 0.01$. **b**. Change in mean BMI from baseline for the same period

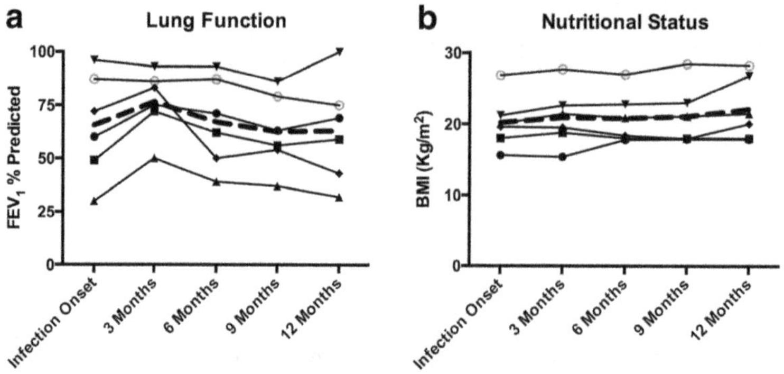

Fig. 2 a. Trends in lung function (FEV_1% predicted) for each eradication group subject over time ($n = 6$ patients). **b**. Trends in nutritional status (BMI) for each eradication group subject over time ($n = 6$ patients). Dashed lines represent the trend of the group mean over time in each graph

this small group. Although no significant difference in lung function or BMI was observed at one year of follow-up between the eradication and control groups, the eradication group demonstrated universal *Bcc* clearance (100% as compared to 25% in the control group), stable lung function and nutritional status, and no treatment-related adverse events. We recognize the limitations of the small chronic Bcc case controls. This data is illustrative that chronically infected patients may have greater risk for exacerbation as well as increased CF-related morbidity. However, we acknowledge that these comparisons are not directly associated with the interventions outlined in our protocol. The protocol was relatively unbiased to patient selection, as all patients with newly discovered *Bcc* entered the protocol, with the exception of a single patient who was actively being treated for additional pulmonary pathogens, which precluded utilizing certain antibiotics.

It is important to note that a subset of patients, particularly younger patients, have been shown to spontaneously clear *Bcc* from sputum cultures suggesting that aggressive eradication may not always be necessary [13, 16]. Although it is not clear which patients are most likely to benefit from *Bcc* eradication, early eradication is likely to be clinically significant given the general association between *Bcc* colonization and progressive clinical decline [10, 17].

The protocol was, by intention, aggressive and it is not known whether this intensive therapy is required for successful *Bcc* eradication. Also note, this protocol demonstrated successful eradication of three different *Bcc* strains, some of which have not been previously associated with outcomes similar to an epidemic strain. Alternative protocols in pediatric patients with newly isolated *Bcc* have been described with some success and have utilized similarly aggressive regimens combining inhaled and intravenous Tobramycin, Ceftazidime and Temocillin [18]. The patients described by that series were not complicated by chronic *PsA* co-infection. An additional case-series described combination of inhaled amiloride and tobramycin with eradication of initial colonization in 3 of 4 patients but was unsuccessful in chronically infected patients [19, 20].

Conclusion

This study has several limitations including a small sample size, retrospective single-center design, and a control group that consisted of chronically infected patients who might have a different course of disease progression. Therefore, a multi-center, prospective study is warranted to evaluate the efficacy of aggressive *Bcc* eradication and provide a more definitive evaluation for treatment of this severe complication of CF lung disease and associated potential benefits on CF-related morbidity and exacerbation frequency we observed compared to case controls.

Abbreviations

Bcc: *Burkholderia cepacia complex*; BMI: Body mass index; CF: Cystic fibrosis; FEV_1: Forced expiratory volume in 1 s; PsA: *Pseudomonas aeruginosa*

Acknowledgments

None applicable.

Funding

No funding source was utilized for the current study.

Summary at a glance

Burkholderia cepacia complex (*Bcc*) results in worsened clinical course in cystic fibrosis patients. Previously described *Bcc* eradication protocols have resulted in limited success. We describe an intensive *Bcc* eradication protocol that resulted in a high rate of *Bcc*-free cultures for one year of follow up.

Authors' contributions

BG participated in study design, data collection and analysis, initial manuscript production, editing, and final manuscript. JC, DG, TS participated in data collection, manuscript editing, and final manuscript production. AG, KL, VA, SMR, and GMS participated in data analysis, initial manuscript preparation, manuscript editing, and final manuscript production. All authors read and approved the final manuscript.

Consent for publication
No individual patient data is presented in this study and thus consent to publish is not applicable.

Competing interests
The authors declare that they have no competing interests.

References

1. Rommens JM, Iannuzzi MC, Kerem B, Drumm ML, Melmer G, Dean M, Rozmahel R, Cole JL, Kennedy D, Hidaka N, et al. Identification of the cystic fibrosis gene: chromosome walking and jumping. Science. 1989;245:1059–65.
2. Balough K, McCubbin M, Weinberger M, Smits W, Ahrens R, Fick R. The relationship between infection and inflammation in the early stages of lung disease from cystic fibrosis. Pediatr Pulmonol. 1995;20:63–70.
3. Ogrinc G, Kampalath B, Tomashefski JF Jr. Destruction and loss of bronchial cartilage in cystic fibrosis. Hum Pathol. 1998;29:65–73.
4. Kosorok MR, Zeng L, West SE, Rock MJ, Splaingard ML, Laxova A, Green CG, Collins J, Farrell PM. Acceleration of lung disease in children with cystic fibrosis after pseudomonas aeruginosa acquisition. Pediatr Pulmonol. 2001; 32:277–87.
5. Kerem E, Viviani L, Zolin A, MacNeill S, Hatziagorou E, Ellemunter H, Drevinek P, Gulmans V, Krivec U, Olesen H, Group EPRS. Factors associated with fev1 decline in cystic fibrosis: analysis of the ecfs patient registry. Eur Respir J. 2014;43:125–33.
6. Taccetti G, Campana S, Festini F, Mascherini M, Doring G. Early eradication therapy against pseudomonas aeruginosa in cystic fibrosis patients. Eur Respir J. 2005;26:458–61.
7. Proesmans M, Vermeulen F, Boulanger L, Verhaegen J, De Boeck K. Comparison of two treatment regimens for eradication of pseudomonas aeruginosa infection in children with cystic fibrosis. J Cyst Fibros. 2013; 12:29–34.
8. Mayer-Hamblett N, Kloster M, Rosenfeld M, Gibson RL, Retsch-Bogart GZ, Emerson J, Thompson V, Ramsey BW. Impact of sustained eradication of new pseudomonas aeruginosa infection on long-term outcomes in cystic fibrosis. Clin Infect Dis. 2015;61:707–15.
9. Gibson RL, Burns JL, Ramsey BW. Pathophysiology and management of pulmonary infections in cystic fibrosis. Am J Respir Crit Care Med. 2003; 168:918–51.
10. Frangolias DD, Mahenthiralingam E, Rae S, Raboud JM, Davidson AG, Wittmann R, Wilcox PG. Burkholderia cepacia in cystic fibrosis. Variable disease course. Am J Respir Crit Care Med. 1999;160:1572–7.
11. Courtney JM, Dunbar KE, McDowell A, Moore JE, Warke TJ, Stevenson M, Elborn JS. Clinical outcome of burkholderia cepacia complex infection in cystic fibrosis adults. J Cyst Fibros. 2004;3:93–8.
12. Ledson MJ, Gallagher MJ, Jackson M, Hart CA, Walshaw MJ. Outcome of burkholderia cepacia colonisation in an adult cystic fibrosis centre. Thorax. 2002;57:142–5.
13. Horsley A, Webb K, Bright-Thomas R, Govan J, Jones A. Can early burkholderia cepacia complex infection in cystic fibrosis be eradicated with antibiotic therapy? Front Cell Infect Microbiol. 2011;1:18.
14. Regan KH, Bhatt J. Eradication therapy for burkholderia cepacia complex in people with cystic fibrosis. Cochrane Database Syst Rev. 2014;10:CD009876.
15. Flume PA, Mogayzel PJ Jr, Robinson KA, Goss CH, Rosenblatt RL, Kuhn RJ, Marshall BC. Clinical practice guidelines for pulmonary therapies C. Cystic fibrosis pulmonary guidelines: treatment of pulmonary exacerbations. Am J Respir Crit Care Med. 2009;180:802–8.
16. Ramsay KA, Butler CA, Paynter S, Ware RS, Kidd TJ, Wainwright CE, Bell SC. Factors influencing acquisition of burkholderia cepacia complex organisms in patients with cystic fibrosis. J Clin Microbiol. 2013;51:3975–80.
17. St Denis M, Ramotar K, Vandemheen K, Tullis E, Ferris W, Chan F, Lee C, Slinger R, Aaron SD. Infection with burkholderia cepacia complex bacteria and pulmonary exacerbations of cystic fibrosis. Chest. 2007;131:1188–96.
18. Kitt H, Lenney W, Gilchrist FJ. Two case reports of the successful eradication of new isolates of burkholderia cepacia complex in children with cystic fibrosis. BMC Pharmacol Toxicol. 2016;17:14.
19. Ball R, Brownlee KG, Duff AJ, Denton M, Conway SP, Lee TW. Can burkholderia cepacia complex be eradicated with nebulised amiloride and tobi? J Cyst Fibros. 2010;9:73–4.
20. Middleton PG, Kidd TJ, Williams B. Combination aerosol therapy to treat burkholderia cepacia complex. Eur Respir J. 2005;26:305–8.

14

The cutoff point of clinical chronic obstructive pulmonary disease questionnaire for more symptomatic patients

Yong Suk Jo[1], Sangshin Park[2,3], Deog Kyeom Kim[4], Chul-Gyu Yoo[1] and Chang-Hoon Lee[1*]

Abstract

Background: An adequate threshold for the Clinical Chronic Obstructive Pulmonary Disease (COPD) Questionnaire (CCQ) defining more symptomatic COPD patients has not been determined. We aimed to determine the efficacy of the CCQ and the appropriate CCQ threshold for more symptomatic COPD patients.

Methods: COPD patients aged > 40 years who smoked/had smoked ≥10 packs/year were prospectively enrolled over 1 year from three South Korean hospitals ($n = 126$). Correlations between the CCQ and St. George's Respiratory Questionnaire (SGRQ), COPD Assessment Test (CAT), the modified Medical Round Council (mMRC) scale, lung function, and exercise capacity were evaluated. "More symptomatic patients" were those with an SGRQ score ≥ 25. Area under the receiver operating curve and classification and regression tree analyses were performed to determine the CCQ threshold equivalent to an SGRQ score ≥ 25.

Results: The CCQ significantly correlated with the SGRQ, CAT, and mMRC scale ($r = 0.76$, 0.69, and 0.53, respectively). A CCQ cutoff of 1.4 predicted an SGRQ score of 25 better than others. A CCQ score of 1.4 was a significant determinant of an SGRQ score ≥ 25 even after adjusting for potential confounders.

Conclusions: The CCQ was correlated with other symptom indicators, lung function, and exercise capacity. A CCQ cutoff of 1.4 agreed better than CCQ cutoff of 1.0, suggested by guideline, and this cutoff value may identify more symptomatic COPD patients well.

Keywords: Chronic Obstructive Pulmonary Disease, Correlation study, Health related quality of life, Clinical Questionnaires

Background

Chronic obstructive pulmonary disease (COPD), characterized by persistent and progressive airflow limitation, is one of the major causes of morbidity and mortality worldwide, and its prevalence is increasing. COPD was previously regarded as a disease mainly characterized by breathlessness, but recently it has been reported that COPD has multiple symptomatic effects on health-related quality of life (HRQOL) [1]. The severity of airflow limitation alone is not strongly correlated with HRQOL in COPD patients [2]; therefore, comprehensive methods to evaluate the COPD-specific health status are needed.

Since 2011, Global Initiative for Chronic Obstructive Lung Disease (GOLD) adopted St. George's Respiratory Questionnaire (SGRQ) as a new assessment tool for COPD patients considering their current respiratory symptoms and future risk of exacerbation. Currently, GOLD emphasizes HRQOL more than dyspnea alone and divides patients into more symptomatic (SGRQ ≥25) and

* Correspondence: kauri670@empal.com
[1]Division of Pulmonary and Critical Care Medicine, Department of Internal Medicine, Seoul National University Hospital, 101 Daehak-Ro Jongno-Gu, Seoul 03080, Republic of Korea
Full list of author information is available at the end of the article

less symptomatic (SGRQ < 25) patients based on previous clinical trials of long-acting bronchodilators [3–5].

SGRQ is the most widely used and valid tool to evaluate the health status of COPD patients [6] and is composed of 50 items with 76 weighted responses. The SGRQ scoring method is a bit difficult considering the amount of items and weighted responses required, and many COPD patients may find it difficult to complete without any help [7]. Thus, the COPD Assessment Test (CAT) was developed to compensate for the complexity of SGRQ [8, 9], and many studies which have evaluated the distribution of patients of GOLD grading classification according to the tool used to assess symptoms, found a different proportion of patients in each category using CAT score ≥ 10. With this background, GOLD recommended that the equivalent point of CAT for SGRQ of 25 is 10 [8–12].

Clinical COPD Questionnaire (CCQ), which has a good correlation with SGRQ [13, 14], is also thought to be a good instrument for assessing health status in COPD patients and is simple to use [13]. However, although studies have reported that a CCQ score range of 1.0–1.5 is consistent with an SGRQ score of 25 [14], until now, a clear CCQ cutoff point that is equivalent to an SGRQ score of 25 has not been determined. Furthermore, to date, the CCQ has not been sufficiently validated for evaluating health status in COPD patients in Asia [15].

Therefore, the present study aimed (i) to assess whether the CCQ correlates well with other health status measures, lung function, and exercise capacity in Korean COPD patients, and (ii) to determine the CCQ cutoff point that corresponds well with the SGRQ cutoff point of 25, considered the standard representing more symptomatic patients.

Methods

Study design and participants

The Seoul National University Airway Registry is a prospective observational cohort study that enrolls patients with chronic airway disease, including COPD.(ClinicalTrials.gov Identifier: NCT02527486). Among the participants in the cohort, patients aged 40 years or more who were diagnosed as having COPD between April 2013 and December 2015 at Seoul National University Hospital, a tertiary care hospital, and between March 2014 and December 2015 at Boramae Medical center, a municipal hospital, and Seoul National University Bundang Hospital, were included in our study. A COPD case was defined as a current or former smoker (≥10 packs/year) with chronic respiratory symptoms who had a post-bronchodilator forced expiratory volume in 1 s (FEV_1) to forced vital capacity ratio < 0.7. Participants who were not assessed either by SGRQ, the CAT, or the CCQ at the baseline visit were excluded. All patients signed the informed consent form to participate in this observational cohort. This study was approved by the Institutional Review Board (IRB) of Seoul National University Hospital (IRB no. 1602-122-743).

For COPD patients, a previous history of symptoms, exposure to smoking and biomass smoke, experiencing exacerbation, and comorbidities were evaluated at baseline. Pulmonary function tests including spirometry and lung volume measurements were performed at least annually. Spirometry was performed by standardized equipment, and lung volume was measured following the American Thoracic Society/European Respiratory Society guidelines [16, 17]. Spirometry was repeated at least three times to verify the reproducibility and validity, and assessments of the pulmonary function test results were performed using computer programs and reviewed by highly qualified physicians. The spirometric reference value was calculated by Morris's predictive equation [18, 19].

Acute exacerbations were evaluated based on self-reported symptom aggravation requiring modification of current treatment. Severe exacerbation was defined as an acute exacerbation event requiring a visit to the emergency room or hospitalization, and moderate exacerbation was defined as an acute exacerbation requiring a visit to an outpatient clinic and treatment with short-term systemic corticosteroids or antibiotics. Our definition of exacerbation was mainly based on a modified respiratory questionnaire from the Epidemiology Standardization Project questionnaire [20].

Clinical assessment instruments

The SGRQ total score ranges from 0 to 100 where 100 indicates the worst quality of life, and its minimum clinically important difference (MCID) value is 4 units [21]. The CAT total score ranges from 0 to 40, and 2.0 units is suggested as its MCID value [22]. The modified British Medical Research Council (mMRC) questionnaire total score ranges from 0 to 4 where 4 means most severe dyspnea, and an mMRC score ≥ 2 is used as a cutoff point for dividing patients with less dyspnea from those with more dyspnea [23]. The 6-min walk test was performed to measure exercise capacity and assessed according to the American Thoracic Society guidelines, and its MCID value is 30 m [24].

The CCQ consists of 10 questions distributed in three domains (symptom, functional state, and mental state) assessed by a seven-point scale from 0 to 6, which indicate the best (asymptomatic and no limitation) and the worst conditions (extremely symptomatic and limited), respectively [13]. The CCQ total score is calculated by summing the scores of the 10 questions and dividing it by the number of items [25]. The Korean version of the CCQ was used in the present study [26].

Statistical analysis

Descriptive data are expressed as mean ± standard deviation or number (%) unless otherwise specified. To evaluate the correlation between questionnaires (CCQ vs. SGRQ, CCQ vs. CAT, and CCQ vs. mMRC) and between CCQ and lung function indexes (FEV_1% and 6-min walk distance), we used Pearson correlation analyses. The degree of agreement between two indexes is expressed as the correlation coefficient, r, where a positive value means positive correlation and the higher the value, the stronger the correlation.

We used several CCQ cutoff scores based on an SGRQ score of 25 and a CAT score of 10, to indicate more symptomatic patients according to guidelines. We also applied a CCQ score that is equivalent to an SGRQ score of 20, which is better than suggesting an SGRQ score of 25 for a CAT score of 10 [27]. To determine which CCQ cutoff score was the most equivalent to an SGRQ score of 25, an area under the receiver operating curve (AUROC) analysis was performed. A classification and regression tree (CART) analysis, a type of decision tree methodology for the identification of mutually exclusive subgroups of at-risk persons who share common characteristics related to particular health-related behavior, was also performed. Then, the Cohen's kappa coefficient was calculated to compare the degree of agreement between the CCQ cutoff points and an SGRQ score of 25.

All analyses were two-sided and performed at a significance level of 0.05 unless otherwise noted. A *P*-value <.05 was considered statistically significant. All analyses were carried out using STATA version 13.1 (StataCorp, College Station, Texas, USA).

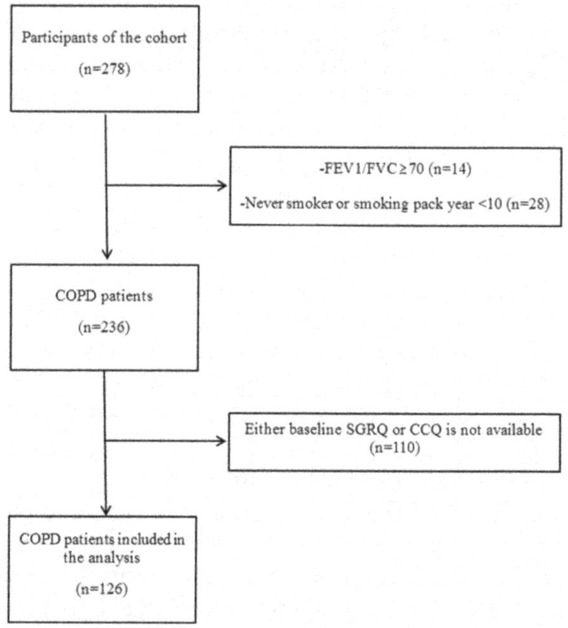

Fig. 1 Patient disposition. Abbreviations: CCQ, Clinical COPD Questionnaire; COPD, chronic obstructive pulmonary disease; FEV_1, forced expiratory volume in 1 s; FVC, forced vital capacity; SGRQ, St. George's Respiratory Disease Questionnaire

Results

Patient characteristics

Among 278 patients enrolled in the prospective cohort, we excluded 42 patients based on their spirometry and smoking pack/year and 110 patients whose health status indexes were not recorded (Fig. 1). Consequently, 126 patients aged 40 years or older who answered the questionnaires and agreed to regular follow-up at an outpatient clinic were finally enrolled.

The mean SGRQ, CAT, and CCQ scores were 38.04 ± 18.18, 17.76 ± 7.68, and 2.03 ± 0.94, respectively. Among 126 patients, 46 (36.51%) patients recalled that they experienced at least one acute exacerbation event 1 year before enrollment and 17 (13.49%) patients recalled more than two acute exacerbation events during the past year. The mean frequency of severe and moderate exacerbation was 1.4 ± 0.52 and 2.05 ± 2.01 events per year, respectively (Table 1). As can be seen in Figs. 2a and b, the CCQ values corresponding to the SGRQ scores of 25, 20, and a CAT score of 10 were 1.2, 1.0, and 0.7, respectively.

Correlation between the CCQ and other health status questionnaires, lung function, and exercise capacity

The CCQ significantly correlated well with SGRQ, the CAT, and the mMRC (r = 0.76, 0.69, and 0.53, respectively) (Fig 2). The CCQ showed a significant negative correlation with FEV_1 and 6-min walk distance (r = – 0.40 and – 0.42, respectively) (Fig. 3).

CCQ cutoff point to identify more symptomatic patients

A cutoff point of 1.4 showed the highest AUROC for identifying more symptomatic patients with SGRQ ≥25 (AUROC = 0.605, 0.633, 0.681, 0.762, and 0.711 for the CCQ cutoff points of 0.7, 1.0, 1.2, 1.4, and 1.6, respectively) (Fig. 4). The categorization based on the CCQ cutoff point of 1.4 showed the highest agreement with the SGRQ 25-based categorization (CCQ cutoff point = 0.7: agreement rate = 75.61% and κ value = 0.27; CCQ cutoff point = 1: agreement rate = 76.42% and κ value = 0.33; CCQ cutoff point = 1.4: agreement rate = 82.11% and κ value = 0.56) (Table 2). Even when adjusting for age, sex, body mass index, and FEV_1, a CCQ score ≥ 1.4 was the good determinant of an SGRQ score ≥ 25 in the CART analysis (relative hazard risk, 1.23) (Fig. 5).

Discussion

This study demonstrated that the CCQ is well correlated with other health status measurements including SGRQ, pulmonary function, and exercise capacity in Korean COPD patients. In our study, based on AUROC and CART analyses, the CCQ cutoff point that best corresponds to an SGRQ score of 25 was 1.4, which showed a better agreement rate and a higher classification power compared with other cutoff points.

Table 1 Baseline characteristics of patients

Characteristics	N = 126
Age (years)	68.83 ± 7.23
Sex: Male	123 (97.62)
BMI (kg/m^2)	22.97 ± 3.27
Smoking status	
Ex-smoker	88 (69.84)
Current smoker	38 (30.16)
Packs per/year	54.47 ± 64.46
History of exacerbations in the past year	
Unplanned visit to an outpatient clinic (no./year)	2.05 ± 2.01
Unplanned visit to an emergency department or hospital admission (no./year)	1.4 ± 0.52
≥ 2 events in the past year (n, %)	17 (13.49)
FEV1 (L)	1.65 ± 0.53
FEV1 (%)	65.35 ± 19.42
FVC (L)	3.59 ± 0.79
FVC (%)	97.15 ± 17.10
FEV1/FVC	45.95 ± 11.55
GOLD stage	
1 (FEV1 > 80% predicted)	23 (18.25)
2 (FEV1 50%–79% predicted)	76 (60.32)
3 (FEV1 30%–49% predicted)	23 (18.25)
4 (FEV1 < 30% predicted)	4 (3.17)
SGRQ score	38.04 ± 18.18
CAT score	17.76 ± 7.68
mMRC dyspnea score	1.44 ± 0.92
CCQ score	2.03 ± 0.94
6MWT (m)	444.39 ± 103.85

Data are presented as mean ± standard deviation or n (%)
Abbreviations: *BMI* body mass index, *CAT* Chronic Obstructive Pulmonary Disease Assessment Test, *CCQ* Clinical Chronic Obstructive Pulmonary Disease Questionnaire, *FEV1* forced expiratory volume in 1 s, *FVC* forced vital capacity, *GOLD* Global Initiative for Chronic Obstructive Lung Disease, *mMRC* modified Medical Research Council, *SGRQ* St. George's Respiratory Disease Questionnaire, *6MWT* 6-min walk test

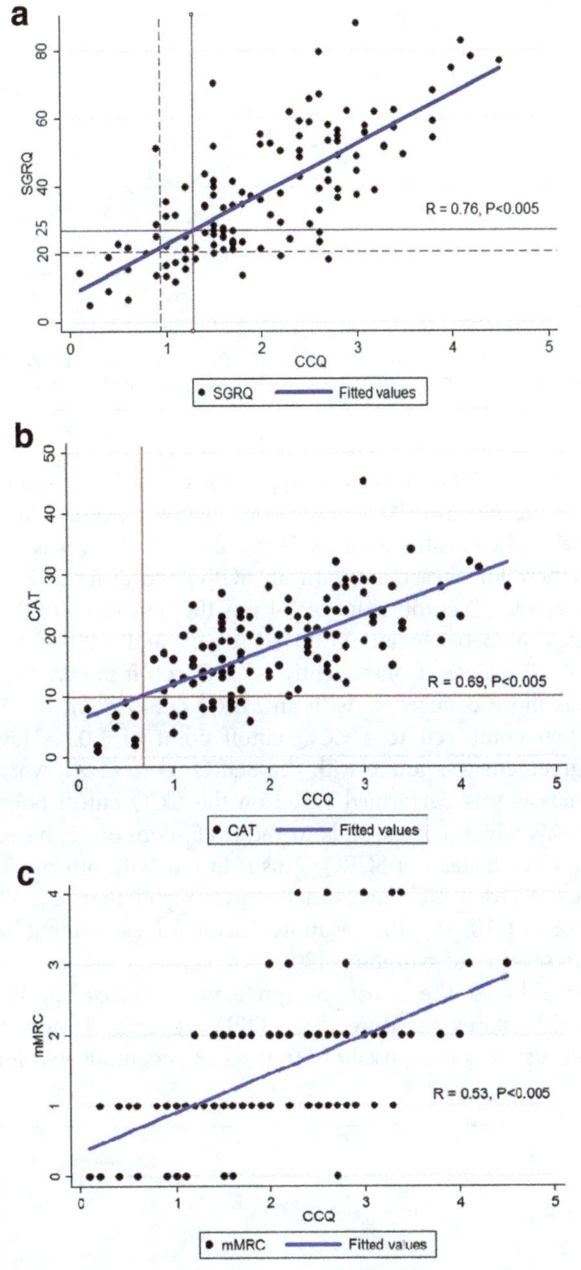

Fig. 2 Correlation between the CCQ and the (**a**) SGRQ, (**b**) CAT, and (**c**) mMRC. **a**, **b** CCQ value for SGRQ score of 25, 20 and for CAT score of 10 determined by an area under the receiver operating curve (AUROC) analysis

GOLD recommends a comprehensive approach to assess and adequately manage symptoms in COPD patients and proposes the mMRC, CAT, and CCQ as interchangeable instruments for evaluation of health status. However, despite the potential clinical importance, the CCQ has not been widely used in clinical practice because there is no known precise CCQ cutoff point that correlates with an SGRQ cutoff point of 25 (considered the standard marker of more symptomatic patients) and also CAT has been preferred than CCQ because CAT is more widely implemented and recommended by GOLD. GOLD guidelines recently set a CCQ score range of 1.0–1.5 as being equivalent to an SGRQ score of 25 [23], and recent studies suggest that the MCID value for the CCQ is approximately 0.4 [28, 29]. However, this wide range seems to be impractical for use in the clinical setting. In addition, GOLD tends to focus more on the CAT rather than the CCQ.

Based on the findings of the present study, we suggest that a CCQ cutoff point of 1.4 is appropriate for dividing

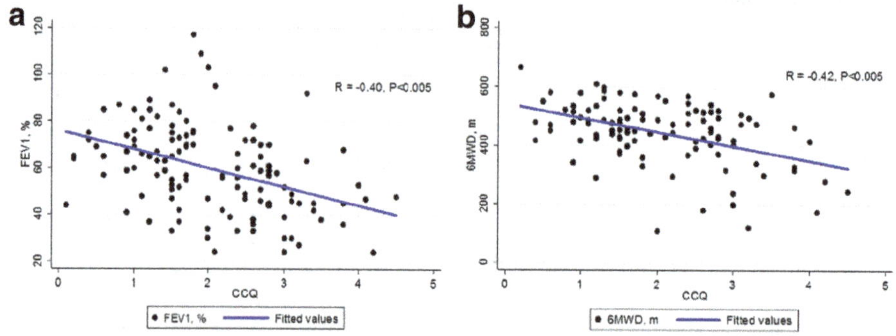

Fig. 3 Correlation between the CCQ and the (**a**) FEV_1% and (**b**) 6MWD. Abbreviations: CCQ, Clinical Chronic Obstructive Pulmonary Disease Questionnaire; FEV_1, forced expiratory volume in 1 s; 6MWT, 6-min walk test

COPD patients into more symptomatic and less symptomatic patients. This was based on two analyses. First, the AUROC value for a CCQ cutoff point of 1.4 was the highest for agreement with an SGRQ score of 25. Second, a CCQ cutoff point of 1.4 was the best value to distinguish between an SGRQ score ≥ 25 and < 25 in the CART analysis. Consequently, a CCQ cutoff point of 1.4 was more concordant with an SGRQ cutoff point of 25, when compared to a CCQ cutoff point of 1.0. A low agreement was found with the SGRQ score of 25, when analysis was performed based on the CCQ cutoff point of 0.7, which corresponds to the CAT score of 10, based on CAT instead of SGRQ. This is in line with our previous report, which states that scores higher than a CAT score of 10, say 15, are more useful for assessment of the severity of symptoms [30].

SGRQ is the most comprehensive disease-specific health status measure for COPD patients. However, because it is composed of 50 items, it is complicated for older COPD patients to answer without any help, and it takes a relatively long time to complete [7]. The CCQ is thought to be an alternative to SGRQ and consists of only 10 questions assessed by a seven-point scale from 0 to 6. Because the CCQ is a simple tool, it takes about 2 min to complete, and subjects require no specific help to complete it [13]. Along with its simplicity, the CCQ is a comprehensive tool to evaluate the health status in COPD patients because it has three domains (symptoms, functional state, and mental state), which means that the CCQ has psychometric properties that make it more useful [13]. CAT, one of the symptom and HRQOL measurement proposed by GOLD, is one-dimensional tool, while CCQ is similar to SGRQ, which is the most comprehensive tool. Further, CCQ is more simple and easy to use than SGRQ. Since it contains the description for each score, patients can sassily respond to the questions by themselves. In this aspect, the present study is focused on CCQ.

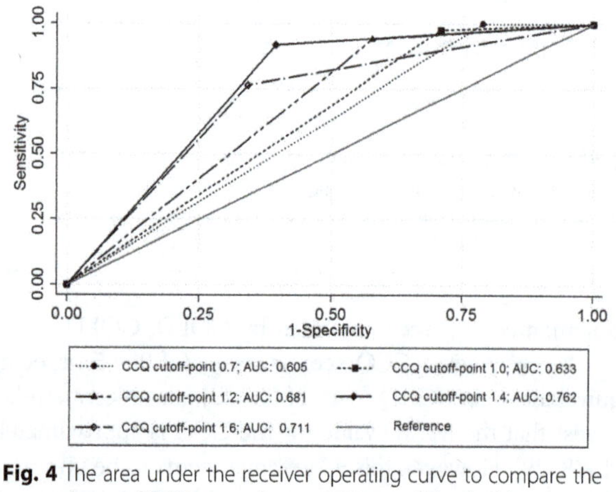

Fig. 4 The area under the receiver operating curve to compare the concordance of SGRQ according to CCQ cut-off level. Abbreviations: AUC, area under curve; CCQ, Clinical Chronic Obstructive Pulmonary Disease Questionnaire; SGRQ, St. George's Respiratory Disease Questionnaire

Table 2 Agreement between SGRQ and the CCQ based on the new GOLD classification of the CCQ cutoff value

	CCQ < 1	CCQ ≥1
SGRQ < 25	11	27
SGRQ ≥25	2	83
Agreement: 76.42%; kappa value, 0.33		
	CCQ < 1.4	CCQ ≥1.4
SGRQ < 25	23	15
SGRQ ≥25	7	78
Agreement: 82.11%; kappa value, 0.56		
	CCQ < 0.7	CCQ ≥0.7
SGRQ < 25	8	30
SGRQ ≥25	0	85
Agreement: 75.61%; kappa value, 0.27		

Abbreviations: *CCQ* Clinical Chronic Obstructive Pulmonary Disease Questionnaire, *GOLD* Global Initiative for Chronic Obstructive Lung Disease, *SGRQ* St. George's Respiratory Disease Questionnaire

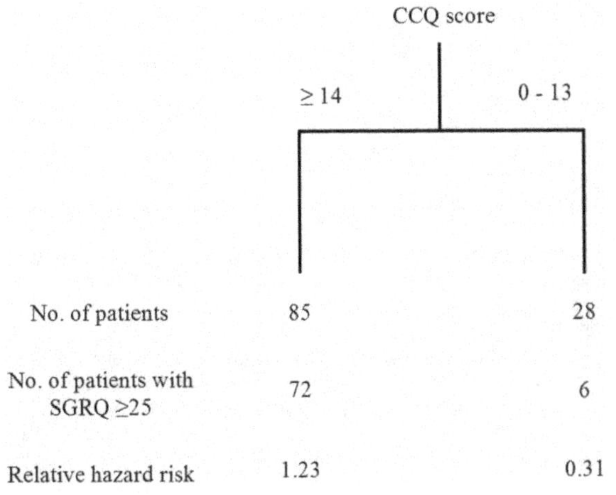

Fig. 5 Classification and regression tree analysis of agreement with an SGRQ score ≥ 25 (adjusted by age, sex, body mass index, and FEV_1). Abbreviations: FEV_1, forced expiratory volume in 1 s; SGRQ, St. George's Respiratory Disease Questionnaire

This study confirmed the clinical efficacy of the CCQ for evaluating the health status of COPD patients. The CCQ correlates well with other health status measures, lung function, and exercise capacity. In addition, recent studies have suggested that an upward revised CAT as a symptom threshold could reflect health status more accurately than the existing CAT cutoff point (≥10), which was previously regarded as a surrogate of the SGRQ [30–32]. Furthermore, our study determined a new and clear CCQ threshold for categorizing COPD patients as more or less symptomatic.

The present study has several limitations to consider. First, we conducted a cross-sectional analysis and did not investigate the predictive value of CCQ for lung function decline or future exacerbation risk. Second, although the CCQ consists of three domains (symptoms, functional state, and mental state), we did not record the three subcategories separately, but rather evaluated the CCQ as a whole. Third, only small number of women were included because of the low prevalence of female smokers, therefore there may be a limitations in external validity. Fourth, the gold standard of cutoff points to measure symptoms in COPD remained open for discussion. Thus, we also showed results of applying the CAT score of 10 as a standard for the symptom criteria. Lastly, the suggested CCQ cutoff point of 1.4 needs to be externally validated.

Conclusions

The CCQ showed significant clinical value for assessing the health status of patients with COPD and showed good correlation with other questionnaires including SGRQ and the CAT as well as lung function and exercise capacity. Although the gold standard tool for assessing the severity of symptom in COPD patients may still be debated, CCQ threshold 1.4 showed a better agreement with SGRQ threshold of 25, suggested by GOLD.

Abbreviations

6MWT: 6-min walk test; BMI: Body mass index;; CAT: Chronic Obstructive Pulmonary Disease Assessment Test; CCQ: Clinical Chronic Obstructive Pulmonary Disease Questionnaire; FEV_1: Forced expiratory volume in 1 s; FVC: Forced vital capacity; GOLD: Global Initiative for Chronic Obstructive Lung Disease; mMRC: Modified Medical Research Council; SGRQ: St. George's Respiratory Disease Questionnaire

Funding

The authors received no funding for this study.

Authors' contributions

YSJ and CHL made substantial contributions to the conception and design of the study, as well as to the acquisition of the data, drafting of the manuscript, and revising the study. YSJ drafted and revised the manuscript, and CHL verified its intellectual merit. We appreciate Professor SSP at the Center for International Health Research, Medical School of Brown University, for the statistical review. DKK, SSP, CGY and CHL read and approved the final manuscript. The decision to submit the report for publication was made by CHL.

Consent for publication

Not applicable.

Competing interests

The authors declare that they have no competing interests.

Author details

[1]Division of Pulmonary and Critical Care Medicine, Department of Internal Medicine, Seoul National University Hospital, 101 Daehak-Ro Jongno-Gu, Seoul 03080, Republic of Korea. [2]Center for International Health Research, Rhode Island Hospital, The Warren Alpert Medical School of Brown University, Providence, RI 02903, USA. [3]Department of Pediatrics, The Warren Alpert Medical School of Brown University, Providence, RI 02903, USA. [4]Division of Pulmonary and Critical Care Medicine, Department of Internal Medicine, Seoul Metropolitan Government-Seoul National University Boramae Medical Center, Seoul, Republic of Korea.

Reference

1. Jones PW. Health status measurement in chronic obstructive pulmonary disease. Thorax. 2001;56(11):880–7.
2. Ioanna T, Kocks J, Tzanakis N, Siafakas N, van der Molen T. Factors that influence disease-specific quality of life or health status in patients with COPD: a systematic review and meta-analysis of Pearson correlations. Prim Care Respir J. 2011;20(3):257–68.
3. Vincken W, Van Noord J, Greefhorst A, Bantje TA, Kesten S, Korducki L, Cornelissen P. Improved health outcomes in patients with COPD during 1 yr's treatment with tiotropium. Eur Respir J. 2002;19(2):209–16.
4. Jones PW, Singh D, Bateman ED, Agusti A, Lamarca R, de Miquel G, Segarra R, Caracta C, Gil EG. Efficacy and safety of twice-daily aclidinium bromide in COPD patients: the ATTAIN study. Eur Respir J. 2012;40(4):830–6.

5. Kerwin EM, D'Urzo AD, Gelb AF, Lakkis H, Gil EG, Caracta CF. Efficacy and safety of a 12-week treatment with twice-daily aclidinium bromide in COPD patients (ACCORD COPD I). COPD: J Chron Obstruct Pulmon Dis. 2012;9(2):90–101.
6. Jones PW, Quirk FH, Baveystock CM, Littlejohns P. A self-complete measure of health status for chronic airflow limitation: the St. George's respiratory questionnaire. Am Rev Respir Dis. 1992;145(6):1321–7.
7. Ferrer M, Alonso J, Prieto L, Plaza V, Monsó E, Marrades R, Aguar M, Khalaf A, Antó J. Validity and reliability of the St George's respiratory questionnaire after adaptation to a different language and culture: the Spanish example. Eur Respir J. 1996;9(6):1160–6.
8. Jones PW, Brusselle G, Dal Negro RW, Ferrer M, Kardos P, Levy ML, Perez T, Cataluña JS, van der Molen T, Adamek L. Properties of the COPD assessment test in a cross-sectional European study. Eur Respir J. 2011;38(1):29–35.
9. Jones P, Harding G, Berry P, Wiklund I, Chen W, Leidy NK. Development and first validation of the COPD assessment test. Eur Respir J. 2009;34(3):648–54.
10. Rieger-Reyes C, García-Tirado FJ, Rubio-Galán FJ, Marín-Trigo JM. Classification of chronic obstructive pulmonary disease severity according to the new Global initiative for chronic obstructive lung disease 2011 guidelines: COPD assessment test versus modified Medical Research Council scale. Archivos de Bronconeumología (English Edition). 2014;50(4):129–34.
11. Jones PW, Nadeau G, Small M, Adamek L. Characteristics of a COPD population categorised using the GOLD framework by health status and exacerbations. Respir Med. 2014;108(1):129–35.
12. Han J, Dai L, Zhong N, Young D. Breathlessness or health status in chronic obstructive pulmonary disease: the impact of different definitions. COPD: J Chron Obstruct Pulmon Dis. 2015;12(2):115–25.
13. Van der Molen T, Willemse BW, Schokker S, Ten Hacken NH, Postma DS, Juniper EF. Development, validity and responsiveness of the clinical COPD questionnaire. Health Qual Life Outcomes. 2003;1(1):1.
14. Sundh J, Ställberg B, Lisspers K, Kämpe M, Janson C, Montgomery S. Comparison of the COPD assessment test (CAT) and the clinical COPD questionnaire (CCQ) in a clinical population. COPD: J Chron Obstruct Pulmon Dis. 2016;13(1):57–65.
15. Lin W-C, Huang T-Y, Liu C-Y, Yeh M-L, Yu C-H, Hwang S-L. Validation of the clinical COPD questionnaire in Taiwan. COPD: J Chron Obstruct Pulmon Dis. 2016;13(3):360–6.
16. American Thoracic Society. Single-breath carbon monoxide diffusing capacity (transfer factor). Recommendations for a standard technique–1995 update. Am J Respir Crit Care Med. 1995;152(6 Pt 1):2185–98.
17. Wanger J, Clausen J, Coates A, Pedersen O, Brusasco V, Burgos F, Casaburi R, Crapo R, Enright P, Van Der Grinten C. Standardisation of the measurement of lung volumes. Eur Respir J. 2005;26(3):511.
18. Morris JF, Koski A, Johnson LC. Spirometric standards for healthy nonsmoking adults 1–3. Am Rev Respir Dis. 1971;103(1):57–67.
19. LEE CH, LEE JY, JANG EJ, PARK KY, HAN HW. New predictive equations for spirometric reference values and comparison with Morris equation in a Korean population. Respirology. 2008;13(3):365–71.
20. Ferris BG. Epidemiology standardization project (American Thoracic Society). Am Rev Respir Dis. 1978;118(6 Pt 2):1.
21. Mahler DA, Wells CK. Evaluation of clinical methods for rating dyspnea. CHEST J. 1988;93(3):580–6.
22. Kon SS, Canavan JL, Jones SE, Nolan CM, Clark AL, Dickson MJ, Haselden BM, Polkey MI, Man WD. Minimum clinically important difference for the COPD assessment test: a prospective analysis. Lancet Respir Med. 2014;2(3):195–203.
23. Global strategy for the diagnosis, management, and prevention of chronic obstructive pulmonary disease. http://www.goldcopd.org/. Accesse 18 Nov 2017.
24. Laboratories ACoPSfCPF. ATS statement: guidelines for the six-minute walk test. Am J Respir Crit Care Med. 2002;166(1):111.
25. Canavan JL, Dilaver D, Clark AL, Jones SE, Nolan CM, Kon SS, Man WDC. Clinical COPD questionnaire in patients with chronic respiratory disease. Respirology. 2014;19(7):1006–12.
26. CCQ Korean version. Available from: http://ccq.nl/?wpsc-product=ccq-korean-korean-24h-version. Accesse 18 Nov 2017.
27. Tsiligianni IG, Alma HJ, de Jong C, Jelusic D, Wittmann M, Schuler M, Schultz K, Kollen BJ, van der Molen T, Kocks JW. Investigating sensitivity, specificity, and area under the curve of the clinical COPD questionnaire, COPD assessment test, and modified Medical Research Council scale according to GOLD using St George's respiratory questionnaire cutoff 25 (and 20) as reference. Int J Chron Obstruct Pulmon Dis. 2016;11:1045–52.
28. Kon SS, Dilaver D, Mittal M, Nolan CM, Clark AL, Canavan JL, Jones SE, Polkey MI, Man WD. The clinical COPD questionnaire: response to pulmonary rehabilitation and minimal clinically important difference. Thorax. 2014;69(9):793–8.
29. Kocks JW, Tuinenga M, Uil S, Van den Berg J, Stahl E, Van der Molen T. Health status measurement in COPD: the minimal clinically important difference of the clinical COPD questionnaire. Respir Res. 2006;7(62):1465–993.
30. Lee C-H, Lee J, Park YS, Lee S-M, Yim J-J, Kim YW, Han SK, Yoo C-G. Chronic obstructive pulmonary disease (COPD) assessment test scores corresponding to modified Medical Research Council grades among COPD patients. Korean J Intern Med. 2015;30(5):629.
31. Pillai AP, Turner AM, Stockley RA. Global initiative for chronic obstructive lung disease 2011 symptom/risk assessment in α1-antitrypsin deficiency. CHEST J. 2013;144(4):1152–62.
32. Karloh M, Mayer AF, Maurici R, Pizzichini MM, Jones PW, Pizzichini E. The COPD assessment test: what do we know so far?: a systematic review and meta-analysis about clinical outcomes prediction and classification of patients into GOLD stages. CHEST J. 2016;149(2):413–25.

15

Pulmonary actinomycosis mimicking a lung metastasis from esophageal cancer

Munemasa Nagao[1*], Akihisa Fukuda[1], Takeshi Matsumura[2], Toshiyuki Kimura[2] and Hiroshi Seno[1]

Abstract

Background: Actinomycosis is a rare bacterial infection caused by *Actinomyces*. The symptom of actinomycosis is nonspecific and radiological images present as a slow-progressive mass lesion similarly to malignancies. Thus, it is difficult to distinguish pulmonary actinomycosis from malignancies.

Case presentation: A 74-year-old male who had esophageal cancer and a pulmonary mass that was positive for ^{18}F–fluorodeoxyglucose positron emission tomography/computed tomography was initially diagnosed with esophageal cancer with a lung metastasis because he was asymptomatic. However, aspiration of pleural effusion revealed that the pulmonary lesion was actinomycosis.

Conclusion: We present a case of pulmonary actinomycosis mimicking a lung metastasis from esophageal cancer. Diagnosis of asymptomatic pulmonary actinomycosis is difficult, and needle aspiration could be useful for a definitive diagnosis of pulmonary actinomycosis.

Keywords: Actinomycosis, Esophageal cancer, Infection

Background

Actinomycosis is a rare chronic granulomatous infection caused by *Actinomyces* species. *Actinomyces* are facultative anaerobic Gram-positive bacteria [1]. The symptom of actinomycosis is nonspecific and similar to those of other chronic suppurative chest diseases. On computed tomography (CT) and ^{18}F–fluorodeoxyglucose positron emission tomography/computed tomography (PET/CT), pulmonary actinomycosis presents as a slow-progressive mass lesion similarly to malignancies. Non-specific symptoms and radiological images make diagnosis of pulmonary actinomycosis difficult [2, 3]. In previous case reports, pulmonary actinomycoses were occasionally resected as pulmonary neoplasms because of its difficult diagnosis [4]. Here we report a case of pulmonary actinomycosis mimicking a lung metastasis from esophageal cancer.

* Correspondence: ds110559@kuhp.kyoto-u.ac.jp
[1]Department of Gastroenterology and Hepatology, Graduate School of Medicine, Kyoto University, 54 Kawahara-cho, Syogoin, Sakyo-ku, Kyoto 606-8507, Japan
Full list of author information is available at the end of the article

Case presentation

A 74-year-old male was admitted to our hospital for the treatment of esophageal cancer. The patient had no symptoms with normal temperature at the time of admission. His past medical history included diabetes mellitus for 24 years. He underwent endoscopic submucosal dissection for early gastric cancer 4 years ago and video-assisted thoracic surgery for pulmonary adenocarcinoma in the right upper lobe 5 years ago. He occupation was making metal molds. He was ex-smoker: Brinkman index was 980. Laboratory studies showed white blood cells of 10.0×10^3/L, C-reactive protein of 6.07 mg/dL, hemoglobin A1c test of 8.8%, fasting blood sugar of 237 mg/dL on admission. Serum tumor markers, including CEA, CA19–9, SCC, CYFRA, were unremarkable. He underwent esophago-gastro-duodenoscopy for follow-up after endoscopic submucosal dissection for early gastric cancer. The upper endoscopy showed a 0-IIa lesion with relatively large granular nodules on the lower thoracic esophagus (Fig. 1). The pathologic assessment of the biopsy revealed squamous cell carcinoma of the esophagus. The esophageal 0-IIa lesion with relatively large granular nodules let us consider the depth of esophageal cancer was deeper than

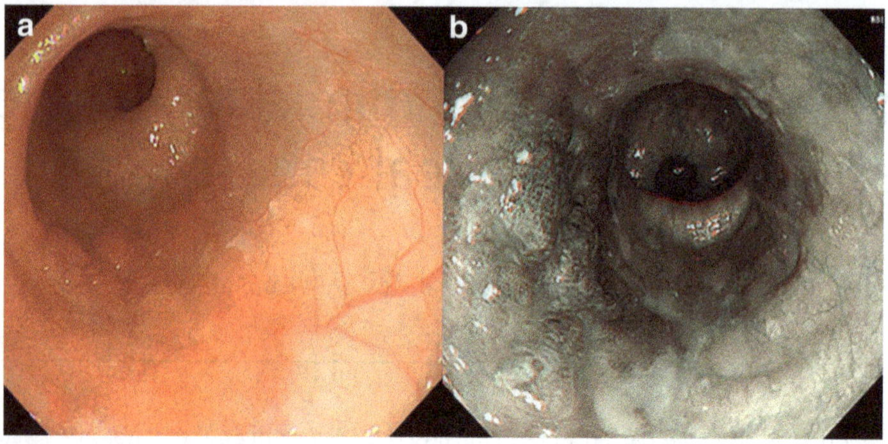

Fig. 1 Images of esophago-gastro-duodenoscopy (EGD). **a** White Light Imaging. EGD showed a 0-IIa lesion with granular nodules on the lower thoracic esophagus. **b** Narrow Band Imaging. The lesion showing the brownish area was predicted to be squamous cell carcinoma

M3/SM1. Chest X-Ray was normal, however, chest CT revealed a 1.3 cm × 0.9 cm pulmonary mass in the lower lobe of the right lung a month before admission (Fig. 2a). PET/CT showed the pulmonary mass had maximal standardized uptake value (SUVmax) of 3.88 (arrow) and part of the lower thoracic esophagus had SUVmax of 2.37 (arrowhead) 2 weeks before admission (Fig. 2b and c). Because the image of pulmonary mass had not changed between CT and PET/CT for 2 weeks and because he had no fever, even though he had inflammation reaction on laboratory studies, pulmonary mass was considered to be unlikely due to infection. Thus, he was initially diagnosed with esophageal cancer with a pulmonary metastasis or recurrence of a pulmonary adenocarcinoma. Considering the both possibilities, we started chemotherapy with cisplatin (CDDP) 70 mg/m^2 day1 plus 5-fluorouracil (5-FU) 700 mg/m^2 day1–4 on the day 4 after admission. On the day 8, CT revealed a slight pleural effusion in the right side (Fig. 3a and b). On the day 9, to rule out carcinomatous pleurisy, an ultrasound-guided aspiration of pleural effusion was performed. The effusion was serous and contained no malignant cells. After the aspiration, the patient got a high fever. Laboratory test showed white blood cells of 18.6 × 103/L (90.8% of Neutrophil), CRP of 25.87 mg/dL.

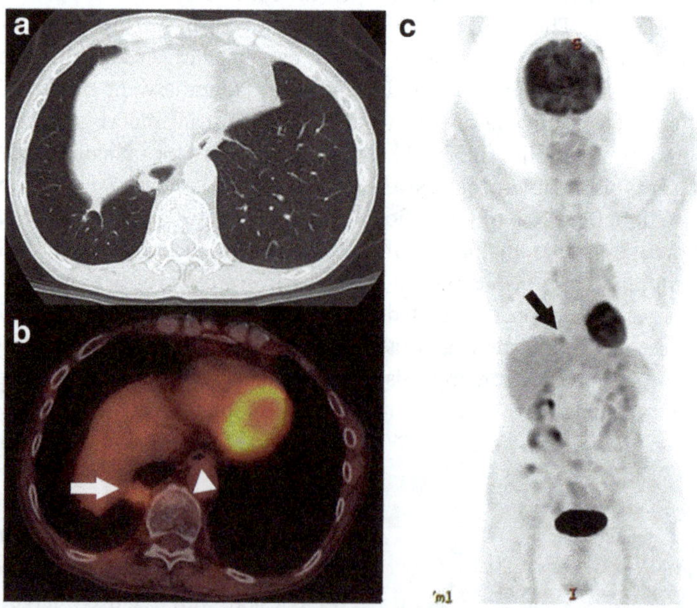

Fig. 2 Images of computed tomography (CT) and Positron emission tomography (PET) /CT before admission to the hospital. **a** CT showing a pulmonary mass in the right lower lobe. **b** and **c**: PET/CT showed the pulmonary mass had maximal standardized uptake value (SUVmax) of 3.88 and the lower thoracic esophagus had SUVmax of 2.37

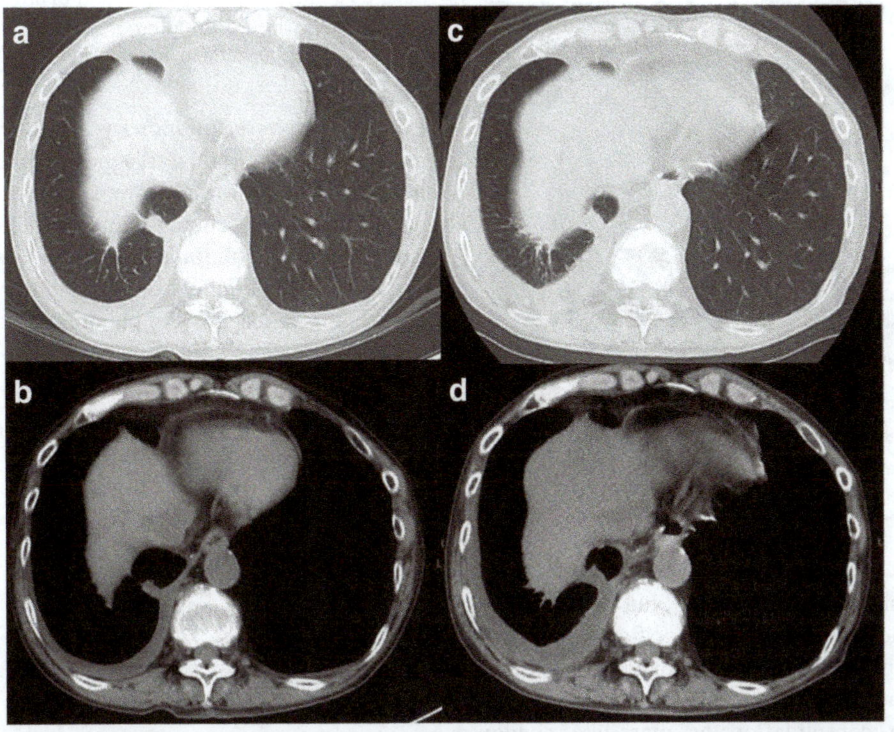

Fig. 3 Images of CT after admission to the hospital. **a** and **b** on the day 8, (**c**) and (**d**) on the day 14. CT revealed an increased amount of pleural effusion

Considering that fever was due to respiratory infection after the aspiration, intravenous Sulbactam/Ampicillin (6 g/day) was administered. On the day14, his fever was persistent and he also had a cough. Because CT revealed an increased amount of pleural effusion (Fig. 3c and d), we considered the mass was lung abscess. By the second ultrasound-guided aspiration of the pleural effusion, we got a 50 ml of white suppurative effusion. The effusion turned out to contain *Actinomyces israelii* (Fig. 4), and proved pulmonary mass-like lesion was pulmonary actinomycosis. The patient received intravenous penicillin G (24 million units/day) for 4 weeks, followed by oral amoxicillin 2250 mg/day for 6 months. The patient received four courses of chemotherapy (CDDP/5-FU) and curative radiotherapy (1.8Gy/total 50.4Gy) as esophageal cancer deeper than M3/SM1. The pulmonary actinomycosis disappeared six months after the treatment with antibiotics (Fig. 5). After the chemoradiation therapy without any complications, the esophageal cancer was in complete remission.

Discussion

Actinomycosis is a rare and chronic bacterial infection caused by *Actinomyces* species. *Actinomyces israelii* is one of the *Actinomyces* species. *Actinomyces* can colonize the cervicofacial, thoracic, abdominal, pelvic lesions, skin, brain and other organs. Pulmonary actinomycosis accounts for 15% of all actinomycoses [5], and is mainly caused by aspiration of oral saphrophytes into respiratory tracts [3]. As actinomycosis can develop after dental care or aspiration, careful history taking is necessary for old ages. Sputum examination and culture is difficult to detect pathogenic bacteria, because *Actinomyces* are anaerobic and exist in normal oral cavity. Clinical symptoms of pulmonary actinomycosis include chest pain, chronic

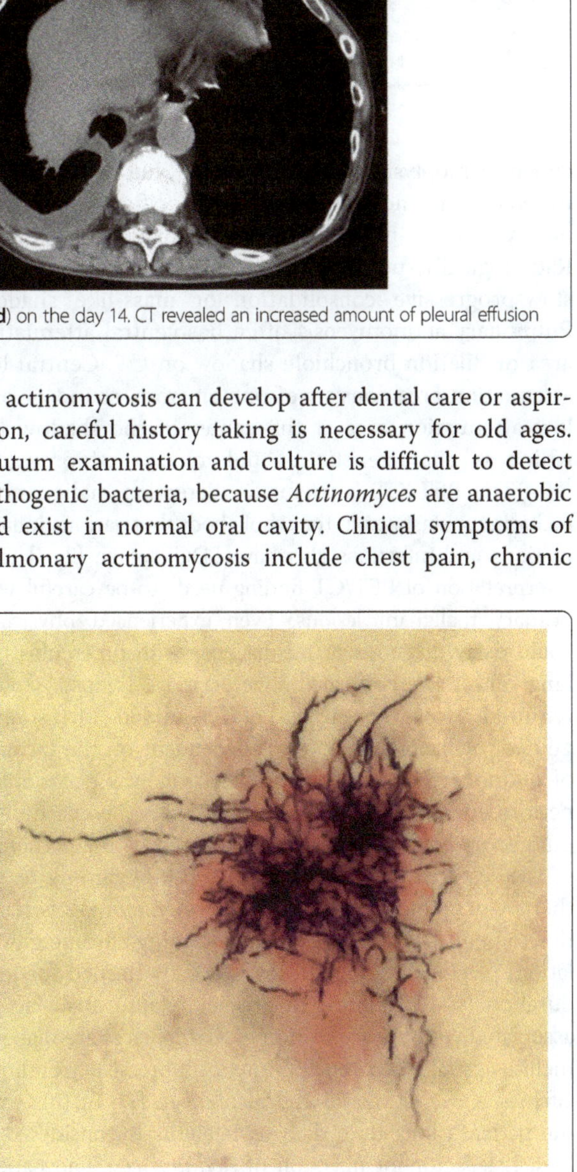

Fig. 4 Gram stain of aspirate from pleural effusion. Gram stain of aspirate from pulmonary mass revealed *Actinomyces israelii* as bronching, gram-positive filaments

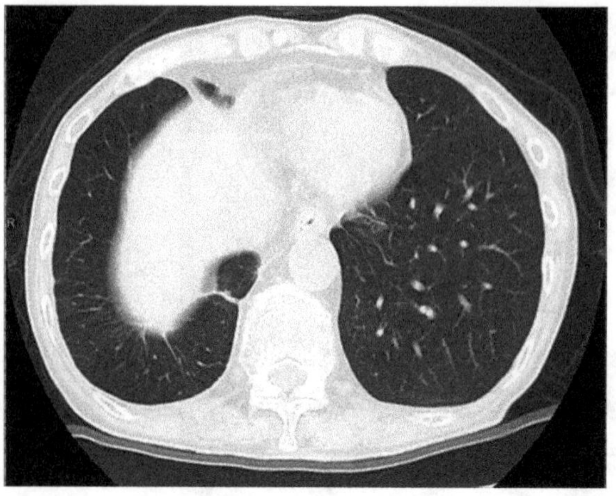

Fig. 5 Image of chest CT 6 months after the treatment with antibiotics. The pulmonary actinomycosis disappeared

cough, hemoptysis, fever and chill [1], but actinomycosis frequently has no symptoms. Nonspecific symptoms or no symptoms make a definitive diagnosis difficult. Radiologically, pulmonary actinomycosis presents as a slow-progressive consolidation or mass-like shadow. Pulmonary actinomycosis often has central attenuation area or dilation bronchiole shadow on CT. Central low attenuation area consists of one or more, round or oval low attenuation area at the center of the shadow [6], which is characteristic of pulmonary actinomycosis. ^{18}F–FDG PET/CT is useful for detecting malignancies including metastases in the whole body, but various inflammations and infections also have FDG uptake [2, 3]. The interpretation of PET/CT finding needs to be careful with primary malignant lesions. Even experienced physicians could delay diagnosis or misdiagnose with tuberculosis or lung cancer [7]. For a definitive diagnosis, biopsy is often required. However, success of CT-guided, ultrasound-guided, or bronchial biopsy is dependent on the location of pulmonary mass [8]. Lung resection was occasionally performed as a diagnosis of pulmonary neoplasm and pulmonary actinomycosis was diagnosed by the pathology of the resected lung specimens [9, 10]. Regarding to the therapy of actinomycoces, almost all *Actinomyces* is sensitive to penicillin. For *Actinomyces* forming chronic granulation, penicillin in high doses is usually needed for long duration (6–12 months) to prevent relapse. Risk factors associated with the acquisition of *Actinomyces* are diabetes mellitus, male sex, and immunosuppressive condition such as a use of steroid and alcoholism [7]. In this case, the patient's long-term diabetes mellitus is considered to be a risk factor for infection of *Actinomyces*. The patient had primary esophageal cancer and past history of primary pulmonary adenocarcinoma, which made a diagnosis difficult. However, a high fever after starting chemotherapy gave us a clue of the infection and prompted us to perform needle aspiration of the pleural effusion.

Conclusion

Even though rare, pulmonary actinomycosis should be included in differential diagnosis of PET/CT positive pulmonary mass without any symptoms. Especially, if a patient has other primary malignant lesions, it is difficult to distinguish pulmonary actinomycosis from a lung metastasis. If available, needle aspiration could be useful for a definitive diagnosis of pulmonary actinomycosis.

Acknowledgements

We thank Dr. Matsuo for advices on diagnosis of asymptomatic pulmonary actinomycosis.

Funding

None (for all authors).

Authors' contributions

MN participated in diagnosis and drafted the manuscript. TM and TK participated in diagnosis. AF and HS supervised this manuscript. All authors read and approved the final manuscript.

Consent for publication

Written informed consent was obtained from the patient for publication of this case report and any accompanying images.

Competing interests

The authors declare that they have no competing interests.

Author details

[1]Department of Gastroenterology and Hepatology, Graduate School of Medicine, Kyoto University, 54 Kawahara-cho, Syogoin, Sakyo-ku, Kyoto 606-8507, Japan. [2]Department of Gastroenterology and Hepatology, Hyogo Prefectural Amagasaki General Medical Center, Amagasaki, Japan.

References

1. Hsieh MJ, Liu HP, Chang JP, Chang CH. Thoracic actinomycosis. Chest. 1993; 104(2):366–70.
2. Andreani A, Rossi G, Giovannini M, Cappiello GF. Unexpected positron emission tomography-positive *Actinomyces*-related mass of the bronchial stump. Can Respir J. 2012;19(2):77–9.
3. Qiu L, Lan L, Feng Y, Huang Z, Chen Y. Pulmonary Actinomycosis imitating lung cancer on 18F-FDG PET/CT: a case report and literature review. Korean J Radiol. 2015;16(6):1262–5.
4. Sakon M, Mikami K, Seki H, Munakata Y, Saitoh G, Nishimura H, Hosaka N. A case report of pulmonary actinomycosis radiologically mimicking lung metastasis from rectal cancer. Nihon Rinsho Geka Gakkai Zasshi. 2008;69(1): 38–43. (in Japanese)
5. Colmegna I, Rodriguez-Barradas M, Young EJ, Rauch R, Clarridge J. Disseminated *Actinomyces meyeri* infection resembling lung cancer with brain metastases. Am J Med Sci. 2003;326(3):152–5.
6. Mato N, Oshikawa K, Sakuma Y, Sawai T, Ohno S, Sugiyama Y. Thoracic actinomycosis: clinical, radiological, and pathological findings in 11 cases. Nihon Kokyuki Gakkai Zasshi. 2003;41(8):514–20. (in Japanese)

7. Wong VK, Turmezei TD, Weston VC. Actinomycosis. BMJ. 2011;343:d6099.
8. Nagaoka T, Setoguchi Y, Muramatsu M, Honma N, Danbara T, Miyamoto H, Fukuchi Y. A case of pulmonary squamous cell carcinoma coexisting with pulmonary Actinomycosis. Nihon Kokyuki Gakkai Zasshi. 2002;40(6):525–9. (in Japanese)
9. Matzumura-Kuan M, Jennings J. Aggregatibacter actinomycetemcomitans infection mimicking lung cancer: a case report. Scand J Infect Dis. 2014; 46(9):669–72.
10. Weese WC, Smith IM. A study of 57 cases of actinomycosis over a 36-year period. Arch Intern Med. 1975;135:1562–8.

16

Aspergillus fumigatus during COPD exacerbation

Xunliang Tong[1†], Anqi Cheng[2†], Hongtao Xu[3], Jin Jin[4], Yimeng Yang[4], Sainan Zhu[5] and Yanming Li[4*]

Abstract

Background: Recently awareness of the importance of Aspergillus colonization in the airway of patients with chronic obstructive pulmonary disease (COPD) was rising. The aim of this study was to investigate the clinical features and short-term outcomes of COPD patients with Aspergillus colonization during acute exacerbation.

Methods: A pair-matched retrospective study on patients presenting with COPD exacerbation was conducted from January 2014 to March 2016 in Beijing Hospital, China.

Results: Twenty-three patients with Aspergillus colonization and 69 patients as controls, diagnosed of COPD exacerbation, were included in this study at a pair-matched ratio of 1:3. In stable stage, the percentage of patients with high-dose corticosteroids inhalation in the Aspergillus colonization group is higher than that of in control group (65.5% vs 33.3%, $p = 0.048$). Multivariate analysis showed that corticosteroids use was the risk factor for isolation of Aspergillus. In acute exacerbation stage, patients in Aspergillus colonization group received higher dose of inhaled corticosteroids and more types of antibiotics than control group. The short-time outcome hinted that the remission time and the duration of hospitalization were longer in the Aspergillus colonization group than in the control group (remission time: 11 ± 4 days vs 7 ± 4 days, $p = 0.001$; duration: 15 ± 5 days vs 12 ± 4 days, $p = 0.011$).

Conclusions: Aspergillus colonization in the lower respiratory tract of COPD patients showed typical clinical manifestations, affected their short time outcome and provided a dilemma of clinical treatment strategy.

Keywords: COPD, Aspergillus fumigatus, Fungal colonization

Background

The prevalence of chronic obstructive pulmonary disease (COPD) is rapidly growing and is associated with significant morbidity and mortality, which increases economic health burden [1–3]. COPD is characterized by irreversible airflow obstruction with underlying emphysema and small airway obliteration, which commonly co-exist. Pathogenic microorganisms, such as bacteria, are commonly colonized in the airways of COPD patients, possibly contributing to increased airway inflammation, and have been implicated in COPD exacerbations [4–6]. However, fungal colonization and its potential role in acute exacerbations of COPD (AECOPD) are poorly understood.

Aspergillus spp. is a ubiquitous fungus in the environment with high sporulation capacity [7, 8]. After Aspergillus sporulates, conidia with a diameter of 2–3 μm are released into the air, enter the airway, and reach alveoli [9]. Therefore, the lung is the main organ affected by Aspergillus. Isolation of Aspergillus spp. from lower respiratory tract (LRT) samples (e.g. sputum, bronchial aspirate, or bronchoalveolar lavage) provides important etiologic evidence for its identification. Aspergillus spp. causes various diseases in lungs, such as Aspergillus colonization, Aspergillus infection and allergic bronchopulmonary aspergillus [10]. In COPD patients, impairment of the defense mechanisms of airways facilitates the binding of conidia to epithelial cells, which may cause Aspergillus colonization in the airway [11]. Positive isolation of Aspergillus spp. in LRT samples from COPD patients is common, and a previous study reported that the positive identification rate was nearly 29%

* Correspondence: lymyl@263.net
[†]Equal contributors
[4]Department of Respiratory and Critical Care Medicine, Beijing Hospital, Beijing 100730, People's Republic of China
Full list of author information is available at the end of the article

[12]. However, clinical manifestations of COPD patients with Aspergillus spp. colonization from LRT have rarely been summarized and are difficult to distinguish, often leading to debate in clinical practice. Consequently, it is difficult for clinicians to make treatment strategies for Aspergillus colonization. The aims of this study were to investigate the clinical features of COPD patients with Aspergillus colonization in LRT, to analyze the risk factors that could predict the possibility of Aspergillus spp. isolation and to summarize the clinical treatment choices and outcomes of COPD patients with Aspergillus colonization.

Methods

Study design

This pair-matched study was conducted from January 2014 to March 2016 in the Department of Respiratory and Critical Care Medicine in Beijing Hospital, China. Patient data were collected from the electronic medical records system of our hospital and by additional chart review. The data used was part of our project "Study on Aspergillus of COPD patients", which was approved by the ethics committee of Beijing Hospital (Approval notice number 2013BJYYEC-024-01). The informed consent was obtained from all participants in written form.

Mentioned conditions

	Conditions
A	Age between 18 and 90 years old.
B	The diagnosis of COPD was based on the Global Initiative for GOLD guidelines. COPD exacerbations are defined as an acute worsening of respiratory symptoms that result in additional therapy.
C	Positive isolation of Aspergillus spp. in an LRT sample by microbiologic examination. LRT samples included sputum, bronchial aspirate, and bronchoalveolar lavage fluid (BALF).
D	Patients without any chest CT findings of chronic pulmonary aspergillosis (CPA), invasive pulmonary aspergillosis (IPA), allergic bronchopulomnary aspergillosis (ABPA), pneumonia.

Inclusion criteria

	Definition
Aspergillus colonization	fulfilled above condition C and D above.
Aspergillus colonization group	fulfilled all conditions above, including A, B, C and D.
Control group	COPD patients who were admitted a day before or after the Aspergillus colonization group patients were recruited to the control group. At the same time, patients fulfilled above conditions A, B and D.

Exclusion criteria

(1) Immunocompromised patients, including those with allogeneic or autologous hematopoietic stem cell transplantation, neutropenia, hematologic malignant disease and solid tumor, hematologic stem cell or solid-organ transplantation, and AIDS, as were patients receiving high-dose immunosuppressive agents (e.g. for connective tissue disease and vasculitis).
(2) Patients with chest CT findings of CPA, IPA, ABPA, pneumonia.
(3) Patients with other underlying lung diseases.

Microbiological examination

When patients admitted into hospital, their LRT samples were delivered for microbiological examination the next day. Microbiological examination included direct microscopy and bacterial and fungal pathogen cultvation. All samples were cultured on conventional media, including blood agar, chocolate agar, MacConkey agar and Sabouraud's dextrose agar. Bacterial infection was defined as a colony count $\geq 10^5$ cfu/mL. Aspergillus and other fungal isolates were identified using microculture and standard morphological procedures.

Data collection

Following information was collected from the electronic medical records system of our hospital: patient characteristics (sex, age, etc.), lung function, administration of corticosteroids and nutritional status before admission, clinical symptoms and signs, chest imaging and CT scan data, laboratory test results (IgE, eosinophil counts, etc.), microbiologic findings of LRT samples, treatment during hospitalization, remission time (defined as the duration of stabilization of clinical symptoms and disappearance of signs, like the typical symptoms of cough, sputum, wheeze, and the typical signs of wheezing rale), length of hospitalization or ICU stay, and mortality.

Statistical analysis

Normally distributed continuous variables were expressed as the mean ± standard deviation and were compared with a *t*-test. Non-normally distributed continuous variables were expressed as medians and quartiles and were compared with the Mann-Whitney *U*-test. Categorical variables were compared with chi-square test or Fisher's exact test. Logistic regression was used to identify independent risk factors for Aspergillus colonization. The first logistic regression analysis univariately considered the explanatory variables in stable stage. Only variables with p value < 0.10 in univariate analysis were entered in the multivariate analysis, using a backward stepwise method, with a probability value for the entry of $p = 0.10$ and removal of $p = 0.05$. Kaplan-Meier method was used to estimate the time from admission to remission of symptoms. P values < 0.05 were considered statistically significant. The statistical analysis was performed using SPSS 19.0.0 (IBM Corporation, Armonk, NY, USA).

Results

Study performance

A total of 504 patients diagnosed with AECOPD were admitted to hospital from January 2014 to March 2016. Aspergillus spp. was identified in the LRT samples of 42 patients (all from qualified sputum specimen), resulting in a detection rate of 8.33%. According to the exclusion criteria, 19 patients with Aspergillus spp. in their sputum samples were excluded from this study, including 9 patients with IPA infection, 5 patients with other pulmonary diseases (asthma: 4 cases, bronchiectasis: 1 case), 2 patients with cancer (lung cancer: 1 case, prostate cancer: 1 case), 1 patient being treated with immunosuppressive agents for connective tissue disease, 1 patient with agranulocytosis and 1 patient who was unable to participate lung function test. Finally, 23 patients with Aspergillus colonization were included in the study group. After performing matching at a ratio of 1:3 (one study group patient to three control group patients), a total of 92 patients were enrolled in this study shown in Fig. 1.

Demographic characteristics and treatment during stable stage

Patients in Aspergillus colonization group consisted of 20 men and 3 women with a median age of 76 ± 7 years. Most of these patients were current smokers with a smoking duration of more than 40 pack-years. All patients were classified by GOLD stage severity. The forced expiratory volume 1 (FEV_1) of patients in Aspergillus colonization group was worse according to GOLD severity classification than that of patients in control group (FEV_1% predicted: 40.0% ± 16.0% vs 44.5% ± 16.8%). Patients in Aspergillus colonization group also had more underlying diseases, including hypertension, diabetes mellitus and coronary heart disease, than patients in control group. The percentage of inhaled corticosteroid (ICS) use during the stable stage was higher in Aspergillus colonization group than that of control group (73.9% vs 40.6%, $p = 0.008$). Besides, more patients received a daily dose of beclomethasone greater than 1000 μg (30.4% vs 11.6%, $p = 0.048$), which was significantly different from patients in control group. The demographic characteristics of patients in Aspergillus colonization and control groups were listed in Table 1.

Univariable baseline analysis showed that smoking history, chronic heart failure and corticosteroids use were risk factors for Aspergillus colonization in COPD patients' LRT. After multivariable adjustment, only corticosteroids use was independently associated with Aspergillus colonization in COPD patients' LRT (OR 4.685, 95% CI 1.529–14.355), shown in Table 2.

Clinical manifestations in the exacerbation stage

The clinical characteristics and selected laboratory abnormalities of included patients were shown in Table 3. Most patients exhibited fever, cough, dyspnea and wheezing. Wheezing and wheezing rales were the most specific symptom and sign, which were significantly common in Aspergillus colonization group (wheezing: 52.2% vs 15.9%, $p = 0.001$; wheezing rales: 65.2% vs 38.2%, $p = 0.031$). Laboratory results showed that the number

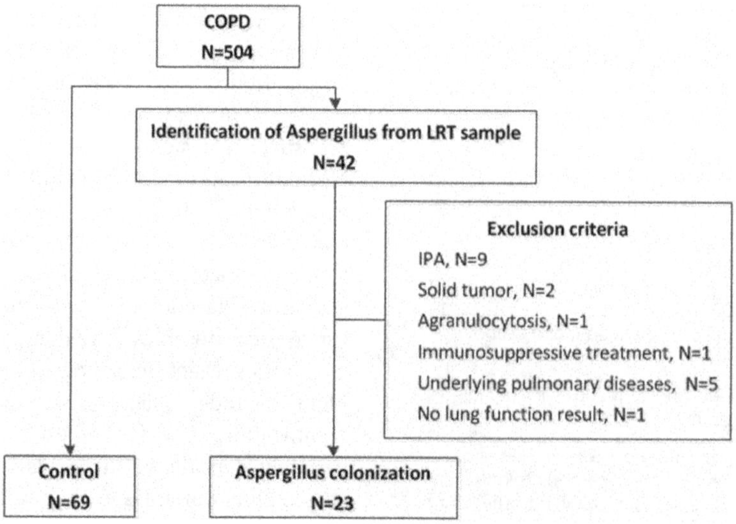

Fig. 1 Study population selection

Table 1 Basic information of COPD patients in stable stage

	Aspergillus colonization, $n = 23$	Control, $n = 69$	*p* value
Demographics			
Age, yr (IQR)	76 ± 7	75 ± 8	0.741
Gender (male/female)	20/3	60/9	1.000
BMI(kg/m^2)	22.4 ± 4.1	23.4 ± 3.7	0.266
Smoking history, n (%)	17 (73.9%)	63 (91.3%)	0.091
Pack-years (IQR)	58 ± 39	47 ± 36	0.291
COPD characteristics (post bronchodilators)			
FEV$_1$% (IQR)	40.0 ± 16.0	44.5 ± 16.8	0.261
GOLD grade			
Grade I	4 (17.4%)	15 (21.7%)	
Grade II	5 (21.7%)	21 (30.4%)	
Grade III	12 (54.5%)	30 (51.7%)	
Grade IV	2 (9.1%)	3 (5.2%)	
GOLD grade ≥ 3, n (%)	14 (63.6)	33 (56.9)	0.744
Underlying conditions, n (%)			
Hypertension	15 (65.2%)	41 (59.4%)	0.806
Diabetes mellitus	7 (31.8%)	7 (15.9%)	0.201
Coronary heart disease	7 (30.4%)	16 (23.2%)	0.580
Cerebral vascular disease	4 (17.4%)	10 (14.5%)	0.774
Chronic heart failure	8 (34.8%)	12 (17.4%)	0.089
Peptic ulcer	0	6 (8.7%)	0.331
Chronic renal failure	2 (8.7%)	3 (4.4%)	0.597
Stable period treatment			
Corticosteroids use, n (%)	17 (73.9%)	28 (40.6%)	*0.008*
daily dose of inhaled corticosteroid >1000μg (Betamethasone equal dosage)	56.5%	33.3%	*0.048*
Long term oxygen therapy	3 (13.0%)	12 (17.4%)	0.753
Times of AECOPD in previous year	1.7 ± 1.3	1.3 ± 1.1	0.186

Italicized *p*-values are statistically significant, ie. $p < 0.05$

and percentage of eosinophils (EOS) were significantly decreased in patients in Aspergillus colonization group compared to those in control group (EOS% > 5%: 4.3% vs 23.2%, $p = 0.044$). Arterial blood gas was measured in all patients, but no significant differences were observed between two groups. Some inflammatory markers, such as C-reactive protein (CRP) and erythrocyte sedimentation rate (ESR), and total IgE levels, were not significantly different between two groups.

Detection of pathogenic bacteria and other fungi

To investigate whether Aspergillus colonization was associated with combined identification of other specific microbial pathogens, we compared the cultivation results of LRT samples from the Aspergillus colonization group and control group. Particular attention was paid to pathogenic bacteria identification, including Acinetobacter baumannii, methicillin-resistant *Staphylococcus aureus* (MRSA), Pseudomonas aeruginosa, Klebsiella pneumonia, Stenotrophomonas maltophilia and Enterococcus faecium. The percentage of pathogens identification in two groups showed no statistical difference (Additional file 1: Table S1). Besides, some of other fungi were also detected in our microbiologic cultivation, especially Saccharomycetes.

Patient treatment during hospitalization and short-term outcomes

The Aspergillus colonization group included a higher percentage of patients who received more than one class of antibiotics (52.2% vs 20.3%, $p = 0.006$) and had a longer duration of antibiotic usage (13 ± 5 vs 10 ± 4 days, $p = 0.003$) than that of the control group. In addition to

Table 2 Univariate and multivariate logistic analysis for Aspergillus colonization

Characteristics	Univariate analysis		Multivariate analysis	
	OR (95% CI)	*p* value	OR (95% CI)	*p* value
BMI	0.929 (0.817–1.057)	0.264		
Smoking history	0.270 (0.077–0.944)	*0.040*	0.275 (0.073–1.036)	0.056
Pack-years	1.008 (0.994–1.022)	0.291		
FEV_1% pre (post bronchodilators)	0.982 (0.951–1.014)	0.259		
GOLD grade	1.968 (0.638–6.075)	0.239		
Hypertension	1.280 (0.479–3.424)	0.622		
Diabetes mellitus	1.719 (0.593–4.983)	0.319		
Coronary heart disease	1.449 (0.507–4.139)	0.488		
Cerebral vascular disease	1.242 (0.349–4.421)	0.738		
Chronic heart failure	2.533 (0.878–7.313)	0.086	3.147 (0.978–10.130)	0.055
Chronic renal failure	2.095 (0.328–13.397)	0.435		
Corticosteroids use	4.149 (1.456–11.825)	*0.008*	4.685 (1.529–14.355)	*0.007*
Long term oxygen therapy	0.713 (0.182–2.787)	0.626		
Times of AECOPD in previous year	1.299 (0.880–1.918)	0.188		

Italicized *p*-values are statistically significant, ie. $p < 0.05$

Table 3 Characteristics and examination results of COPD patients in acute exacerbation stage

	Aspergillus colonization, $n = 23$	Control, $n = 69$	*p* value
Symptom and sign			
cough	20 (87.0%)	61 (88.4%)	1.000
dyspnea	14 (60.9%)	53 (76.8%)	0.177
wheezing	12 (52.2%)	11 (15.9%)	*0.001*
fever	12 (52.2%)	28 (40.6%)	0.344
moist rale	13 (56.5%)	27 (39.1%)	0.156
wheezing rale	15 (65.2%)	26 (38.2%)	*0.031*
Blood routine			
WBC count ($\times 10^9$/L)	6.45 ± 2.23	7.25 ± 3.57	0.319
NEUT count ($\times 10^9$/L)	4.73 ± 2.07	4.94 ± 3.28	0.771
NEUT% (%)	71.2 ± 13.2	65.7 ± 13.0	0.092
EOS% < 0.5%	30.4%	23.2%	0.487
EOS% > 5%	4.3%	23.2%	*0.044*
Arterial blood gas			
Pa/Fi	317 ± 42	324 ± 59	0.625
pH	7.41 ± 0.03	7.38 ± 0.72	0.063
$PaCO_2$ (mmHg)	40.3 ± 6.3	44.5 ± 10.6	0.088
PaO_2 (mmHg)	70.5 ± 10.9	76.8 ± 15.5	0.102
Biomarker			
CRP (mg/dl)	3.23 ± 3.51	2.53 ± 3.12	0.412
ESR (mm/h)	25.3 ± 28.2	20.0 ± 20.3	0.436
Total IgE (IU/ml)	441 ± 1075	282 ± 362	0.386

Italicized *p*-values are statistically significant, ie. $p < 0.05$

antibiotic treatment, systemic corticosteroids and/or ICS were used to control wheezing symptom. The percentage of patients in Aspergillus colonization group who use high dose of inhaled corticosteroids (accumulated budesonide dose: no less than 40 mg) were higher than that of control group (30.4% vs 5.8%, $p = 0.002$). Remission time curve was estimated by Kaplan-Meier analysis. Median remission time was 10 days in the Aspergillus colonization group and 6 days in the control group (log-rank test $p = 0.004$) (Fig. 2). The duration of hospitalization were longer in the Aspergillus colonization group than it is in the control group (15 ± 5 days vs 12 ± 4 days, $p = 0.011$), shown in Table 4.

Discussion

AECOPD is often associated with infectious agents, including bacteria, virus and fungi. A previous study was conducted in critically ill patients with isolation of Aspergillus spp. from the respiratory tract, with mortality rates of 50% in the colonization group and 80% in the invasive infection group after 9 months of follow-up [13]. Therefore, clinicians usually focus on infection when a positive Aspergillus spp. culture is obtained from the LRT. However, the significance of a more frequent clinical phenomenon, Aspergillus spp. colonization, has yet to be clarified. In this research, a pair-matched observational study was conducted to investigate the differences in the clinical manifestations and short-term outcomes between COPD patients with and without Aspergillus colonization in LRT.

Cigarette smoking, one of the major risk factors for the development of COPD, induces structural and functional changes in airway epithelium in vitro and in vivo [14–16]. In our study, the number of patients with a history of smoking was higher in the Aspergillus colonization group than in the control group, which indicated that smoking is a potential risk for Aspergillus colonization. Cigarette smoking and repeated airway inflammation could alter the structure and function of lung and injure a profound effect on the host defense against invading pathogens and particulates, thus impairing the airway epithelium [17, 18] and mad COPD patients more susceptible to Aspergillus colonization. Meanwhile, most patients in the Aspergillus colonization group received higher doses of ICS during stable stage treatment, in contrast to the control group. Our findings were consistent with a previous study that suggested that high-dose corticosteroids use was a risk for Aspergillus colonization or positive Aspergillus culture [19, 20].

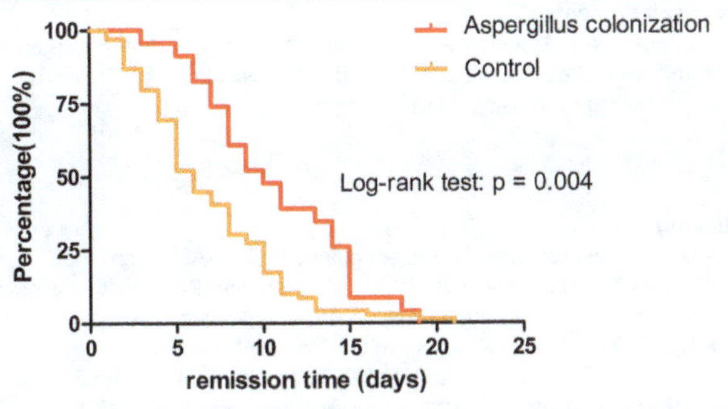

Fig. 2 Remission time curve estimated by Kaplan-Meier analysis

In our study, Aspergillus-colonized patients presented with wheezing and wheezing rales in the acute exacerbation period. More than half of the patients received systemic corticosteroids and/or ICS. The percentage of corticosteroid usage in the two groups was similar, but in the Aspergillus colonization group, patients received higher doses of ICS. This finding suggested that Aspergillus colonization contributed to an increased severity of exacerbations in COPD patients. These phenomena suggested that high-dose ICS treatment was related to Aspergillus colonization and induced similar clinical manifestations to allergic reactions due to Aspergillus colonization. A previous study on the mechanism involved in Aspergillus-related allergic reactions was based on the Aspergillus hyphae and involved antigen-triggered mast cell degranulation and release of histamine and inflammatory factors [21–24]. These data showed that Aspergillus colonization may aggravate airway hyper-responsiveness and worsen airway inflammation and bronchoconstriction. But no cohort study of patients with repeated cultures of Aspergillus have been done in COPD patients, it is unclear whether fungal colonization contributes to lower lung function or is a marker of more severe lung disease and aggressive therapy. In our study, patients with Aspergillus colonization had a longer time to be stable and a longer duration of hospitalization, which indicated that Aspergillus colonization was related with clinical manifestations and short-term outcomes of COPD patients.

After demonstrating the significance of Aspergillus colonization in the airways of COPD patients, we highlighted an essential clinical treatment dilemma: whether to eliminate colonization with anti-fungal therapy or to stabilize wheezing with continuous ICS. Because Aspergillus colonization is clinically significant, the treatment strategy should aim to eliminate colonization. However, a previous study showed that the removal of Aspergillus colonization did not improve lung function in a long-term observation; this finding cast doubt on the value of anti-fungal therapy. Due to the lack of research on the effect of Aspergillus colonization on AECOPD and stable COPD, challenges remain for clinical decision making. The relationship between colonization and invasive infection is unclear. Whether increasing the fungal load of colonization in the airway could result in invasive pulmonary mycosis

Table 4 Clinical treatment and short-term outcomes in AECOPD patients

	Aspergillus colonization, $n = 23$	Control, $n = 69$	p value
Admitted in ICU	4 (17.4%)	11 (15.9%)	1.000
Machined ventilation	3 (13.0%)	9 (13.0%)	0.906
Antibiotics	21 (95.5%)	66 (95.7%)	1.000
More than 1 class	52.2%	21.7%	*0.006*
Duration of treatment (days)	13 ± 5	10 ± 4	*0.003*
Corticosteroid use	17 (77.3%)	42 (60.9%)	0.204
Systemic only	0	2 (2.90%)	1.000
Inhalation only	8 (34.8%)	20 (29.0%)	0.601
Dose of usage			
Budesonide (inhaled,≥40 mg)	30.4%	5.8%	*0.002*
Methylprednisolone (iv,≥120 mg)	39.1%	31.9%	0.524
Bronchodilators (aerosol inhalation)	21 (91.3%)	57 (82.6%)	0.505
Ipratropium Bromide (mg)	16.3 ± 11.6	14.8 ± 8.2	0.631
Salbutamol (mg)	115 ± 98	83 ± 53	0.308
Remission time (days)	11 ± 4	7 ± 4	*0.001*
Duration of hospitalization (days)	15 ± 5	12 ± 4	*0.011*

Italicized p-values are statistically significant, ie. $p < 0.05$

has not been determined. Aspergillus colonization induces sustainable inflammation in the airway, which leads to worsening lung function. Meanwhile, poorer lung function is significantly associated with Aspergillus colonization. However, in clinical practice, ICS are commonly used to control wheezing and airway inflammation, which could also enhance the risk of Aspergillus colonization in the airway. It is concerning that once Aspergillus colonization in the airways of COPD patients is identified, a vicious cycle is established. Unfortunately, no accurate timing, biomarker, or scoring system exists that could determine the optimal antifungal therapy.

There were some limitations to this study: (1) we could not determine the timing of Aspergillus colonization: the acute exacerbation or stable stage; (2) we only conducted this retrospective study without a long-term observation from the beginning of Aspergillus colonization to its causing symptomatic clinical manifestation. Thus, whether Aspergillus colonization could affect the clinical process was still unknown, including lung function decline, the frequency of acute exacerbation, and daily symptoms; and (3) we performed this research in a single center and recruited a small sample of patients.

Conclusions

Our findings show that Aspergillus colonization in the airway could cause significant change in clinical manifestations and treatment outcome of COPD patients. This study provides new insight for clinicians when managing patients with fungal colonization and also indicates the directions for future comprehensive studies, including the development of a reliable and rapid method to accurately identify infection and colonization and to develop a full-scale investigation and treatment strategy of COPD patients with Aspergillus colonization.

Abbreviations

ABPA: Allergic bronchopulomnary aspergillosis; AECOPD: Acute exacerbation of chronic obstructive pulmonary disease; BALF: Bronchoalveolar lavage fluid; COPD: Chronic obstructive pulmonary disease; CPA: Chronic pulmonary aspergillosis; CRP: C-reactive protein; CT: Computed tomography; EOS: Eosinophils; ESR: Erythrocyte sedimentation rate; FEV_1: Forced expiratory volume 1; GOLD: Global initiative for chronic obstructive lung disease; ICS: Inhaled corticosteroids; ICU: Intensive care unit; IPA: Invasive pulmonary aspergillosis; LRT: Lower respiratory tract

Acknowledgments

The authors thank Academician Chen Wang for his guidance and assistance with this work. We acknowledge the China National Center for Protein Sciences Beijing for providing facility support.

Funding

This project was supported by project grant 2012AA02A511 from the National High Technology Research and Development Program, China; grant 2012BAI05B02 from the National Key Technology Research and Development Program, China; grant 81400037 from the National Natural Science Foundation of China; and grant 201302017 from the Public Health Special Research of the Ministry of Health of the People's Republic of China.

Authors' contributions
YL and XT contributed to the conception and design of the study, acquisition of the data, and interpretation of the results and drafted the manuscript. AC contributed to the acquisition of the mycological data and revision of the manuscript for important intellectual content. HX contributed to the acquisition of the bacteriological data and revision of the manuscript for important intellectual content. SZ performed the statistical analysis and revised the manuscript for important intellectual content. All authors read and approved the final manuscript.

Consent for publication
Not applicable.

Competing interests
The authors declare that they have no competing interests.

Author details
[1]Department of Geriatrics, Beijing Hospital, National Center of Gerontology, Beijing 100730, People's Republic of China. [2]Tobacco Medicine and Tobacco Cessation Centre, Center of Respiratory Medicine, China-Japan Friendship Hospital; WHO Collaborating Centre for Tobacco Cessation and Respiratory Diseases Prevention; National Clinical Research Center for Respiratory Diseases, Beijing 100029, People's Republic of China. [3]Department of Laboratory Medicine, Beijing Hospital, Beijing 100730, People's Republic of China. [4]Department of Respiratory and Critical Care Medicine, Beijing Hospital, Beijing 100730, People's Republic of China. [5]Statistics Department, First Hospital of Peking University, Beijing 100034, People's Republic of China.

References
1. WHO. The top 10 causes of death. http://www.who.int/mediacentre/factsheets/fs310/en/. Date last updated: 27 Oct 2016.
2. WHO. Burden of COPD. http://www.who.int/respiratory/copd/burden/en/. Date last updated: 15 Mar 2017.
3. Mathers CD, Loncar D. Projections of global mortality and burden of disease from 2002 to 2030. PLoS Med. 2006;3(11):e442.
4. Banerjee D, Khair OA, Honeybourne D. Impact of sputum bacteria on airway inflammation and health status in clinical stable COPD. Eur Respir J. 2004; 23(5):685–91.
5. Patel IS, Seemungal TAR, Wilks M, Lloyd-Owen SJ, Donaldson GC, Wedzicha JA. Relationship between bacterial colonisation and the frequency, character, and severity of COPD exacerbations. Thorax. 2002;57(9):759–64.
6. Wedzicha JA, Donaldson GC. Exacerbations of chronic obstructive pulmonary disease. Respir Care. 2003;48(12):1204–13.
7. Streifel AJ, Lauer JL, Vesley D, Juni B, Rhame FS. Aspergillus fumigatus and other thermotolerant fungi generated by hospital building demolition. Appl Environ Microbiol. 1983;46(2):375–8.
8. Latgé JP. The pathobiology of aspergillus fumigatus. Trends Microbiol. 2001; 9(8):382–9.
9. Bulpa P, Dive A, Sibille Y. Invasive pulmonary aspergillosis in patients with chronic obstructive pulmonary disease. Eur Respir J. 2007;30(4):782–800.
10. Soubani AO, Chandrasekar PH. The clinical spectrum of pulmonary aspergillosis. Chest. 2002;121(6):1988–99.
11. Latgé JP. Aspergillus fumigatus and aspergillosis. Clin Microbiol Rev. 1999; 12(2):310–50.
12. Pashley CH, Fairs A, Morley JP, et al. Routine processing procedures for isolating filamentous fungi from respiratory sputum samples may underestimate fungal prevalence. Med Mycol. 2012;50(4):433–8.
13. Garnacho-Montero J, Amaya-Villar R, Ortiz-Leyba C, et al. Isolation of Aspergillus spp. from the respiratory tract in critically ill patients: risk factors, clinical presentation and outcome. Crit Care. 2005;9(3):R191–9.
14. Kohansal R, Martinez-Camblor P, Agustí A, Buist AS, Mannino DM, Soriano JB. The natural history of chronic airflow obstruction revisited: an analysis of the Framingham offspring cohort. Am J Respir Crit Care Med. 2009;180(1):3–10.
15. Nyunoya T, Mebratu Y, Contreras A, Delgado M, Chand HS, Tesfaigzi Y. Molecular processes that drive cigarette smoke-induced epithelial cell fate of the lung. Am J Respir Cell Mol Biol. 2014;50(3):471–82.
16. Amitani R, Murayama T, Nawada R, et al. Aspergillus culture filtrates and sputum sols from patients with pulmonary aspergillosis cause damage to human respiratory ciliated epithelium in vitro. Eur Respir J. 1995;8(10):1681–7.
17. Jones JG, Minty BD, Lawler P, Hulands G, Crawley JC, Veall N. Increased alveolar epithelial permeability in cigarette smokers. Lancet. 1980;1(8159):66–8.
18. Hulbert WC, Walker DC, Jackson A, Hogg JC. Airway permeability to horseradish peroxidase in guinea pigs: the repair phase after injury by cigarette smoke. Am Rev Respir Dis. 1981;123(3):320–6.
19. Muquim A, Dial S, Menzies D. Invasive aspergillosis in patients with chronic obstructive pulmonary diseases. Can Respir J. 2005;12(4):199–204.
20. Bafadhel M, McKenna S, Agbetile J, et al. Aspergillus fumigatus during stable state and exacerbations of COPD. Eur Respir J. 2014;43(1):64–71.
21. Urb M, Snarr BD, Wojewodka G, et al. Evolution of the immune response to chronic airway colonization with Aspergillus fumigatus hyphae. Infect Immun. 2015;83(9):3590–600.
22. Saluja R, Metz M, Maurer M. Role and relevance of mast cells in fungal infections. Front Immunol. 2012;3:146.
23. Urb M, Pouliot P, Gravelat FN, Olivier M, Sheppard DC. Aspergillus fumigatus induces immunoglobulin E-independent mast cell degranulation. J Infect Dis. 2009;200(3):464–72.
24. Chaudhary N, Marr KA. Impact of Aspergillus fumigatus in allergic airway diseases. Clin Transl Allergy. 2011;1(1):4.

17

Serum (1→3)-β-D-glucan and galactomannan levels in patients with cystic fibrosis

Johannes Träger[1†], Volker Otto Melichar[2†], Renate Meyer[1], Manfred Rauh[2], Christian Bogdan[1] and Jürgen Held[1*]

Abstract

Background: *Aspergillus fumigatus* is frequently encountered in sputum samples of patients with cystic fibrosis (CF), which traditionally has been interpreted as saprophytic airway colonization. However, this mere bystander role has been challenged by recent data. There is now evidence that *Aspergillus fumigatus* accelerates the decline of pulmonary function. (1→3)-β-D-glucan (BDG) and galactomannan (GM) are highly sensitive fungal biomarkers that are used to diagnose invasive fungal disease. However, their diagnostic value in CF patients is largely unknown.

Methods: We conducted a retrospective cohort study on 104 CF patients to determine whether serum BDG and GM levels correlate with parameters such as *Aspergillus*-positive sputum cultures and lung function.

Results: *Aspergillus fumigatus* was persistently detected in 22 of the 104 CF patients (21%). Mean serum BDG and GM levels in the *Aspergillus*-positive patients were significantly higher than in those without persistent *Aspergillus* detection (89 versus 40 pg/ml [$p = 0.022$] and 0.30 versus 0.15 ODI [$p = 0.013$], respectively). 27 and 7 patients had elevated BDG (≥ 60 pg/ml) or GM levels (> 0.5 ODI), respectivly. BDG and GM levels showed a significant correlation ($p = 0.004$). Patients with increased serum concentrations of BDG were more frequently *Aspergillus*-positive (40.7 versus 14.3%, p = 0.004) and had a significantly lower forced expiratory volume in one second (FEV1) than patients with a normal BDG (61.6 versus 77.1%, $p = 0.007$). In the multivariate analysis, BDG but not GM or the growth of *A. fumigatus*, proved to be an independent predictor for the FEV1.

Conclusions: CF patients with persistent *Aspergillus* detection have elevated BDG and GM levels which ranged between healthy and invasively infected patients. Serum BDG may be superior to GM and fungal culture in predicting an impaired lung function in CF patients.

Keywords: (1→3)-β-D-glucan, Galactomannan, Biomarker, Cystic fibrosis, *Aspergillus*, Allergic bronchopulmonary aspergillosis, ABPA, Aspergillosis, Lung function, FEV1

Background

Cystic fibrosis (CF) is the most frequent lethal autosomal recessive disorder in Caucasians. It is caused by mutations in the cystic fibrosis transmembrane conductance regulator (CFTR) gene leading to impaired ion transport across epithelial cells. The disease affects primarily the exocrine glands, resulting in pancreatic insufficiency and progressive pulmonary disease; the latter is the major cause of morbidity and mortality in CF patients. Within the lungs, highly viscous sputum facilitates the colonization and infection of the lower respiratory tract with various microorganisms [1].

While the role of bacterial pathogens, like *Staphylococcus aureus*, *Pseudomonas aeruginosa* or *Burkholderia cepacia* complex, for the progression of the disease is well established, far less is known about the impact of chronic airway colonization with fungi. *Aspergillus fumigatus*, *Scedosporium* species, *Candida albicans* and *Exophiala dermatitidis* are frequently encountered in sputum samples of CF patients [2]. In particular, the traditional view on *A. fumigatus,* which has been regarded as saprophytic microorganism with doubtful clinical significance, is challenged by recent data. There

* Correspondence: juergen.held@uk-erlangen.de
†Equal contributors
[1]Mikrobiologisches Institut - Klinische Mikrobiologie, Immunologie und Hygiene, Universitätsklinikum Erlangen und Friedrich-Alexander-Universität (FAU) Erlangen-Nürnberg, Wasserturmstr. 3/5, 91054 Erlangen, Germany
Full list of author information is available at the end of the article

is evidence that chronic *A. fumigatus* colonization is associated with an increased risk of hospitalization for pulmonary exacerbation and lower lung function and that this effect is aggravated by *P. aeruginosa* co-infection [3, 4]. Furthermore, it seems that antifungal therapy is of benefit for patients who are non-responsive to antibiotics and that the administration of itraconazole to *A. fumigatus*-sensitized CF patients can improve lung function [5, 6].

Galactomannan (GM) is a major component of the fungal cell wall. It is primarily detected in the serum or bronchoalveolar lavage fluid specimens of patients with invasive aspergillosis [7]. Another fungal antigen used for this purpose is (1→3)-β-D-glucan (BDG). BDG differs in several aspects from GM. Firstly, it is produced by all medically relevant fungi (e.g. *Candida* spp., *Aspergillus* spp., *Pneumocystis jirovecii*) apart from zygomycetes and *Cryptococcus neoformans* which contain no or only low amounts of BDG in their cell walls [8]. Secondly, BDG has superior sensitivity for diagnosis of invasive aspergillosis compared to serum GM [9].

Only little is known about serum BDG and GM levels in patients with CF. Because of their high sensitivity, BDG and/or GM measurements might help to identify patients with fungus-associated morbidity. Therefore, we initiated a retrospective study in order to analyze causal relationships between clinical and microbiological parameters and BDG- as well as GM-antigenemia.

Methods

Study population

We conducted a retrospective cohort study at the University Hospital Erlangen, Germany, a 1400-bed tertiary care hospital. All patients with CF (children, adolescents and adults), who presented to the CF outpatient clinic between September 2015 and October 2016, were enrolled. Patients with a history of lung transplantation were excluded. As part of the routine diagnostic workup paired respiratory and serum samples were taken.

Microbiological analyses

Respiratory samples were analyzed for the growth of bacteria (e.g. *S. aureus, P. aeruginosa*) and fungi (e.g. *A. fumigatus*) using Columbia blood agar plates, chocolate agar plates, endo agar plates and Sabouraud dextrose agar plates with 0.5 mg/ml chloramphenicol. If necessary, the samples were pretreated with dithiothreitol at a final concentration of 50 µg/ml. The agar plates were then incubated for at least seven days at 37 °C in ambient air with 5% CO_2 for the culture of bacteria and at 28 °C in ambient air for the culture of fungi. Relevant microorganisms were differentiated to the species level by Matrix Assisted Laser Desorption Ionization - Time of Flight Mass Spectrometry (MALDI-TOF-MS; Bruker Daltonik GmbH, Germany). Filamentous fungi were differentiated by microscopy of a lactophenol cotton blue wet mount preparation.

Serum samples were tested for *Aspergillus*-specific antibodies (Aspergillose Fumouze, Fumouze Diagnostics, France), *Aspergillus*-specific IgE, recombinant *Aspergillus* antigens f4 and f6 [rAsp f4 IgE, rAsp f6 IgE] (ImmunoCAP 250, Thermo Fisher Scientific, Sweden) and IgG against alkaline protease, elastase and exotoxin A of *P. aeruginosa* (Mediagnost GmbH, Germany). The sera were then stored at – 20 °C. In October 2016, the stored samples were tested in batch for their content of BDG (Fungitell® assay; Associates of Cape Cod, USA) and GM (Platelia™ *Aspergillus* Ag assay; Bio-Rad, France). Both assays were performed according to the manufacturer's instructions. BDG levels above the upper validation limit were diluted and retested. BDG levels below the lower validation limit were calculated by extrapolation. In July 2017, the same serum samples were tested for human fatty acid binding protein 2 (FABP2) using the Quantikine ELISA human FABP2/I-FABP kit (R&D Systems Europe, UK) according to the manufacturer's instructions. The use of these sera was approved by the local ethics committee (application number 7-17B).

Clinical data and classification of patients

Demographic data and clinical information (body mass index [BMI], cough frequency, sputum production, annual number of pulmonary exacerbations, anti-infective therapy, corticosteroid use, exocrine pancreatic insufficiency, CF-related *Diabetes mellitus* [CFRD], CF-related liver disease [CFLD], forced expiratory volume in 1 s [$FEV1_{predicted}$] at serum sampling, and immunological results (C-reactive protein [CRP], leucocyte count [WBC], total serum IgG and IgE) were obtained from all patients analyzed. Following the Global Initiative for Chronic Obstructive Lung Disease (GOLD) classification of severity of airflow obstruction, the study population was divided into patients with mild or no airflow limitation ($FEV1_{predicted} \geq 80\%$) and patients with moderate to very severe airflow limitation ($FEV1_{predicted} < 80\%$) at the time of serum sampling. Furthermore, on the basis of the Leed's criteria for chronic *P. aeruginosa* infection [10], patients were classified according to their respiratory culture results during the past two years in persistently colonized (growth of *A. fumigatus* in > 50% of total samples or at least in all of the last three samples before serum sampling), intermittently colonized (detection of *A. fumigatus* that does not fulfil the criteria for persistently colonized patients) and not colonized (no detection of *A. fumigatus*).

Statistical analysis

Statistical analysis was performed using SPSS-V24 (SPSS Inc., USA) and MedCalc Statistical Software-V16.8 (MedCalc Software bvba, Belgium). Data are given as mean +/–

standard deviation (SD) or median with interquartile range (IQR). Receiver-operating-characteristic (ROC)-analysis was used to evaluate the ability of BDG and GM to distinguish between *Aspergillus*-positive and *Aspergillus*-negative patients. The highest Youden index indicated the optimal cut-off. As BDG and GM values were not normally distributed, the chi-square test, the Mann-Whitney-U test and the Spearman coefficient of correlation were used for comparison of variables. Differences were considered significant when p values were < 0.05.

Results

Study population

The local cystic fibrosis cohort consisted of 137 patients. Archived serum samples were available from 107 patients. Three patients had to be excluded, because BDG-testing repeatedly produced discrepant results ($n = 2$) or a respiratory tract specimen for microbiological analysis was not taken at the day of serum sampling ($n = 1$). Thus, 104 patients were included in the study.

Demographic data, clinical and microbiological results for all patients as well as for subgroups (stratified according to $FEV1_{predicted}$ values at the time of serum sampling, the growth of *A. fumigatus* and the concentration of serum BDG and GM) are shown in Tables 1 and 2. Correlations of $FEV1_{predicted}$ values, BDG and GM concentrations with continuous clinical and microbiological parameters are given in Table 3 and Fig. 1.

Microbiological predictors of an impaired $FEV1_{predicted}$ value

Fifty-five patients (56.7%) of our CF cohort suffered from moderate to very severe airflow limitation ($FEV1_{predicted} < 80\%$), whereas 42 patients (43.3%) had only mild or no airflow limitation ($FEV1_{predicted} \geq 80\%$). In the univariate analysis, the group of patients with a $FEV1_{predicted} < 80\%$ was significantly older (24.0 versus 15.7 years, $p < 0.001$), had a significantly higher serum concentration of BDG (68 versus 32 pg/ml, $p = 0.003$), but not of GM (0.22 versus 0.14 optical density index [ODI], $p = 0.150$), and contained a higher percentage of patients with an elevated BDG (34.5% versus 14.3%, $p = 0.024$). In addition, this group had higher levels of *A. fumigatus*-specific IgE and there was a trend towards a higher percentage of patients with persistent *A. fumigatus* detection (29.1 versus 14.3%, $p = 0.084$) (Table 1).

Patients with a $FEV1_{predicted} < 80\%$ were more often colonized by *P. aeruginosa* and less likely colonized by *S. aureus*. *Pseudomonas aeruginosa*-specific antibodies, WBC, CRP, total IgG and IgE, cough frequency, number of pulmonary exacerbations within the last 12 months and consumption of systemic and nebulized antibiotics before and after serum sampling were also significantly elevated in this group (Table 1).

To examine, which parameters are independent predictors of the lung function, we performed a multivariate analysis with $FEV1_{predicted}$ as dependent variable and all parameters with a significant difference in the univariate analysis as independent variables. The results are shown in Table 4. BDG, WBC, *S. aureus*- and *P. aeruginosa*-colonization turned out to be independent predictors of the $FEV1_{predicted}$ in the multivariate analysis. These parameters were able to explain 52.6% of the variation of $FEV1_{predicted}$ which corresponds to a strong effect according to Cohen [11]. An increase of the BDG concentration of 10 pg/ml was associated with an average loss in $FEV1_{predicted}$ of 1%.

Characteristics of patients positive for *A. fumigatus*

Analysis of fungal cultures revealed that 22 patients (21.2%) were persistently colonized/infected with *A. fumigatus*, whereas one patient was only transiently colonized and 81 patients (77.9%) were negative for *A. fumigatus* (Table1). In addition, *Candida* spp. were detected in 55 patients (52.9%), *Penicillium* spp. in three patients (2.9%), *Scedosporium* sp. in two patients (1.9%) and *Lomentospora prolificans, Exophiala dermatitidis* and *Trichosporon asahii* in one patient each.

The mean serum concentrations of BDG and GM in patients that were persistently positive for *A. fumigatus* were significantly higher (89 pg/ml and 0.30 ODI, respectively) than in patients without persistent growth of *A. fumigatus* (40 pg/ml [$p = 0.022$] and 0.15 ODI [$p = 0.013$], respectively) (Fig. 2). Although the difference in BDG concentrations between the two subgroups was small, there were significantly more patients with elevated BDG levels ($\geq$ 60 pg/ml) in the *A. fumigatus*-positive subgroup (50.0 versus 19.5%, $p = 0.004$) (Table 1). ROC-analysis for discrimination between *A. fumigatus*-positive and -negative patients gave an area under the ROC curve (AUC) of 0.658 (95%-CI: 0.559–0.748) for BDG and 0.635 (0.535–0.727) for GM (Fig. 3). The AUC of BDG and GM was not significantly different ($p = 0.760$). The cut-off with the highest Youden index was $\geq$60 pg/ml for BDG (sensitivity 50.0%, specificity 80.5%) and $>$ 0.1 ODI for GM (sensitivity 45.5%, specificity 78.0%). In addition, patients with persistent *A. fumigatus* detection were significantly older (24.8 versus 17.9 years, $p = 0.001$), had a higher BMI (21.6 versus 19.2 kg/m^2, $p = 0.006$) and were more often colonized with *P. aeruginosa* (59.1 versus 26.8%, 0.004) (Table 1). The $FEV1_{predicted}$ was lower in patients with a positive culture for *A. fumigatus* (64.2 versus 75.7%, $p = 0.057$) and they were treated more frequently with nebulized antibiotics in the year before, at and during the 6 months after serum sampling. Although the frequency of systemic antibiotic therapy was also higher in the *A. fumigatus*-positive subgroup, these differences were not statistically significant.

Table 1 Patient demographics, microbiological and clinical results stratified after FEV_1 at serum sampling and persistent *A. fumigatus* detection

	All patients	FEV_1 at serum sampling			Persistent *A. fumigatus* detection		
	(*n* = 104)	(< 80% pred.) (*n* = 55)	(≥80% pred.) (*n* = 42)	*P* value	No (*n* = 82)	Yes (*n* = 22)	*P* value
Age [years (min-max)]	19.3 (4–51)	24.0 (6–51)	15.7 (7–31)	< 0.001	17.9 (4–51)	24.8 (10–51)	0.001
Sex [female/male]	43/61	22/33	17/25	0.962	32/50	11/11	0.353
BMI [kg/m^2 (± STD)]	19.7 (± 3.9)	20.4 (± 3.6)	19.2 (± 3.6)	0.114	19.2 (± 3.7)	21.6 (± 3.8)	0.006
Mean BDG [pg/ml (± STD)]	50 (± 84)	68 (± 100)	32 (± 57)	0.003	40 (± 63)	89 (± 131)	0.022
Median BDG [pg/ml (IQR)]	22 (3–62)	37 (12–82)	11 (0–42)		18 (2–48)	50 (14–115)	
BDG [normal/elevated, (% elevated)]	77/27 (26.0%)	36/19 (34.5%)	36/6 (14.3%)	0.024	66/16 (19.5%)	11/11 (50.0%)	0.004
Mean GM [ODI (± STD)]	0.18 (± 0.22)	0.22 (± 0.28)	0.14 (± 0.10)	0.150	0.15 (± 0.12)	0.30 (± 0.40)	0.013
Median GM [ODI (IQR)]	0.10 (0.1–0.2)	0.10 (0.1–0.2)	0.10 (0.1–0.1)		0.10 (0.1–0.1)	0.10 (0.1–0.3)	
GM [normal/elevated, (% elevated)]	97/7 (6.7%)	49/6 (10.9%)	41/1 (2.4%)	0.108	78/4 (4.9%)	19/3 (13.6%)	0.145
Persistent *A. fumigatus* detection [no. of patients (%)]	22 (21.2%)	16 (29.1%)	6 (14.3%)	0.084	–	–	–
A. fumigatus-specific antibodies [normal/elevated, (% elevated)]	100/4 (3.8%)	52/3 (5.5%)	41/1 (2.4%)	0.451	78/4 (4.9%)	22/0 (0%)	0.291
A. fumigatus-specific IgE level [kU/l, (± STD)]	3.8 (± 9.9)	5.2 (± 11.3)	2.3 (± 8.2)	0.004	4.5 (± 10.9)	1.1 (± 2.0)	0.687
rAsp f4-IgE level [kUA/l, (± STD)]	0.5 (± 2.5)	0.7 (± 3.1)	0.3 (± 1.5)	0.073	0.6 (± 2.7)	0.1 (± 0.2)	0.879
rAsp f6-IgE level [kUA/l (± STD)]	0.5 (± 2.3)	0.7 (± 3.0)	0.1 (± 0.7)	0.245	0.6 (± 2.5)	0.0 (± 0.0)	0.118
S. aureus detection [no. of patients (%)]	11 (10.6%)	2 (3.6%)	7 (16.7%)	0.028	10 (12.2%)	1 (4.5%)	0.300
P. aeruginosa detection [no. of patients (%)]	35 (33.7%)	31 (56.4%)	4 (9.5%)	< 0.001	22 (26.8%)	13 (59.1%)	0.004
P. aeruginosa-specific antibodies [normal/elevated, (% elevated)]							
against alkaline protease	70/14 (16.7%)	26/12 (31.6%)	38/1 (2.6%)	0.001	62/10 (13.9%)	8/4 (33.3%)	0.094
against elastase	69/15 (17.9%)	25/13 (34.2%)	38/1 (2.6%)	< 0.001	60/12 (16.7%)	9/3 (25.0%)	0.485
against exotoxin A	65/19 (22.6%)	24/14 (36.8%)	34/5 (12.8%)	0.015	58/14 (19.4%)	7/5 (41.7%)	0.088
WBC [× 10^3/μl (± STD)]	9.1 (± 4.3)	10.1 (± 5.2)	7.5 (± 2.4)	0.002	8.8 (± 3.3)	10.1 (± 7.0)	0.891
CRP [mg/l (± STD)]	6.5 (± 19.1)	11.6 (± 25.1)	0.7 (± 1.0)	< 0.001	4.6 (± 12.2)	13.6 (± 33.6)	0.114
Total IgG [lowered/normal/elevated]	12/62/25	3/26/21	7/31/4	0.002	12/49/19	0/13/6	0.187
Total IgE level [normal/elevated, (% elevated)]	65/37 (36.3%)	27/26 (49.1%)	33/9 (21.4%)	0.006	54/27	11/10	0.225
Fatty acid-binding protein 2 [pg/ml (± STD)]	2407 (± 1471)	2279 (± 1429)	2565 (± 1524)	0.248	2540 (± 1574)	1889 (± 871)	0.115
FEV_1 at serum sampling [% predicted (± STD)]	73.1 (± 24.1)	55.8 (± 15.9)	95.8 (± 9.9)	–	75.7 (± 23.9)	64.2 (± 23.1)	0.057
Cough frequency [none/temporarily/permanently/at night]	11/64/19/6	1/33/14/4	8/28/4/1	0.007	11/50/16/4	0/14/3/2	0.278
Number of pulmonary exacerbations within the last 12 months	0.56 (± 0.77)	0.76 (± 0.90)	0.40 (± 0.55)	0.044	0.52 (± 0.72)	0.74 (± 0.93)	0.293
Systemic antibiotic therapy at serum sampling [no. of patients (%)]	30 (28.8%)	19 (34.5%)	10 (23.8%)	0.252	23 (28.0%)	7 (31.8%)	0.729
Systemic antibiotic therapy courses (no. (± STD)							
12 month before serum sampling	1.6 (± 2.0)	2.2 (± 2.3)	0.9 (± 1.1)	< 0.001	1.4 (± 1.6)	2.2 (± 3.0)	0.477
6 month after serum sampling	1.0 (± 1.4)	1.3 (± 1.7)	0.5 (± 0.8)	0.008	0.8 (± 1.1)	1.5 (± 2.4)	0.314

Table 1 Patient demographics, microbiological and clinical results stratified after FEV_1 at serum sampling and persistent *A. fumigatus* detection *(Continued)*

	All patients	FEV_1 at serum sampling			Persistent *A. fumigatus* detection		
	(*n* = 104)	(< 80% pred.) (*n* = 55)	(≥80% pred.) (*n* = 42)	*P* value	No (*n* = 82)	Yes (*n* = 22)	*P* value
Nebulized antibiotic [none/temporarily/permanently]							
12 month before serum sampling	58/16/30	18/9/28	33/7/2	< 0.001	54/11/17	4/5/13	< 0.001
at serum sampling	51/38	14/34	30/4	< 0.001	48/23	3/15	< 0.001
6 month after serum sampling	57/21/26	17/14/24	33/7/2	< 0.001	52/16/14	5/5/15	0.001
Inhaled corticosteroids [no. of patients (%)]	14 (14.6%)	9 (18.4%)	5 (12.5%)	0.449	9 (11.7%)	5 (26.3%)	0.106
Exocrine pancreatic insufficiency [no. of patients (%)]	93 (89.4%)	50 (90.9%)	39 (92.9%)	0.730	72 (87.8%)	21 (95.5%)	0.300
CF-related diabetes mellitus [no. of patients (%)]	11 (10.6%)	8 (14.5%)	3 (7.1%)	0.255	9 (11.0%)	2 (9.1%)	0.799
CF-related liver disease [no. of patients (%)]	30 (28.8%)	16 (29.1%)	14 (33.3%)	0.654	22 (27.8%)	8 (32.0%)	0.729

FEV1 **forced expiratory volume in 1 s,** ***BMI*** **body mass index,** ***STD*** **standard deviation,** ***BDG*** **(1→3)-β-D-glucan,** ***IQR*** **interquartile range,** ***GM*** **galactomannan,** ***ODI*** **optical density index,** ***WBC*** **white blood cell count,** ***CRP*** **C-reactive protein,** ***no*** **number,** ***CF*** **cystic fibrosis**

Table 2 Patient demographics, clinical and microbiological results stratified after serum BDG and GM positivity

	All patients	Serum BDG level			Serum GM level		
	(n = 104)	Normal (< 60) (*n* = 77)	Elevated (≥60) (*n* = 27)	*P* value	Normal (< 0.5) (*n* = 97)	Elevated (≥0.5) (n = 7)	*P* value
Age [years (min-max)]	19.3 (4–51)	18.1 (4–48)	22.7 (4–51)	0.079	18.6 (4–51)	29.6 (14–51)	0.047
Sex [female/male]	43/61	31/46	12/15	0.704	40/57	3/4	0.933
BMI [kg/m^2 (± STD)]	19.7 (± 3.9)	19.8 (± 3.9)	19.4 (± 3.9)	0.739	19.8 (± 3.9)	19.3 (± 2.7)	0.897
Mean BDG [pg/ml (± STD)]	50 (± 84)	16 (± 17)	148 (± 116)	–	50 (± 86)	57 (± 26)	0.044
Median BDG [pg/ml (IQR)]	22 (3–62)	11 (0–28)	108 (69–179)		20 (3–56)	59 (48–68)	
BDG [normal/elevated, (% elevated)]	77/27 (26.0%)	–	–	–	73/24 (24.7%)	4/3 (42.9%)	0.291
Mean GM [ODI (± STD)]	0.18 (± 0.22)	0.15 (± 0.17)	0.24 (± 0.32)	0.013	0.13 (± 0.1)	0.89 (± 0.4)	–
Median GM [ODI (IQR)]	0.10 (0.1–0.2)	0.10 (0.10)	0.10 (0.10)		0.10 (0.10)	0.70 (0.6–1.2)	
GM [normal/elevated, (% elevated)]	97/7 (6.7%)	73/4 (5.2%)	24/3 (11.1%)	0.291	–	–	–
Persistent *A. fumigatus* detection [no. of patients (%)]	22 (21.2%)	11 (14.3%)	11 (40.7%)	0.004	19 (19.6%)	3 (42.9%)	0.145
S. aureus colonization/infection [no. of patients (%)]	11 (10.6%)	10 (13.0%)	1 (3.7%)	0.177	11 (11.3%)	0 (0.0%)	0.346
P. aeruginosa colonization/infection [no. of patients (%)]	35 (33.7%)	23 (29.9%)	12 (44.4%)	0.168	30 (30.9%)	5 (71.4%)	0.029
P. aeruginosa-specific antibodies [normal/elevated, (% elevated)]							
against alkaline protease	70/14 (16.7%)	52/11 (17.5%)	18/3 (14.3%)	0.735	67/12 (15.2%)	3/2 (40.0%)	0.149
against elastase	69/15 (17.9%)	52/11 (17.5%)	17/4 (19.0%)	0.869	67/12 (15.2%)	2/3 (60.0%)	0.011
against exotoxin A	65/19 (22.6%)	48/15 (23.8%)	17/4 (19.0%)	0.651	65/14 (17.7%)	0/5 (100.0%)	< 0.001
A. fumigatus-specific antibodies [normal/elevated, (% elevated)]	100/4 (3.8%)	74/3 (3.9%)	26/1 (3.7%)	0.964	93/4 (4.1%)	7/0 (0.0%)	0.584
A. fumigatus-specific IgE level [kU/l, (± STD)]	3.8 (± 9.9)	3.6 (± 9.5)	4.4 (± 11.2)	0.777	4.0 (± 10.2)	1.8 (± 1.7)	0.051
rAsp f4-IgE level	0.5 (± 2.5)	0.2 (± 1.1)	1.3 (± 4.5)	0.768	0.5 (± 2.5)	0.3 (± 0.4)	0.048
rAsp f6-IgE level	0.5 (± 2.3)	0.2 (± 0.8)	1.2 (± 4.3)	0.930	0.5 (± 2.4)	0.0 (± 0.0)	0.391
WBC [$\times10^3$/μl (± STD)]	9.1 (± 4.3)	8.6 (± 3.3)	10.3 (± 6.3)	0.183	9.0 (± 4.5)	9.2 (± 2.3)	0.529
CRP [mg/l (± STD)]	6.5 (± 19.1)	4.5 (± 12.2)	12.1 (± 30.9)	0.125	6.5 (± 19.6)	6.6 (± 9.0)	0.506
Total IgG [lowered/normal/elevated]	12/62/25	9/49/17	3/13/8	0.553	12/58/22	0/4/3	0.392
Total IgE level [normal/elevated]	65/37	53/24	12/13	0.060	61/34	4/3	0.707
Fatty acid-binding protein 2 [pg/ml (± STD)]	2411 (± 1481)	2468 (± 1588)	2236 (± 1105)	0.712	2373 (± 1469)	2917 (± 1673)	0.392
FEV_1 at serum sampling [% predicted (± STD)]	73.1 (± 24.1)	77.1 (±22.8)	61.6 (±25.5)	0.007	73.6 (± 24.7)	66.1 (± 14.1)	0.407
Cough frequency [none/temporarily/permanently/at night]	11/64/19/6	11/49/11/3	0/15/8/3	0.038	11/58/18/6	0/6/1/0	0.589
Number of pulmonary exacerbations within the last 12 months	0.56 (± 0.77)	0.46 (± 0.72)	0.85 (± 0.83)	0.008	0.57 (± 0.78)	0.43 (± 0.54)	0.762
Systemic antibiotic therapy at serum sampling [no. of patients (%)]	30 (28.8%)	18 (23.4%)	12 (44.4%)	0.038	28 (28.9%)	2 (28.6%)	0.987
Systemic antibiotic therapy courses (no. (± STD)							
12 month before serum sampling	1.6 (± 2.0)	1.4 (± 1.8)	2.0 (± 2.4)	0.415	1.5 (± 2.0)	2.1 (± 1.6)	0.120
6 month after serum sampling	1.0 (± 1.4)	0.8 (± 1.1)	1.5 (± 2.1)	0.047	1.0 (± 1.5)	1.0 (± 1.0)	0.619

Table 2 Patient demographics, clinical and microbiological results stratified after serum BDG and GM positivity *(Continued)*

	All patients	Serum BDG level			Serum GM level		
	(n = 104)	Normal (< 60) (*n* = 77)	Elevated (≥60) (*n* = 27)	*P* value	Normal (< 0.5) (*n* = 97)	Elevated (≥0.5) (n = 7)	*P* value
Nebulized antibiotic [none/temporarily/permanently]							
12 month before serum sampling	58/16/30	49/10/18	9/6/12	0.024	56/16/25	2/0/5	0.032
at serum sampling	51/38	43/25	8/13	0.042	49/33	2/5	0.109
6 month after serum sampling	57/21/26	46/15/16	11/6/10	0.173	55/20/22	2/1/4	0.124
Inhaled corticosteroids [no. of patients (%)]	14 (14.6%)	10 (13.0%)	4 (14.8%)	0.662	13 (13.4%)	1 (14.3%)	0.982
Exocrine pancreatic insufficiency [no. of patients (%)]	93 (89.4%)	67 (87.0%)	26 (96.3%)	0.177	86 (88.7%)	7 (100%)	0.346
CF-related diabetes mellitus [no. of patients (%)]	11 (10.6%)	7 (9.1%)	4 (14.8%)	0.405	9 (9.3%)	2 (28.6%)	0.109
CF-related liver disease [no. of patients (%)]	30 (28.8%)	25 (32.5%)	5 (18.5%)	0.169	28 (28.9%)	2 (28.6%)	0.987

BDG (1→3)-β-D-glucan, *GM* galactomannan, *BMI* body mass index, *STD* standard deviation, *IQR* interquartile range, *ODI* optical density index, *WBC* white blood cell count, *CRP* C-reactive protein, *no* number, *FEV1* forced expiratory volume in 1 s, *CF* cystic fibrosis

Table 3 Correlation of FEV_1 at serum sampling, BDG and GM with continuous clinical and microbiological parameters (Spearman-Rho test)

	FEV_1 at serum sampling			BDG			GM		
	Correlation Coefficient r	Significance level *p*-value	Coefficient of determination r^2	Correlation Coefficient r	Significance level *p*-value	Coefficient of determination r^2	Correlation Coefficient r	Significance level p-value	Coefficient of determination r^2
Age	−0.382	< 0.001	0.146	0.187	0.057	0.035	0.186	0.058	0.035
BMI	−0.028	0.787	0.001	- 0.075	0.452	0.006	−0.041	0.682	0.002
FEV_1 at serum sampling	–	–	–	- 0.460	< 0.001	0.212	−0.213	0.037	0.045
No. of pulmonary exacerbations (last 12 month)	−0.301	0.004	0.091	0.266	0.009	0.071	0.024	0.818	0.001
Systemic antibiotic therapy courses									
12 month before serum sampling	−0.438	< 0.001	0.192	0.281	0.004	0.079	0.186	0.059	0.035
6 month after serum sampling	−0.338	0.001	0.114	0.277	0.005	0.077	0.232	0.019	0.054
WBC	−0.450	< 0.001	0.203	0.246	0.012	0.061	0.168	0.091	0.028
CRP	−0.621	< 0.001	0.386	0.267	0.006	0.071	0.131	0.188	0.017
BDG	−0.460	< 0.001	0.212	–	–	–	0.281	0.004	0.079
GM	− 0.213	0.037	0.045	0.281	0.004	0.079	–	–	–
A. fumigatus-specific IgE level	−0.311	0.002	0.097	0.181	0.070	0.033	0.062	0.154	0.004
rAsp f4-IgE level	−0.203	0.051	0.041	0.151	0.134	0.023	0.041	0.688	0.002
rAsp f6-IgE level	−0.066	0.532	0.004	0.051	0.613	0.003	−0.179	0.074	0.032
Fatty acid-binding protein 2	0.159	0.125	0.025	0.044	0.666	0.002	0.072	0.475	0.005

FEV1 forced expiratory volume in 1 s, *BDG* (1→3)-β-D-glucan, *GM* galactomannan, *BMI* body mass index, *no* number, *WBC* white blood cell count, *CRP* C-reactive protein

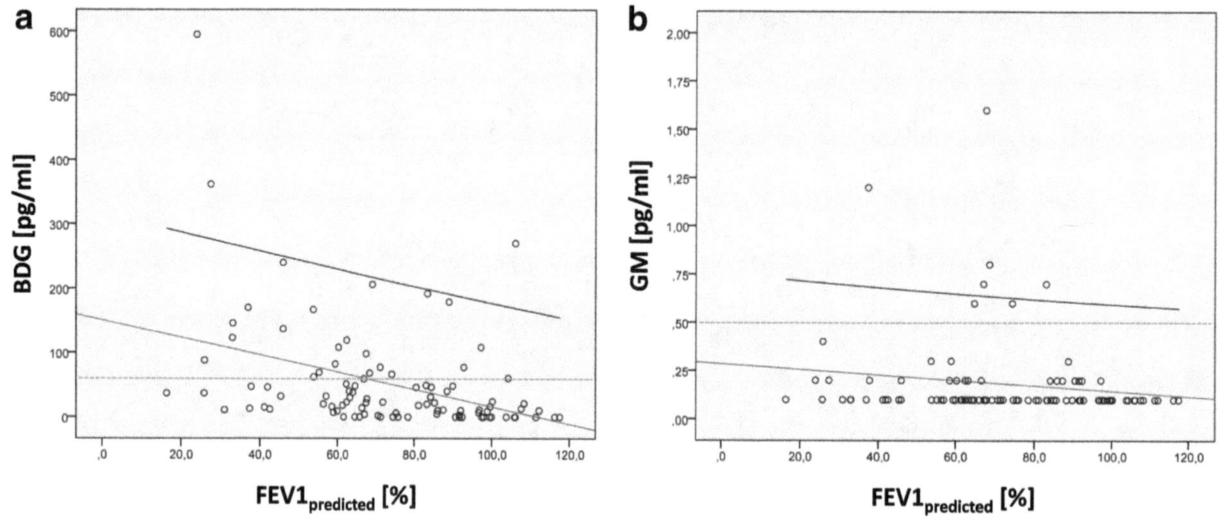

Fig. 1 Correlation of the FEV1 at serum sampling with BDG and GM. BDG (**a**.) and GM (**b**.) show a significant correlation with the FEV1 ($p < 0.001$ and 0.037, respectively). The effect size is 0.5 for BDG and 0.2 for GM, respectively. This corresponds to a medium effect for BDG and a small effect for GM according to Cohen [11]. The regression line is depicted in red, the 95%-confidence interval in black and the manufacturer's cut-off value for invasive fungal disease in green. FEV1: forced expiratory volume in 1 s; BDG: (1→3)-β-D-glucan; GM: galactomannan

Interestingly, none of the *Aspergillus*-specific antibodies was significantly elevated in *A. fumigatus*-positive patients (Table 1).

Characteristics of patients with elevated BDG and GM serum concentrations

To further investigate possible differences in the diagnostic value of fungal cultures versus biomarker measurements, we also analyzed the association of BDG and GM with clinical parameters. Of our CF cohort, 27 patients (26.0%) had elevated BDG levels (median 108 pg/ml, IQR 69–179) and 7 patients (6.7%) elevated GM levels (median ODI 0.7, IQR 0.6–1.2). Patients with an elevated serum BDG (≥ 60 pg/ml) had a significantly higher serum GM (0.24 versus 0.15, $p = 0.013$) than patients with a normal BDG and vice versa ($p = 0.044$) (Table 2). BDG and GM levels showed a significant correlation but with a very weak effect size (Table 3).

Patients with an elevated serum BDG were more frequently *A. fumigatus*-positive (40.7 versus 14.3%, $p = 0.004$). They had a significantly lower $FEV1_{predicted}$ than patients with a normal BDG (61.6 versus 77.1%, $p = 0.007$) and BDG levels correlated inversely with the paired $FEV1_{predicted}$ (Table 4). Furthermore, patients with an elevated BDG tended to be older (22.7 versus 18.1 years, $p = 0.079$), had a significantly higher cough rate and more pulmonary exacerbations during the last year. They had received more frequently a nebulized antibiotic, had a higher probability of systemic and nebulized antibiotic therapy at serum sampling and were treated more often with systemic antibiotics during the 6 months follow-up (Table 2).

Table 4 Multivariate analysis with $FEV1_{predicted}$ at serum sampling as dependent variable

Independent variables	Regression coefficient	*p*-value	R^2 corr.	Effect size f
Age	−0.073	0.772	52.6%	1.05 (strong effect)
BDG	−0.098	0.002		
Persistent *A. fumigatus* detection	−2.951	0.562		
A. fumigatus-specific IgE level	0.045	0.810		
S. aureus detection	16.337	0.011		
P. aeruginosa detection	−13.628	0.023		
WBC	−2.911	< 0.001		
CRP	−0.015	0.933		
Systemic antibiotic therapy within the last 12 month	− 1.939	0.115		
Nebulized antibiotic within the last 12 month	0.890	0.832		

FEV1 forced expiratory volume in 1 s, *BDG* (1→3)-β-D-glucan, *WBC* white blood cell count, *CRP* C-reactive protein, R^2 coefficient of determination

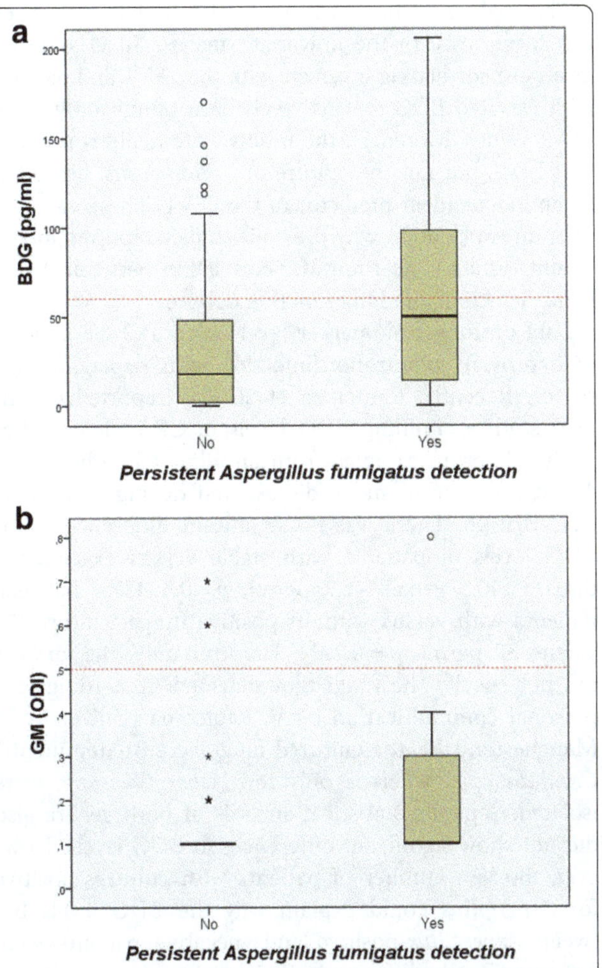

Fig. 2 Box-Plots of BDG (**a**) and GM (**b**) results stratified by persistent *A. fumigatus* detection. The red dotted line indicates the manufacturer's cut-off value for the biomarker. The small circles depict outliers and the stars extreme outliers. For better display not all extreme outliers are shown. BDG: (1→3)-β-D-glucan; GM: galactomannan

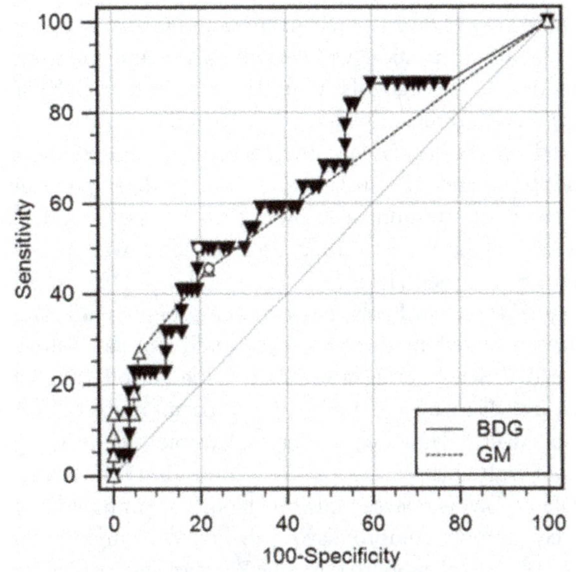

Fig. 3 Receiver-operating-characteristic (ROC)-analysis for discrimination between *A. fumigatus*-positive and -negative patients. The cut-off with the highest Youden index (black circles) was ≥60 pg/ml for BDG (sensitivity 50.0%, specificity 80.5%) and > 0.1 ODI for GM (sensitivity 45.5%, specificity 78.0%). The area under the ROC-curve was not significantly different for BDG and GM (0.658 versus 0.635, $p = 0.760$). BDG: (1→3)-β-D-glucan; GM: galactomannan

Patients with elevated GM levels (> 0.5 ODI) were also older and received more often nebulized antibiotics during the last year. However, in contrast to BDG, patients with an elevated serum concentration of GM showed higher levels of *A. fumigatus*-specific IgE and significantly lower levels of rAsp f4-IgE. Interestingly, patients with an elevated GM were more frequently colonized/infected with *P. aeruginosa* and showed more often elevated antibody levels against *P. aeruginosa* elastase and exotoxin A (Table 2).

Most importantly, patients with elevated GM levels did not have significantly reduced $FEV1_{predicted}$ values (66.1% versus 73.6%, $p = 0.407$). However, this was only the case if the cut-off value was used that is recommended for the diagnosis of invasive fungal disease (ODI ≥ 0.5). After applying the cut-off calculated by our ROC-analysis (ODI > 0.1), patients with elevated GM levels ($n = 18$) showed significantly reduced $FEV1_{predicted}$ values (65.4% versus 76.1%, $p = 0.042$).

Discussion

Aspergillus fumigatus is cultured from respiratory samples of CF patients with a prevalence of 6–57% [2]. There is an ongoing debate whether its presence is contributing to the decline of pulmonary function in these patients [12]. If this were the case, it would have far-reaching implications because CF patients might profit from antifungal therapy.

In our cohort, 21.2% of patients were persistently colonized or infected with *A. fumigatus*. Univariate analysis revealed that these patients were in a more advanced stage of disease, i.e. they were older, had a higher BMI, were more often colonized or infected with *P. aeruginosa*, were treated more frequently with nebulized but not systemic antibiotics and, most importantly, had a lower $FEV1_{predicted}$ at serum sampling. Similar findings concerning the association between culture positivity for *Aspergillus* and increasing age [13–15], lower BMI [13], detection of *P. aeruginosa* [13, 16], exposure to nebulized antibiotics [13, 14, 17–19] and reduced FEV1 [3, 4, 13] were reported in the past. However, there are also studies that could not find such an association between the detection of *Aspergillus* spp. and lung function [18, 20]. So far, the reasons for these conflicting results are unclear.

In the present study, we performed for the first time a detailed correlative analysis of BDG and GM antigenemia, colonization/infection with *A. fumigatus* and pulmonary function in CF patients. Our data shows that BDG and GM were significantly higher in *Aspergillus*-positive compared to *Aspergillus*-negative patients (BDG 89 versus 40 pg/ml and GM 0.3 versus 0.15 ODI, respectively). These concentrations are lower than the BDG and GM levels that have been observed in patients with invasive pulmonary aspergillosis (186 pg/ml and 0.70 ODI, respectively) [21]. Accordingly, most of our patients with *Aspergillus* detected in their airways would not fall into the category "serum antigen positive" if the cut-off values for invasive disease were applied ($\geq$ 80 pg/ml and $\geq$ 0.5 ODI, respectively). However, it seems plausible that in CF patients with chronic *Aspergillus* colonization/infection less BDG or GM is released into the blood as compared to severely immunocompromised patients with angioinvasive disease. This is supported by our ROC analysis which gave optimal BDG and GM cut-off values for discrimination between *Aspergillus*-positive and *Aspergillus*-negative patients of $\geq$60 pg/ml and > 0.1 ODI, respectively. After applying these cut-offs to our study population, there were significantly more patients with elevated BDG and GM levels in the *Aspergillus*-positive than in the *Aspergillus*-negative subgroup. Interestingly, in case of BDG there is an "indeterminate" range between 60 and 80 pg/ml defined by the manufacturer and patients without invasive fungal disease have BDG-levels below 60 pg/ml. Thus, it seems that CF-patients with persistent *Aspergillus* detection have BDG and GM levels that range between healthy and invasively infected patients.

The diagnostic performance of BDG and GM to distinguish between *Aspergillus*-positive and *Aspergillus*-negative patients was, despite the optimized cut-offs, rather low. The sensitivity and specificity were around 50% or 80%, respectively, for both biomarkers. This means that half the patients with respiratory cultures positive for *Aspergillus* did not have elevated biomarker levels. However, it also means that 80% of patients with elevated biomarker levels were *Aspergillus*-positive. This constellation of low sensitivity and high specificity could be explained by the existence of two subgroups within the *Aspergillus*-positive patients. One subgroup consists of patients that are merely colonized with *A. fumigatus* (exhibiting normal biomarker levels) and the other of patients with true *A. fumigatus* infection (exhibiting elevated biomarker levels). If this is the case, BDG and GM could potentially differentiate between these two subgroups. If one further assumes that only infected but not colonized patients will develop an *Aspergillus*-associated impairment of their lung function, it would imply that biomarkers are superior to culture in predicting the FEV1 evolution.

The analysis of the FEV1 in our CF population supports this hypothesis. In the univariate analysis BDG and GM levels are correlating inversely with the FEV1 and patients with elevated BDG or GM levels have significantly lower FEV1 values. Moreover, the multivariate analysis revealed that BDG, but not the culture of *A. fumigatus,* proved to be an independent predictor of the FEV1. These data also offer an explanation why previous studies reported inconsistent results concerning the correlation between *Aspergillus* detection and lung function decline.

Data on fungal biomarker levels in sera of CF patients with proven colonization/infection with *Aspergillus* are scarce. Recently, Rautemaa et al. [22] reported on the only study examining BDG levels in CF patients. They analyzed serum samples from an adult CF cohort (n = 46) at the time of stable disease and during pulmonary exacerbation. There was no significant difference in the BDG levels of patients with stable versus exacerbated disease (40.2 versus 48.7 pg/ml, $p = 0.544$) or between patients with versus without positive fungal culture (76 versus 37 pg/ml, $p = 0.227$). Unfortunately, the authors did not specify the fungi they detected. According to a personal communication by V. Rauteema (University of Manchester, UK), the cultured fungi were predominantly *Candida* spp., whereas only few *Aspergillus* spp. were isolated. Separate statistical analysis of both genera also did not show significant differences in BDG levels. However, the low number of patients with cultures positive for *Aspergillus* could explain why the BDG levels between *Aspergillus*-positive and -negative patients were not significantly different in their study.

Furthermore, Rautemaa et al. [22] reported that multiple serum samples collected over a period of 13 months from 6 patients showed that BDG-positive patients stayed positive and BDG-negative patients remained negative. This would support our hypothesis that BDG-antigenemia in CF patients is not a transient phenomenon but rather the consequence of a persistent condition like chronic *Aspergillus* infection.

Interestingly, Rautemaa et al. [22] found significantly elevated BDG-levels in patients with exocrine pancreatic insufficiency (PI) and CF-related diabetes (CFRD) and hypothesized that the chronically inflamed intestinal epithelium in CF could allow a translocation of BDG from the gut into the blood. However, we were not able to confirm this data. BDG levels were independent of PI and CFRD (data not shown). To further examine the gut as possible source of serum BDG, we measured intestinal fatty acid binding protein 2 (FABP2), a specific marker for gut mucosal injury [23–25], in the serum of our CF population. FABP2 was not elevated in patients with positive BDG levels arguing against an intestinal source of BDG.

So far, the only study on GM and the detection of *Aspergillus* in CF patients was performed by Warren et al.

[26]. They analyzed GM levels from 138 CF patients. 43% of patients were persistently and 23% transiently colonized/infected with *Aspergillus*, whereas 34% of the patients were negative for *Aspergillus*. The GM levels of these three groups were identical and none of the patients had GM levels above an ODI of 0.5. These results are contradictory to our findings. Comparing the findings by Warren et al. [26] with our data, it is striking that 43% and 23% of their patients were persistently or intermittently culture-positive for *Aspergillus*, whereas in our cohort only 21% of patients were persistently and 1% were transiently *Aspergillus*-positive. This suggests that there were either profound differences in the study populations or in the diagnostic methodology. Patient recruitment and the utilized GM assay were identical. Unfortunately, the authors did not specify their fungal culture methodology. Also, the definitions for persistent and transient detection of *Aspergillus* were different. Warren et al. [26] defined ≥2 positive *Aspergillus* cultures in the last year as persistent colonization/infection, whereas we required > 50% positive cultures in the past 2 years. Essentially, this could mean that our patients were more heavily colonized/infected and therefore had higher GM levels. Interestingly, in the study by Warren et al. [26], patients colonized with *Aspergillus* were significantly younger than patients without. Again, this finding contrasts with our result (colonized patients were older), which is in accordance with other data showing that higher age is as a risk factor for *Aspergillus* colonization [13, 15].

Our study has some limitations. The retrospective and cross-sectional design leads to difficulties in distinguishing between cause and effect. It is currently unclear, whether colonization/infection with *Aspergillus* leads to a more rapid decline in lung function or whether patients with more severe disease exhibit an increased susceptibility to *Aspergillus*. Furthermore, we did not use culture media selective for *Scedosporium* spp.. Consequently, the number of patients with *Scedosporium* spp. present in respiratory samples might be underestimated. Since *Scedosporium* spp. also produce BDG, we cannot exclude the possibility that part of the BDG detected in the patients′ sera was derived from fungi other than *A. fumigatus*. Finally, it has been shown that the overall sensitivity of fungal culture is rather poor and that sputum GM or nucleic acid amplification techniques (NAT) are able to detect *Aspergillus* DNA in a considerable number of samples that were culture-negative [27]. In this context it seems plausible that patients with a negative *Aspergillus* culture but a positive sputum GM or NAT test are less heavily colonized than culture-positive patients. This would implicate that most *Aspergillus*-positive patients of our study were heavily colonized and that we might have missed the low-level colonized patients. Further research has to investigate whether these patients are serum BDG and GM positive and if low-level colonization will have an effect on pulmonary function. Therefore, prospective and longitudinal studies using sputum GM and NAT-assisted *Aspergillus* detection together with serum biomarker measurement are necessary to confirm and expand our data.

Conclusions

We have shown that serum BDG and GM levels are significantly elevated in CF patients with persistent detection of *A. fumigatus* in respiratory specimens. BDG-, GM- and *Aspergillus*-positive patients were in a more advanced stage of disease. However, only BDG proved to be an independent predictor of the FEV1. Our data suggest that the serum level of BDG rather than the level of GM or the detection of *Aspergillus* by culture, might allow to predict the decline of lung function in CF and to identify patients that would profit from antifungal therapy.

Abbreviations

AUC: Area under the ROC curve; BDG: (1→3)-β-D-glucan; BMI: Body mass index; CF: Cystic fibrosis; CFLD: CF-related liver disease; CFRD: CF-related Diabetes mellitus; CFTR: Cystic fibrosis transmembrane conductance regulator; CRP: C-reactive protein; FABP2: Fatty acid binding protein 2; FEV1: Forced expiratory volume in 1 s; GM: Galactomannan; GOLD: Global Initiative for Chronic Obstructive Lung Disease; Ig: Immunoglobulin; IQR: Interquartile range; MALDI-TOF-MS: Matrix Assisted Laser Desorption Ionization-Time of Flight Mass Spectrometry; NAT: Nucleic acid amplification techniques; ODI: Optical density index; PI: Exocrine pancreatic insufficiency; ROC: Receiver-operating-characteristic; SD: Standard deviation; WBC: Leucocyte count

Acknowledgments

We would like to thank Sebastian Meyer from the Department of Medical Informatics, Biometry & Epidemiology of the Friedrich-Alexander-Universität (FAU) Erlangen-Nürnberg for his assistance with the statistical analysis and the team of the cystic fibrosis outpatient clinic for the diagnostic work-up and the treatment of the patients.

Funding

No specific funding.

Authors' contributions

JT collected clinical data, performed BDG and FABP2 tests and analyzed the data. VOM aquired clinical data and critically revised the manuscript, RM and MR performed diagnostic tests, CB critically revised the manuscript, JH planned the study, analyzed the data and drafted the manuscript. All authors read and approved the final manuscript. All authors agreed to be accountable for all aspects of the work.

Consent for publication

Not applicable.

Competing interests

JH received royalties for lectures from MSD as well as lecture royalties and a research grant from Pfizer. The remaining authors declare no conflict of interest.

Author details
[1]Mikrobiologisches Institut - Klinische Mikrobiologie, Immunologie und Hygiene, Universitätsklinikum Erlangen und Friedrich-Alexander-Universität (FAU) Erlangen-Nürnberg, Wasserturmstr. 3/5, 91054 Erlangen, Germany. [2]Kinder- und Jugendklinik, Universitätsklinikum Erlangen und Friedrich-Alexander-Universität (FAU) Erlangen-Nürnberg, Erlangen, Germany.

References

1. Rowe SM, Miller S, Sorscher EJ. Cystic fibrosis. N Engl J Med. 2005;352:1992–2001.
2. Pihet M, Carrere J, Cimon B, Chabasse D, Delhaes L, Symoens F, Bouchara JP. Occurrence and relevance of filamentous fungi in respiratory secretions of patients with cystic fibrosis–a review. Med Mycol. 2009;47:387–97.
3. Amin R, Dupuis A, Aaron SD, Ratjen F. The effect of chronic infection with aspergillus fumigatus on lung function and hospitalization in patients with cystic fibrosis. Chest. 2010;137:171–6.
4. Fillaux J, Bremont F, Murris M, Cassaing S, Rittie JL, Tetu L, Segonds C, Abbal M, Bieth E, Berry A, et al. Assessment of aspergillus sensitization or persistent carriage as a factor in lung function impairment in cystic fibrosis patients. Scand J Infect Dis. 2012;44:842–7.
5. Shoseyov D, Brownlee KG, Conway SP, Kerem E. Aspergillus bronchitis in cystic fibrosis. Chest. 2006;130:222–6.
6. Kanthan SK, Bush A, Kemp M, Buchdahl R. Factors effecting impact of aspergillus fumigatus sensitization in cystic fibrosis. Pediatr Pulmonol. 2007; 42:785–93.
7. Mennink-Kersten MA, Donnelly JP, Verweij PE. Detection of circulating galactomannan for the diagnosis and management of invasive aspergillosis. Lancet Infect Dis. 2004;4:349–57.
8. Finkelman MA. Pneumocystis jirovecii infection: cell wall (1-3)-ß-D-glucan biology and diagnostic utility. Crit Rev Microbiol. 2010;36:271–81.
9. Sulahian A, Porcher R, Bergeron A, Touratier S, Raffoux E, Menotti J, Derouin F, Ribaud P. Use and limits of (1-3)-beta-d-glucan assay (Fungitell), compared to galactomannan determination (Platelia aspergillus), for diagnosis of invasive aspergillosis. J Clin Microbiol. 2014;52:2328–33.
10. Lee TW, Brownlee KG, Conway SP, Denton M, Littlewood JM. Evaluation of a new definition for chronic Pseudomonas aeruginosa infection in cystic fibrosis patients. J Cyst Fibros. 2003;2:29–34.
11. Cohen J. A power primer. Psychol Bull. 1992;112:155–9.
12. Chotirmall SH, McElvaney NG. Fungi in the cystic fibrosis lung: bystanders or pathogens? Int J Biochem Cell Biol. 2014;52:161–73.
13. de Vrankrijker AM, van der Ent CK, van Berkhout FT, Stellato RK, Willems RJ, Bonten MJ, Wolfs TF. Aspergillus fumigatus colonization in cystic fibrosis: implications for lung function? Clin Microbiol Infect. 2011;17:1381–6.
14. Cheer SM, Waugh J, Noble S. Inhaled tobramycin (TOBI): a review of its use in the management of Pseudomonas aeruginosa infections in patients with cystic fibrosis. Drugs. 2003;63:2501–20.
15. Milla CE, Wielinski CL, Regelmann WE. Clinical significance of the recovery of aspergillus species from the respiratory secretions of cystic fibrosis patients. Pediatr Pulmonol. 1996;21:6–10.
16. Baxter CG, Rautemaa R, Jones AM, Webb AK, Bull M, Mahenthiralingam E, Denning DW. Intravenous antibiotics reduce the presence of aspergillus in adult cystic fibrosis sputum. Thorax. 2013;68:652–7.
17. Burns JL, Emerson J, Stapp JR, Yim DL, Krzewinski J, Louden L, Ramsey BW, Clausen CR. Microbiology of sputum from patients at cystic fibrosis centers in the United States. Clin Infect Dis. 1998;27:158–63.
18. Bargon J, Dauletbaev N, Kohler B, Wolf M, Posselt HG, Wagner TO. Prophylactic antibiotic therapy is associated with an increased prevalence of aspergillus colonization in adult cystic fibrosis patients. Respir Med. 1999;93: 835–8.
19. Hodson ME, Gallagher CG, Govan JR. A randomised clinical trial of nebulised tobramycin or colistin in cystic fibrosis. Eur Respir J. 2002;20:658–64.
20. Jubin V, Ranque S, Stremler Le Bel N, Sarles J, Dubus JC. Risk factors for aspergillus colonization and allergic bronchopulmonary aspergillosis in children with cystic fibrosis. Pediatr Pulmonol. 2010;45:764–71.
21. Cai X, Ni W, Wei C, Cui J. Diagnostic value of the serum galactomannan and (1, 3)-beta-D-glucan assays for invasive pulmonary aspergillosis in non-neutropenic patients. Intern Med. 2014;53:2433–7.
22. Rautemaa V, Green HD, Jones AM, Rautemaa-Richardson R. High level of beta-(1,3)-d-glucan antigenaemia in cystic fibrosis in the absence of invasive fungal disease. Diagn Microbiol Infect Dis. 2017;
23. Schurink M, Kooi EM, Hulzebos CV, Kox RG, Groen H, Heineman E, Bos AF, Hulscher JB. Intestinal fatty acid-binding protein as a diagnostic marker for complicated and uncomplicated necrotizing enterocolitis: a prospective cohort study. PLoS One. 2015;10:e0121336.
24. Schellekens DH, Grootjans J, Dello SA, van Bijnen AA, van Dam RM, Dejong CH, Derikx JP, Buurman WA. Plasma intestinal fatty acid-binding protein levels correlate with morphologic epithelial intestinal damage in a human translational ischemia-reperfusion model. J Clin Gastroenterol. 2014;48:253–60.
25. Kanda T, Fujii H, Tani T, Murakami H, Suda T, Sakai Y, Ono T, Hatakeyama K. Intestinal fatty acid-binding protein is a useful diagnostic marker for mesenteric infarction in humans. Gastroenterology. 1996;110:339–43.
26. Warren TA, Yau Y, Ratjen F, Tullis E, Waters V. Serum galactomannan in cystic fibrosis patients colonized with aspergillus species. Med Mycol. 2012; 50:658–60.
27. Nagano Y, Elborn JS, Millar BC, Walker JM, Goldsmith CE, Rendall J, Moore JE. Comparison of techniques to examine the diversity of fungi in adult patients with cystic fibrosis. Med Mycol. 2010;48:166–76. e161

IFNΛ3/4 locus polymorphisms and IFNΛ3 circulating levels are associated with COPD severity and outcomes

Adrian Egli[1,2], Jyotshna Mandal[3], Desiree M. Schumann[3*], Michael Roth[3], Brad Thomas[4], D. Lorne Tyrrell[4], Francesco Blasi[5], Kostantinos Kostikas[3], Wim Boersma[6], Branislava Milenkovic[7], Alicia Lacoma[8], Katharina Rentsch[9], Gernot G. U. Rohde[10], Renaud Louis[11], Joachim G. Aerts[12], Tobias Welte[13], Antoni Torres[14], Michael Tamm[3] and Daiana Stolz[3]

Abstract

Background: Interferon lambdas (IFNLs) have important anti-viral/bacterial and immunomodulatory functions in the respiratory tract. How do IFNLs impact COPD and its exacerbations?

Methods: Five hundred twenty eight patients were recruited in a prospective observational multicentre cohort (PROMISE) study. The genetic polymorphisms (rs8099917 and rs12979860) within the IFNL3/4 gene region and circulating levels of IFNL3 in COPD patients were determined and associated with disease activity and outcome during a median follow-up of 24 months.

Results: The GG genotype significantly influenced severe exacerbation rate (42 vs. 23%; $p = 0.032$) and time to severe exacerbation (HR = 2.260; $p = 0.012$). Compared to the TT or TG genotypes, the GG genotype was associated with severe dyspnoea (modified medical research council score ≥ median 3; 22 vs 42%, $p = 0.030$). The CC genotype of the rs12979860 SNP was associated with a poorer prognosis (body mass index, airflow obstruction, dyspnea and exercise capacity index ≥ median 4; 46 vs. 36% TC vs. 20.5% TT; $p = 0.031$). Patients with stable COPD and at exacerbation had significantly lower circulating IFNL3 compared to healthy controls ($p < 0.001$ and $p < 0.001$, respectively). Circulating IFNL3 correlated to post-bronchodilator FEV_1%predicted and the tissue maturation biomarker Pro-collagen 3.

Conclusion: IFNL3/4 polymorphisms and circulating IFNL3 may be associated with disease activity and outcomes in COPD.

Keywords: Interleukin 28B, Cohort, Mortality, Biomarker, Single nucleotide polymorphisms

Background

Interferons (IFN) are known to have important direct anti-viral and anti-bacterial effects, as well as potent modulatory effects on the adaptive immune response via the induction of hundreds of IFN-stimulated genes (ISGs) [1, 2] The newest discovered class of IFN, the IFN lambda (IFNL) family, has four members: IFNL1–4 [3]. The IFNL receptor consists of a heterodimer with an alpha subunit (IL28RA) and a beta subunit (IL10RB). IL10RB is ubiquitously expressed, whereas IL28RA expression is restricted and interestingly, it is highly expressed on lung epithelial cells [4] and alveolar macrophages [5]. When a virus is seen by the pattern recognition receptors which are found on macrophages and epithelial cells, IFNL gene expression is stimulated via various signalling pathways [6]. This leads to increased circulating IFNL3 which interacts with the IFNL receptor expressed on lung, intestinal and liver cells, and via the JAK-STAT signalling cascade induces interferon stimulated genes which in turn influence viral

* Correspondence: desiree.schumann@usb.ch
[3]Clinic of Pneumology and Pulmonary Cell Research, University Hospital Basel, Petersgraben 4, 4031 Basel, Switzerland
Full list of author information is available at the end of the article

replication [6]. A series of single nucleotide polymorphisms (SNPs) in the IFNL3/4 gene region have been described [7–9] and associated with variable IFNL3/4 gene expression [10–13]. The variability of IFNL3 during viral or bacterial infections may lead to significant differences in the subsequent immune response and thus variable clinical outcomes [3].

IFNL3 has immune-modulatory and anti-tumorigenic effects and is induced by viral infections [6, 14]. Viral infections play an important role in the exacerbation of asthma [15–17] and COPD [18–20]. Reduced interferon activity during a respiratory syncytial virus infection has been linked to the later development of asthma in children [20, 21]. The mechanism of virus-induced exacerbations of COPD is not well-defined. Recently, the role of IFNLs in the exacerbation of asthma has been explored [22–24]. However, no data are available regarding the effect of IFNL3 or its polymorphisms on the exacerbation and further clinical outcomes of COPD. COPD patients exposed to rhinovirus consistently showed a trend towards less IFNL expression in bronchoalveolar lavage fluid [25] and in animal models it has been shown that IFNL plays a role in viral (influenza A, coronavirus and rotavirus) modulation [6].

We hypothesize, that in patients with COPD, SNPs in the IFNL3/4 gene will impact clinical outcomes such as exacerbation and that they might be associated with circulating markers of inflammation and tissue remodelling. Therefore, we aimed to explore the IFNL3/4 polymorphisms (rs8099917 and rs12979860) and circulating IFNL3 in association with the occurrence of exacerbation of COPD and all-cause mortality in a multinational, multicenter, prospective, longitudinal, observational cohort study of patients with clinically stable and exacerbated COPD.

Methods

Study overview

Patients in stable state COPD with GOLD II to IV were enrolled for an observational prospective trial (PROMISE-COPD; www.controlled-trials.com identifier ISRCTN9 9586989). The study details have been published previously [26]. For the current nested biomarker study, 638 patients were consecutively recruited and followed at 11 European hospital pneumology departments from November 2008 to October 2011 (Fig. 1). Details of inclusion and exclusion criteria were previously published [27]. We analysed data from 528 patients, who completed the first 6 month-follow-up of the study and for whom serum samples from visit 1 were available. We used serum samples at the stable phase and during the first episode of exacerbation of COPD.

For each patient, a physical examination was performed, vital signs were registered, and a detailed history

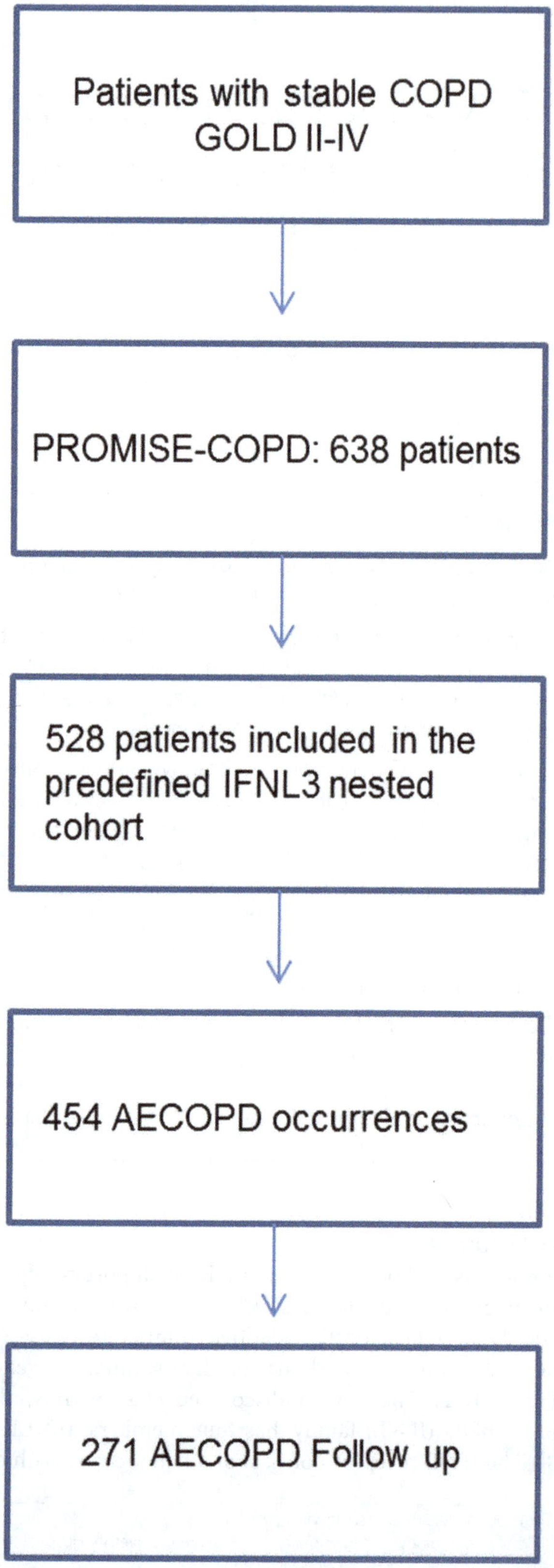

Fig. 1 Flow chart of the patient cohort selection criteria

obtained. Spirometry and 6-min walk tests (6MWTs) were performed following American Thoracic Society guidelines [24, 25]. One- and two-year follow-up in a stable phase, including a series of outcome markers were determined as previously published [26]. Additionally, patients treated for infection-triggered exacerbation of COPD had a scheduled follow-up four weeks post-exacerbation onset. Acute exacerbations were defined as an acute sustained worsening of dyspnoea, cough and/or sputum beyond normal day-to-day variations in a patient with underlying COPD; severe exacerbations were defined as an exacerbation requiring hospitalisation [28]. A total of 30 age and gender unmatched healthy controls were included in the study.

Ethics

The study was an observational study without specific intervention. The IFNL3 genotypes and serum levels were retrospectively determined and had no impact on the treatment decisions. The study was approved by the respective participating local IRBs in all centers (Ethikkommission beider Basel EKBB/295707, Medical Ethical Committee Amphia Ziekenhuis 958, Medical Ethical Committee North Holland M08–016, Klinicki Centar Srbije Eticki Odbor, Clinical Research Ethics Committee Germans Trias I Pujol Hospital, Medizinische Hochschule Hannover Ethikkommission 5071, Ethics committee of the Hospital Clinic of Barcelona, Ethics committee of the Policlinico of Milan, Ethics committee in Greece). All patients provided a written informed consent.

IFNL3 ELISA assay

IFNL3 serum levels were determined in the stable phase and during exacerbation of COPD. A commercially available sandwich immunoassay ELISA kit that showed no cross-reactivity with IFNL2 (IL28A) or IFNL4 (IL29; Human IL-28B/IFN-lambda 3 DuoSet ELISA, DY5259, R&D Systems Minneapolis, MN, USA) was used, according to the manufacturer's instructions. The IFNL3 assay had a linear range of detection from 31.20–2000 pg/ml.

IFNL genotyping

Two common SNPs, rs8099917 and rs12979860, in the IFNL3/L4 gene regions were determined as previously described [11]. The distribution of minor and major allele genotypes is comparable to previous publications in European populations [29, 30].

Collagen markers

As previously described [31], serum levels of fragments of collagen type III (C3M), fragments of collagen type VI (C6M), pro-form of collagen type III (Pro-C3) and pro-form of collagen type VI (Pro-C6) were measured with Nordic Bioscience assays according to the manufacturer's instructions.

Inflammatory markers

Procalcitonin, Copeptin, pro-adrenomedullin (ADM), and atrial natriuretic polypeptide (ANP) were measured as previously described [32].

Statistics

Differences in dichotomous variables were evaluated using the Chi-square test or Fischer's exact test, as appropriate. Normally distributed parameters were analyzed using the Student's t-test for equality of means. All other continuously non-normally distributed parameters were evaluated using the non-parametric Mann-Whitney U test or Kruskal-Wallis test, as appropriate. If the IFNL3 was below the detection level, the sample was assigned the value 31.20 pg/ml which is the lowest detectable value with the assay used in this study. Kaplan Meier curves were created to determine survival within 2 years and overall survival, occurrence of exacerbation and occurrence of severe exacerbation. The log-rank test was used to compare differences between survival curves. The Statistical Package for Social Sciences Program (SSPS Inc., version 22 for Windows) was used. All tests are two-tailed; a p-value of < 0.05 was considered significant. Results are expressed as mean (standard deviation) or median (interquartile range), unless otherwise stated.

Results

Five hundred twenty eight patients were included in this nested study (Fig. 1). The majority of the patients were male (71%) and the average age was 66.9 years (Table 1). 70% of the patients were past smokers and 50% of the patients were classified as GOLD II.

IFNL3 genotyping

The distribution of both rs8099917 and rs12979860 SNPs adhered to the Hardy Weinberg Equilibrium with the $\chi 2$ test for deviation equalling 2.21 for rs8099917 and 0.781 for rs12979860. Both values were less than 3.84 which represents the 5% significance level for 1 degree of freedom and therefore the null hypothesis that the population is in the Hardy-Weinberg frequencies is not rejected [33]. The most common genotype rs8099917 TT (65%) was followed by TG (30%) and GG (5%; Table 1).

Patients with the rs8099917 GG genotype had a significantly shorter time to severe exacerbation than patients with the TT or TG genotype (Fig. 2; $p = 0.037$). Significantly more severe exacerbations occurred in patients with rs8099917 GG genotype compared to patients with rs8099917 TT or rs8099917 TG genotype (42

Table 1 Baseline characteristics of patients included in the study

	Mean (SD), *n* (%)
Gender: Male	377 (71)
Age, years	66.9 (9.3)
Current smoker, n (%)	157 (30)
BMI (kg/m2)	26.00 (5.13)
Unadjusted Charlson Score (*n* = 528)	1.82 (1–16)
BODE index (median; IQR)	3 (1–4)
6MWT (m)	380.61 (104.69)
Exacerbation rate	2.05 (0–15)
Severe exacerbation rate	0.39 (0–8)
Lung function (post-brd)	
FEV_1, in L	1.40 (0.71)
FVC, in L	2.81 (0.89)
FEV_1/FVC%	47.87 (13.97)
FEV_1, % predicted	49.89 (16.8)
FVC, % predicted	80.70 (21.21)
Collagen markers [ng/ml]	
C3M	30.54 (12.61)
C6M	15.25 (8.62)
Pro-C3	13.29 (10.03)
Pro-C6	8.76 (4.31)
EL-NE	7.78 (6.78)
GOLD Grade[a]	
GOLD II	262 (50)
GOLD III	180 (35)
GOLD IV	80 (15)
rs8099917 genotypes	
TT	339 (65)
GG	26 (5)
TG	155 (30)
rs12979860 genotypes	
CC	76 (30)
TT	45 (18)
TC	131 (52)
MMRC score (median; IQR)	2 (1–2)
Inflammation markers at baseline	
Copeptin, pMol/L	12.57 (16.66)
Adrenomedullin, nMol/L	0.69 (0.38)
Atrial Natriuretic Peptide, pMol/L	113.67 (101.03)
Procalcitonin, μg/l	0.09 (0.14)
SF-36	
Physical function	51.54 (25.94)
Role physical	51.05 (43.48)
Role emotional	66.26 (43.52)
Social Functioning	69.49 (28.56)

Table 1 Baseline characteristics of patients included in the study *(Continued)*

	Mean (SD), *n* (%)
Mental Health	64.89 (20.07)
Body Pain	74.19 (27.94)
Vitality	51.79 (21.00)
General Health	47.88 (22.90)
SGRQ	
Symptoms score	49.30 (22.65)
Activity score	57.22 (22.90)
Impacts score	32.11 (18.66)
Total score	42.39 (18.11)

Continuous data are shown as mean (SD) or median (interquartile range) and categorical variables as No. (%). BMI = body mass index; brd = bronchodilator; BODE = BMI, airflow obstruction, dyspnea and exercise capacity; 6MWD = 6-min walk distance; C3M = fragments of collagen type III; C6M = fragments of collagen type VI; Pro-C3 = pro-forms of collagen type III; Pro-C6 = pro-forms of collagen type VI; EL-NE = neutrophil elastase-generated fragments of elastin; GOLD = Gold Initiative for Chronic Obstructive Lung Disease; MMRC = modified Medical Research Council; SF-36 = 36-item Short-Form Health Survey; SGRQ = St. George's Respiratory Questionnaire
[a]GOLD grades are based on FEV1% predicted: 50% ≤ II ≤ 80%; 30% ≤ III ≤ 50%; and IV ≤ 30%

vs 23%, respectively; chi-squared p = 0.032). The rs8099917 genotypes had no significant effect on mortality (p = 0.726). There was a significant association between MMRC and the rs8099917 GG genotype with 42% (11/26) of patients with the GG genotype having an MMRC more than the median compared to 22% (107/479) of patients with rs8099917 TT or rs8099917 TG

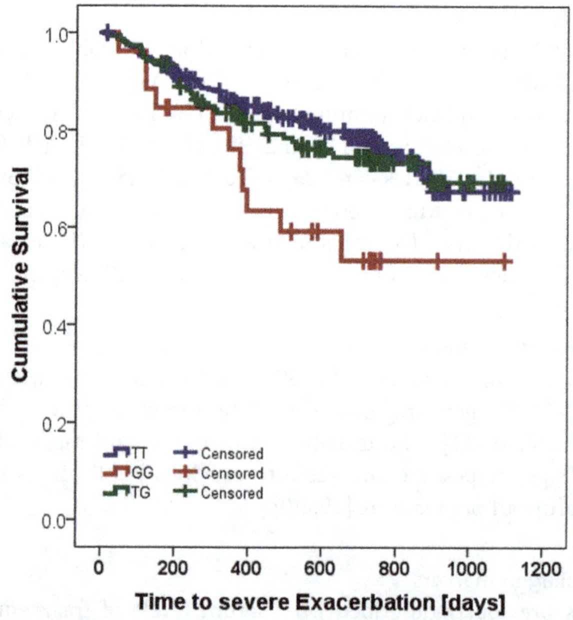

Fig. 2 Kaplan Meier curve showing the significant effect of the rs8099917 GG genotype on time to severe exacerbation; p = 0.037. GG p = 26, 11 events; TT n = 335, events = 73; TG n = 154, events = 39

genotype (Table 2; chi-squared, p = 0.030). Although there was no difference in the unadjusted Charlson score (p = 0.705), suggesting a similar distribution of comorbidities and life expectancy between the groups, five times the number of patients with rs8099917 GG genotype had been diagnosed with a malignancy at the start of the study compared to patients with rs8099917 TT or rs8099917 TG genotype (chi-squared, p = 0.014). The association between rs8099917 GG genotype and having a malignancy remained after adjusting for age and smoking (OR = 6.726, p = 0.003). Mann-Whitney-U-Test showed a significant difference in C6M between rs8099917 GG genotype and rs8099917 TT/TG genotype (Table 2).

The rs12979860 genotypes had no effect on mortality (p = 0.703), exacerbation rate (p = 0.946) or time to exacerbation (p = 0.324). The rs12979860 CC genotype was associated with BODE index with 46% (30/65) of the patients with a BODE index more than the median compared to 36% (44/122) of patients with the rs12979860 TC and 20.5% (8/39) of patients with the rs12979860 TT genotype (p = 0.031).

Circulating IFNL3 in serum

Circulating IFNL3 was detectable in 3.6% (19/528) of the COPD patients during stable phase and in 7.2% (32/446) of the COPD patients during the exacerbation phase whereas it was detectable in 80% (24/30) of the blood samples from healthy controls. The level of IFNL3 was higher in the controls compared to the COPD patients during stable phase, exacerbation phase and follow-up to the exacerbation (Fig. 3).

There was no association between the rs8099917 (chi-square test; p = 0.392) or rs12979860 genotypes (chi-square test; p = 0.733) and whether IFNL3 was detectable or not during the stable phase.

Circulating IFNL3 during stable COPD phase

None of the patients with a GOLD IV classification had detectable circulating IFNL3 during stable phase. 3% (5/180) of the patients classified as GOLD III and 5% (14/262) of the patients classified as GOLD II had detectable circulating IFNL3 levels. GOLD II (31.2 pg/ml; Range = undetectable – 661.83) and GOLD III (31.2 pg/ml; Range = undetectable – 122.26) patients had similar levels of circulating IFNL3, which was less than in healthy controls (82.7 pg/ml; IQR = 81.9–83.4). Using a Mann-Whitney-U-test, patients with detectable circulating IFNL3 had significantly better post-bronchodilator FEV_1%predicted than patients with undetectable IFNL3 (57.97 vs. 49.62; p = 0.035). We found a significant correlation between circulating IFNL3 and post bronchodilator FEV_1%predicted (Spearman Rho = 0.098; p = 0.034). There was no significant difference in other variables, including quality of life, between patients with detectable circulating IFNL3 and patients with non-detectable circulating IFNL3.

Circulating IFNL3 and collagen biomarkers

There was a significant association between circulating IFNL3 and Pro-C3 (Linear regression, Beta = 0.099 95% CI 0.037–0.634; p = 0.028) but no association with C3M, C6Mor Pro-C6. Patients with detectable circulating IFNL3 had significantly more Pro-C3 than patients with undetectable levels of IFNL3 (Mann-Whitney U-Test, median 16.1 [IQR = 8.0] vs 10.7 [IQR = 5.6] ng/ml, respectively; p = 0.003). There was no significant difference in the other collagen biomarkers between the two groups of patients.

Discussion

Viral infections are thought to play a role in the exacerbation of COPD [18, 19]. IFNL3, a member of the interferon lambda family, has immune-modulatory and anti-tumorigenic effects and is induced by viral infections [14]. This is the first study evaluating the association between IFNL circulating levels and its polymorphisms in patients with COPD.

The distribution of both rs8099917 and rs12979860 SNPs adhered to the Hardy Weinberg Equilibrium. Ethnic background strongly impacts SNP distribution, however, people with Caucasian ancestry (the main ethnic background of the present cohort) have a more balanced distribution of genetic polymorphisms [9, 34]. In our COPD cohort, the SNP rs8099917 GG genotype significantly influenced the severe exacerbation rate, and the time to severe exacerbation and it was associated with a higher MMRC score. Conversely, SNP rs12979860 had no effect on exacerbations or death. This is in line with what is known for hepatitis and diabetes, where the SNP rs8099917 GG genotype is considered to be the risk genotype and the SNP rs12979860 CC genotype the protective genotype [35–37]. The IFNL3 polymorphisms predict response to treatment in patients with hepatitis C [27, 30, 31]. We found that the prevalence of malignancy was increased among patients with the rs8099917 GG genotype. This was also seen in patients with chronic hepatitis C, where more patients with the rs8099917 GG or non-TT genotype had hepatocellular carcinoma [38]. In antiretroviral-treated HIV-infected patients, however, the SNP rs12979860 CC genotype was associated with higher mortality and thus it was not protective [39]. In COPD patients, we found that the SNP rs12979860 CC genotype was associated with a higher BODE index, and thus possibly a higher risk of mortality, though the rs12979860 CC genotype did not associate with mortality directly in this study.

Table 2 A comparison of the patient baseline characteristics according to their rs8099917 genotype

	GG (median, IQR)	TT/TG (median, IQR)	*p*-value
Gender: Male (n,%)	16 (61.5)	355 (71.9)	0.269
Age, years	70.50 (14.50)	67.00 (13)	0.139
Current smoker (n, %)	4 (15.4)	149 (30.3)	0.125
PY, months	40.00 (36.75)	45.00 (35)	0.261
BMI, kg/m2	27.29 (7.83)	25.86 (6.14)	0.339
Unadjusted Charlson Score	1.00 (2.00)	1.00 (1.00)	0.305
6MWT, m	375 (161.25)	395 (120)	0.362
Exacerbation rate (number of exacerbations/year)	2.00 (3.00)	1.00 (3.00)	0.935
Severe exacerbation rate (number of severe exacerbations/year)	0.58 (0–3)	0.37 (0–8)	*0.033*
Lung function (post-brd)			
FEV_1, in L	1.31 (0.8)	1.32 (0.74)	0.749
FVC, in L	2.53 (1.95)	2.69 (1.07)	0.688
FEV_1/FVC%	49.38 (27.47)	47.00 (22.91)	0.723
FEV_1, % predicted	56.50 (28.17)	49.50 (25.15)	0.314
FVC, % predicted	82.40 (42.75)	80.00 (26.22)	0.349
BODE index			0.659
≤ median of 3	15 (62.5)	302 (67.3)	
> median of 3	9 (37.5)	147 (32.7)	
Collagen markers [ng/ml]			
C3M	25.3 (14.5)	28.6 (11.6)	0.302
C6M	11.0 (9.7)	13.3 (8.1)	*0.032*
Pro-C3	12.1 (6.1)	10.8 (5.6)	0.684
Pro-C6	8.1 (3.7)	8.0 (0.535)	1.000
GOLD Grade[a] (n,%)			0.699
GOLD II	15 (57.7)	242 (49.6)	
GOLD III	8 (30.8)	169 (34.6)	
GOLD IV	3 (11.5)	77 (15.8)	
MMRC Test (n,%)			*0.030*
≤ median of 2	15 (57.7)	372 (77.7)	
> median of 2	11 (42.3)	107 (22.3)	
Inflammation markers			
Copeptin, pMol/l	8.24 (10.45)	8.57 (12.53)	0.465
Adrenomedullin, nMol/l	0.60 (0.28)	0.60 (0.3)	0.929
ANP, pMol/l	91.38 (52.43)	83.47 (83.18)	0.408
Procalcitonin, µg/l	0.08 (0.03)	0.08 (0.03)	0.862
SF-36			
Physical function	45 (47.5)	50 (45)	0.346
Role physical	50 (100)	50 (100)	0.742
Role emotional	100 (75)	100 (100)	0.518
Social Functioning	75 (65.6)	75 (50)	0.852
Mental Health	67.50 (36.25)	65 (27.50)	0.780
Body Pain	80 (58)	80 (48)	0.720
Vitality	46.88 (32.81)	50 (31.25)	0.403
General Health	37.50 (42.5)	50 (36.69)	0.570

Table 2 A comparison of the patient baseline characteristics according to their rs8099917 genotype *(Continued)*

	GG (median, IQR)	TT/TG (median, IQR)	*p*-value
SGRQ			
Symptoms score	46.60 (26.87)	49.72 (34.44)	0.356
Activity score	66.19 (31.99)	54.43 (31.81)	0.607
Impact score	29.16 (25.68)	29.39 (26.46)	0.802
Total score	44.15 (31.27)	39.03 (27.54)	0.892

Continuous data are shown as median (interquartile range) and categorical variables as No. (%). Italicized *p*-values are statistically significant, ie. $p < 0.05$. *BMI* body mass index, *brd* bronchodilator, *BODE* BMI, airflow obstruction, dyspnea and exercise capacity; *6MWD* 6-min walk distance, *C3M* fragments of collagen type III, *C6M* fragments of collagen type VI, *Pro-C3* pro-forms of collagen type III, *Pro-C6* pro-forms of collagen type VI, *GOLD* Gold Initiative for Chronic Obstructive Lung Disease, *MMRC* modified Medical Research Council, *ANP* Atrial Natriuretic Peptide, *SF-36* 36-item Short-Form Health Survey, *SGRQ* St. George's Respiratory Questionnaire
[a]GOLD grades are based on FEV1% predicted: 50% ≤ II ≤ 80%; 30% ≤ III ≤ 50%; and IV ≤ 30%

We found no association between the genotype and the circulating IFNL3 levels. In the literature, the association between genotype and circulating IFNL3 levels varies according to illness and group. Arpaci et al. [40] found no association between genotype and circulating IFNL3 in patients with Hashimoto's Thyroiditis. Langhans et al. [41] found that hepatitis C patients with the protective SNP rs12979860 CC genotype had more circulating IFNL3 compared to patients with the SNP rs12979860 TT genotype whereas Alborzi A., et al. [42] found no association between circulating IFNL3 and genotype.

Less IFNL3 is secreted by primary cells from asthmatic patients compared to cells from healthy controls infected with a virus but the basal levels are similar between the two groups [22]. Bullens et al. [43] found increased basal IFNL3 mRNA in the sputum of asthmatic patients compared to controls. Thus far there is no literature regarding basal serum IFNL3 levels in asthma patients compared to controls. Circulating IFNL3 levels were similar between hepatitis C patients and healthy controls [41] and Arpaci et al. [40] found increased basal circulating IFNL3 in patients with Hashimoto's thyroiditis compared to healthy controls. In our cohort of COPD patients, basal circulating IFNL3 levels were significantly less compared to controls. The circulating IFNL3 levels increased during an exacerbation, as was also seen in vitro in the cells from asthmatic patients that were infected with virus [22], and then returned to basal levels after the patient had recovered from the exacerbation. In COPD, the basal circulating IFNL3 levels were associated with the severity of airflow limitation. We hypothesise that the difference in circulating IFNL3 between healthy donors, GOLD II, GOLD III and GOLD IV patients may be due not only to the association between IFNL3 and FEV1, but also due to remodelling of the extracellular matrix in the lungs. This hypothesis is in part corroborated by the fact that there is a strong association between circulating IFNL3 and Pro-C3. Pro-C3 is the N-protease cleavage site of type III collagen and is a marker of tissue formation [44]. Low levels of Pro-C3 is associated with worse lung function [31, 45] and with a shorter time to severe exacerbation [31]. It is therefore possible that changes in the cell structure of the lung results in decreased secreted IFNL3 which causes an impaired immune response to infection. More exacerbations occur resulting in more remodelling of the cells and less IFNL3 secretion, both of which are associated with impaired lung function, and a vicious cycle is continued. It is also possible that the decreased circulating IFNL3 facilitates viral infection leading to less Pro-C3 which results in worse lung function and shorter time to exacerbation. We are unable to determine which element is the catalyst therefore further studies are required to explore the association between IFNL3 polymorphisms and the remodelling of the extra-cellular matrix in stable and exacerbated COPD.

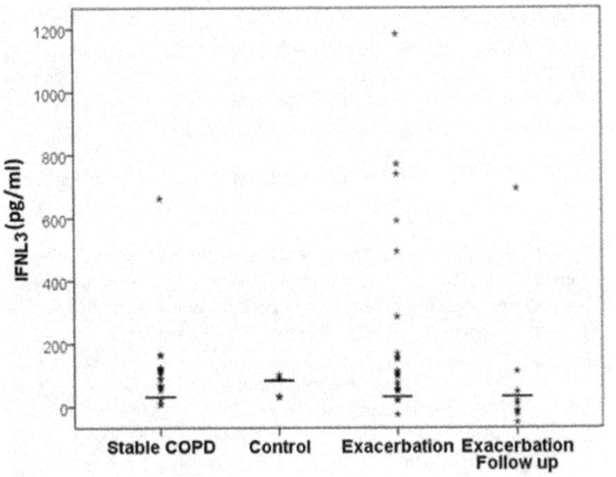

Fig. 3 Circulating IFNL3 during stable COPD, in healthy controls, during exacerbation and during follow up to exacerbation 4 weeks later

We found no association between circulating IFNL3 levels and disease outcome as is also evident in patients with hepatitis C [41].

The main limitation to this study is that there are no genotyping results for healthy controls and the SNP data was not validated in a separate cohort. We only investigated two SNPs, further studies are needed to investigate other SNPs related to IFNL3. In addition, the circulating IFNL3 was measured from unmatched blood donor samples. However, we found no association between circulating IFNL3 levels and gender or age, so the differences seen between the healthy controls and the COPD patients probably are not due to gender or age differences. The clinical value of IFNL3 alone or in combination with other biomarkers has to be assessed in conformational and randomized clinical trials.

Strengths of the study include the originality, longitudinal design assessing clinically relevant end-points and the fact that both genotypes and circulating IFNL3 were determined in a large multicentric cohort.

Conclusions

IFNL3 polymorphisms may play a role in disease activity and outcomes in COPD and circulating IFNL3 may be associated with disease severity and stability. Further investigations are required to determine the underlying mechanisms.

Abbreviations

6MWT: 6Minute walk test; ADM: Pro-adrenomedullin; ANP: Atrial natriuretic polypeptide; BMI: Body mass index; BODE: Body mass index, airflow obstruction, dyspnea and exercise capacity; C3M: Collagen type III; C6M: Collagen type VI; GOLD: Gold Initiative for Chronic Obstructive Lung Disease; IFNL: Interferon lambda; MMRC: Modified medical research council; Pro-C3: Pro-form of collagen type III; Pro-C6: Pro-form of collagen type VI; QoL: Quality of life; SNPs: Single nucleotide polymorphisms

Acknowledgments

We thank all general physicians for providing follow-up information. We thank Anja Meyer RN for her outstanding contribution in data management and patient follow-up.

Funding

D.S. was supported by the Swiss National Science Foundation (PP00P3_128412/1). A.E. was supported by a grant from the University of Basel "Nachwuchsförderung" and the Swiss National Science Foundation (Ambizione, PZ00P3_154709/1).

Authors' contributions

Data collection, accuracy of data, contributed to discussion of results, statistical analysis, writing of the manuscript, finalization of the manuscript, and approval of the submitted article: AE, JM, DMS, MR; Data collection, integrity and accuracy of data, revision and approval of the submitted article: BT, DLT, KK, FB, WB, BM, AL, KR, GR, RL, JA, TW, AT, MT. Conceived the research project, contributed in clinical work, integrity and accuracy of data, preparing, and approval of the submitted article: DS. All authors read and approved the final manuscript.

Consent for publication

Not applicable.

Competing interests

The authors declare that they have no competing interests.

Author details

[1]Applied Microbiology Research, Department of Medicine, University of Basel, Basel, Switzerland. [2]Clinical Microbiology, University Hospital Basel, Basel, Switzerland. [3]Clinic of Pneumology and Pulmonary Cell Research, University Hospital Basel, Petersgraben 4, 4031 Basel, Switzerland. [4]Li Ka Shing Institute for Virology, University of Alberta, Edmonton, Canada. [5]Department of Pathophysiology and Transplantation, Università degli Studi di Milano, Milan, Italy. [6]Department of Pneumology, Medisch Centrum Alkmaar, Alkmaar, The Netherlands. [7]Department of Pneumology, Institute for Pulmonary Diseases, Belgrade, Serbia. [8]Department of Microbiology, Hospital Universitari Germans Trias i Pujol, Badalona, Spain. [9]Laboratory Medicine, University Hospital Basel, Basel, Switzerland. [10]Department of Respiratory Medicine, Maastricht University Medical Center, Maastricht, The Netherlands. [11]Department of Pneumology, CHU Liege, University of Liege, GIGAI Research Group, Liege, Belgium. [12]Department of Pneumology, Amphia Hospital/Erasmus MC, Breda, The Netherlands. [13]Department of Pneumology, Medizinische Hochschule Hannover, Hannover, Germany. [14]Department of Pneumology, Hospital Clinic, Barcelona, Spain.

References

1. Decker T, Muller M, Stockinger S. The yin and yang of type I interferon activity in bacterial infection. Nat Rev Immunol. 2005;5:675–87.
2. McNab F, Mayer-Barber K, Sher A, Wack A, O'Garra A. Type I interferons in infectious disease. Nat Rev Immunol. 2015;15:87–103.
3. Egli A, Santer MD, O'Shea D, Tyrrell DL, Houghton M. The impact of the interferon-lambda family on the innate and adaptive immune response to viral infections. Emerg Infect Dis. 2014:e51.
4. Mordstein M, Neugebauer E, Ditt V, Jessen B, Rieger T, Falcone V, Sorgeloos F, Ehl S, Mayer D, Kochs G, et al. Lambda interferon renders epithelial cells of the respiratory and gastrointestinal tracts resistant to viral infections. J Virol. 2010;84:5670–7.
5. Koltsida O, Hausding M, Stavropoulos A, Koch S, Tzelepis G, Ubel C, Kotenko SV, Sideras P, Lehr HA, Tepe M, et al. IL-28A (IFN-lambda2) modulates lung DC function to promote Th1 immune skewing and suppress allergic airway disease. EMBO Mol Med. 2011;3:348–61.
6. Syedbasha M, Egli A. Interferon lambda: modulating immunity in infectious diseases. Front Immunol. 2017;8
7. Ge D, Fellay J, Thompson AJ, Simon JS, Shianna KV, Urban TJ, Heinzen EL, Qiu P, Bertelsen AH, Muir AJ, et al. Genetic variation in IL28B predicts hepatitis C treatment-induced viral clearance. Nature. 2009;461:399–401.
8. Rauch A, Kutalik Z, Descombes P, Cai T, Di Iulio J, Mueller T, Bochud M, Battegay M, Bernasconi E, Borovicka J, et al. Genetic variation in IL28B is associated with chronic hepatitis C and treatment failure: a genome-wide association study. Gastroenterology. 2010;138:1338–45. 1345 e1331-1337
9. Tanaka Y, Nishida N, Sugiyama M, Kurosaki M, Matsuura K, Sakamoto N, Nakagawa M, Korenaga M, Hino K, Hige S, et al. Genome-wide association of IL28B with response to pegylated interferon-alpha and ribavirin therapy for chronic hepatitis C. Nat Genet. 2009;41:1105–9.
10. Dill MT, Duong FH, Vogt JE, Bibert S, Bochud PY, Terracciano L, Papassotiropoulos A, Roth V, Heim MH. Interferon-induced gene expression is a stronger predictor of treatment response than IL28B genotype in patients with hepatitis C. Gastroenterology. 2011;140:1021–31.
11. Egli A, Levin A, Santer DM, Joyce M, O'Shea D, Thomas B, Lisboa LF, Barakat K, Bhat R, Fischer KP, et al. Immunomodulatory function of interleukin-28B during primary infection with cytomegalovirus. J Infect Dis. 2014;
12. Honda M, Sakai A, Yamashita T, Nakamoto Y, Mizukoshi E, Sakai Y, Nakamura M, Shirasaki T, Horimoto K, Tanaka Y, et al. Hepatic ISG expression is

associated with genetic variation in interleukin 28B and the outcome of IFN therapy for chronic hepatitis C. Gastroenterology. 2010;139:499–509.
13. Rallon NI, Soriano V, Naggie S, Restrepo C, McHutchison J, Vispo E, Benito JM. Impact of IL28B gene polymorphisms on interferon-lambda3 plasma levels during pegylated interferon-alpha/ribavirin therapy for chronic hepatitis C in patients coinfected with HIV. J Antimicrob Chemother. 2012; 67:1246–9.
14. Galani IE, Koltsida O, Andreakos E. Type III interferons (IFNs): emerging master regulators of immunity. In: Schoenberger SP, Katsikis PD, Pulendran B, editors. Crossroads between innate and adaptive immunity V. Volume 850: Springer; 2015.
15. Kling S, Donninger H, Williams Z, Vermeulen J, Weinberg E, Latiff K, Ghildyal R, Bardin P. Persistence of rhinovirus RNA after asthma exacerbation in children. Clin Exp Allergy. 2005;35:672–8.
16. Heymann PW, Platts-Mills TA, Johnston SL. Role of viral infections, atopy and antiviral immunity in the etiology of wheezing exacerbations among children and young adults. Pediatr Infect Dis J. 2005;24:S217–22.
17. Steinke JW, Borish L. Immune responses in rhinovirus-induced asthma exacerbations. Curr Allergy Asthma Rep. 2016;16:78.
18. Kherad O, Kaiser L, Bridevaux P-O, Sarasin F, Thomas Y, Janssens J-P, Rutschmann OT. Upper-respiratory viral infection, biomarkers and COPD exacerbation. Chest. 2010;138:896–904.
19. Biancardi E, Fennell M, Rawlinson W, Thomas PS. Viruses are frequently present as the infecting agent in acute exacerbations of chronic obstructive pulmonary disease in patients presenting to hospital. Intern Med J. 2016;46: 1160–5.
20. Proud D, Chow C-W. Role of viral infections in asthma and chronic obstructive pulmonary disease. Am J Respir Cell Mol Biol. 2006;35:513–8.
21. Singanayagam A, Joshi PV, Mallia P, Johnston SL. Viruses exacerbating chronic pulmonary disease: the role of immune modulation. BMC Med. 2012;10
22. Contoli M, Message SD, Laza-Stanca V, Edwards MR, Wark PA, Bartlett NW, Kebadze T, Mallia P, Stanciu LA, Parker HL, et al. Role of deficient type III interferon-lambda production in asthma exacerbations. Nat Med. 2006;12: 1023–6.
23. Koch S, Finotto S. Role of interferon-lambda in allergic asthma. J Innate Immun. 2015;7:224–30.
24. Schwantes EA, Denlinger LC, Evans MD, Gern JE, Jarjour NN, Mathur SK. Severity of virus-induced asthma symptoms is inversely related to resolution IFN-lambda expression. J Allergy Clin Immunol. 2015;135:1656–9.
25. Mallia P, Message SD, Gielen V, Contoli M, Gray K, Kebadze T, Aniscenko J, Laza-STanca V, Edwards MR, Slater L, et al. Experimental rhinovirus infection as a human model of chronic obstructive pulmonary disease exacerbation. Am J Respir Crit Care Med. 2011;183:734–42.
26. Mandal J, Roth M, Costa L, Boeck L, Rakic J, Scherr A, Tamm M, Stolz D. Vasoactive intestinal peptide for diagnosing exacerbation in chronic obstructive pulmonary disease. Respiration. 2015;90:357–68.
27. Boeck L, Mandal J, Costa L, Roth M, Tamm M, Stolz D. Longitudinal measurement of serum vascular endothelial growth factor in patients with chronic obstructive pulmonary disease. Respiration. 2015;90:97–104.
28. Boeck L, Soriano JB, Brusse-Keizer M, Blasi F, Kostikas K, Boersma W, Milenkovic B, Louis R, Lacoma A, Djamin R, et al. Prognostic assessment in COPD without lung function: the B-AE-D indices. Eur Respir J. 2016;47:1635–44.
29. Derbala M, Rizk NM, Al-Kaabi S, John A, Sharma M, El-dweik N, Yakoob R, Pasic F, Almohanadi M, Alejji K, et al. The predictive value of IL28B rs12979860, rs11881222 and rs8099917 polymorphisms and IP-10 in the therapeutic response of Egyptian genotype 4 patients. Virology. 2013;444: 292–300.
30. Sedighimehr P, Irani S, Sakhaee F, Vaziri F, Aghasadeghi M, Sadat SM, Jamnani FR, Fateh A, Siadat SD. IL28B rs12980275 and HLA rs4273729 genotypes as a powerful predictor factor for rapid, early, and sustained virologic response in patients with chronic hepatitis C. Arch Virol. 2017;162: 181–9.
31. Stolz D, Leeming DJ, Kristensen JH, Karsdal MA, Boersma W, Louis R, Milenkovic B, Kostikas K, Blasi F, Aerts J, et al. Systemic biomarkers of collagen and elastin turnover are associated with clinically relevant outcomes in COPD. Chest. 2017;151:47–59.
32. Stolz D, Christ-Crain M, Morgenthaler NG, Leuppi J, Miedinger D, Bingisser R, Müller C, Struck J, Müller B, Tamm M. Copeptin, C-reactive protein, and procalcitonin as prognostic biomarkers in acute exacerbation of COPD. Chest. 2007;131:1058–67.
33. Hardy-Weinberg principle. https://en.wikipedia.org/wiki/Hardy%E2%80%93Weinberg_principle.
34. Suppiah V, Moldovan M, Ahlenstiel G, Berg T, Weltman M, Abate ML, Bassendine M, Spengler U, Dore GJ, Powell E, et al. IL28B is associated with response to chronic hepatitis C interferon-alpha and ribavirin therapy. Nat Genet. 2009;41:1100–4.
35. Dong ZX, Zhou HJ, Xiang XG, Guo SM, Zhuang Y, Zhao GD, Xie Q. IL28B genetic variations are associated with treatment response of patients with chronic hepatitis C in a Chinese Han population. J Dig Dis. 2015;16:90–7.
36. Moran-Auth Y, Penna-Martinez M, Perner D, Susser S, Wicker S, Zeuzem S, Sarrazin C, Badenhoop K. IL28B gene variants and glucose metabolism in type 2 diabetes. Hum Immunol. 2016;77:1280–3.
37. Tillmann HL, Patel K, Muir AJ, Guy CD, Li JH, Lao XQ, Thompson A, Clark PJ, Gardner SD, McHutchison JG, McCarthy JJ. Beneficial IL28B genotype associated with lower frequency of hepatic steatosis in patients with chronic hepatitis C. J Hepatol. 2011;55:1195–200.
38. Asahina Y, Tsuchiya K, Nishimura T, Muraoka M, Suzuki Y, Tmaki N, Yasui Y, Hosokawa T, Ueda K, Nakanishi H, et al. Genetic variation near interleukin 28B and the risk of hepatocellular carcinoma in patients with chronic hepatitis C. J Gastroenterol. 2014;49:1152–62.
39. Parczewski M, Bander D, Leszczyszyn-Pynka M, Urbanska A, Socha L, Boron-Kaczmarska A. IL28B CC genotype is associated with higher all-cause mortality in antiretroviral-treated HIV-infected patients. AIDS Res Hum Retrovir. 2012;28:1640–6.
40. Arpaci D, Karakas CS, Can M, Cakmak GG, Kuzu F, Unal M, Bayraktaroglu T. Increased serum levels of IL-28 and IL-29 and the protective effect of IL28B rs8099917 polymorphism in patients with Hashimoto's thyroiditis. Immunol Investig. 2016;45:668–78.
41. Langhans B, Kupfer B, Braunschweiger I, Arndt S, Schulte W, Nischalke HD, Nattermann J, Oldenburg J, Sauerbruch T, Spengler U. Interferon-lambda serum levels in hepatitis C. J Hepatol. 2011;54:859–65.
42. Alborzi A, Hashempour T, Moayedi J, Musavi Z, Pouladfar G, Merat S. Role of serum level and genetic variation of IL-28B in interferon responsiveness and advanced liver disease in chronic hepatitis C patients. Med Microbiol Immunol. 2017;206:165–74.
43. Bullens DMA, Decraene A, Dilissen E, Meyts I, De Boeck K, Dupont LJ, Ceuppens JL. Type III IFN-lambda mRNA expression in sputum of adult and school-aged asthmatics. Clin Exp Allergy. 2008;38:1459–67.
44. Nielsen MJ, Veidal SS, Karsdal MA, Orsnes-Leeming DJ, Vainer B, Gardner SD, Hamatake R, Goodman ZD, Schuppan D, Patel K. Plasma pro-C3 (N-terminal type III collagen propeptide) predicts fibrosis progression in patients with chronic hepatitis C. Liver Int. 2015;35:429–37.
45. Sand JMB, Knox AJ, Lange P, Sun S, Kristensen JH, Leeming DJ, Karsdal MA, Bolton CE, Johnson SR. Accelerated extracellular matrix turnover during exacerbations of COPD. Respir Res. 2015;16

The association between circulating adiponectin levels, lung function and adiposity in subjects from the general population; data from the Akershus Sleep Apnea Project

Nina F. Caspersen[1,2], Helge Røsjø[1,2], Allan Flyvbjerg[3], Mette Bjerre[4], Anna Randby[1], Harald Hrubos-Strøm[5], Torbjørn Omland[1,2] and Gunnar Einvik[1,2*]

Abstract

Background: Circulating adiponectin (ADPN) levels are inversely associated with disease severity in patients with chronic obstructive pulmonary disease (COPD), while studies assessing the relationship between ADPN and lung function in subjects from the general population have shown diverging results. Accordingly, we hypothesized that ADPN would be associated with lung function in a population-based sample and tested how abdominal adiposity, metabolic syndrome, and systemic inflammation influenced this association.

Methods: We measured total ADPN in serum, forced vital capacity (FVC) and forced expiratory volume during the 1st second (FEV_1) in 529 participants (median 50 years, 54.6% males) recruited from the general population. We assessed the association between ADPN and lung function by multivariate linear regression analyses and adjusted for age, gender, height, smoking habits, weight, body mass index, waist-hip ratio, metabolic syndrome, obstructive sleep apnoea (OSA) and C-reactive protein.

Results: The median (interquartile range) level of serum ADPN was 7.6 (5.4–10.4) mg/L. ADPN levels were positively associated with FVC % of predicted (beta 3.4 per SD adiponectin, $p < 0.001$)) in univariate linear regression analysis, but the association was attenuated in multivariate analysis (standardized beta 0.03, $p = 0.573$)). Among co-variates only WHR significantly attenuated the relationship. ADPN levels were also associated with FEV_1% of predicted in bivariate analysis that adjusted for smoking (beta 1.4, $p = 0.042$)), but this association was attenuated and no longer significant in multivariate analysis (standardized beta -0.06, $p = 0.254$)).

Conclusion: In this population-based sample no association between ADPN and lung function was evident after adjustment for covariates related to adiposity.

Keywords: Adiponectin, Chronic obstructive pulmonary disease, Adiposity, Lung function

* Correspondence: gunnar.einvik@medisin.uio.no
[1]Division of Medicine, Akershus University Hospital, Lørenskog, Norway
[2]Institute of Clinical Medicine, University of Oslo, Oslo, Norway
Full list of author information is available at the end of the article

Background

Chronic obstructive pulmonary disease (COPD) is a heterogeneous disease characterized by chronic airway inflammation and reduced lung function [1]. The effects of current treatment options are modest, and COPD is one of the leading causes of morbidity and mortality worldwide [2]. Few serologic biomarkers are currently available for guiding diagnosis, providing prognostic information or evaluating treatment response in COPD [3].

Among proposed serologic biomarkers is adiponectin (ADPN); a protein abundant in serum, which is produced in adipocytes, but also in other tissues including macrophages and airway epithelium [4]. ADPN levels have been found to vary with age, gender, smoking, adiposity and the presence of metabolic syndrome [5–7], some of which may also influence pulmonary function [8]. ADPN is involved in several physiological processes and predominantly exerts anti-inflammatory effects [9, 10]. Previous observations in COPD patients indicate that elevated ADPN levels are associated with accelerated lung function impairment and respiratory mortality [11–13]. In contrast, only limited and contrasting results are currently available regarding the association between ADPN levels and indices of lung function in subjects from the general population [14, 15]. Accordingly, we aimed to assess the association between adiponectin and lung function in a general population sample. We hypothesized that we would find an inverse association between ADPN levels and lung function. We also aimed to assess the impact of adiposity, metabolic syndrome and systemic inflammation on the association between ADPN levels and indices of lung function.

Methods

Study design and participants

This is a substudy of the Akershus Sleep Apnea Project (ASAP), a two-phased clinical epidemiological study designed to examine sleep apnea in a general population. The recruitment protocol and inclusion/exclusion criteria have previously been reported [16]. In brief, 30,000 subjects between 30 and 65 years, randomly drawn from the Norwegian Personal Registry, received the Berlin Questionnaire by mail in the first phase of the study (Fig. 1). Among the 16,302 respondents, a clinical sample of 535 persons was drawn from pre-specified strata based on equilibrium of age and gender, as well as 2/3 of persons with at least 2 positive risk categories of the Berlin Questionnaire [17].

The study was conducted in accordance with the amended Declaration of Helsinki, and the Regional Committee for Medical Research Ethics in Eastern Norway approved the protocol (1.2005.839). We obtained written informed consent from all participants prior to study commencement.

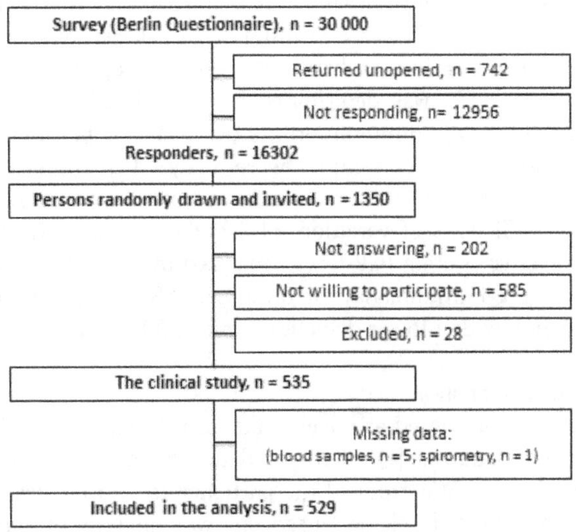

Fig. 1 Study flow in the Akershus Sleep Apnea Project

Data collection

During an overnight hospital stay, the participants underwent standardized data collection that included medical history, clinical examination, venous blood sampling, polysomnography and spirometry. Tobacco use was categorized as current, former and never. Height, weight, waist and hip circumference were recorded as the mean of three measurements with less than 10% variation, and were used to calculate the body mass index (BMI; weight (kg)/ height $[cm]^2$) and the waist-hip-ratio (WHR). Lung function was assessed by Spirosoft spirometry and CardioSoft software (GE HealthCare, Munich, Germany) and recorded as the best performance for forced vital capacity (FVC) and forced expiratory volume during 1st second (FEV_1) from at least 3 attempts with < 15% variation. FEV_1 and FVC in percent of predicted [18] were calculated and used as lung function variables in the analyses. Metabolic syndrome was defined according to the National Cholesterol Educational Program criteria [19], based on measurements of systolic blood pressure, total cholesterol, low-density lipoprotein cholesterol, glucose and WHR. Polysomnography was performed and analyzed by two US board-certified polysomnography technicians (Somnologica 3.2 software package (Flaga-Medcare, Buffalo, NY, USA)). Obstructive sleep apnoea (OSA) was defined as an apnoea-hypopnoea index (AHI) equal to or higher than five.

Biochemical analysis

Venous blood samples were collected in the fasting state in the morning, immediately prepared by centrifugation and separation into plasma and serum samples that were frozen at − 20 °C for a maximum of 1 week before stored at − 80 °C pending analyses, as previously reported [20]. Serum ADPN was determined by a validated in-house time-resolved immunofluorometric assay as previously described [21]. All samples were analyzed in duplicate, with a detection limit of 1.5 μg/L and intra- and interassay coefficients of variation < 5% and < 7%, respectively. C-reactive protein (CRP) was analyzed by a highly sensitive latex immunoassay-kit on a COBAS INTEGRA400 (Roche), with a lower detection limit of 0.1 mg/L.

Statistical analysis

Data are presented as mean ± standard deviation (SD) or median (quartile [Q] 1–3) for data with a non-normal distribution. We grouped the participants into tertiles of serum ADPN levels and used one-way analysis of variance, Kruskal-Wallis test or chi-square tests to compare clinical data between the groups. We applied multivariate linear regression to explore the association between ADPN and chosen covariates. Linear regression was also used to examine the univariate association between lung function and ADPN, as well as the covariates smoking status, weight, BMI, WHR, metabolic syndrome and CRP. We used FEV_1 and FVC in percent of predicted as dependent variables, thus, additional adjustment for the covariates age, gender, ethnicity and height were not considered. The multivariate analyses were performed in two stages; we first added adiposity variables, metabolic syndrome and CRP one-by-one to separately evaluate the impact of these features on the association between ADPN and lung function. In the final multivariate linear regression analysis all covariates were first entered simultaneously followed by a stepwise removal of the covariate with the highest p-value until all covariates were significantly associated with lung function. Adiponectin was kept in all steps independently of p-value. All regression models were assessed for collinearity. The statistical analyses were performed with Statistical Package for Social Sciences 22, and a p-value < 0.05 was regarded as statistical significant.

Results

The median (Q 1-3) ADPN level in the total population was 7.6 (5.4–10.4) mg/L. Indices of lung function, demographic and clinical characteristics, and laboratory data of the participants are presented stratified according to tertiles of serum ADPN concentrations in Table 1.

The absolute values of FEV_1 and FVC decreased by increasing ADPN tertiles. For FEV_1% of predicted, there was no significant difference between ADPN tertiles, while FVC% of predicted increased by increasing ADPN levels (Fig. 2). Age and proportion of females increased across tertiles of serum ADPN, while height, weight, BMI, WHR, CRP and the proportion of participants with metabolic syndrome decreased. Smoking status and prevalence of OSA did not differ significantly between the groups. Univariate and multivariate analysis of the association between ADPN and selected covariates are shown in Additional file 1: Table S1. All variables except smoking were significantly correlated with ADPN in univariate analysis, while age, gender, WHR and metabolic syndrome remained significantly associated with ADPN in multivariate analyses.

The crude associations between FEV_1 or FVC % of predicted and ADPN, smoking status, anthropometric parameters, metabolic syndrome, OSA and CRP are shown in Table 2.

There was no significant association between FEV_1% of predicted and ADPN. A positive association with ADPN was found after adjustment for smoking, while the models including each of the other co-variates found no associations between FEV_1% of predicted and ADPN. In contrast, FVC% of predicted was significantly associated with ADPN, measures of adiposity, metabolic syndrome, OSA and CRP, but not with smoking. The association between ADPN and FVC in % of predicted remained positive after adjusting for smoking status, weight, BMI, metabolic syndrome, OSA and CRP one by one in separate linear regression models. However, the association was attenuated and no longer significant when adjusting for WHR (Table 3).

In the final multivariate models that included smoking status, BMI, WHR, metabolic syndrome, OSA and CRP, ADPN was not associated with any of the lung function variables (Table 4).

Discussion

In the present population-based sample, we found that ADPN was positively associated with lung function after adjustment for age, gender, height and smoking, but this association was attenuated and not significant when adjusting also for indices of adiposity, metabolic syndrome, CRP and OSA. This result reflects the negative impact of adiposity on both lung function and serum ADPN levels.

The negative association between ADPN and severity of COPD previously observed in clinical cohorts has no established pathophysiological explanation, but could imply that ADPN is linked to disease development and progression. In the present study, we investigated whether a negative association between ADPN and lung function was present in a Caucasian general-population sample, hypothetically reflecting ADPN as an early marker of obstructive airway limitation. The two previous population-based studies assessing the relationship between ADPN and lung function have reported diverging results. A Japanese study reported a negative

Table 1 Characteristics of the participants according to tertiles of serum adiponectin levels

Variables	Total	ADPN tertiles			p
		Tertile 1	Tertile 2	Tertile 3	
	$n = 529$	$n = 176$	$n = 176$	$n = 177$	
ADPN, mg/L[d]	7.6 (5.4, 10,4)	4.6 (3.8, 5.4)	7.6 (6.7, 8.3)	12.6 (10.3, 15.4)	N/A
Age, years	48.6 (11.3)	46.4 (11.2)	48.6 (10.9)	50.7(11.0)	0.002[a]
Female gender	240 (45.4)	40 (22.7)	74 (42.0)	126 (71.2)	< 0.001[b]
Height, cm	173 (9)	176 (8)	174 (9)	170 (8)	< 0.001[a]
Smoking status					0.860[b]
Current smokers	138 (26.8)	45 (25.9)	50 (29.1)	43 (25.4)	
Previous smokers	184 (35.7)	64 (36.8)	62 (36.0)	58 (31.5)	
Never smokers	193 (37.5)	65 (37.4)	60 (34.9)	68 (40.2)	
Weight, kg	86.7 (17.3)	94.2 (15.4)	88.3 (17.2)	77.6 (15.2)	< 0.001[a]
BMI, kg/m^2	28.9 (4.98)	30.5 (4.6)	29.2 (5.0)	26.9 (4.6)	< 0.001[a]
WHR	0.94 (0.1)	0.99 (0.08)	0.95 (0.09)	0.88 (0.09)	< 0.001[a]
Metabolic syndrome	174 (32.9)	89 (50.6)	58 (33.0)	27 (15.5)	< 0.001[b]
OSA	293 (55.6)	71 (30.3)	75 (32.1)	88 (37.6)	0.167[b]
CRP, mg/L[d]	1.26 (0.65, 2.94)	1.48 (0.78, 3.20)	1.44 (0.69, 3.28)	0.92 (0.50, 2.09)	0.001[c]
FEV$_1$	3.41 (0.88)	3.64 (0.89)	3.51 (0.93)	3.09 (0.77)	< 0.001[c]
FVC	4.15 (1.03)	4.37 (0.99)	4.27 (1.08)	3.81 (0.93)	< 0.001[c]
FEV$_1$, % of predicted	103.25 (16.11)	101.19 (16.11)	104.45 (16.66)	104.09 (15.44)	0.115[a]
FVC, % of predicted	103.96 (16.33)	99.52 (15.78)	104.79 (16.22)	107.53 (16.05)	< 0.001[a]

ADPN adiponectin, *FEV$_1$* forced expiratory volume during 1st second, *FVC* forced vital capacity, *BMI* body mass index, *WHR* waist-hip ratio, *OSA* obstructive sleep apnoea, *CRP* C-reactive protein
[a]analyses of variance, [b]chi-square tests, [c]Kruskal-Wallis
Continuous variables are expressed as mean (standard deviation) or [d]median (interquartile range) and categorical variables are expressed as number (%).
Metabolic syndrome is defined according to the National Cholesterol Education Program criteria. OSA, Obstructive Sleep apnoea is defined as apnoea-hypopnoea index ≥5

association between ADPN and FEV$_1$/FVC in unadjusted analyses, as well as accelerated decline in FEV$_1$ with higher ADPN levels after adjustment for age, gender, height, smoking and BMI. In contrast, the CARDIA study, like the present study, observed an inverse association between ADPN and lung function in unadjusted analyses, but this association was attenuated and no longer significant in analysis that adjusted also for insulin resistance and systemic inflammation [14]. Thus, we find it plausible that circulating ADPN levels are primarily associated with indices of adiposity, and that univariate associations between ADPN levels and pulmonary function reflect an inverse association between adiposity and pulmonary function.

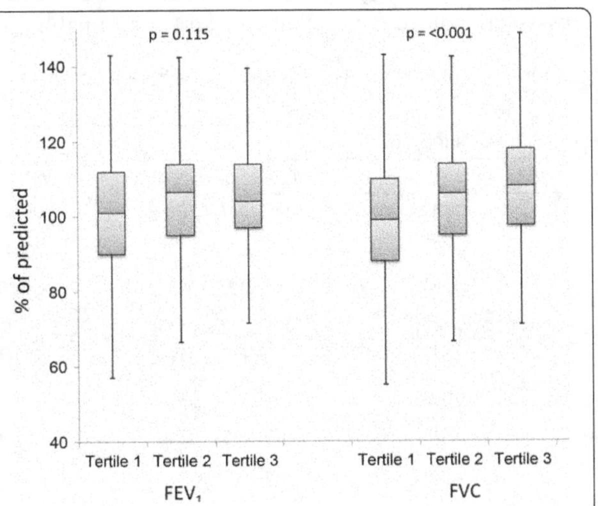

Fig. 2 Lung function in % of predicted according to tertiles of adiponectin

A novel finding in the present study is the important role of WHR as a confounder in the association between ADPN and lung function. While previous studies and the present study found that BMI alone did not attenuate the association between ADPN and lung function, WHR alone attenuated the association between ADPN and FVC in the present study. WHR also remained significantly associated with both FEV$_1$% of predicted and FVC % of predicted in multivariate analysis. Abdominal adiposity is a surrogate marker of visceral adiposity and is associated with serum levels of adiponectin, metabolic disease and systemic inflammation, but also results in mechanical restriction that may affect lung function and

Table 2 Univariate associations between lung function expressed as FEV_1 and FVC in percent of predicted, adiponectin, smoking status, indices of adiposity, metabolic syndrome, obstructive sleep apnoea and C-reactive protein

	FEV_1% predicted		FVC % predicted	
	Unstandardized beta (CI)	p	Unstandardized beta (CI)	p
ADPN (per SD)	1.012 (− 0.365, 2.388)	0.149	3.414 (2.047, 4.781)	< 0.001
Current smoking	−5.444 (−8.483, − 2.406)	< 0.001	−2.219 (−5.410, 0.972)	0.173
Previous smoking	0.645 (− 2.197, 3.487)	0.656	− 1.143 (−4.096, 1.811)	0.448
Weight (per 5 kg)	−0.661 (− 1.055, − 0.268)	0.001	− 1.119 (− 1.510, − 0.728)	< 0.001
BMI kg/m^2	−0.466 (− 0.740, − 0.192)	0.001	−0.647 (− 0.922, − 0.371)	< 0.001
WHR	−38.297 (− 52.041, − 24.553)	< 0.001	−62.199 (−75.488, − 48.909)	< 0.001
Metabolic syndrome	−4.905 (−7.808, − 2.001)	0.001	− 7.375 -10.289, − 4.471)	< 0.001
OSA	−2.143 (− 4.911, 0.625)	0.129	− 3.923 (− 6.725, − 1.120)	0.006
CRP (per SD)	− 2.157 (− 3.524, − 0.791)	0.002	− 2.071 (− 3.457, − 0.685)	0.003

FEV_1 forced expiratory volume during 1st second, *FVC* forced vital capacity, *CI* confidence interval, *ADPN* adiponectin, *SD* standard deviation, *BMI* body mass index, *WHR* waist-hip ratio, *OSA* obstructive sleep apnoea, *CRP* C-reactive protein

FVC in particular. The results from the present study indicate that the role of mechanic restriction from abdominal obesity contributes more to lung function than the changes in ADPN secretion and metabolic disease associated with this condition,

Interestingly, there were differences between FEV_1 and FVC in % of predicted as dependent variables. While FVC is a measure of lung volume, FEV_1 is also an indicator of airway obstruction. In our study, ADPN was only associated with FVC % of predicted in univariate analyses. Also, while all types of adiposity-related factors further attenuated the association between ADPN and FEV_1% of predicted, only WHR attenuated the positive association between FVC % of expected and ADPN. This might reflect that CRP and metabolic syndrome, as indicators of inflammatory and metabolic consequences of adiposity, are more important for FEV_1 than for FVC. This is in accordance with results in the CARDIA-study, which found metabolic syndrome and insulin resistance as well as systemic inflammation to attenuate the relationship between FEV_1 and adiponectin. These factors will be important to include in multivariate analysis when evaluating the relationship between ADPN and lung function.

There are several differences in the three presented population-based studies, besides the choice of covariates, which could explain the discrepant conclusions. One factor that could impact the result is ethnic variations with our study including primarily Caucasian subjects, the CARDIA study including a mixed American population while the third study examined a Japanese population. The CARDIA study also included younger individuals (mean age 40 years), the present study subjects with mean age of 50 years, and the Japanese study subjects with mean age of ~ 60 years. As ADPN levels are known to increase with age [22], different age groups could potentially also contribute to the diverging results between these three general population-based cohorts.

A limitation compared to previous studies is the cross-sectional design that makes us unable to

Table 3 The associations between adiponectin (ADPN) and lung function in percent of predicted adjusting for different covariates one by one

		Unstandardized beta (95% CI) ADPN (per SD)			
		FEV1% of predicted	p	FVC % of predicted	p
Unadjusted		1.012 (− 0.365, 2.388)	0.149	3.414 (2.047, 4.781)	< 0.001
Adjusted for	Weight (per 5 kg)	0.060 (− 1.445, 1.566)	0.937	2.166 (0.681, 3.651)	0.004
	BMI	0.303 (− 1.139, 1.744)	0.680	2.658 (1.229, 4.087)	< 0.001
	WHR	− 1.213 (− 2.771, 0.345)	0.127	0.425 (− 1.085,1.935)	0.581
	Current smoking	1.393 (0.048, 2.739)	0.042	3.556 (2.172, 4.941)	< 0.001
	Previous smoking	1.380 (0.017, 2.742)	0.047	3.529 (2.141, 4.917)	< 0.001
	Metabolic syndrome	0.353 (−1.078, 1.785)	0.628	2.610 (1.195, 4.025)	< 0.001
	OSA	1.090 (−0.299, 2.480)	0.124	3.282 (1.90, 4.664)	< 0.001
	CRP(per SD)	0.834 (−0.537, 2.206)	0.232	3.262 (1.897, 4.626)	< 0.001

FEV_1 forced expiratory volume during 1st second, *FVC* forced vital capacity, *CI* confidence interval, *ADPN* adiponectin, *BMI* body mass index, *WHR* waist-hip ratio, *OSA* obstructive sleep apnoea, *CRP* c-reactive protein

Table 4 The association between lung function and serum adiponectin levels adjusted for multiple covariates

	FEV1% of predicted Standardized B (CI)	*p*	FVC % of predicted Standardized B (CI)	*p*
Adiponectin/SD	−0.056 (−2.390, 0.632)	0.254	0.027 (−1.083, 1.956)	0.573
WHR	−0.264 (−58.269, −27.208)	< 0.001	− 0.360 (−76.027, −44.799)	< 0.001
Current smoking	− 0.170 (−8.940, −3.075)	< 0.001	−0.083 (−6.010, − 0.113)	0.042
CRP/SD	− 0.125 (− 3.235, − 0.660)	0.003	−0.103 (− 2.957, − 0.368)	0.012

FEV_1 forced expiratory volume during 1st second, *FVC* forced vital capacity, *CI* confidence interval, *ADPN* adiponectin, *SD* standard deviation, *WHR* waist-hip ratio, *CRP* c-reactive protein

evaluate changes in lung function and causal pathways. On the other hand, compared to CARDIA, we were able to analyze ADPN samples obtained at the same time point as the spirometry. The ASAP cohort consisted of individuals with more risk factors for obstructive sleep apnoea than a strict general population sample and were as a group more obese, more sleepy and had a higher rate of diabetes and prior myocardial infarction than the general population sample responding to the Berlin questionnaire in the first part of the study. OSA is associated with lower ADPN levels and is a possible confounder in the examined relationship between ADPN and lung function. However, the prevalence of OSA did not differ between the tertiles of ADPN and the association between FVC% of predicted and ADPN remained significant after adjustment for OSA and metabolic syndrome. Also mean ADPN levels and measures of lung function in the study sample were comparable to those observed in previous general population studies [15, 23]. Based on this we believe our results are valid also for subjects from the general population. Finally, only total ADPN levels were measured and therefore information regarding different isoforms is not available.

Conclusions

In this population-based study, we found a positive association between ADPN and FEV_1 and FVC after adjustment for age, gender, height and smoking that was attenuated after additional adjustment for indices of abdominal adiposity. Accordingly, future assessment of the association between ADPN and lung function should take both multiple indices of adiposity and its metabolic consequences into consideration.

Abbreviations

ADPN: Adiponectin; ASAP: Akershus Sleep Apnea Project; BMI: Body mass index; CARDIA: Coronary artery risk development in young adults; COPD: Chronic obstructive pulmonary disease; CRP: C-reactive protein; FEV_1: Forced expiratory volume in 1 second; FVC: Forced vital capacity; SD: Standard deviation; WHR: Waist-hip ratio

Acknowledgements

We thank the staff at Stensby Hospital and the Clinical Trial Unit, Division of Medicine, Akershus University Hospital for performing the spirometry. We also thank Silje Kjeka Namtvedt for contributing to data collection and Fredrik A. Dahl for statistical advice.

Funding

The Akershus Sleep Apnea Project was supported by the South-Eastern Norway Regional Health Authority (grant number 2004219, 2007048) and the University of Oslo. The study was conducted at Akershus University Hospital. NFC has received a grant (2015/FO7781) from Extrastiftelsen initiated in collaboration with the Norwegian Heart and Lung Association (LHL).

Authors' contributions

TO had the original idea of ASAP, while the concept of the current study was conceived by NFC and GE. HHS and AR contibuted to the study design and performed the data collection. AF and MB were responsible for the biomarker substudy of adiponectin including laboratory analyses. HR contributed with critical revision of the manuscript and data interpretation. NFC and GE had the full responsibility for the statistical analyses. NFC performed the drafting of the manuscript, while all authors contributed significantly and approved the final version.

Consent for publication

Not applicable

Competing interests

TO has received speaker and/or consultancy honoraria from Abbott Diagnostics, Roche Diagnostics, Novartis and research support from Abbott Diagnostics, AstraZeneca, Thermo Fisher Scientific, and Biomedica. GE has received research grants from Astra Zeneca and speaker honorarium from Takeda. The other authors declare no reported conflicts of interest.

Author details

[1]Division of Medicine, Akershus University Hospital, Lørenskog, Norway. [2]Institute of Clinical Medicine, University of Oslo, Oslo, Norway. [3]Steno Diabetes Center Copenhagen (SDCC), the Capital Region of Denmark and

University of Copenhagen, Copenhagen, Denmark. [4]Medical Research Laboratory, Department of Clinical Medicine, Aarhus University, Aarhus, Denmark. [5]Department of Otorhinolaryngology, Division of Surgery, Akershus University Hospital, Lørenskog, Norway.

References

1. Global Strategy for the Diagnosis, Management and Prevention of COPD. Global Initiative for Chronic Obstructive Lung Disease (GOLD). 2017. http://www.goldcopd.org.
2. Murray CJ, Lopez AD. Alternative projections of mortality and disability by cause 1990-2020: Global Burden of Disease Study. Lancet. 1997;349(9064): 1498–504.
3. Agusti A, Sin DD. Biomarkers in COPD. Clin Chest Med. 2014;35(1):131–41.
4. Miller M, Cho JY, Pham A, Ramsdell J, Broide DH. Adiponectin and functional adiponectin receptor 1 are expressed by airway epithelial cells in chronic obstructive pulmonary disease. J Immunol. 2009;182(1):684–91.
5. Obata Y, Yamada Y, Takahi Y, Baden MY, Saisho K, Tamba S, et al. Relationship between serum adiponectin levels and age in healthy subjects and patients with type 2 diabetes. Clin Endocrinol. 2013;79(2):204–10.
6. Tilg H, Moschen AR. Adipocytokines: mediators linking adipose tissue, inflammation and immunity. Nat Rev Immunol. 2006;6(10):772–83.
7. Kotani K, Hazama A, Hagimoto A, Saika K, Shigeta M, Katanoda K, et al. Adiponectin and smoking status: a systematic review. J Atheroscler Thromb. 2012;19(9):787–94.
8. Chen WL, Wang CC, Wu LW, Kao TW, Chan JY, Chen YJ, et al. Relationship between lung function and metabolic syndrome. PLoS One. 2014;9(10): e108989.
9. Xu A, Vanhoutte PM. Adiponectin and adipocyte fatty acid binding protein in the pathogenesis of cardiovascular disease. Am J Physiol Heart Circ Physiol. 2012;302(6):H1231–H40.
10. Yamauchi T, Kamon J, Waki H, Terauchi Y, Kubota N, Hara K, et al. The fat-derived hormone adiponectin reverses insulin resistance associated with both lipoatrophy and obesity. Nat Med. 2001;7(8):941–6.
11. Tomoda K, Yoshikawa M, Itoh T, Tamaki S, Fukuoka A, Komeda K, et al. Elevated circulating plasma adiponectin in underweight patients with COPD. Chest. 2007;132(1):135–40.
12. Yoon HI, Li Y, Man SF, Tashkin D, Wise RA, Connett JE, et al. The complex relationship of serum adiponectin to COPD outcomes COPD and adiponectin. Chest. 2012;142(4):893–9.
13. Carolan BJ, Kim YI, Williams AA, Kechris K, Lutz S, Reisdorph N, et al. The association of adiponectin with computed tomography phenotypes in chronic obstructive pulmonary disease. Am J Respir Crit Care Med. 2013; 188(5):561–6.
14. Thyagarajan B, Jacobs DR Jr, Smith LJ, Kalhan R, Gross MD, Sood A. Serum adiponectin is positively associated with lung function in young adults, independent of obesity: the CARDIA study. Respir Res. 2010;11:176.
15. Sato K, Shibata Y, Abe S, Inoue S, Igarashi A, Yamauchi K, et al. Association between plasma adiponectin levels and decline in forced expiratory volume in 1 s in a general Japanese population: the Takahata study. Int J Med Sci. 2014;11(8):758–64.
16. Hrubos-Strom H, Randby A, Namtvedt SK, Kristiansen HA, Einvik G, Benth J, et al. A Norwegian population-based study on the risk and prevalence of obstructive sleep apnea. The Akershus Sleep Apnea Project (ASAP). J Sleep Res. 2011;20(1 Pt 2):162–70.
17. Netzer NC, Stoohs RA, Netzer CM, Clark K, Strohl KP. Using the Berlin Questionnaire to identify patients at risk for the sleep apnea syndrome. Ann Intern Med. 1999;131(7):485–91.
18. Quanjer PH, Tammeling GJ, Cotes JE, Pedersen OF, Peslin R, Yernault JC. Lung volumes and forced ventilatory flows. Report working party standardization of lung function tests, European Community for steel and coal. Official statement of the European Respiratory Society. Eur Respir J Suppl. 1993;16:5–40.
19. Executive summary of the third report of the National Cholesterol Education Program (NCEP) expert panel on detection, evaluation, and treatment of high blood cholesterol in adults (Adult Treatment Panel III). JAMA. 2001;285(19):2486–97.
20. Einvik G, Rosjo H, Randby A, Namtvedt SK, Hrubos-Strom H, Brynildsen J, et al. Severity of obstructive sleep apnea is associated with cardiac troponin I concentrations in a community-based sample: data from the Akershus sleep apnea project. Sleep. 2014;37(6):1111–6.
21. Frystyk J, Tarnow L, Hansen TK, Parving HH, Flyvbjerg A. Increased serum adiponectin levels in type 1 diabetic patients with microvascular complications. Diabetologia. 2005;48(9):1911–8.
22. Marques-Vidal P, Bochud M, Paccaud F, Mooser V, Waeber G, Vollenweider P. Distribution of plasma levels of adiponectin and leptin in an adult Caucasian population. Clin Endocrinol. 2010;72(1):38–46.
23. Hayashikawa Y, Iwata M, Inomata M, Kawagishi Y, Tokui K, Taka C, et al. Association of serum adiponectin with asthma and pulmonary function in the Japanese population. Endocr J. 2015;62(8):695–709.

20

MDA-5 associated rapidly progressive interstitial lung disease with recurrent Pneumothoraces

Safi Alqatari[1*], Peter Riddell[2], Sinead Harney[3], Michael Henry[2] and Grainne Murphy[2]

Abstract

Background: Clinically hypomyopathic dermatomyositis is a rare disease that is important to recognize, investigate and treat early as it is associated with poor prognosis. In a proportion of patients, myositis specific antibodies could be negative, but with high clinical suspicion, myositis associated antibodies should be ordered. Anti-MDA-5 antibodies was reported in literature to be associated with severe and rapidly progressive interstitial lung disease, with few case reports of pneumothorax and/or pneumomediastinum.

Case presentation: A 49-year-old previously healthy lady, presented with a 6 week history of skin rash, photosensitivity, mouth ulcers, fatiguability, arthralgia and myalgia. She denied subjective weakness, respiratory symptoms or dysphagia. She had Raynaud's phenomenon affecting her fingers only. Initial examination showed synovitis in her hands with skin rash. Autoimmune screen was negative. She was started on hydroxychloroquine. 4 weeks later on follow-up, she developed proximal muscle pain, dysphagia, dyspnea and dry cough. Examination showed mild proximal muscle weakness and bi-basal crackles. She was admitted and extended myositis screen was sent. She had mild anemia, lymphopenia and neutropenia, normal inflammatory markers, liver and renal panels. Capillaroscopy showed pattern of systemic sclerosis. CT chest showed early ILD. Electromyography and MRI showed features of mild myositis. PFT showed muscle weakness with low DLCO. She was given intravenous steroid and Rituximab. As she continued to deteriorate, intravenous immunoglobulins and cyclophosphamide were given. There was a brief clinical response that was short-lived with increasing oxygen dependency necessitating transfer to the ICU. At this point, the extended myositis screen confirmed the presence of anti-MDA-5 antibodies. She commenced plasmapharesis and required intubation. Unfortunately, she developed multiple pneumothoraces, and was transferred urgently for ECMO. Subsequent immunosuppression included rituximab and tacrolimus. There was progression of her ILD and recurrent pneumothoraces and pneumomediastinum. Unfortunately, she passed away as a consequence of her disease.

Conclusion: This case highlights a number of considerations in approaching patients with inflammatory myositis, particularly to pulmonary involvement. It is important to highlight the utility of extended myositis antibody testing in predicting disease phenotypes and its impact on therapeutic decisions. From a management perspective, aggressive immunosuppression should be considered with potential need of earlier utilization of ECMO.

Keywords: Myositis, Interstitial lung disease, MDA-5

* Correspondence: alqatarisafi@hotmail.com
[1]Royal College of Physicians of Ireland, Rheumatology Department, Cork University Hospital, Wilton, Cork, IrelandT12 DC4A
Full list of author information is available at the end of the article

Background

Clinically hypomyopathic DM is a rare disease that is important to recognize, investigate and treat early as it is associated with poor prognosis. In a proportion of patients, myositis specific antibodies are negative, but with high clinical suspicion, myositis associated antibodies should be ordered. Hypomyopathic dermatomyositis with positive anti-MDA-5 antibodies was reported in literature to be associated with severe and rapidly progressive interstitial lung disease. There are a limited number of case reports of associated pneumothorax and/or pneumomediastinum largely in an Asian population. We present a challenging case of rapidly progressive interstitial lung disease (ILD) and pneumothorax/ pneumomediastinum in an Irish/Caucasian patient with hypomyopathic MDA-5 positive dermatomyositis.

Case presentation

A 49-year-old lady was referred to the rheumatology services with a 6-week history of an erythematous rash on her face, fingers and feet which was painful, desquamative and itchy. This was photosensitive in nature and accompanied by painful mouth ulcers. More recently she had noticed generalized myalgia, widespread joint pain especially in her small joints, easy fatiguability and malaise. She reported symptoms of Raynaud's phenomenon on exposure to cold two years prior. She denied respiratory symptoms, dysphagia or odynophagia. Examination was remarkable for puffy fingers with polyarthritis (MCPs, PIPs, DIPs, wrists and toes), peri-ungual erythema and a desquamative rash. Power on initial presentation was normal and there were no clinical findings to suggest ILD. She was commenced on low dose prednisolone and hydroxychloroquine and serological testing was requested. A standard screen was negative (RF, ACPA, ANA, ENA, ANCA). She had no family history of autoimmune disorders.

Over the ensuing 4 weeks she experienced a significant deterioration. She developed new progressive proximal muscle pain with no subjective weakness. She also reported dysphagia to solids as well as dyspnea on minimal exertion associated with a dry cough. Clinical examination revealed a mild proximal myopathy and end inspiratory bi-basal crackles. At that point, she was admitted for investigation and management including an extended myositis antibody panel. Results of her initial investigations are summarized in Table 1.

Echocardiography was normal. Capillaroscopy showed early and active pattern of systemic sclerosis. CT chest showed early ILD in the form of non-specific interstitial pneumonia (NSIP) (Fig. 1a, b). Electromyography showed features of mild non-necrotic myopathy in the quadriceps muscles. MRI of bilateral humeri and femora showed features of myositis involving multiple muscle groups (Fig. 1c, d). PFT showed restrictive pattern with moderate DLCO reduction (DLCO 11.8 (predicted = 20), FEV1 1.7 L (predicted = 2.02), FVC 2.1 (predicted = 2.4), FEV//FVC = 80.95%).

She was commenced on methylprednisolone 500 mg intravenously for 3 days and received Day 1 Rituximab 1 g, with a plan to retreat on Day 14. Unfortunately, she developed a steroid-induced psychosis, necessitating a reduction in subsequent prednisolone dosing. Over the ensuing days she further deteriorated with radiological progression of her ILD. In the context of progressive dysphagia, she commenced IV Immunoglobulin and received cyclophosphamide (15 mg/kg). There was a brief clinical response following this combination but this was short-lived with increasing oxygen dependency necessitating transfer to the ICU for initial non-invasive ventilation. At this point, the extended myositis screen detected the presence of anti-MDA-5 antibodies confirming the diagnosis of hypomyopathic dermatomyositis. She commenced plasmapharesis for 5 days. She required intubation due to respiratory fatigue and increasing oxygen requirements. She developed multiple pneumothoraces, and due to ventilatory difficulties was transferred urgently for ECMO. Subsequent immunosuppression included day 14 rituximab and the addition of tacrolimus. Despite aggressive immunosuppression and prolonged ECMO therapy there was further progression of her interstitial lung disease, recurrent pneumothoraces and pneumomediastinum. Unfortunately, she passed away as a consequence of her disease.

Table 1 Results of blood tests

Test	Result	Test	Result	Test	Result
WBCs	2.25/ L (4.4–11.3/L)	Urea	2.4 mmol/L (2.8–8.4 mmol/L)	Urinalysis	Negative
Neutrophils	1.2/ L (1.4–6.6/L)	Creatinine	54 micromol/L (49–90 micromol/L)	ANA and ENA	Negative
Lymphocytes	0.6/ L (0.9–3.2/L)	ALT	48 U/L (0–34 U/L)	DsDNA	Negative
Hemoglobin	10.1 g/dl (11.7–15.9 g/dl)	AST	78 U/L (6–42 U/L)	C3	1.15 g/L (normal)
Platelets	420,000/L (140–440 X10*9/L	LDH	1531 U/L (220–450 U/L)	C4	0.30 g/L (normal)
ESR	7 mm (0–20 mm)	CPK	208 U/L (40–180 U/L)	RF and Anti-CCP	Negative
CRP	2 mg/L (0–10 mg/L)	Albumin	25 g/L (35–52 g/L)	ANCA	Negative

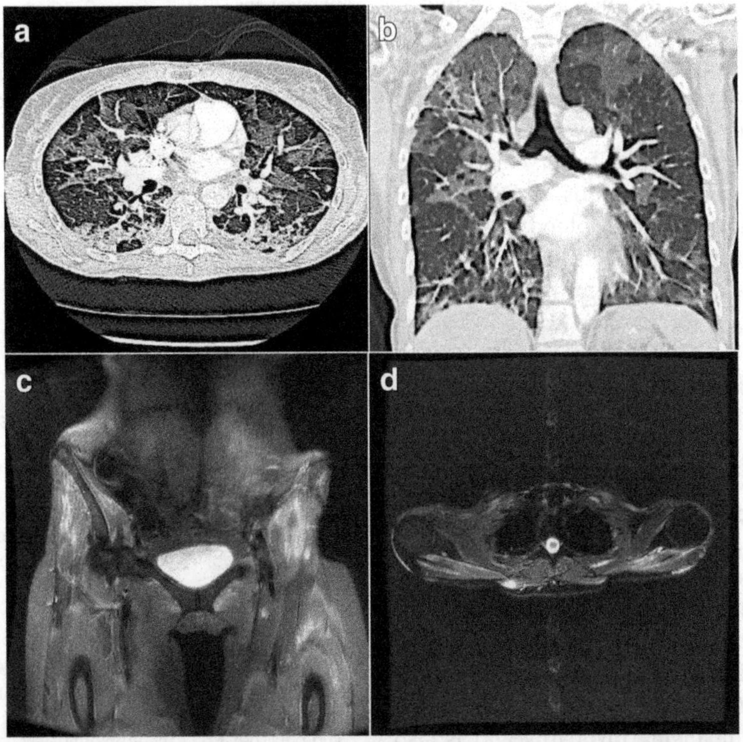

Fig. 1 Axial (**a**) and Coronal (**b**) CT (lung windows). Multifocal ground glass opacity progressing to consolidation in the dependent lungs. (**d**) Coronal STIR Pelvis: T2 hyperintensity in gluteal, quadriceps and adductor musculature in keeping with myositis. (**e**) Axial T2FS Upper limbs: Further oedema within trapezius, deltoid and rotator cuff musculature

Discussion and conclusion

Idiopathic inflammatory myopathies (IIMs) are a heterogeneous group of diseases [polymyositis (PM), dermatomyositis (DM), inclusion body myositis (IBM), necrotizing autoimmune myositis (NAIM)], characterized by myositis. Other organs such as the skin in DM and the lungs, heart, joints and gastrointestinal tract can be affected. Classification of IIMs is important as different phenotypes and serotypes are caused by different presentations, suggesting the need for targeted therapies [1]. Autoantibody testing has become crucial for the assessment of patients with IIM (as described by Betteridge and McHugh) [2].

Auto-antibodies can be generally classified into myositis-associated and myositis-specific antibodies. The recognition of specific clinical phenotypes associated with individual antibodies has had significant clinical impact. Notable examples include the association of antibodies directed at TIF-1gamma with malignancy. Antisynthetase antibodies are strongly associated with ILD, especially non-Jo-1 (anti-PL-7 and anti-PL-12) where the association approaches 90–100% [3]. A rare form of ILD with a very poor prognosis, is strongly associated with CADM and the novel MDA- 5/anti-CADM-140 auto-antibody. A combination of anti-Jo-1 and anti-SSA/Ro antibodies also indicates severe pulmonary involvement [3].

The strong association between ILD and myositis has been recognized for many years and has led to the routine screening for ILD in individuals presenting with an inflammatory myopathy. Clinically amyopathic or hypomyopathic dermatomyositis however may initially present to a variety of specialties and ultimately this can lead to diagnostic delay. These individuals may present initially to respiratory services with symptoms and signs of ILD. The advent of EMA testing has suggested that particular antibodies segregate with propensity for ILD, such as PL-7 and PL-12. Interestingly these individuals who may present with imaging in keeping with established fibrosis may respond to immunosuppression [3]; highlighting the importance of requesting extended antibody testing, even in the absence of circulating antinuclear antibodies. In the case of MDA-5 antibodies in particular, ILD can be rapidly progressive and, as in the case discussed above, refractory to intensive immunosuppression, suggesting its valuable utility as a prognostic indicator of disease severity.

In our case, it is probably the high pressure from ventilatory support that caused the pneumothoraces but it is important to highlight an interesting and perhaps less recognized phenomenon, which is the potential for pneumothoraces and pneumomediastinum. Both can occur spontaneously as published in previous case reports/series [4]. The aetiopathogeneis is poorly understood but multiple theories have been proposed. These include the presence of raised intra-alveolar pressure which leads to rupture of previously damaged alveoli, or rupture of subpleural cyst(s) that developed from co-existing interstitial fibrosis. Another factor could be the presence of an underlying lung vasculitis, as DM is associated with inflammation of small blood vessels [4]. Many patients with rapidly progressive ILD and amyopathic myositis needed a combination of multiple immunosuppressives and steroids for a prolonged period (up to twelve months in some reports) highlighting the aggressive nature of ILD in this cohort.

Given the rarity of individuals with myositis associated antibodies, trials aiming to target a particular therapy by antibody type do not exist. Existing reports suggest that initial high dose steroids are the most common initial therapy used and perhaps the most effective medication in controlling acute disease. They are used in conjunction with a variety of additional immunosuppressives including cyclophosphamide, mycophenolate mofetil, ciclosporin and tacrolimus and biologic medication, commonly rituximab. Of note, rituximab offers dual benefit in treating accompanying myopathy and is also gaining increasing attention in treating ILD in the context of connective tissue disorders. Some studies suggested that the addition of tacrolimus improved the disease free survival of PM/DM as will as ILD. However, the number of patients involved in those studies were small [5].

Finally, the impact of ECMO therapy merits discussion and particularly its role in reducing the risk of pneumothorax in this setting. In the case of rapidly progressive ILD associated with CADM, the use of ECMO should be considered early in the disease process, especially in potentially reversible conditions to avoid the need for mechanical ventilation [6].

In conclusion, this case highlights a number of critical considerations in approaching patients with inflammatory myositis, particularly in relation to associated pulmonary involvement. While ILD has long been recognized as a potential complication of myositis, the potential for ILD to be the prominent feature of presentation is now well described particularly in a subgroup of patients with little clinical evidence of myopathy. We wish to highlight the importance of clinical surveillance for the development of myopathy in individuals with amyopathic or hypomyopathic dermatomyositis; the utility of extended myositis antibody testing in predicting disease phenotypes and the potential impact on subsequent management in this cohort. Of particular significance, this case emphasized the importance of early consideration of ECMO to decrease the risk of pneumothorax/ mediastinum.

Abbreviations

ACPA: Anti-cetrullinated peptide antibody; ANA: Anti-nuclear antibody; ANCA: Anti-neutrophilic cytoplasmic antibody; CADM: Clinically amyopathic dermatomyositis; DIPs: Distal inter-phalangeal joints; DLCO: Diffusion carbon monoxide; DM: Dermatomyositis; ECMO: Extra-corporeal membrane oxygenation; ENA: Extractable nuclear antibody; FEV1: Forced expiratory volume in 1 s; FVC: Forced vital capacity; IBM: Inclusion body myositis; IIMs: Idiopathic interstitial myopathies; ILD: Interstitial lung disease; MCPs: Meta-carpo-phalangeal joints; MDA-5: melanoma differentiation-associated gene 5; MRI: Magnetic resonance imaging; NAIM: Necrotizing autoimmune myositis; NSIP: Non-specific interstitial pneumonia; PFT: Pulmonary function test; PIPs: Proximal inter-phalangeal joints; Anti-PL-7: Anti-Threonyl-tRNA Synthetase; Anti-PL-12: anti-alanyl-tRNA synthetase; PM: Polymyositis; RF: Rheumatoid factor

Funding

We received no funding to work on or publish this case report.

Authors' contributions

SQ, PR wrote the manuscript of this case report including the case report and discussion. SH, MH and GM reviewed the manuscript and added to the discussion. All authors have read and agreed on the manuscript.

Consent for publication

Consent was obtained from the patient's husband. He signed a consent form indicating that he is aware of this case report and the possibility of it being published (the patient unfortunately passed away).

Competing interests

There is no financial or non-financial conflict of interest with any person or organization.

Author details

[1]Royal College of Physicians of Ireland, Rheumatology Department, Cork University Hospital, Wilton, Cork, IrelandT12 DC4A. [2]Rheumatology Department, Cork University Hospital, Wilton, Cork, Ireland. [3]Internal Medicine and Rheumatology Consultant Rheumatology Department, Cork University Hospital, Wilton, Cork, Ireland.

References

1. Lundberg IE, Miller FW, Tjearnlund A, Bottai M. Diagnosis and classification of idiopathic inflammatory myopathies. J Intern Med. 2016;280:39–51. https://doi.org/10.1111/joim.12524.
2. Moghadam-Kia S, Oddis CV, Sato S, Kuwana M, Aggarwal R. Anti–melanoma differentiation–associated gene 5 is associated with rapidly progressive lung disease and poor survival in US patients with Amyopathic and Myopathic dermatomyositis. Arthritis Care & Research. May 2016;68(5):689–94. https://doi.org/10.1002/acr.22728.
3. Solomon J, Swigris JJ, Brown KK. Myositis-related interstitial lung disease and antisynthetase syndrome. J Bras Pneumol. 2011;37(1):100–9. https://doi.org/10.1590/S1806-37132011000100015.
4. Bradley JD. Spontaneous pneumomediastinum in adult dermatomyositis. Ann Rheum Dis. 1986;45:780–2. https://doi.org/10.1136/ard.45.9.780.
5. Kurita T, Yasuda S, Oba K, Odani T, Kono M, Kotaro O, et al. The efficacy of tacrolimus in patients with interstitial lung diseases complicated with polymyositis or dermatomyositis. Rheumatology. 2015, 54:39–44. https://doi.org/10.1093/rheumatology/keu166.
6. MacLare G, Combes A, Bartlett RH. Contemporary extracorporeal membrane oxygenation for adult respiratory failure: life support in the new era. Intensive Care Med. February 2012;38(2):210–20. https://doi.org/10.1007/s00134-011-2439-2.

21

Is daily physical activity affected by dynamic hyperinflation in adults with cystic fibrosis?

Daniela Savi[1,2*], Marcello Di Paolo[1], Nicholas J. Simmonds[3], Chiara Pascucci[4], Serena Quattrucci[5] and Paolo Palange[1,6]

Abstract

Background: The aim of this study was to investigate the relationship between dynamic hyperinflation and daily physical activity (DPA) in adults with cystic fibrosis (CF).

Methods: Thirty-four clinically stable CF were studied. All patients undertook incremental cardiopulmonary exercise testing (CPET). CPET-related measurements included: oxygen uptake ($V'O_2$), carbon dioxide production ($V'CO_2$), ventilatory profile, work rate (W), inspiratory capacity (IC), end-expiratory lung volume (EELV). PA was assessed using the accelerometer SenseWear Pro3 Armband.

Results: Exercise tolerance was reduced in most of patients and the mean $V'O_{2,peak}$ value was 75.2% of predicted (28.5 ± 4.8 ml/min/kg). Seventy % of patients responded to CPET with dynamic hyperinflation. Higher incidence of dynamic hyperinflation was found in CF males compared to CF females ($p = 0.026$). Patients who developed dynamic hyperinflation during CPET had higher vigorous PA ($p = 0.01$) and more total energy expenditure ($p = 0.006$) than patients who did not. EELVΔ was related to activities requiring vigorous intensity and total energy expenditure ($R = 0.46$, $p = 0.001$; $R = 0.57$, $p < 0.001$).

Conclusions: In adults with CF and mild to moderate lung impairment, DPA might not be limited by dynamic hyperinflation.

Keywords: Cystic fibrosis, Daily physical activity, Dynamic hyperinflation, Exercise intolerance

Background

The assessment of daily physical activity (DPA) is a parameter of increasing interest in the clinical evaluation of patients with cystic fibrosis (CF). Despite the well-recognized physical and psychological benefits of exercise in maintaining health in CF, exercise participation is often below recommended levels [1] especially in CF females [2]. Recently, two studies showed that activity levels in daily life correlate significantly with exercise tolerance in CF adults [3, 4]. It is important to identify significant factors related to aerobic capacity because peak oxygen uptake ($V'O_{2,peak}$) is a prognostic factor in CF [5, 6]. Maintaining high levels of physical activity is an important objective in the management of CF.

Many studies have investigated exercise intolerance in CF and have showed multiple compromised mechanisms [7]. These include musculoskeletal abnormalities [8, 9], abnormal oxygen delivery and gas exchange [10], deconditioning [11] and finally lung dynamic hyperinflation [12]. In chronic obstructive pulmonary disease (COPD) breathing at higher lung volumes increases respiratory work and thus potentiates the perception of breathlessness, which may discourage patients from taking part in DPA and become responsible for a decrease in DPA [13].

In the past, Alison et al. measured changes in end-expiratory lung volume (EELV) during leg and arm exercise in 22 CF patients [14]. They observed that CF patients with FEV1 < 90% predicted were likely to dynamically hyperinflate during arm cranking. This is

* Correspondence: danielasavi1@virgilio.it
[1]Department of Public Health and Infectious Diseases, Adult Cystic Fibrosis Center, Sapienza University of Rome, 00185 Rome, Italy
[2]Cystic Fibrosis Unit, Bambino Gesù Children's Hospital, Rome, Italy
Full list of author information is available at the end of the article

particularly interesting if we consider that the ability to perform upper-limb exercise is important for daily activities. More recently, a larger study showed that dynamic hyperinflation during cardiopulmonary exercise testing (CPET) is almost common in adult patients with mild-to-moderate CF [12]. To date, although the impact of dynamic hyperinflation on exercise is recognized [12], little information on the effect of dynamic hyperinflation on DPA is available in CF. Several studies have found that the level of DPA is independent of lung function in CF [15, 16] suggesting that high activity levels do not necessarily reflect the level of lung function [16]. Whether DPA level in adult CF can be associated with a development of dynamic hyperinflation warrants further investigations.

The aim of the present study was to investigate the relationship between dynamic hyperinflation developed during CPET and DPA levels in a cohort of adults with mild-to-moderate airflow obstruction. Specifically, we wished to evaluate if the identification of dynamic hyperinflation with exercise may correlate with daily life activities in these CF patients.

Methods

Study design

Thirty-four adults with CF were recruited consecutively between January 2012 and December 2013 from the Policlinico Umberto I Hospital, Sapienza University of Rome, Italy. The study was approved by the Ethics Committee of Policlinico Umberto I Hospital, with approval number 582/11. Data on demographic and clinical characteristics, baseline spirometry and CPET-related measurements were collected at the time of enrolment. The patients were equipped with a physical activity monitor. Their habitual physical activities were assessed for a period of 5 days. Medical management of the CF patients was carried out as normal, including use of bronchodilators. Subjects with CF were asked to continue any respiratory-related medications before the visits. The estimation of the calculation for sample size was done using a previous study by Lahaije Anke JMC, et al. [17] who showed a $r = 0.42$ for the relation between dynamic hyperinflation and physical activity. For this study, assuming $\alpha = 0.05$ and 0.80 power with r between 0.40 and 0.50, our effect size would require a number of patients between 30 and 47. We therefore recruited 34 CF patients in total.

Patients and data collection

Patients attending a CF outpatient clinic were approached for participation in the study. Patients were included if they were ≥ 18 years of age, with mild-to-moderate pulmonary impairment based on FEV_1 (i.e., mild = FEV_1 > 80% predicted; moderate = FEV_1 40 to 80% predicted) and had a confirmed diagnosis of CF based on genetic testing showing two CF-causing mutations and/or two documented sweet chloride values > 60 mEq/l. Patients were excluded if they had unstable medical conditions that could cause or contribute to breathlessness (i.e cardiovascular, metabolic, or other respiratory diseases) or other disorders that could interfere with exercise testing, such as neuromuscular diseases or musculoskeletal problems. Patients with a pulmonary exacerbation in the 4 weeks prior to the study, with acute respiratory failure, on oxygen therapy, on the waiting list for lung transplantation or post- transplant were excluded from the study. Baseline data were collected at the time of study entry.

After obtaining written informed consent and appropriate screening of medical history, we collected data on age, sex, height, weight, body mass index (BMI), chronic infections and CF comorbidity (pancreas insufficiency and CF-related diabetes). At the time of study entry all patients underwent spirometry, nitrogen washout and single-breath diffusing capacity (DLCO) which were performed by standardized techniques using an automated pulmonary function testing system (COSMED PFT, Pavona Italy) [18–20]. All pulmonary function data were standardized as percentages of predicted normal values [21, 22]. Maximal voluntary ventilation (MVV) was estimated using the formula $FEV_1 \times 40$.

A maximal incremental CPET was conducted. We used an electronically-braked cycle ergometer (Ergoline-800, Ergoline GmbH, Bitz, Germany) and the Quark b^2 system (COSMED, Rome, Italy) according to recommended guidelines [23]. CPET consisted of a steady-state resting period, then 2 min of warm-up at 10 watt followed by a stepwise protocol in which the work rate was increased in 1-min intervals by increments of 20 W. The test was continued until exhaustion and subjects were encouraged throughout the test. Subjects rated the magnitude of their perceived breathing and leg discomfort at rest, every two minutes during exercise and at peak exercise by pointing a modified Borg scale [24]. Oxygen saturation (SpO_2) by pulse oximetry on the finger, electrocardiographic monitoring of heart rate (HR), rhythm and ST-segment changes, minute ventilation (V'E), oxygen uptake ($V'O_2$), carbon dioxide production ($V'CO_2$) were measured at rest and during CPET. Peak $V'O_2$ ($V'O_{2,peak}$) was normalized for body weight and was also expressed as percentage of the predicted value [25]. The inspiratory capacity (IC) maneuver was performed by patients at rest, at the end of each increment of exercise and at peak of exercise. The IC represents the volume inhaled from the end of normal exhalation to maximal inhalation (i.e., total lung capacity). EELV was calculated by subtracting the IC from the total lung capacity (EELV = TLC-IC) [26]. It is assumed that total lung capacity remains unchanged during exercise, which is supported by literature in health [27] and COPD [28]. The change in the IC from rest to peak exercise was calculated (ICΔ) and consequently, the change in EELV from rest to peak exercise was also calculated (EELVΔ). Based on previous studies in CF [12, 29], patients were categorized into the dynamic hyperinflation group if they showed evidence of decreasing in IC from rest to peak exercise (ICΔ) ≥ 100 mL.

Assessment of daily physical activity

DPA was assessed at the time of the study enrollment, using a multi-sensor armband (SenseWear Pro3 Armband (SWA), BodyMedia, Pittsburgh, USA) which has been validated in CF [30, 31]. Patients wore the armband for at least five full consecutive typical days (including 3 weekdays and 2 weekend days) when they were at home. Data are reported as the average of 5 days. It was reported in CF that 5 days monitoring was enough to assess DPA and that DPA levels were similar through the week (i.e., weekdays versus weekend days) [3, 4]. The characteristics of the device have been previously described [2]. The outputs obtained from the armband were the detection of energy expenditure (EE), including total energy expenditure (TEE) and active energy expenditure (AEE), total physical activity duration, number of steps, time lying down, sleep duration and intensity of PA, expressed in metabolic equivalents (METS). The time (min) spent in PA at different intensities (mild, moderate, vigorous) and the definitions for activity levels based on METS were those used by Troosters et al. [3]. See Additional file 1.

Statistical analysis

Data obtained from CF patients with dynamic hyperinflation and non-dynamic hyperinflation were compared. Categorical data are presented as percentages, and comparisons were performed using the χ^2 or *Fisher's exact test.* Parametric data are presented as mean ± standard deviation (SD) and comparisons were made using the two-sample independent *t test.* Non-parametric data are presented as median and interquartile range and comparisons were performed using the *Mann–Whitney U test.* Correlations were identified between PA measurements and CPET parameters through the use of the *Pearson's R correlation coefficient* or the *Spearman's rank correlation coefficient* according to parametric or non-parametric distribution of data, respectively and corrected for gender. Significant contributors (gender, $V'O_{2,peak}$ $ml \cdot min^{-1}$, EELVΔ in absolute value and % of TLC) were introduced into a stepwise multiple linear regression analysis to identify independent determinants of PA.

All statistical tests were two-sided, and significance was reported at $p < 0.05$. Analyses were performed using the SPSS Statistics version 22.0 software package (IBM, Armonk, New York, USA).

Results

Study population characteristics and daily physical activity

Baseline characteristics and pulmonary function data for the group as a whole and the dynamic ($n = 24$) and non-dynamic hyperinflation ($n = 10$) groups are shown in Table 1. The study group comprised CF patients with a good nutritional status and a mild to moderate lung impairment based on FEV1 as a percentage of predicted. (Table 1). Seventy percent (24/34) of patients demonstrated evidence of dynamic hyperinflation during CPET. There was no difference for age, BMI, airways infection, pulmonary function and oxygen saturation between the dynamic hyperinflation and non-dynamic hyperinflation groups. However, the frequency distribution of males in the dynamic hyperinflation group was significantly greater than females ($p < 0.05$).

Physiological responses to CPET in the dynamic and non-dynamic hyperinflation groups are presented in Table 2. Exercise tolerance was reduced in most of patients. Their mean $V'O_{2,peak}$ value was 75.2% of predicted (28.5 ± 4.8 ml/min/kg). The majority of CF patients (24 of 34) increased their EELV back toward resting levels at maximal exercise and did increase EELV beyond resting values, demonstrating evidence of dynamic hyperinflation during CPET. In the dynamic hyperinflation group, the IC from rest to peak exercise decreased by 0.5 ± 0.3 l as showed in Table 3 by EELVΔ value.

When we analyzed dynamic hyperinflation at submaximal level of exercise (i.e. at lactic threshold, LT), there was no difference for EELVΔ value between hyperinflated and not hypeinflated CF patients (− 0.09 ± 0.22 l versus − 0.11 ± 0.09 respectively, $p = 0.50$).

Patients with evidence of dynamic hyperinflation had similar $V'O_2$, work-rate and heart rate at peak exercise to those without evidence of dynamic hyperinflation. Both groups achieved maximal heart rates above 80% of predicted. In dynamic hyperinflation group we found higher values of $V\ E_{peak}$ ($p < 0.05$) and lower values of breathing reserve (BR) even if did not achieve the statistical significance ($p = 0.2$). For both groups, mean maximal ventilation was less than the predicted MVV and breathing reserve was always preserved, suggesting that ventilation limit was not a main limiting factor. Both CF groups stopped exercise primarily because of leg discomfort. No differences were found in the ventilatory equivalents for carbon dioxide ($V'E/V'CO_2$) at peak exercise; no differences were detected for $V'E/V'CO_2$ slope and $PETCO_2$, indicating similar ventilatory efficiency and gas exchange functionality. There was a fall in mean SpO_2 from rest to peak exercise ($SpO_2\Delta$) in hyperinflated

Table 1 Demographic characteristics and pulmonary function of the study group

Characteristics	All ($n = 34$)	Dynamic hyperinflation ($n = 24$)	Non-dynamic hyperinflation ($n = 10$)	p value
Age, years	33.1 ± 8.5	34.2 ± 9.0	30.5 ± 6.7	0.322
BMI, kg/m^2	22.6 ± 2.6	23.0 ± 2.3	21.5 ± 3.0	0.093
Male, %	67	79	40	0.026
Pseudomonas aeruginosa infection, %	64.7	70.8	50.0	0.247
Staphylococcus aureus infection, %	67.6	62.5	80.0	0.320
Burkholderia cepacia infection, %	2.9	4.2	0	0.512
Pancreatic insufficiency, %	73.5	75.0	70.0	0.763
F508 del homozygous/heterozygous	6/21	5/14	1/7	0.731
Lung function				
FEV_1, % of predicted	69.6 ± 19.0	68.3 ± 19.2	72.9 ± 19.3	0.532
FVC, % of predicted	86.1 ± 17.2	85.9 ± 17.6	86.5 ± 17.2	0.921
FEV_1/FVC, %	67.9 ± 10.9	63.3 ± 10.7	71.8 ± 11.1	0.189
IC, % of predicted	100.8 ± 23.3	102.8 ± 24.2	96.1 ± 21.9	0.478
TLC, % of predicted	95.6 ± 15.9	96.9 ± 17.4	92.5 ± 11.9	0.473
RV, % of predicted	112.2 ± 45.2	117.9 ± 51.0	98.6 ± 23.7	0.183
RV/TLC,%	31.6 ± 9.4	32.4 ± 10.0	29.8 ± 8.3	0.483
FRC, % of predicted	93.5 ± 27.5	95.7 ± 31.9	88.5 ± 12.9	0.859
DL_{CO}, % of predicted	81.3 ± 13.7	82.1 ± 13.2	79.1 ± 15.7	0.612
MVV, l·min^{-1}	104.6 ± 31.3	107.5 ± 32.5	97.4 ± 28.3	0.396
SpO_2, %	96.8 ± 1.6	96.7 ± 1.7	97.2 ± 1.3	0.445

Definition of abbreviations: *BMI* body mass index, *FEV_1* forced expiratory volume in one second, *FVC* forced vital capacity, *FEV_1/FVC* forced expiratory volume in one second and forced vital capacity ratio, *TLC* total lung capacity, *RV* residual volume, *IC* inspiratory capacity, *FRC* functional residual capacity, *DL_{CO}* diffusion lung capacity for carbon monoxide, *MVV* estimated maximal voluntary ventilation, *SpO_2* arterial oxygen saturation, *% of predicted* percentage of predicted normal values
Data are presented as mean ± SD. p values are differences between the dynamic hyperinflation and non-dynamic hyperinflation groups

patients (– 3.5%) which exceeded that seen in non-hyperinflated patients (– 2.5%) but was not statically different.

DPA is shown in Table 3. Patients with evidence of dynamic hyperinflation demonstrated higher total energy expenditure and higher daily time spent in activities above vigorous intensity. Similarly, there was a trend for more activities above moderate intensity ($p = 0.1$) and active energy expenditure ($p = 0.09$) in the dynamic hyperinflation group.

Correlation analysis was done for the group as a whole. DPA above moderate intensity was related to $V'O_{2,peak}$ expressed as ml·min^{-1} ($R = 0.44$, $p = 0.002$) and as ml·min^{-1}.kg^{-1} ($R = 0.52$, $p < 0.001$). Interestingly, daily activity measures were related to the development of dynamic hyperinflation. We found a relationship between total energy expenditure and $EELV_{peak}$ ($R = 0.56$, $p < 0.001$), $EELV_{peak}$ expressed as % of TLC ($R = -0.47$, $p = 0.001$). Moreover, we found a positive relationship between total

Table 2 Daily physical activity of the study group

Variable	All ($n = 34$)	Dynamic hyperinflation ($n = 24$)	Non-dynamic hyperinflation ($n = 10$)	p value
Total energy expenditure, kcal	2577 (2395–3014)	2785 (2513–3093)	2260 (2018–2541)	0.006
Active Energy expenditure, kcal	695 (497–1327)	744 (541–1516)	580 (376–1044)	0.109
Duration Physical Activity, min/day	179 (116–310)	187 (111–321)	168 (116–313)	0.849
Average METs, kcal·kg^{-1}·h^{-1}	1.8 (1.6–2.0)	1.8 (1.6–2.0)	1.7 (1.6–2.0)	0.994
Steps, number/day	8784 (6533–11,321)	8784 (7031–11,763)	8647 (5172–11,427)	0.624
Mild intensity activities, min/day	160 (106–253)	167 (93–268)	151 (106–287)	0.944
Moderate intensity activities, min/day	14 (9–29)	15 (9–32)	12 (5–24)	0.270
Vigorous intensity activities, min/day	1 (0–3)	1 (1–4)	0	0.010
Moderate+Vigorous intensity activities, min/day	16 (9–29)	16 (10–35)	12 (5–24)	0.196

Definition of abbreviations: *CF* Cystic Fibrosis, *METs* Metabolic Equivalents of Task
Data are presented as median (interquartile range). p values are differences between the dynamic hyperinflation and non-dynamic hyperinflation groups

Table 3 Cardiopulmonary exercise testing data of the study group

CPET variables at peak exercise	All ($n = 34$)	Dynamic hyperinflation ($n = 24$)	Non-dynamic hyperinflation ($n = 10$)	p value
Work rate, % of predicted maximum	87.5 ± 18.4	85.2 ± 14.7	93.2 ± 25.2	0.365
$V'O_2$, ml·min^{-1}·kg^{-1}	28.5 ± 4.8	28.7 ± 4.6	27.8 ± 5.6	0.639
$V'O_2$, % of predicted maximum	75.2 ± 13.3	75.2 ± 13.5	75.0 ± 13.4	0.960
HR, beats·min^{-1}	155.4 ± 12.4	155.0 ± 12.5	156.3 ± 12.6	0.785
HR, % of predicted maximum	83.3 ± 7.4	83.6 ± 7.9	82.5 ± 6.4	0.697
$V'O_2$/HR, ml·beat^{-1}	12.2 ± 3.1	12.9 ± 3.0	10.5 ± 2.5	0.037
SpO_2, %	93.6 ± 3.3	93.2 ± 3.4	94.7 ± 3.0	0.254
$SpO_2\Delta$, %	−3.2 ± 3.2	−3.5 ± 3.3	−2.5 ± 2.8	0.467
V_T, l	1.9 ± 0.6	2.0 ± 0.5	1.6 ± 0.6	0.040
Respiratory rate, breaths·min^{-1}	37.8 ± 7.6	37.4 ± 6.7	38.8 ± 10.0	0.655
V'E, l·min^{-1}	68.8 ± 19.9	73.2 ± 19.1	58.2 ± 18.7	0.042
BR, %	31.2 ± 19.6	28.8 ± 18.7	36.7 ± 21.6	0.292
$V'E/V'CO_2$ slope	27.4 ± 5.3	28.2 ± 5.9	25.5 ± 2.8	0.181
PET_{CO2}, mmHg	40.1 ± 5.5	39.5 ± 5.8	41.3 ± 4.8	0.304
EELV, l	3.8 ± 1.4	4.3 ± 1.2	2.7 ± 1.3	0.001
EELVΔ, l	0.2 ± 0.6	0.5 ± 0.3	− 0.5 ± 0.6	< 0.001
EELVΔ, % of TLC	2.6 ± 12.5	8.0 ± 5.4	− 10.4 ± 15.3	< 0.001
Dyspnea, modified Borg scale	4.7 ± 2.5	5.1 ± 2.5	4.0 ± 2.4	0.183
Leg discomfort, modified Borg scale	6.3 ± 2.1	6.6 ± 2.2	5.6 ± 1.8	0.223

Definition of abbreviations: *CF* Cystic Fibrosis, *$V'O_2$* oxygen uptake, *HR* heart rate, *SpO_2* arterial oxygen saturation, *V_T* tidal volume, *V'E* minute ventilation, *BR* breathing reserve, *$V'E/V'CO_2$* ventilatory equivalent for carbon dioxide, *PET_{CO2}* partial pressure of end-tidal CO_2, *EELV* end-expiratory lung volume, *EELVΔ* end-expiratory lung volume delta from rest to peak exercise, *TLC* total lung capacity

Data recorded at peak exercise. Data are presented as mean ± SD, unless otherwise stated. p values are differences between the dynamic hyperinflation and non-dynamic hyperinflation groups

energy expenditure and change in EELV from rest to peak exercise (EELVΔ) ($R = 0.57$, $p < 0.001$, Fig. 1). A relationship was also found between activities requiring vigorous intensity and $EELV_{peak}$ ($R = 0.59$, $p < 0.001$) and EELVΔ ($R = 0.46$, $p = 0.001$).

Among these significant contributors to DPA, the multivariate linear regression analysis identified $V'O_{2,peak}$ and gender as independent predictor of DPA and excluded the role of dynamic hyperinflation in predicting DPA levels (Table 4). Specifically, EELVΔ (l) and EELVΔ (% of TLC) were discarded as not significant predictors: EELVΔ (l) p values were 0.412, 0.513 and 0.719 for model 1, 2 and 3, respectively; EELVΔ (% of TLC) p values were 0.796, 0.581 and 0.691 for model 1, 2 and 3, respectively (Table 4).

Discussion

The main finding of this study is that DPA levels of patients with mild-to moderate CF might not be correlated with the development of dynamic hyperinflation. Specifically, the variance in DPA within these CF patients cannot be explained by the dynamic hyperinflation that occurs during CPET. Patients who responded to exercise with dynamic hyperinflation performed higher daily activity requiring vigorous intensity and had more total energy expenditure than those without dynamic hyperinflation.

It is well known that the development of dynamic hyperinflation makes patients breathe at increased operational lung volumes, resulting in a higher respiratory effort and oxygen requirement of breathing [32]. Dynamic hyperinflation leaves less room for the expansion of tidal volume that comes with increasing minute ventilation. Several studies are available for COPD patients, which observed that dynamic hyperinflation is likely to lead to such mechanical constraints on tidal volume [26, 33]. At some point, further increase in the effort to breathe does not result in an equal increase in tidal volume, known as neuromechanical dissociation [33]. This causes an increase in symptoms and impairments that patients experience [33]. As consequence, in moderate-severe COPD patients, reduced DPA might be partially explained by the development of dynamic hyperinflation during CPET [13]. Although extrapolation of data from COPD to CF is not appropriate, the COPD model is used to explain some physiological mechanisms during exercise mainly because the study of dynamic hyperinflation and its clinical utility in CF is limited. Specifically,

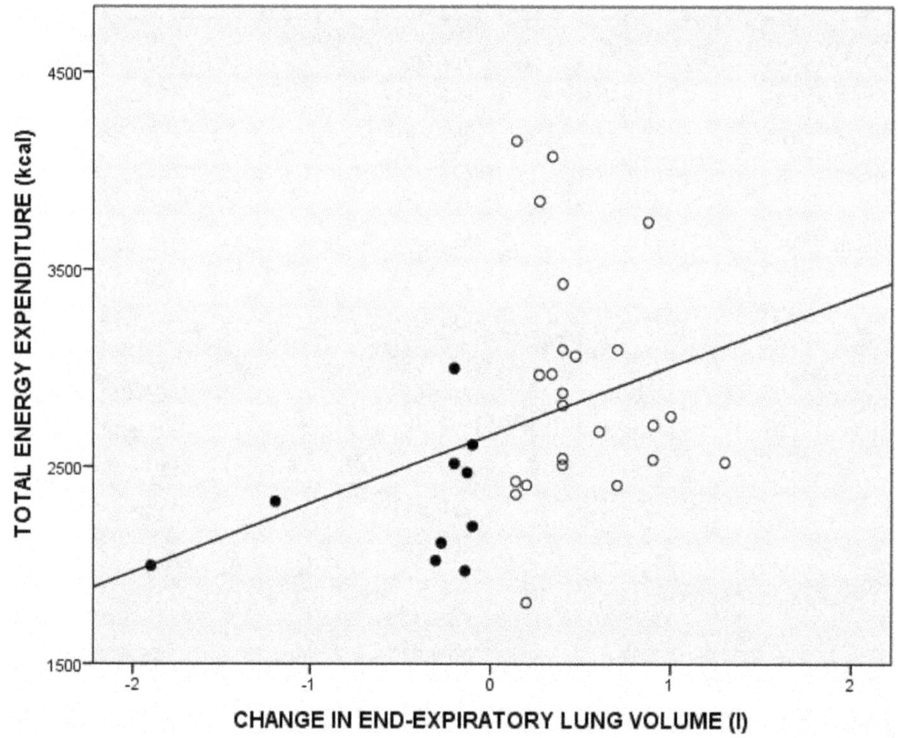

Fig. 1 Relationship between total energy expenditure in daily living recorded by accelerometer and change in end-expiratory lung volume (EELV) in patients with cystic fibrosis ($R = 0.57$, $p < 0.001$). In this figure, the most hyperinflated CF patients, those with the highest EELV, also showed the highest physical activity parameter represented as total energy expenditure. Open circles = CF patients with dynamic hyperinflation, closed circles = CF patients without dynamic hyperinflation

the aspects of lung mechanics related to daily activity have not been studied in detail in patients with CF, who are younger and less likely to be smokers [34]. In our mild-to moderate CF who developed dynamic hyperinflation during exercise, this neuromechanical dissociation did not happen, because their IC value at peak exercise was still large. We found that dynamic hyperinflation did not limit exercise tolerance on CPET in this CF group examined. The hyperinflated group reported symptoms of muscle effort equal or in excess of dyspnea.

Table 4 Independent predictors of physical activity level in a multivariate linear regression analysis

Model	Dependent	Predictors	Unstandardized coefficients		Standardized coefficients	95% CI	p	R^2
			T	SE	β			
1	Total Energy Expenditure	(Constant)	1582.144	302.285		966.334 to 2197.955	< 0.001	
		Gender	450.965	184.121	0.412	75.877 to 826.054	0.020	
		V'O2 peak	0.450	0.200	0.378	0.042 to 0.857	0.032	
								52.9%
2	Vigorous PA	(Constant)	0.091	0.523		−0.973 to 1.155	0.863	
		Gender	3.040	0.856	0.526	1.297 to 4.782	0.001	
								27.7%
3	Moderate + Vigorous PA	(Constant)	−11.567	11.908		−35.797 to 12.663	0.338	
		V'O2 peak	0.018	0.007	0.418	0.004 to 0.032	0.013	
								17.5%

Definition of abbreviations: *CF* Cystic Fibrosis, *V'O*$_2$ oxygen uptake, *PA* physical activity, *CI* confidence interval. For every model: included independent variables were: gender (male), V'O2 peak (ml·min^{-1}), EELVΔ (l) and EELVΔ (% of TLC)

For every model: EELVΔ (l) and EELVΔ (% of TLC) were discarded as not significant predictors. For model 2 and 3: V'O2 peak (ml·min^{-1}) and gender (male) were discarded as not significant predictors, respectively

One explanation could be that the occurrence of hyperinflation during CPET played a minor role in limiting exercise tolerance in our CF patients, likely because of mild lung function impairment. This is in keeping with Moorcroft et al.' conclusions that non pulmonary factors predominate in limiting patients with mild to moderate disease [35].

We were able to demonstrate a positive correlation between changes in EELV from rest to peak exercise and levels of DPA, expressed both as energy expenditure and activities requiring vigorous intensity. These features described that CF patients with the highest EELV also showed the highest physical activity parameters, suggesting that DPA might not be limited by the occurrence of dynamic hyperinflation. There are different procedures to estimate DPA using accelerometers. One of the most common is estimating the energy expenditure of the activity performed. Several studies have highlighted the accuracy of SWA on estimate energy expenditure in CF. It was found an agreement between energy expenditure measures estimated by the SWA and indirect calorimetry during daily activities [31]. Furthermore, the hypersalinity of sweat in people with CF had no significant negative impact on the accuracy of SWA estimate of energy expenditure [30].

In our patients, the multiple regression analysis did not identify dynamic hyperinflation as an independent variable. Aerobic capacity and gender were found significant predictor of DPA, explaining almost 53% of the variance in DPA of our patients with mild-to moderate lung disease. The DPA that a subject does throughout her/his habitual life can be influenced by many aspects. Except physical capabilities, whether a lifestyle is less or more active is determined by social, behavioural and psychological factors. We were also able to confirm previous results describing that the level of physical activity was independently related to gender in CF population [2, 16]. Recently, Stevens et al. studied for the first time the prevalence of dynamic hyperinflation in a large CF population with a broad range of lung disease severity [12]. The authors demonstrated that dynamic hyperinflation during CPET is common among CF patients with mild-to moderate lung impairment. In our study, we confirmed the fact that CF patients are likely to hyperinflate during exercise and our EELV values were comparable to those of Stevens et al. [12] (EELVΔ: 0.5 ± 0.3 l in our study vs. 0.44 ± 0.26 in Stevens' study). They also showed that patients who developed dynamic hyperinflation had lower lung function, lower exercise tolerance and greater breathlessness at peak exercise than patients without dynamic hyperinflation. By contrast, we found no significant differences on aerobic capacity between CF patients with evidence of dynamic hyperinflation and patients without hyperinflation. One explanation could be that, in both studies, there was a greater gender difference on the distribution of males versus females in hyperinflated or not hyperinflated CF group. This may have possibly affected the exercise testing parameters. Specifically, in Stevens's study the frequency distribution of males in the non-dynamic hyperinflation group was significantly greater than females (88%, $p < 0.05$) while in our study was significantly lower (40%, $p = 0.02$) [12]. For comparison, we retained that it would be more appropriate to scale the values for % of predicted and then analyse if there are differences between hyperinflated and not hypeinflated CF patients. Conversely, Stevens et al. presented their CPET results as absolute values rather than percentage of predicted [12]. The lower CPET parameters observed in their dynamic hyperinflated group might have been influenced by the fact that subjects were almost CF females and that the non-dynamic hyperinflation group was composed mainly by males. In this kind of gender distribution, we retain that should not be used the absolute values for CPET parameters to observe differences between dynamic hyperinflation and non-dynamic hyperinflation groups, because these parameters depend strongly on anthropometric features (i.e., height and sex) [25].

Following up on these results, the present study now confirms the high prevalence of dynamic hyperinflation in CF adult patients and adds that dynamic hyperinflation may not influence mild CF from taking part in DPA.

There is evidence that submaximal exercise related data (also known as lactate threshold-LT measures) are more reflective of exercise fitness [36] and would be more appropriate for comparison with DPA in order to investigate the possible effects of the latter on exercise tolerance. When we analyzed the EELVΔ value at submaximal level of exercise (i.e. at LT), which in turn should reflect more closely normal daily activities, there was no difference for EELVΔ value between hyperinflated and not hypeinflated CF patients. It seems that in patients with mild to moderate lung obstruction, dynamic hyperinflation started during an incremental CPET where the intensity of exercise become closer to the zone/range of the maximal effort. So, if we consider that activities of daily life are of sub-maximal intensity, they are also likely not to be limited by dynamic hyperinflation.

We recognize that detecting the occurrence of dynamic hyperinflation during daily life activities is important, but may be unfeasible in clinical practice. However, this can be determined alternatively during CPET. More studies may be interesting to evaluate the role of dynamic hyperinflation induced by exercise on daily activities, especially in CF patients with more advanced disease. In agreement with Stevens' comment [12], we would expect a greater incidence of dynamic hyperinflation during exercise in patients with severe CF (i.e., $FEV_1 < 30\%$pred).

The study has important limitations. Firstly, the cohort is small and from a single centre so it has limited generalizability to the whole CF population. Secondly, more males than females were recruited. This was unintentional and a result of patient enthusiasm to participate at the study, but we recognise this may affect the interpretation of the results. Finally, because it is a cross-sectional study, it cannot establish a causal relationship, but instead an association between dynamic hyperinflation and PA.

Conclusion

In CF patients with mild to moderate lung impairment, dynamic hyperinflation during exercise is very common and seems not to be a limiting factor for daily physical activity. More research is needed to study directly the development of dynamic hyperinflation during daily life activities and to establish whether hyperinflation could influence habitual PA in more advanced CF disease.

Abbreviations

BMI: Body mass index; BR: Breathing reserve; CF: Cystic Fibrosis; EELV: End-expiratory lung volume; FEV1: Forced expiratory volume in 1 s; FVC: Forced vital capacity; IC: Inspiratory capacity; PA: Physical activity; PET_{CO2}: Partial pressure of end-tidal CO_2; SpO_2: Arterial oxygen saturation; TLC: Total lung capacity; V'E: Minute ventilation; V'E/V'CO_2: Ventilatory equivalent for carbon dioxide; VO_2: Oxygen uptake; V_T: Tidal volume

Acknowledgements

The authors would like to thank Professor E. Bonci for his help with the statistical analysis and the "Lega Italiana Fibrosi Cistica - Associazione Laziale Onlus" for the support of the Cystic Fibrosis Center. NJS is supported by the National Institute of Health Research Respiratory Disease Biomedical Research Unit, Royal Brompton Hospital NHS Foundation Trust, London.

Authors' contributions

Conception and design: DS, MDP, NJS, PP. Acquisition of data: DS, MDP, CP, SQ. Analysis and interpretation: DS, MDP, NJS, CP, SQ, PP. Drafting the manuscript: DS, MDP. All authors revised the work for important intellectual content and gave final approval for the version to be published. All authors agree to be accountable for the all aspects of the work in ensuring that questions related to the accuracy or integrity of any part of the work are appropriately investigated and resolved.

Competing interests

The authors declare that they have no competing interests.

Author details

[1]Department of Public Health and Infectious Diseases, Adult Cystic Fibrosis Center, Sapienza University of Rome, 00185 Rome, Italy. [2]Cystic Fibrosis Unit, Bambino Gesù Children's Hospital, Rome, Italy. [3]Department of Cystic Fibrosis, Royal Brompton Hospital and Imperial College, London SW3 6NP, UK. [4]Department of Experimental Medicine, Sapienza University of Rome, 00185 Rome, Italy. [5]Department of Pediatrics, Cystic Fibrosis Center, Sapienza University of Rome, 00185 Rome, Italy. [6]Eleonora Lorrillard-Spencer Cenci Foundation, 00185 Rome, Italy.

References

1. White D, Stiller K, Haensel N. Adherence of adult cystic fibrosis patients with airway clearance and exercise regimens. J Cyst Fibros. 2007;6(3):163–70.
2. Savi D, Simmonds N, Di Paolo M, Quattrucci S, Palange P, Banya W, et al. Relationship between pulmonary exacerbations and daily physical activity in adults with cystic fibrosis. BMC Pulm Med. 2015; https://doi.org/10.1186/s12890-015-0151-7.
3. Troosters T, Langer D, Vrijsen B, Segers J, Wouters K, Janssens W, et al. Skeletal muscle weakness, exercise tolerance and physical activity in adults with cystic fibrosis. Eur Respir J. 2009;33:99–106.
4. Savi D, Quattrucci S, Internullo M, De Biase RV, Calverley P, Palange P. Measuring habitual physical activity in adults with cystic fibrosis. Respir Med. 2013;107(12):1888–94.
5. Nixon PA, Orenstein DM, Kelsey SF, Doershuk CF. The prognostic value of exercise testing in patients with cystic fibrosis. N Engl J Med. 1992;327(25):1785–8.
6. Moorcroft AJ, Dood ME, Webb AK. Exercise testing and prognosis in adult cystic fibrosis. Thorax. 1997;52(3):291–3.
7. Almajed A, Lands LC. The evolution of exercise capacity and its limiting factors in cystic fibrosis. Paediatr Respir Rev. 2012;13(4):195–9.
8. Moorcroft AJ, Dodd ME, Webb AK. Exercise limitations and training for patients with cystic fibrosis. Disabil Rehabil. 1998;20(6–7):247–53.
9. Gruet M, Troosters T, Verges S. Peripheral muscle abnormalities in cystic fibrosis: etiology, clinical implications and response to therapeutic interventions. J Cyst Fibros. 2017; https://doi.org/10.1016/j.jcf.2017.02.007.
10. Selvadurai HC, Allen J, Sachinwalla T, Macauley J, Blimkie CJ, Van Asperen PP. Muscle function and resting energy expenditure in female athletes with cystic fibrosis. Am J Respir Crit Care Med. 2003;168(12):1476–80.
11. Moser C, Tirakitsoontorn P, Nussbaum E, Newcomb R, Cooper DM. Muscle size and cardiorespiratory response to exercise in cystic fibrosis. Am J Respir Crit Care Med. 2000;162(5):1823–7.
12. Stevens D, Stephenson A, Faughnan ME, Leek E, Tullis E. Prognostic relevance of dynamic hyperinflation during cardiopulmonary exercise testing in adult patients with cystic fibrosis. J Cyst Fibros. 2013;12(6):655–61.
13. Garcia-Rio F, Lores V, Mediano O, Rojo B, Hernanz A, López-Collazo E, et al. Daily physical activity in patients with chronic obstructive pulmonary disease is mainly associated with dynamic hyperinflation. Am J Respir Crit Care Med. 2009; https://doi.org/10.1164/rccm.200812-1873OC.
14. Alison JA, Regnis JA, Donnelly PM, Adams RD, Sullivan CE, Bye PT. End-expiratory lung volume during arm and leg exercise in normal subjects and patients with cystic fibrosis. Am J Respir Crit Care Med. 1998;158:1450–8.
15. Boucher GP, Lands LC. Hay ja, et al. activity levels and the relathionship to lung function and nutritional status in children with cystic fibrosis. Am J Phys Med Rehab. 1977;76:311–5.
16. Selvadurai HC, Blimkie CJ, Cooper PJ, Mellis CM, Van Aspern PP. Gender differences in habitual activity in children with cystic fibrosis. Arch Dis Child. 2004;89:928–33.
17. Lahaije AJMC, van Helvoort HAC, Dekhuijzen PNR, Vercoulen JH, Heijdra YF. Resting and ADL-induced dynamic hyperinflation explain physical inactivity in COPD better than FEV1. Respir Med. 2013;107:834–40.
18. Miller MR, Hankinson J, Brusasco V, Burgos F, Casaburi R, Coates A, et al. ATS/ERS task force: standardisation of spirometry. Eur Respir J. 2005;26:319–38.
19. Wanger J, Clausen JL, Coates A, Pedersen OF, Brusasco V, Burgos F, et al. Standardisation of measurements of lung volumes. Eur Respir J. 2005;26:511–22.
20. MacIntyre N, Crapo RO, Viegi G, Johnson DC, van der Grinten CP, Brusasco V, et al. Standardisation of the single-breath determination of carbon monoxide uptake in the lung. Eur Respir J. 2005;26:720–35.
21. Morris JF, Koski A, Temple WP, Claremont A, Thomas DR. Fifteen-year interval spirometric evaluation of the Oregon predictive equations. Chest. 1998;93:123–7.
22. Crapo RO, Morris AH, Clayton PD, Nixon CR. Lung volumes in healthy nonsmoking adults. Bull Eur Physiopathol Respir. 1982;18:419–25.

23. American Thoracic Society, American College of Chest Physicians. ATS/ACCP statement on cardiopulmonary exercise testing. Am J Respir Crit Care Med. 2003;167:211–77.
24. Borg GA. Psychophysical basis of perceived exertion. Med Sci Sports Exerc. 1982;14:377–81.
25. Jones NL, Makrides L, Hitchcock C, Chypchar T, McCartney N. Normal standards for an incremental progressive cycle ergometer test. Am Rev Respir Dis. 1985; 131:700–8.
26. O'Donnel DE, Revill SM, Webb KA. Dynamic hyperinflation and exercise intolerance in chronic obstructive pulmonary disease. Am J Respir Crit Care Med. 2001;164:770–7.
27. Stubbing DG, Pengelly LD, Morse JL, Jones NL. Pulmonary mechanics during exercise in normal males. J Appl Physiol. 1980;49:506–10.
28. Stubbing DG, Pengelly LD, Morse JL, Jones NL. Pulmonary mechanics during exercise in subjects with chronic airflow obstruction. J Appl Physiol. 1980;49:511–5.
29. Donnelly PM, Robinson M, Alison JA, Bye PTP. Ventilatory mechanics at rest and during exercise in patients with cystic fibrosis. Am J Respir Crit Care Med. 1996;154:1418–25.
30. Dwyer T, Alison JA, McKeough Z, Elkins MR, Bye PT. Evaluation of the SenseWear activity monitor during exercise in cystic fibrosis and in health. Respir Med. 2009;103:1511–7.
31. Cox NS, Alison JA, Button BM, Wilson JW, Morton JM, Dowman LM, et al. Validation of a multi-sensor armband during free-living activity in adults with cystic fibrosis. J Cyst Fibros. 2014;13:347–50.
32. O'Donnell DE, Lam M, Webb KA. Measurements of symptoms, lung hyperinflation, and endurance during exercise in chronic obstructive pulmonary disease. Am J Respir Crit Care Med. 1998;158:1557–65.
33. O'Donnell DE. Hyperinflation, dyspnea, and exercise intolerance in chronic obstructive pulmonary disease. Proc Am Thorac Soc. 2006;3:180–4.
34. Morrissey BM. Pathogenesis of bronchiectasis. Clin Chest Med. 2007;28(2):289–96.
35. Moorcroft AJ, Dodd ME, Morris J, Webb AK. Symptoms, lactate and exercise limitation at peak cycle ergometry in adults with cystic fibrosis. Eur Respir J. 2005;25(6):1050–6.
36. Wasserman K. The anaerobic threshold measurement to evaluate exercise performance. Am Rev Respir Dis. 1984;129(Suppl):S35–40.

22

NonTuberculous Mycobacteria infection and lung transplantation in cystic fibrosis: a worldwide survey of clinical practice

Adrien Tissot[1,2,3], Matthew F. Thomas[1,2,4], Paul A. Corris[1,2] and Malcolm Brodlie[1,2,4*]

Abstract

Background: In people with cystic fibrosis infection with NonTuberculous Mycobacteria is of increasing prevalence. *Mycobacterium abscessus* complex is of particular concern and has been associated with adverse clinical outcomes. Optimal treatment usually requires multiple antibiotics for over 12 months. When considering lung transplantation for patients with NonTuberculous Mycobacteria potential benefits must be balanced against the risks of uncontrolled infection post-transplant and significant side-effects associated with treatment. In this survey we assessed current international practice with regard to assessing and listing patients for lung transplantation.

Methods: We designed a questionnaire enquiring about local practice regarding screening for NonTuberculous Mycobacteria infection, specific contra-indications to transplantation, management and segregation of patients pre- and post-transplant. The survey was sent via e-mail to 37 paediatric and adult lung transplant centres across Europe, North America and Australia.

Results: We gathered complete questionnaires from 21 centres (57% response rate). Few centres (29%) have a clear written policy regarding NonTuberculous Mycobacteria. Sixteen (76%) centres require molecular identification of NonTuberculous Mycobacteria species. Only four centres would consider infection with *M. abscessus* complex in itself a contra-indication for listing, however 76% regard it as a relative contra-indication. Eighty-six percent require treatment pre-transplantation. Finally, only 61% of centres had a clear policy regarding segration of patients pre-transplant and 48% post-transplant.

Conclusions: The issue of NonTuberculous Mycobacteria infection in people with cystic fibrosis requiring lung transplantation is well-recognized however current international recommendations are not detailed and there is variation in practice between centres. There is an urgent requirement for high quality clinical data to inform decision-making.

Keywords: Cystic fibrosis, Nontuberculous mycobacteria, Lung transplantation, *Mycobacterium abscessus*, *Mycobacterium avium*

* Correspondence: malcolm.brodlie@ncl.ac.uk
[1]Institute of Cellular Medicine, Newcastle University, Medical School, Framlington Place, Newcastle upon Tyne NE2 4HH, UK
[2]Institute of Transplantation, Freeman Hospital, Newcastle upon Tyne Hospitals NHS Foundation Trust, Newcastle upon Tyne NE7 7DN, UK
Full list of author information is available at the end of the article

Background

Pulmonary infection with nontuberculous mycobacteria (NTM) in people with cystic fibrosis (CF) is of increasing importance and concern to both patients and clinicians [1]. Infection with NTM is of particular relevance during the assessment process of suitability for lung transplantation [2].

The incidence of respiratory cultures positive for NTM in people with CF has risen over recent decades [3]. Multicenter studies have reported varying prevalence that ranges from 2.7% across Europe [4], 6.6% in France [5] to 14% throughout the United States (US) [6]. Significant geographical variation has also been identified, for example in the US some states have been found to have a prevalence as high as 20% whereas in others it is much lower at < 5% [6]. Environmental factors are thought to influence this variation but screening practices may also vary between individual CF centres. The most common NTM species isolated from people with CF are *Mycobacterium abscessus* complex and *M. avium* complex (MAC).

The American Thoracic Society/Infectious Disease Society of America definition of NTM pulmonary disease (NTM PD) involves clinical, radiological and microbiological criteria and is widely used clinically [7]. Importantly, pulmonary infection with *M. abscessus* complex in people with CF has been associated with accelerated decline in lung function and is of particular clinical concern [4, 8–10]. There is also emerging evidence to suggest transmission of *M. abscessus* complex between individuals with CF [11, 12]. NTM PD is challenging to treat requiring multiple antibiotic regimes for a prolonged period of at least 12 months [13, 14]. The antibiotics used are frequently associated with adverse effects and represent a significant treatment burden for patients. Ultimately NTM are also often difficult to eradicate from the airways of people with CF despite treatment.

In the past pulmonary NTM infection in patients with CF was considered an absolute contra-indication for lung transplantation by some groups due to poor post-transplant outcomes that were largely attributed to uncontrolled infection in the context of systemic immunosuppression, though the ISHLT guidelines never endorsed NTM infection as an absolute contraindication [15–17]. Soft tissue and wound infections are often particularly challenging to treat post-operatively [18]. Specifically, the presence of *M. abscessus* complex pre-transplant has been associated with severe clinical problems and poor outcomes following lung transplantation [15–17]. The specific subspecies of *M. abscessus* complex may also impact on risk stratification [19]. The isolation of NTM in respiratory samples post-lung transplantation has also been associated with adverse clinical outcomes [18, 20].

However, some single-centre case series have suggested that lung transplantation in people with NTM infection can be associated with comparable outcomes to those free of NTM infection [21–23]. Albeit with the caveat that anti-NTM treatment is likely to need to be prolonged and may be associated with adverse effects and complications.

The 2014 update for the selection of lung transplant candidates from the International Society for Heart and Lung Transplantation (ISHLT) recommends *"controlled chronic infection pre-operatively and a reasonable expectation for adequate control post-operatively"* in order for patients with NTM to be safely listed for transplantation [24]. Recent consensus recommendations from the United States Cystic Fibrosis Foundation (CFF) and the European Cystic Fibrosis Society (ECFS) emphasize the need to thoroughly evaluate patients with CF for NTM as part of the lung transplant assessment process and to start treatment prior to transplant listing but largely leave decision-making open to the individual centre and clinician [14].

The increasing prevalence of NTM in people with CF means that it is becoming more and more of an issue during the process of assessment of suitability for lung transplantation [2]. Anecdotally we have observed different approaches in the global lung transplantation community towards this challenging clinical area and we therefore wished to investigate current practice worldwide with regard to assessing and listing patients for lung transplantation with CF who have NTM infection.

Methods

We designed a survey consisting of 16 questions enquiring about local practice regarding screening for NTM infection, specific contra-indications to transplantation, management and segregation of patients pre- and post-transplant (Fig. 1). This questionnaire was sent via e-mail to 37 adult and pediatric lung transplantation centres across Europe, North America and Australia in April 2016.

Results

We received complete questionnaires from 21 centres (57% response rate).

Screening for NTM during transplant assessment process

All centres specifically screened patients with CF for NTM infection pre-transplant but only a minority (29%) had a clear written policy regarding this issue (Table 1). Sixteen centres (76%) required molecular identification of NTM species. The main respiratory samples (Fig. 1) accepted as relevant were sputum and broncho-alveolar lavage (100 and 95% respectively). Induced sputum was also considered acceptable by 16 centres. Only one centre based decisions on results from cough swabs.

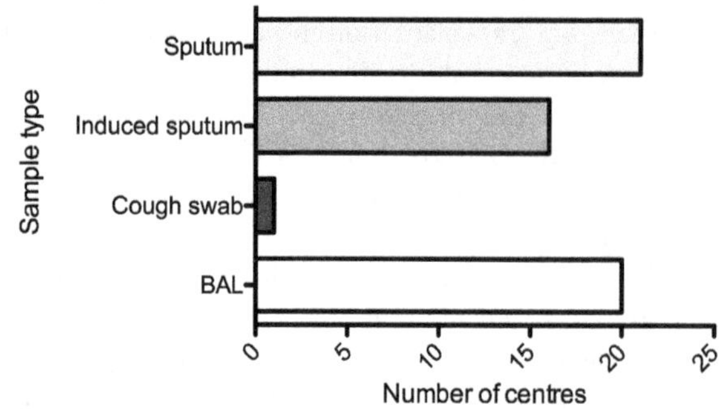

Fig. 1 Type of respiratory samples considered as relevant for NTM screening at assessment for lung transplantation. Total number of centres returning questionnaires = 21. Answers to the question: *"Do you consider the following respiratory samples as relevant for NTM screening?"*. BAL: bronchio-alveolar lavage

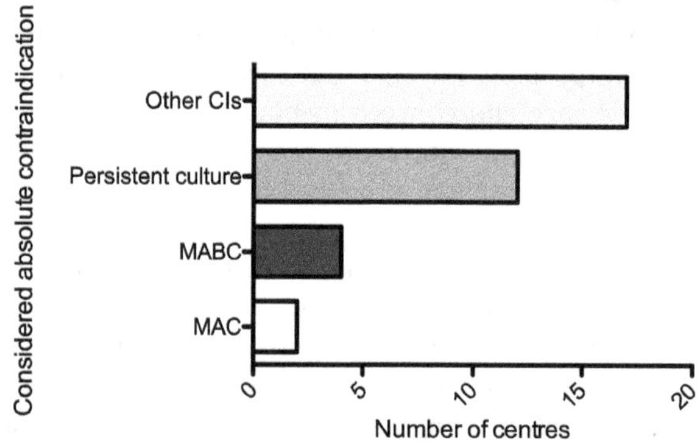

Fig. 2 What is considered a contraindication to lung transplantation at each centre? Total number of centres returning questionnaires = 21. In answer to the question, "are the following considered an absolute contraindication for lung transplantation?": MAC: current infection with *Mycobacterium avium* Complex; MABC: current infection with *Mycobacterium abscessus* complex; Persistent culture: persisting MAC or *M. abscessus* complex infection despite optimal therapy; other CI: Would you regard a patient with persisting *M. abscessus* complex and another relative contraindication as together representing an absolute contraindication?

Policies for suitability of patients with NTM for lung transplantation listing

Only four centers considered infection with *M. abscessus* complex in itself an absolute contra-indication for transplant listing (Fig. 2). More than half (57%) stated they would not list a patient with persisting positive respiratory cultures despite optimal treatment. A majority (76%) of centres considered persistent *M. abscessus* complex infection to be a relative contraindication to listing if other adverse factors are present. Eighteen centres require treatment pre-transplant and 20 (95%) would decide a peri-transplant treatment cocktail at the time of listing.

Table 1 Questionnaire results (n = 21 centres)

Question	Yes n (%)
Do you have a clear written policy regarding the assessment and listing of patients with CF and NTM infection?	6 (29)
During assessment do you require screening for NTM?	21 (100)
Do you require molecular identification of NTM species?	16 (76)
Do you regard current infection with MAC an absolute contraindication?	1 (5)
Do you regard current infection with *M. abscessus* complex as an absolute contraindication?	4 (19)
Do you regard persisting MAC or *M. abscessus* complex infection despite optimal therapy as an absolute contraindication?	12 (57)
Would you regard a patient with persisting *M. abscessus* complex and another relative contraindication as together representing an absolute contraindication?	16 (76)
Do you require specific NTM treatment to be undertaken before listing?	18 (86)
At time of listing is a treatment cocktail decided on for use peri-transplant?	20 (95)
Are patients segregated on the basis of NTM status pre-transplant?	13 (62)
Are patients segregated post-transplant on the basis of NTM status?	10 (48)

Abbreviations: CF Cystic Fibrosis, *NTM* NonTuberculous Mycobacteria, *MAC Mycobacterium avium* Complex, *M. abscessus complex Mycobacteria abscessus* complex

Infection control policies

Finally, 13, centres (61%) apply a segregation policy based on NTM status of patients pre-transplant and 10 (48%) post-transplantation, for example in outpatient clinic waiting areas.

Discussion

This survey captures current practice in the global lung transplant community with regard to patients with CF and NTM infection. This is well recognised to be a challenging issue clinically with a dearth of high quality evidence on which to base decision-making. Most centres do currently consider patients with CF and NTM infection for lung transplantation assessment and potential listing, i.e. it is not considered an absolute contraindication. However, the majority do consider it a relative contraindication if other comorbidities or relative contraindications are present. The specific species of NTM and response to treatment pre-transplant are also taken in to account during the decision-making process at the majority of centres.

In our questionnaire, we asked about isolation of NTM from respiratory samples, i.e. infection rather than patients who fulfil the ATS NTMPD criteria per se. This was because the presence alone of NTM, and *M. abscessus complex* in particular, is a significant potential concern in the context of immunosuppression post-major thoracic surgery as is the case following lung transplantation.

Our findings highlight the importance of further high-quality clinical research to comprehensively investigate the outcomes and international experience of patients with NTM after lung transplantation. Other key questions include risk stratification around specific species and subspecies, resistance profiles, response to treatment and disease-burden pre-transplant. For example, In a single centre paediatric case series adverse outcomes were associated with infection pre-transplant with *M. abscessus* subspecies *abscessus* with improved results in children with *M. abscessus* subspecies *bolletti* or *massilliense* infection [19]. *M. avium* complex is the most prevalent grouping of NTM in North American patients with CF and data is equally lacking around outcomes and best practice in individuals with *M.avium* complex infection.

The variation in international practice that we have identified affirms the current attention being given to NTM infection in respiratory disease and CF in particular. As a poorly-defined strong relative contraindication to lung transplantation NTM and *M. abscessus* complex status in particular is of huge relevance to individual patients in terms of lung transplantation listing being a viable option or not for them, which may be life-changing. Evidence to support an increasing prevalence of NTM in people with CF continues to grow. The proportion of patients affected and the complexity of treatment necessary in terms of length, toxicity and limited efficacy make infection with NTM an issue of major concern for CF clinicians. The specific question of considering lung transplantation for these patients adds a further level of complexity with the added post-transplant threat of systemic immunosuppression and increased risk of drug-related toxicity.

It is clear in both the ISHLT and the CFF/ECFS consensus recommendations that NTM infection has to be looked for and if possible treated pre-transplant. The ISHLT stated that *"chronic infection with highly virulent and/or resistant microbes that are poorly controlled pre-transplant"* is an absolute contraindication, which is a situation that can been seen in NTM infection. In the CFF/ECFS document it is recommended that *"the presence of persistent MABC or MAC infection despite optimal therapy is not an absolute contraindication for lung transplant referral"*. Pragmatically therefore many transplant clinicians firstly evaluate the "controlled" character of the chronic infection or colonization with NTM pre-transplant and then evaluate the post-transplant risk associated with the presence of NTM. It is interesting to note that almost all centres do not consider in itself the presence of NTM as an absolute contraindication but a majority would not list a patient with a failure of an optimal therapy to eradicate NTM or if associated with another relative contraindication. This illustrates in our view the central concern of clinicians to have an available efficient combination of antibiotics that can be tolerated by the patient before moving on to the difficult process of lung transplantation.

Finally, the relatively low rate of centres segregating patients depending on NTM status pre- and post-transplant is concerning when placed in the context of the recent studies suggesting potential transmission of *M. abscessus* complex between patients with CF [11, 12, 25]. Extensive and elaborate infection control measures have been recommended to prevent such transmission events [14]. The likely low number of patients post-transplant with NTM is also a possible explanation for the lower number of centres segregating post-transplant [18, 20].

There are some limitations to our work. Firstly, we did not send the questionnaire to all existing lung transplantation centres. Our objective was not to be exhaustive but to have a representative sample as in an opinion poll. Secondly, we did not adjust the results for the size of centre, which means an answer from a small centre, for example performing less than 20 transplants per year, has the same value as that from a larger centre.

Conclusions

In conclusion, the issue of NTM infection in patients with CF requiring lung transplantation is of current extensive debate and discussion amongst the lung transplantation community. Although many clinicians anecdotally suspected sub-optimal outcomes following transplantation in patients with NTM, most centres do not consider it as an absolute contra-indication unless associated with other comorbidities or in the absence of a suitable cocktail for antimicrobial therapy. Practice is not consistent however between centres and there is an urgent requirement for the collection and analysis of high-quality clinical data followed by development of an evidence-based guideline on this specific issue.

Abbreviations

CF: Cystic fibrosis; CFF: Cystic Fibrosis Foundation; ECFS: European Cystic Fibrosis Society; ISHLT: International Society for Heart and Lung Transplantation; MAC: *Mycobacterium avium* complex; NTM: Nontuberculous mycobacteria; NTMPD: Nontuberculous mycobacterial pulmonary disease

Acknowledgements

We are grateful to those centres and individuals that kindly completed the survey.

Funding

AT was supported by awards from Pays de la Loire and Fondation du Souffle. MB is supported by a Medical Research Council Clinician Scientist Fellowship (MR/M008797/1).

Authors' contributions

All authors have read and agreed to the final version of the paper. AT: was involved in the design of the study, data collection and analysis and wrote the first draft of the manuscript. MFT: was involved in the design of the study and commented on the manuscript. PAC: was involved in the design of the study and commented on the manuscript. MB: was involved in the design of the study and completed the final version of the manuscript.

Authors' information

AT: Is a Consultant Lung Transplant Physician in Nantes, France. MFT: Is a Consultant Paediatric Respiratory Physician in Newcastle upon Tyne, United Kingdom. PAC: Is Professor of Thoracic Medicine at Newcastle University and Consultant Lung Transplant Physician at the Freeman Hospital, United Kingdom; he is past-president of the International Society for Heart and Lung Transplantation (ISHLT) and was invited to debate the issue of lung transplantation in people with CF and infection with *M. abscessus* at the 2017 Annual Meeting of the ISHLT, San Diego, April 2017. MB: Is a MRC Clinician Scientist/Clinical Senior Lecturer at Newcastle University and Honorary Consultant in Paediatric Respiratory Medicine in Newcastle upon Tyne, United Kingdom.

Competing interests

AT: None. MFT: Not related to this work: investigator-led research grant from Pfizer. PAC: Not related to this work: investigator-led research grants from Bayer, Actelion and GSK; advisory boards for Bayer and Actelion. MB: Not related to this work: investigator-led research grants from Pfizer and Roche Diagnostics; speaker fees for educational events paid to Newcastle University from Novartis, Roche Diagnostics and Teva.

Author details

[1]Institute of Cellular Medicine, Newcastle University, Medical School, Framlington Place, Newcastle upon Tyne NE2 4HH, UK. [2]Institute of Transplantation, Freeman Hospital, Newcastle upon Tyne Hospitals NHS Foundation Trust, Newcastle upon Tyne NE7 7DN, UK. [3]Centre Hospitalier Universitaire de Nantes, Nantes, France. [4]Great North Children's Hospital, Newcastle upon Tyne Hospitals NHS Foundation Trust, Level 3, Clinical Resource Building, Queen Victoria Road, Newcastle upon Tyne NE1 4LP, UK.

References

1. Leung JM, Olivier KN. Nontuberculous mycobacteria: the changing epidemiology and treatment challenges in cystic fibrosis. Curr Opin Pulm Med. 2013;19(6):662–9.
2. Lobo LJ, Noone PG. Respiratory infections in patients with cystic fibrosis undergoing lung transplantation. Lancet Respir Med. 2014;2(1):73–82.
3. Prevots DR, Marras TK. Epidemiology of human pulmonary infection with nontuberculous mycobacteria: a review. Clin Chest Med. 2015;36(1):13–34.
4. Martiniano SL, Sontag MK, Daley CL, Nick JA, Sagel SD. Clinical significance of a first positive nontuberculous mycobacteria culture in cystic fibrosis. Ann Am Thorac Soc. 2014;11(1):36–44.
5. Roux AL, Catherinot E, Ripoll F, Soismier N, Macheras E, Ravilly S, Bellis G, Vibet MA, Le Roux E, Lemonnier L, et al. Multicenter study of prevalence of nontuberculous mycobacteria in patients with cystic fibrosis in France. J Clin Microbiol. 2009;47(12):4124–8.
6. Adjemian J, Olivier KN, Prevots DR. Nontuberculous mycobacteria among patients with cystic fibrosis in the United States: screening practices and environmental risk. Am J Respir Crit Care Med. 2014;190(5):581–6.
7. Griffith DE, Aksamit T, Brown-Elliott BA, Catanzaro A, Daley C, Gordin F, Holland SM, Horsburgh R, Huitt G, Iademarco MF, et al. An official ATS/IDSA statement: diagnosis, treatment, and prevention of nontuberculous mycobacterial diseases. Am J Respir Crit Care Med. 2007;175(4):367–416.
8. Qvist T, Taylor-Robinson D, Waldmann E, Olesen HV, Hansen CR, Mathiesen IH, Hoiby N, Katzenstein TL, Smyth RL, Diggle PJ, et al. Comparing the harmful effects of nontuberculous mycobacteria and Gram negative bacteria on lung function in patients with cystic fibrosis. J Cyst Fibros. 2016;15(3):380–5.
9. Oliver A, Maiz L, Canton R, Escobar H, Baquero F, Gomez-Mampaso E. Nontuberculous mycobacteria in patients with cystic fibrosis. Clin Infect Dis. 2001;32(9):1298–303.
10. Griffith DE. Mycobacterium abscessus subsp abscessus lung disease: 'trouble ahead, trouble behind...'. F1000Prime Rep. 2014;6:107.
11. Bryant JM, Grogono DM, Greaves D, Foweraker J, Roddick I, Inns T, Reacher M, Haworth CS, Curran MD, Harris SR, et al. Whole-genome sequencing to identify transmission of Mycobacterium abscessus between patients with cystic fibrosis: a retrospective cohort study. Lancet. 2013;381(9877):1551–60.
12. Bryant JM, Grogono DM, Rodriguez-Rincon D, Everall I, Brown KP, Moreno P, Verma D, Hill E, Drijkoningen J, Gilligan P, et al. Emergence and spread of a human-transmissible multidrug-resistant nontuberculous mycobacterium. Science. 2016;354(6313):751–7.
13. Skolnik K, Kirkpatrick G, Quon BS. Nontuberculous mycobacteria in cystic fibrosis. Curr Treat Options Infect Dis. 2016;8(4):259–74.
14. Floto RA, Olivier KN, Saiman L, Daley CL, Herrmann JL, Nick JA, Noone PG, Bilton D, Corris P, Gibson RL, et al. US Cystic Fibrosis Foundation and European cystic fibrosis society consensus recommendations for the management of non-tuberculous mycobacteria in individuals with cystic fibrosis: executive summary. Thorax. 2016;71(1):88–90.
15. Gilljam M, Schersten H, Silverborn M, Jonsson B, Ericsson Hollsing A. Lung transplantation in patients with cystic fibrosis and Mycobacterium abscessus infection. J Cyst Fibros. 2010;9(4):272–6.
16. Sanguinetti M, Ardito F, Fiscarelli E, La Sorda M, D'Argenio P, Ricciotti G, Fadda G. Fatal pulmonary infection due to multidrug-resistant Mycobacterium abscessus in a patient with cystic fibrosis. J Clin Microbiol. 2001;39(2):816–9.
17. Taylor JL, Palmer SM. Mycobacterium abscessus chest wall and pulmonary infection in a cystic fibrosis lung transplant recipient. J Heart Lung Transplant. 2006;25(8):985–8.
18. Chernenko SM, Humar A, Hutcheon M, Chow CW, Chaparro C, Keshavjee S, Singer LG. Mycobacterium abscessus infections in lung transplant recipients: the international experience. J Heart Lung Transplant. 2006;25(12):1447–55.
19. Robinson PD, Harris KA, Aurora P, Hartley JC, Tsang V, Spencer H. Paediatric lung transplant outcomes vary with Mycobacterium abscessus complex species. Eur Respir J. 2013;41(5):1230–2.
20. Huang HC, Weigt SS, Derhovanessian A, Palchevskiy V, Ardehali A, Saggar R, Saggar R, Kubak B, Gregson A, Ross DJ, et al. Non-tuberculous mycobacterium infection after lung transplantation is associated with increased mortality. J Heart Lung Transplant. 2011;30(7):790–8.
21. Qvist T, Pressler T, Thomsen VO, Skov M, Iversen M, Katzenstein TL. Nontuberculous mycobacterial disease is not a contraindication to lung transplantation in patients with cystic fibrosis: a retrospective analysis in a Danish patient population. Transplant Proc. 2013;45(1):342–5.
22. Lobo LJ, Chang LC, Esther CR Jr, Gilligan PH, Tulu Z, Noone PG. Lung transplant outcomes in cystic fibrosis patients with pre-operative Mycobacterium abscessus respiratory infections. Clin Transpl. 2013;27(4):523–9.
23. Chalermskulrat W, Sood N, Neuringer IP, Hecker TM, Chang L, Rivera MP, Paradowski LJ, Aris RM. Non-tuberculous mycobacteria in end stage cystic fibrosis: implications for lung transplantation. Thorax. 2006;61(6):507–13.
24. Weill D, Benden C, Corris PA, Dark JH, Davis RD, Keshavjee S, Lederer DJ, Mulligan MJ, Patterson GA, Singer LG, et al. A consensus document for the selection of lung transplant candidates: 2014–an update from the Pulmonary Transplantation Council of the International Society for Heart and Lung Transplantation. J Heart Lung Transplant. 2015;34(1):1–15.
25. Aitken ML, Limaye A, Pottinger P, Whimbey E, Goss CH, Tonelli MR, Cangelosi GA, Dirac MA, Olivier KN, Brown-Elliott BA, et al. Respiratory outbreak of Mycobacterium abscessus subspecies massiliense in a lung transplant and cystic fibrosis center. Am J Respir Crit Care Med. 2012;185(2):231–2.

23

NOX4 expression and distal arteriolar remodeling correlate with pulmonary hypertension in COPD

Xiaotong Guo[1†], Yuchun Fan[1†], Jieda Cui[1,2†], Binwei Hao[1], Li Zhu[3], Xiao Sun[3], Jinxi He[4], Jiali Yang[5], Jianda Dong[7], Yanyang Wang[6], Xiaoming Liu[5,1*] and Juan Chen[1*]

Abstract

Background: Pulmonary hypertension (PH) in chronic obstructive pulmonary disease (COPD) is suggested as the consequence of emphysematous destruction of vascular bed and hypoxia of pulmonary microenvironment, mechanisms underpinning its pathogenesis however remain elusive. The dysregulated expression of nicotinamide adenine dinucleotide phosphate (NADPH)-oxidases and superoxide generation by pulmonary vasculatures have significant implications in the hypoxia-induced PH.

Methods: In this study, the involvement of NADPH oxidase subunit 4 (NOX4) in pulmonary arteriolar remodeling of PH in COPD was investigated by ascertaining the morphological alteration of pulmonary arteries and pulmonary blood flow using cardiac magnetic resonance imaging (cMRI), and the expression and correlation of NOX4 with pulmonary vascular remodeling and pulmonary functions in COPD lungs.

Results: Results demonstrated that an augmented expression of NOX4 was correlated with the increased volume of pulmonary vascular wall in COPD lung. While the volume of distal pulmonary arteries was inversely correlated with pulmonary functions, despite it was positively associated with the main pulmonary artery distensibility, right ventricular myocardial mass end-systolic and right ventricular myocardial mass end-diastolic in COPD. In addition, an increased malondialdehyde and a decreased superoxide dismutase were observed in sera of COPD patients. Mechanistically, the abundance of NOX4 and production of reactive oxygen species (ROS) in pulmonary artery smooth muscle cells could be dynamically induced by transforming growth factor-beta (TGF-β), which in turn led pulmonary arteriolar remodeling in COPD lungs.

Conclusion: These results suggest that the NOX4-derived ROS production may play a key role in the development of PH in COPD by promoting distal pulmonary vascular remodeling.

Keywords: Pulmonary hypertension, Chronic obstructive pulmonary disease, Cardiac magnetic resonance imaging, Pulmonary arteriolar remodeling, Nicotinamide adenine dinucleotide phosphate oxidase subunit 4

* Correspondence: liuxiaoming@nxmu.edu.cn; erc1080@163.com; chenjuan7419@163.com
[†]Xiaotong Guo, Yuchun Fan and Jieda Cui contributed equally to this work.
[5]Institute of Human Stem Cell Research, General Hospital of Ningxia Medical University, Yinchuan 750004, Ningxia, China
[1]Department of Pulmonary and Critical Care Medicine, General Hospital of Ningxia Medical University, 804 Shengli South Street, Xingqing District, Yinchuan, Ningxia 750004, People's Republic of China
Full list of author information is available at the end of the article

Background

Chronic obstructive pulmonary disease (COPD) is a complex disease characterized by airflow limitation, inflammation and airway remodeling. It is one of the most important causes of death in aging population, and is associated with a significantly economic burden worldwide [1, 2]. Pulmonary hypertension (PH), an important negative prognostic sign may be developed during the late course of COPD [3]. Despite the pathogenesis of PH in COPD remains incompletely understood, the loss of pulmonary capillary bed in emphysema is suggested to contribute to the increased pressure in pulmonary circulation. In this regard, the pulmonary vascular remodeling is widely recognized as a key factor in development of hypoxic pulmonary hypertension (HPH), and a main cause of COPD. It is worthy to note that the process of pulmonary vascular remodeling includes the proliferation and hypertrophy of pulmonary smooth muscle cells and deposition of extracellular matrixes (ECM) [4].

In patients with COPD, the enlargement of pulmonary artery was found to correlate with right ventricular (RV) dysfunction and loss of blood volume in small pulmonary vessels [5], which precedes the development of PH and cor pulmonale. Both of these two manifestations are independent predictors of poor survival [6]. However, controversial results were also reported in several studies, in which vascular changes in COPD were failed to identify any abnormalities, or found only minimal increased volume of pulmonary arterial walls, even in lungs of patients with severe COPD [7, 8]. These conflicting data indicate a complexity of COPD pathogenesis.

It has been well recognized that the oxidative stress is one of the major causes of COPD [9]. An increase of reactive oxygen species (ROS) production is involved in changes of vasoreactivity, endothelial dysfunction, and vascular remodeling including vascular wall cell proliferation and vasoconstriction [9–11]. In this respect, NADPH oxidases (NOXs) have been recognized as important sources of superoxide production in vasculatures [9, 12]. Indeed, the NOX-mediated redox signaling is implicated in vascular remodeling of human pulmonary artery cells and the PAH development [13–15]. Several lines of studies have revealed that the hypoxia-induced expression of NADPH oxidase subunit 4 (NOX4) played a critical role in the development of PH in mice model [13, 16–19]. Clinically, an increased NOX4 was observed in pulmonary vasculatures of both chronic PH and human idiopathic pulmonary arterial hypertension (PAH) [13–15]. Of importance, the NOX4 was a relevant NOX homolog in human airway, which could be induced by transforming growth factor beta (TGF-β) in human PASMCs (HPASMCs) and had an important implication in pulmonary vascular remodeling [12, 19, 20]. Our previous study also demonstrated that an augmented expression of NOX4 and TGF-β was correlated with the increased volume of airway smooth muscle (ASM) mass and epithelial cells of small airways in patients with COPD [21]. Moreover, the increased expression of NOX4 was accompanied by an up-regulated TGF-β in ASM of small airway in COPD lungs [21]. These studies thus strongly imply a contribution of NOX4 and TGF-β in the development of PH in COPD. However, the regulation of NOX4 in peripheral artery smooth muscle cells of COPD patients and its clinical implications in the pathogenesis of PH in COPD has yet been extensively explored.

Cardiac magnetic resonance imaging (cMRI) enables a combination of morphological and functional assessment of right ventricular (RV) and pulmonary circulation, including left ventricular (LV) and RV chamber sizes, wall thickness and mass, and velocity of flow in blood vessels [22]. Therefore it can be harnessed to detect early RV dysfunction and remodeling in patients with non-severe COPD, and used to noninvasively diagnose PH with high accuracy (92%). For instance, the late gadolinium enhancement, retrograde flow ≥0.3 L/ (min·m^2), and pulmonary artery relative area change ≤15% measured by cMRI were useful parameters for predicting the presence of PH with a high degree of diagnostic certainty in patients with COPD [5, 23, 24]. Equally noteworthy, previous data from cMRI measurements have suggested that the right ventricular ejection fraction (RVEF) and right ventricular myocardial mass (RVMM) were correlated with the severity of airflow limitation in COPD [24].

In view of aforementioned findings, we therefore sought to assess the morphological characteristics of distal pulmonary arteries by cMRI measurement, and investigate the relationship between NOX4 of distal pulmonary arteries and airflow limitation in patients with COPD. In order to better understand the role and mechanism underlying NOX4 in distal pulmonary vascular remodeling, relationships between the NOX4 and distal pulmonary artery remodeling, pulmonary circulation and/or ventricular morphology of COPD patients were explored. In addition, the interaction between NOX4 and TGF-β in human primary artery smooth muscle cells (HPASMCs) was also investigated.

Methods

Ethics statement

Human samples were collected with a protocol approved by the Ethic Committee for the Conduct of Human Research at Ningxia Medical University (NXMU-2015-205). Written consent was obtained from every individual according to the Ethic Committee for the Conduct of Human Research protocol. All participants were above 18 years old, and were provided a written informed consent for the publication of the data. The Ethic Committee the Conduct of Human Research at General Hospital of Ningxia Medical University approved the consent procedure for this study (NXMU-2015-205).

Subjects

A total of 15 patients with COPD (ages range 43–64 years) and 19 of gender- and age- matched individuals (ages range 45–68 years) with normal lung function were recruited in General Hospital of Ningxia Medical University between January 2015 and December 2016. All enrolled individuals who were about to undergo pneumonectomy, or lobectomy for suspected early stage of non-small cell lung cancer (NSCLC). Of the 15 enrolled patients in the COPD group, 8 had lung adenocarcinomas, three had squamous lung cancer (among the 11 lung cancer patients, 6 patients suffered TNM stage I and 5 patients were with stageII cancer), and the rest 4 patients had benign lesions, as confirmed by histology. Of all 19 individuals in non-COPD group, 14 had lung adenocarcinomas, four suffered from squamous lung cancer (among these cancer patients, 9 patients were with TNM stage I and 8 patients with stageII cancer), and 2 had benign lesions. The stages of NSCLC were diagnosed according to the NCCN guideline of TNM staging of NSCLC (2016 version) (https://www.nccn.org/).

Basic demographic information was collected using a specifically designed questionnaire after a written informed consent was obtained. Smoking status was defined as non-smoker (never smoking), ex-smoker (smoking quit for at least 6 months), and current smoker (smoking at least one cigarette daily for more than 6 months). The cigarette consumption was calculated by multiplying the number of pack of cigarette smoked per day by years of smoking (pack-years). Basic data on pulmonary function testing (PFT) [25, 26], echocardiography [27], and 6-min walk distance (6MWD) [28] were also collected (Table 1). All subjects underwent cMRI and echocardiography in General hospital of Ningxia Medical University (Yinchuan, China). Standard pulmonary function testing was performed on all subjects before the surgical performance. The pulmonary function was ascertained by measured the postbronchodilator forced vital capacity (FVC) and forced expiratory volume of one second (FEV1), using a MasterScreen PFT spirometer system (Care Fusion, San Diego, CA, USA). The diagnosis of COPD was essentially according to the criteria of Global Initiative on Obstructive Lung Disease (GOLD 2015) [1]. The exclusive criteria: patients accompanied with 1) other chronic lung diseases, such as bronchial asthma, sleep apnea-hypopnea syndrome, bronchiectasis, pulmonary fibrosis, interstitial lung disease; 2) abnormal liver and kidney function; 3) known ischemic heart disease; 4) congestive heart failure; 5) structural heart disease; 6) PH; 7) prior thromboembolic disease; 8) cerebrovascular disease; 9) peripheral arterial disease; 10) hepatitis and autoimmune

Table 1 Demographics of patients with COPD and non-COPD control subjects

Demographics	Control	Patients with COPD		t/t′	*P*
		Mild (GOLD1)	Moderate (GOLD2)		
Subjects	19	6	9		
Age (s)	55.84±7.82 (45–68)	54.83±7.36 (43–64)	54.11±6.92 (43–64)	0.56	0.58
Gender					
Male	13	6	6	0.74	0.46
Female	6	0	3		
Stature (m)	1.68±0.07	1.70±0.07	1.68±0.05	− 0.45	0.65
Weight (kg)	69.79±11.63	65.33±7.00	55.84±14.38		
BSA (m2)	1.76±0.18	1.72±0.12	1.71±0.22	0.86	0.40
BMI (kg/m^2)	24.69±2.95	22.75±2.25	22.77±3.56	1.87	0.07
Smoking status and cigarette consumption (Pack-years)	9.66±11.83	19.17±14.97	13.33±15.81	−1.296	0.20
Never smoking (n)	9	1	4		
Current smoking (n)	6	4	3		
Ex-smoker (n)	4	1	2		
PO_2 (mmHg)	92.51±7.34	60.85±8.36	63.63±2.72	7.82	0.00
PCO_2 (mmHg)	37.67±2.60	41.20±4.81	41.56±4.53	−2.88	0.01
FEV_1/FVC (%)	76.29±6.04	63.67±3.56	53.22±8.26	7.30	0.00
FEV_1%prep (%)	97.74±18.80	91.00±4.47	62.22±4.09	4.02	0.00
DLCO(%)	87.89 ± 8.43	86.00 ± 8.32	67.89 ± 6.49	3.72	0.00
6MWD (m)	507.00±25.27	422.33±49.94	425.89±37.25	6.84	0.00

6MWD six-Minute Walk Distance, *BSA* body surface area, *BMI* body mass index, *FEV1/FVC* forced expiratory volume in one second/ forced vital capacity, *FEV1%pred* forced expiratory volume in one second total predicted value, *PCO2* partial pressure of carbon dioxide, *PO2* arterial partial pressure of oxygen. Data was presented as mean ± SD, and *P* values were given as COPD versus non-COPD groups

diseases and/or 11) inability to undergo cMRI were excluded in this study. According to the guideline of GOLD 2015, the distribution of spirometric classification in 15 recruited patients with COPD was as follow: 6 out of the 15 patients with mild stage of COPD, 9 with moderate stage (patients with mild stage and moderate stage of COPD were grouped in the moderate COPD for statistics in the study). A portion of grossly normal lung tissue with size of approximately 1.0 cm^2 in area and 0.5 cm of thickness was collected from the distal end of the lesion (≥5.0 cm) during the process of operation. Tissue specimens were harvested after written informed consents for the publication of the data were obtained. The specimen was immediately snap frozen in liquid nitrogen (LN) for protein and RNA analysis, embedded in optimal cutting temperature (OCT) compound, or immerged in 10% buffered formalin fixative.

Cardiac magnetic resonance imaging (cMRI)

The cMRI examination was performed using a 3.0-T MRI scanner (GE Healthcare, Buckinghamshire, UK,). All cMRI images were acquired using an eight-channel heart array coil, followed by electrocardiogram gating and breath-holding, with the patient in a supine position. All subjects needed to repeat breath exercises before being scanned. The axial, sagittal, and coronal planes were scanned and images were acquired in end-expiratory breath-hold. A BH Ax Fiesta sequence was used to collect 10 layers of axial images in the coronal plane at the center of main pulmonary artery. The Oblique Fiesta and Fast Cine PC sequences were used to obtain images of the main pulmonary artery, while the two-dimensional steady-state precession fast acquisition sequence (Fiesta) was used to obtain LV and RV two-chamber and four-chamber heart and short-axis cMRI images. The RV function was analyzed using Fiesta short-axis images. All images were transferred to the Advantage Windows workstation 4.3 (GE Medical Systems, WI, USA) after scanning. The Report Card 4.0 cardiac function analysis software (GE Healthcare, Milwaukee, WI) was used for measuring parameters of heart function. Two professional radiologists blindly evaluated data independently by measuring the maximum and minimum cross-sectional area (CSA) of main pulmonary artery during the cardiac cycle. The main pulmonary artery distensibility (mPAD%) was calculated using the following equation: mPAD% = (CSAmax-CSAmin)/CSAmin × 100% [29]. The epicardial and endocardial contours of RV of systolic and diastolic short-axis images were manually traced on screen. Functional parameters of heart, such as RVEF and left ventricular ejection fraction (LVEF) were automatically calculated. The myocardial mass was assessed using the following equation: myocardial mass = (epicardial volume - endocardial volume) × 1.05 (specific gravity of myocardium). Then, the right ventricular myocardial mass end-diastolic (RVMED), right ventricular myocardial mass end-systolic (RVMES), and right ventricular mass index (RVMI) were obtained as previously described [30, 31].

Cell culture and treatment

Human primary artery smooth muscular cells (HPASMCs) were purchased from ScienCell Research Laboratories (Carlsbad, CA, USA) and cultured in SMCM basic medium (ScienCell Research Laboratories, Carlsbad, CA, USA) supplemented with 10% fetal bovine serum (FBS), 100 U/mL penicillin and 100 μg/mL streptomycin at 37 °C in a humidified atmosphere with 5% CO_2. Cells between passages 3–12 were used in this study. Cells were treated with $TGF\beta_1$ at various concentrations (0–10 ng/mL) for different time periods (0–48 h).

Morphometric studies

Lung tissues were embedded in paraffin or optimal cutting temperature (OCT) compound, and cut at a thickness of 4 μm for hematoxylin and eosin (HE) or Weigert-van Gieson staining (to highlight collagen and elastic fibers). Tissue sections from all subjects were stained with HE for histopathologic examination. Pulmonary vascular elastic fibers and collagen were determined on paraffin sections by Weigert-van Gieson staining using a kit (DC0066B7, Leagene, Beijing, China) [32, 33]. The morphometric characteristics of smooth muscle of distal pulmonary arteries were analyzed in sections immunohistochemically stained with α-smooth muscle actin (α-SMA) and Weigert-van Gieson staining (Fig. 1a). Arteries with an external diameter 100–500 μm and completely elastic laminas were evaluated as previously reported [34–36]. 5–10 arteries with an external diameter 100–500 μm per subject were evaluated in this study. The external and internal elastic lamina and the inner area of the intima were outlined; the area of muscular layer, intimal layer, and lumen were computed; and areas were expressed as a percentage of the total measured area. The stained slide was examined using the Olympus light microscope BX51 (Olympus China, Beijing, China), and images were analyzed using Image-Pro Plus 6.0 (IPP6.0) software (Media Cybernetics, MD, USA). The computer-assisted quantification of the staining in a selected area was performed in images with a magnification of 400×. For measurements, the total area of artery (TA), luminal area of artery (LA), and perimeter of blood vessels (P) were measured using IPP6.0 as outlined in Fig. 1a. The following parameters were further calculated: the blood vessel radius (R) = $P/2\pi$; the external diameter of blood vessels (ED) = R + WT/2; the vascular wall area (WA) = TA-LA; and the thickness of blood vessel wall (WT) = WA/P. The thickness of pulmonary vessel wall was expressed as the percentage of external diameter calculated by the formula as

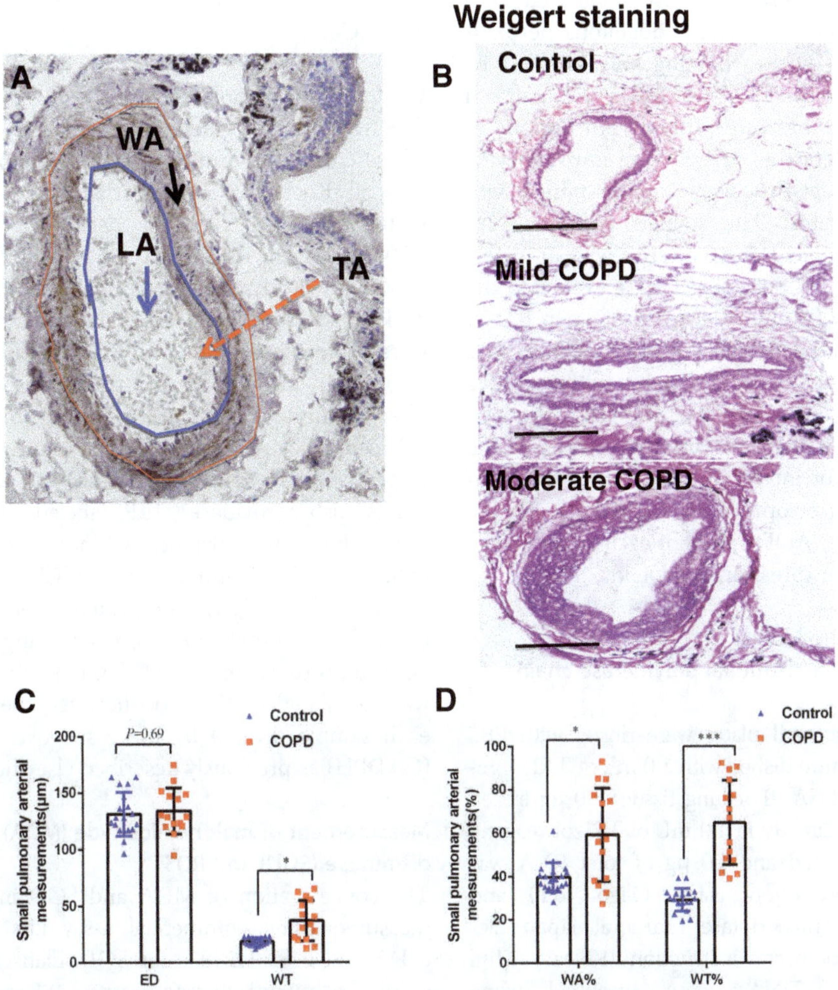

Fig. 1 An increased volume of distal pulmonary arteries in COPD patients. **a** The image illustrates the method for measurement of muscular area of pulmonary arteries in this study (× 400). The total area of artery (TA, area inside the red line), luminal area of artery (LA, area inside the blue line), the vascular wall area (WA, the area between red line and blue line) were measured by Image-Pro Plus software 6.0. **b** Weigert-van Gieson staining showed more abundant collagen and connective tissues in arteries of COPD lung relative to controls; (**c**) comparison of external diameter (ED) and vascular diameter (WT) determined by IHC staining of α-SMA between normal and COPD lungs; (**d**) comparison of the pulmonary artery smooth muscle area accounted for the percentage of total vascular area (WA%) and the pulmonary artery smooth muscle thickness accounted for the percentage of vascular diameter (WT%) determined by IHC staining of α-SMA between non-COPD and COPD lungs. Compared to non-COPD lung, *: $p < 0.05$ 01 ($N = 19$ for non-COPD; $N = 15$ for COPD)

(2×WT/ED)×100% [4, 37]. The thickness of pulmonary vessel wall accounted for the percentage of vascular diameter (WT%), and the area of pulmonary artery smooth muscle accounted for the percentage of total vascular area (WA%) = WA/TA×100% [38].

Immunocytochemical histochemical,and immunohistochemical staining

For immunocytochemical staining, HPASMCs were fixed in 4% paraformaldehyde for 15 min and permeabilized with 0.1% Triton X-100 in PBS for 10 min at room temperature. The cells were blocked with 5% bovine serum albumin (BSA; Sigma Chemical Co., MO, USA) for 1 h at room temperature, washed with PBS, and probed with rabbit anti-NOX4 antibody (1:500, Novus Biotech, CO, USA), mouse anti-collagen I antibody (1:500, Abcam, MA, USA), mouse anti-TGFβ1 antibody (1:1000, Abcam, MA, USA) or mouse anti-α-smooth muscle actin (SMA) antibody (1:200, Abcam, MA, USA) overnight at 4°C. Species-matched normal sera were served as negative controls of antibodies. The cells were rinsed in PBS for 3×5 min and incubated with peroxidase-labeled appropriate secondary antibodies (ZSGB-Bio, Beijing, China) (1:1000 in blocking buffer) for 45 min at room temperature. The signal of interest was developed with 3,3′-diaminobenzidine (DAB) peroxidase substrate.

The immunohistochemical analysis was performed on paraffin-embedded tissues as previously described [21].

Briefly, the deparaffined sections were incubated with 0.3% H_2O_2 in methanol to inhibit endogenous peroxidase activity, and non-specific binding was blocked by incubating sections with 5% BSA for 1 h at room temperature. The sections were probed with antibodies against proteins of interest as described in immunocytochemical staining, except they were counterstained with hematoxylin if applicable. The stained sections were examined and photographed. 5–10 arteries with an external diameter 100–500 μm per subject were evaluated the average optical density (AOD) of target protein in PASM in lung tissue. Five randomly fields of each section at a magnification of 400× were used for analyzing the positive staining as previously reported [21, 33]. The obtained images were then for a semi-quantitative analysis of the expression of protein of interest by measuring the integrated absorbance (IA) or optical density (OD) using the IPP6.0 software, and the AOD values of each sample were used as an index of the expression of proteins.

Quantitative reverse transcriptional polymerase chain reaction (qRT-PCR)

HPASMCs grown in six-well plates were rinsed with PBS and lysed directly in culture dished with 1.0 mL of TRIzol reagent (Invitrogen, CA, USA). For lung tissues, 50 μg frozen lung tissues were lysed directly in 1.0 mL of TRIzol reagent. Total RNAs were extracted and 1.0 μg of total RNA was used for reverse-transcription using Oligo (dT) and Transcriptor Reverse Transcriptase (TaKaRa, Japan) according to the manufacturer's instruction (RNeasy Mini Kit, TaKaRa, Japan). cDNAs were amplified using gene-specific primers from published data or designed using Oligo version 6 (Molecular Biology Insights, CO, USA). Transcripts were amplified by polymerase chain reaction (PCR) using a specific primer for NOX4, α-SMA and glyceraldehyde-3-phosphate dehydrogenase (GAPDH). The quantitative reverse transcriptional PCR (qRT-PCR) was performed using the RT2 SYBR Green qPCR Mastermix (Qiagen, Duesseldorf, Germany) in Lightcycler 480 Real-Time System (Roche, Basel, Switzerland). qRT-PCR was performed with following parameters: 95 °C for 10 min, 45 cycles of 94 °C for 5 s and 60 °C for 30 s, and 60 °C for 5 min followed by a dissociation curve analysis. The expression of transcripts was analyzed using the $^{\Delta\Delta}$CT method [39]. Each sample was examined in triplicate, and the abundance of transcripts was normalized against GAPDH. Primers used in this study were as follows: NOX4 forward: 5'-AGATGTTGGGGCTAGGATTG-3', reverse: 5'TCTCCTGCTTGGAACCTTCT-3'; α-SMA forward: 5'-GACCGAATGCAGAAGGAGAT-3', reverse: 5'-CCAC CGATCCAGACAGAGTA-3'; GAPDH forward: 5'-CAGC CTCAAGATCATCAGCA-3', reverse: 5'-ACAGTCTTC TGGGTGGCAGT-3'. TGFβ1 forward: 5'-GAAATTGAG GGCTTTCGCCT-3', reverse: 5'-AGTGAACCCGTTGA TGTCC-3'.

Western blotting analysis

The frozen lung tissues were stored at − 80 °C and 1.0 ml of ice-cold RIPA buffer containing a protease inhibitor cocktail (Roche, Basel, Switzerland) was added to approximately 300 mg of lung tissue for homogenization. HPMECs were harvested on ice and proteins were extracted with lysis buffer containing a protease inhibitor cocktail as described elsewhere. Protein concentrations were determined by the BCA assay. Proteins were resolved in SDS-PAGE and transferred on nitrocellulose filter membrane, blots were probed for NOX4, TGFβ1, collagen, α-SMA or GAPDH with appropriate antibodies, respectively. Protein of interest was detected using a horseradish peroxidase (HRP)-labeled secondary antibody (ZSGB-Bio Ltd., Beijing, China) and acquired with enhanced chemiluminescence (ECL) (Thermo Fisher Scientific, MA, USA). The protein expression levels were quantified by optical densitometry using NIH ImageJ Fiji Software (https://imagej.net/Fiji) if applicable. Fold change was calculated as the ratio between the net intensity of each sample divided by the respective internal controls (GADPH) as previously described elsewhere [40].

Measurement of malondialdehyde (MDA), superoxide dismutase (SOD) and ROS

The concentration of MDA and SOD in HPASMC were measured using commercial assay kits (E-EL-0060c for MDA and E-EL-H2382c for SOD, Elabscience, China) according to manufacturer's protocols. The concentration of Collagen Type 1 alphal in HPASMC culture supernatants was measured using commercial assay kits (ab210966, Abcam, MA, USA) according to manufacturer's protocols. Intracellular ROS level was determined by accessing the mean fluorescent intensity of 2′-7′-dichlorodihydrofluorescein diacetate (H_2DCFH-DA, Molecular Probes, OR, USA) using a flow cytometric assay with 495-nm excitation and 525-nm emission (BD Biosciences, CA, USA). Briefly, HPASMCs were seeded in six-well plates and cultured for 24 h in SMCM media before they were exposed to media containing different concentrations (0–10 ng/mL) of TGFβ_1 for various time periods (0-48 h). For measurement of MDA and SOD in HPASMC, cells washed twice with cold PBS, then added the protein lysis (RIPA with proteinase inhibitor) on the ice, scraped and collected the lysis, centrifuge at 12000 rpm for 20 min. The supernatant was collected and sample protein concentration in the extract was quantified using a BCA protein assay. The protein expression of MDA and SOD was determined in supernatant of cell lysate using an ELISA kit. For measurement of ROS in HPASMC, the cells were rinsed with warm PBS and incubated in serum-free and phenol red-free DMEM/F-12 medium containing 10μM H_2DCFH-DA at 37°C for 30 min. At the end of incubation, the medium was removed, and the cells were rinsed twice with pre-warm PBS prior to intracellular ROS analysis using a flow cytometer.

Statistical analysis

All data were expressed as mean ± standard error of the mean (SEM). The independent-samples *t* test (for two-group comparison) and one-way analysis of variance (for multiple-group comparison), and least significant difference test were employed to compare between groups using SPSS 19.0 software (Chicago, IL, USA). The Pearson correlation analysis was used to analyze correlations between the pulmonary artery smooth muscle thickness accounting for the percentage of vascular diameter (WT%), the pulmonary artery smooth muscle area accounting for the percentage of total vascular area (WA%), FEV1/FVC, FEV1%pred, and the abundance of NOX4 protein in the pulmonary arteriolar smooth muscles. A *P* value less than 0.05 was considered as a statistical significance.

Results

Demographic data

Fifteen patients with COPD were enrolled in this study, included 3 females and 12 males with a mean age of 54.40 ± 6.84 years (range of 43–64 years). Of these, six were diagnosed with mild COPD (all males; four current smokers, one ex-smoker, and one never smoker) and nine with moderate COPD (six males and three females; three current smokers, two ex-smokers, and four never smokers). The cigarette consumption (pack-years) in the COPD group was 15.67 ± 15.22; of enrolled patients in the COPD group, eight had lung adenocarcinomas, three had squamous lung cancer, and four had benign lesions confirmed by histology. Nineteen non-COPD patients were enrolled in this study, included six females and thirteen males with a mean age of 55.84 ± 7.82 years (range of 45–68 years). Six non-COPD patients were current smokers, four were ex-smokers, and nine were never smokers. The cigarette consumption (pack-years) in non-COPD group was 9.66 ± 11.83. Of all individuals in non-COPD group, thirteen had lung adenocarcinomas, four suffered from squamous lung cancer, and two had benign lesions, as confirmed by histology. No significant difference in age, body mass index (BMI), cigarette consumption (pack-years), and tumor histology was found between patients with COPD and without COPD. But parameters of pulmonary functions FEV1%pred, FEV1/FVC%, and 6MWD were significantly different in patients with COPD compared with non-COPD subjects (Table 1).

Parameters of ventricular dimensions and pulmonary circulation on cMRI

cMRI images showed an enlargement of main pulmonary artery and a reduced left and right ventricle in patients with COPD compared to those without COPD (Fig. 1b). The cMRI parameters of mPAP (22.78 ± 1.6 vs 24.98 ± 3.68, $P = 0.02$), mPADmax (26.96 ± 2.13 vs 30.36 ± 3.34, $P = 0.00$), mPADmin (22.06 ± 2.15 vs 24.91 ± 2.50, $P = 0.00$), CSAmax (5.77 ± 0.99 vs 6.98 ± 0.95, $P = 0.00$), and CSAmin (3.69 ± 0.69 vs 4.91 ± 0.98, $P = 0.00$) exhibited statistical difference between patients with COPD and those without COPD, respectively (Table 2). The average negative flow (ANF) (3.25 ± 2.00 vs 5.27 ± 2.55, $P = 0.01$) and regurgitant fraction (RF%) (4.68 ± 3.04 vs 7.91 ± 3.74, $P = 0.01$) also showed statistically different ($P < 0.05$), despite the positive peak velocity, negative peak velocity, average volume flow, and average positive flow were not statistically different between COPD and non-COPD groups ($P > 0.05$). In addition, cMRI parameters of ventricular dimensions in individuals with COPD and without COPD, including RVMED (32.94 ± 4.31 vs

Table 2 Cardiac magnetic measurement parameters

	Control (*n* = 19)	COPD (*n* = 15)	*t/t'*	*P*
mPAP (mmHg)	22.78±1.62	24.98±3.68	−1.40	0.02
mPADmax (mm)	26.96±2.13	30.36±3.34	−3.61	0.00
mPADmin (mm)	22.06±2.15	24.91±2.50	−3.59	0.00
CSAmax (cm2)	5.77±0.99	6.98±0.95	−3.60	0.00
CSAmin (cm2)	3.69±0.69	4.91±0.98	−4.26	0.00
mPAD (%)	57.29±14.47	43.82±10.87	2.99	0.01
PPV (cm/s)	69.71±15.76	74.71±26.79	−0.68	0.50
PNV (cm/s)	21.42±14.28	27.31±14.81	−1.18	0.25
AF (ml/beat)	70.01±22.00	64.73±17.31	0.76	0.45
APF (ml/beat)	72.93±22.27	68.50±16.75	0.64	0.53
ANF (ml/beat)	3.25±2.00	5.27±2.55	−2.60	0.01
RF (%)	4.68±3.04	7.91±3.74	−2.78	0.01
RVEDV (ml)	124.28±21.53	122.15±25.78	0.26	0.80
REESV (ml)	58.51±14.57	58.63±22.03	−0.02	0.99
RVSV (ml)	65.77±16.68	63.53±13.99	0.42	0.68
RVEF (%)	52.81±10.19	51.27±8.97	0.46	0.65
RVMED (g)	32.94±4.31	40.03±8.55	−2.93	0.00
RVMES (g)	28.05±5.00	32.87±8.10	−2.132	0.04
RVMI (g/m2)	0.38±0.08	0.46±0.13	0.10	0.04

AF average volume flow, *ANF* average negative flow, *APF* average positive flow, *CSAmax* minimum cross-sectional area, *CSAmin* maximum cross-sectional area, *mPAD* main pulmonary artery diameter, *mPADmax* maximum main pulmonary artery diameter, *mPADmin* minimum main pulmonary artery diameter, *mPAP* mean pulmonary artery pressure, *PNV* negative peak velocity, *PPV* positive peak velocity, *RF* regurgitant fraction, *RVEDV* right ventricular end-diastolic volume, *RVEF* right ventricular ejection fraction, *RVMED* right ventricular myocardial mass end-diastolic, *RVMES* right ventricular myocardial mass end-systolic, *RVMI* right ventricular mass index, *RVESV* right ventricular end-systolic volume, *RVSV* right ventricular stroke volume. Data was presented as mean ± SD, and P values were given as COPD versus non-COPD groups

40.03 ± 8.55, $P = 0.01$), RVMES (28.05 ± 5.00 vs 32.87 ± 8.10, $P = 0.04$), and RVMI (0.38 ± 0.08 vs 0.46 ± 0.13, $P = 0.04$) also displayed a statistical difference ($P < 0.05$), respectively. But the RVEDV, RVESV, RVSV, and RVEF were not statistically different between these two groups ($P > 0.05$) (Table 2).

The volume of distal pulmonary arteries was increased in patients with COPD

Morphometric analysis of pulmonary arteries using Weigert-van Gieson staining and α-SMA-IHC staining showed a thicker vessel wall in COPD lungs compared to non-COPD lungs (Fig. 1b). Semi-quantitative analysis of the morphometric study demonstrated that the WT (Fig. 1c), WT% (Fig. 1d), and WA% (Fig. 1d) were significantly greater in COPD lungs (37.07 ± 18.07 μm, 64.76 ± 19.48%, and 55.38 ± 23.46%, respectively) relative to non-COPD lungs (18.71 ± 3.35 μm, 29.17 ± 5.36%, and 39.67 ± 6.78%, respectively), although the ED value was not statistically different between the COPD and the non-COPD lungs ($P = 0.687$, Fig. 1c).

A correlations between the cMRI finding and airway limitation in COPD patients

Next, we sought to analyze whether the cMRI finding had a relationship with pulmonary functions in COPD. The correlation analysis showed that the mPAD% was positively correlated with pulmonary function parameters FEV_1/FVC and FEV_1%pred, with a correlation coefficient of $r = 0.42$ ($P < 0.05$) (Fig. 2b) and $r = 0.50$ ($P < 0.01$), respectively (Fig. 2c). In addition, RVMED was found to positively correlate with PCO_2 ($r = 0.46$, $P < 0.05$) (Fig. 2d), but negatively correlate with PO_2 ($r = -0.36$, $P < 0.05$) (Fig. 2e).

Correlations between the volume of distal pulmonary arteries, cMRI findings, and lung functions

We next further explored whether the volume of distal pulmonary arteries was correlated with cMRI findings and pulmonary functions in COPD. Indeed, the volume of distal pulmonary arteries was inversely correlated with lung functions (FEV_1/FVC and FEV_1%pred) but positively correlated with cMRI findings (mPAD%, RVMES, and RVMED) (Fig. 3). The correlation coefficients between WA% and mPAD, WT% and mPAD%, WA% and FEV_1/FVC, WA% and FEV_1%pred, WT% and FEV1/FVC, WT% and FEV1%pred were $r = -0.42$ ($P < 0.05$) and $r = -0.50$ ($P < 0.01$), $r = -0.35$ ($P < 0.05$), $r = -0.35$ ($P < 0.05$), $r = -0.54$ ($P < 0.05$), and $r = -0.51$ ($P < 0.05$), respectively. The respective correlation coefficients between WA% and RVMES, WA% and RVMED, WT% and RVMES, WT% and RVMED, WA% and RF%, WA% and RF% were $r = 0.34$ ($P < 0.05$), $r = 0.37$ ($P < 0.05$), $r = 0.45$ ($P < 0.01$), $r = 0.52$ ($P < 0.01$), $r = 0.27$ ($P = 0.13$) and $r = 0.49$ ($P < 0.01$), respectively (Fig. 3).

An elevated expression of NOX4 and extracellular matrix deposition in artery smooth muscle (ASM) of distal pulmonary arteries of COPD

In order to investigate whether NOX4 is involved in distal pulmonary artery remodeling, the abundance of NOX4, α-SMA, TGFβ1 and collagen I proteins and transcripts in pulmonary arteries was determined by IHC, Western blot and qRT-PCR. More abundant NOX4, α-SMA, TGFβ1 and collagen I proteins were detected by IHC (Fig. 4), and Western blotting assay (Fig. 5) in pulmonary arteries or lung tissues of COPD compared with non-COPD, respectively. An increased abundance of NOX4, α-SMA and TGFβ1 transcripts was also observed in COPD lungs relative to non-COPD lungs by the RT-PCR assay ($P < 0.05$) (Fig. 5). Moreover, the correlation analysis further demonstrated that the abundance of NOX4 protein in pulmonary arteries was positively correlated with WA% and WT%, but inversely correlated with pulmonary functions. The correlation coefficients between NOX4 and WA%, NOX4 and WT%, NOX4 and FEV1/FVC, NOX4 and FEV1%pred were $r = 0.79$ ($P < 0.01$), $r = -0.41$ ($P < 0.05$), $r = -0.4$ ($P < 0.05$), $r = 0.53$ ($P < 0.01$), respectively (Fig. 6).

TGFβ1 augmented the expression of NOX4, α-SMA, and collagen I in HPASMCs

Previous study has demonstrated that the NOX4 had important implication in pulmonary vascular remodeling and could be induced by TGFβ in HPASMCs [12]. In agreement with this finding, a dynamic induction of NOX4, α-SMA, and collagen I proteins and transcripts of HPASMCs by TGFβ1 was also observed in this study. Significantly more abundant NOX4, α-SMA, and collagen I proteins (Fig. 7) and transcripts (Fig. 8) were induced in HPASMCs by various doses of TGFβ1 for different time periods ($P < 0.05$). Interestingly, the TGFβ1-induced NOX4 expression was dynamic but not in a time- or dose-dependent manner in this cell type, i.e. the most induction of NOX4 was observed in HPASMCs exposed to 2.0–5.0 ng/mL of TGF-β1 at 24 h (Fig. 7), although a time- and dose-dependent induction of α-SMA, and collagen I was found in cells treated with 0.0–10.0 ng/mL of TGFβ1 (Fig. 7). The induction of NOX4, α-SMA, and collagen I proteins in HPASMCs was further confirmed by RT-PCR assay (Fig. 8). Of interest, TGFβ1 also exhibited a capacity to significantly induce the expression of Collagen type 1 alphal in HPASMCs as determining their concentrations in supernatants of cell cultures (Fig. 9d).

TGFβ1 altered the production of MDA, SOD and ROS in HPASMCs

To investigate whether the imbalance of oxidant/antioxidants is involved in the development of COPD, contents

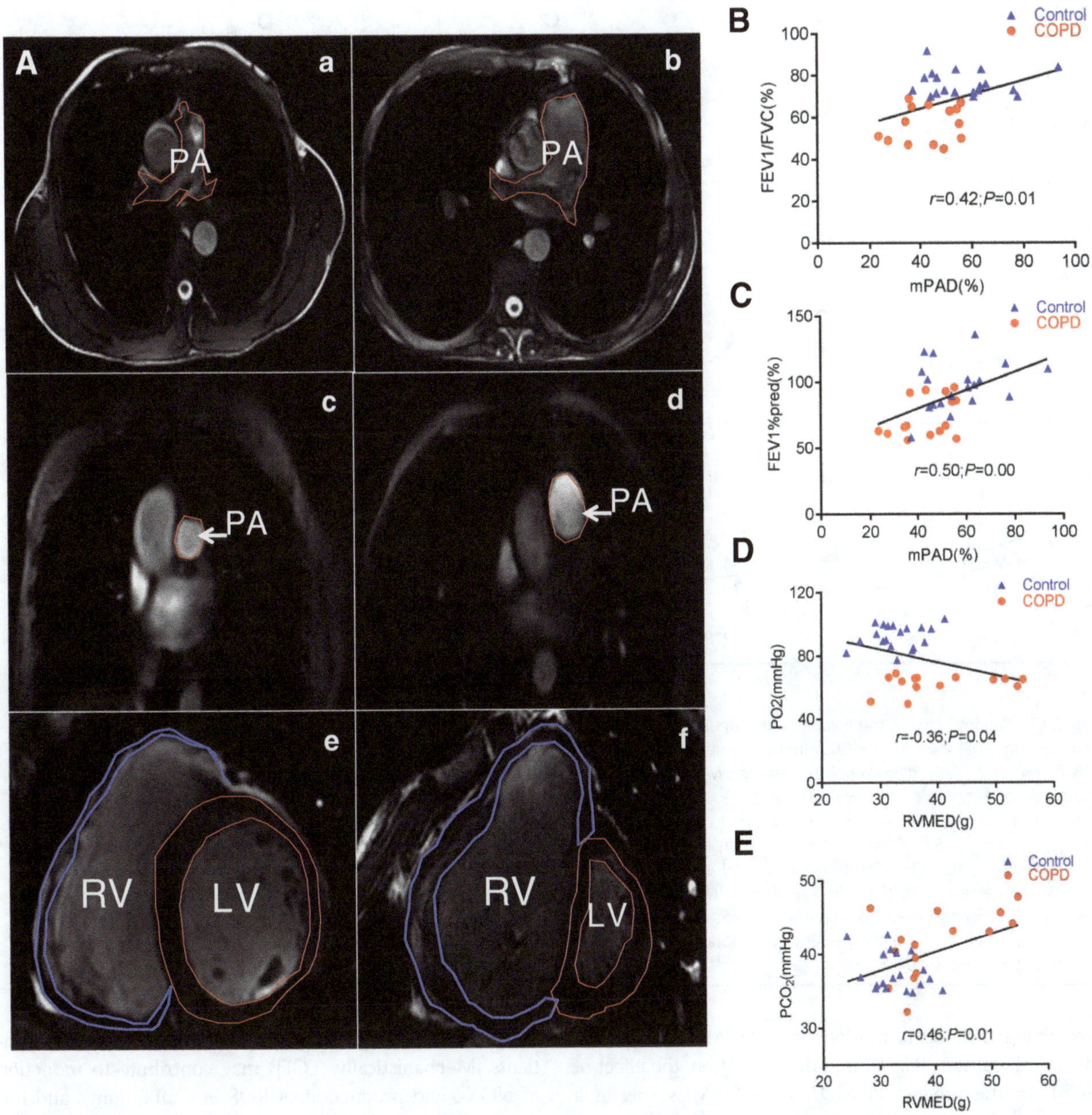

Fig. 2 Ventricular dimensions and pulmonary circulation parameters on cMRI. (**a**) Representative images of cMRI movie showed the main pulmonary artery and ventricle. (a) A main pulmonary artery FIESTA short axis image of non-COPD patients; (b) a main pulmonary artery FIESTA short axis image of COPD patients; (c) a main pulmonary artery vertical position image of non-COPD patients; (d) a main pulmonary artery vertical position image of COPD patients; (e) a left and right ventricle short axis image of non-COPD patients; (f) a left and right ventricle short axis image of COPD patients. (**b-e**) Correlations between pulmonary artery parameters and pulmonary functions. (**b**) Correlation between mPAD and FEV1/FVC; (**c**) correlation between mPAD and FEV1%pred: (**d**) correlation between RVMED and PO2; (**e**) correlation between RVMED and PCO2. PA: main pulmonary artery; REMED: right ventricular myocardial mass end diastolic; RV: right ventricle; LV: left ventricle; mPAD%: the main pulmonary artery distensibility; PO_2: arterial partial pressure of oxygen; PCO_2: partial pressure of carbon dioxide; FEV_1/FVC: forced expiratory volume in one second/forced vital capacity; FEV1%pred: forced expiratory volume in one second total predicted value

of oxidants (MDA, lipid hydroperoxide) and antioxidants enzymes (SOD) were evaluated in sera of patients with COPD and non-COPD, and HPASMCs exposed to TGFβ1. As expected, a respective higher and lower concentrations of serum MDA and SOD were determined in the sera of COPD patients as compared with those of non-COPD individuals ($P < 0.05$) (Fig. 9b). In consistent with above result of sera of COPD patients, TGFβ1 also exhibited a capacity to significantly induce HPASMCs produce MDA, but have no effect on SOD production as

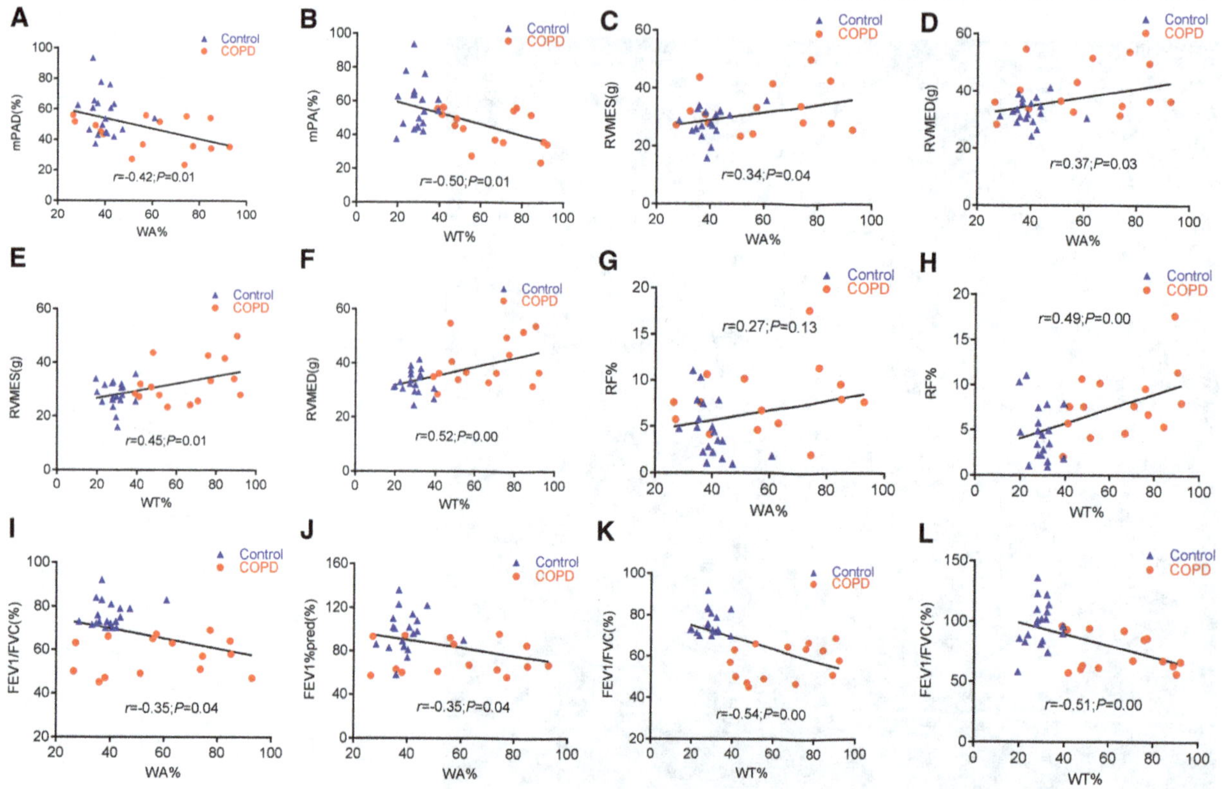

Fig. 3 Correlations between the volume of distal pulmonary arteries and cMRI findings and pulmonary functions. **a** The correlation between WA% and mPAD% ($r = -0.42, P < 0.05$); (**b**) the correlation between WT% and mPAD% ($r = -0.50, P < 0.01$); (**c**) the correlation between WA% and RVMES ($r = 0.34, P < 0.05$); (**d**) the correlation between WA% and RVMED ($r = 0.37, P < 0.05$); (**e**) the correlation between WT% and RVMES ($r = 0.45, P < 0.01$); (**f**) the correlation between WT% and RVMED ($r = 0.52, P < 0.01$); (**g**) the correlation between WA% and RF% ($r = 0.27, P = 0.13$); (**h**) the correlation between WT% and RF ($r = 0.49, P < 0.01$); (**i**) the correlation between WA% and FEV_1/FVC ($r = -0.35, P < 0.05$); (**j**) the correlation between WA% and FEV_1%pred ($r = -0.35, P < 0.05$); (**k**) the correlation between WT% and FEV1/FVC ($r = -0.54$, $P < 0.05$); (**l**) the correlation between WT% and FEV1%pred ($r = -0.51$, $P < 0.05$). FEV_1/FVC: forced expiratory volume in one second/ forced vital capacity; FEV1%pred: forced expiratory volume in one second total predicted value; mPAD%: the main pulmonary artery distensibility; RF%: regurgitant fraction; RVMED: right ventricular myocardial mass end-diastolic; RVMES: right ventricular myocardial mass end-systolic; WA%: the pulmonary artery smooth muscle area accounted for the percentage of total vascular area; WT%: the pulmonary artery smooth muscle thickness accounted for the percentage of vascular diameter

determining their concentrations in HPASMC or supernatants of cell cultures (Fig. 9c and d). In addition, the effect of TGFβ1 on the production MDA in HPASMCs was in a time- and dose-dependent manner (Fig. 9c and d). In addition, the exposure of HPASMCs to TGFβ1 led an increased ROS production in vitro (Fig. 10), suggesting the involvement of imbalance of oxidant-antioxidants in HPASMC remodeling. These results clearly suggest an implication of TGFβ1/NOX4-mediated ROS production and oxidant/antioxidant imbalance in the development of COPD and distal pulmonary artery remodeling.

Discussion

In the present study, morphological changes of pulmonary arteries and pulmonary blood flow, and the expression of NOX4 in distal pulmonary arteries in COPD lungs were investigated. The results demonstrated an involvement of NOX4, the imbalance of oxidant/antioxidants in pulmonary vascular remodeling and pulmonary functions in COPD patients. Mechanistically, TGFβ may contribute to induction of NOX4 and production of ROS in COPD lungs and human pulmonary arterial smooth muscle cells, suggesting the occurrence of distal pulmonary vascular remodeling during the early stage of COPD development. The remodeling of distal pulmonary vessels may affected the morphology and function of pulmonary artery and RV, and become a main cause of PAH in patients with severe COPD.

The pathogenic characteristic of COPD is a chronic inflammatory damage of airway and/or alveoli, which gradually leads to airway obstruction and alveolar structure disruption and the reduction of gas exchange. Moreover, the chronic hypoxia and persistent oxidative damage result in alveolar hypoxia and pulmonary vascular remodeling, thereby promoting pulmonary vascular resistance (PVR) and the increase of pulmonary arterial pressure in patients with COPD, which eventually may

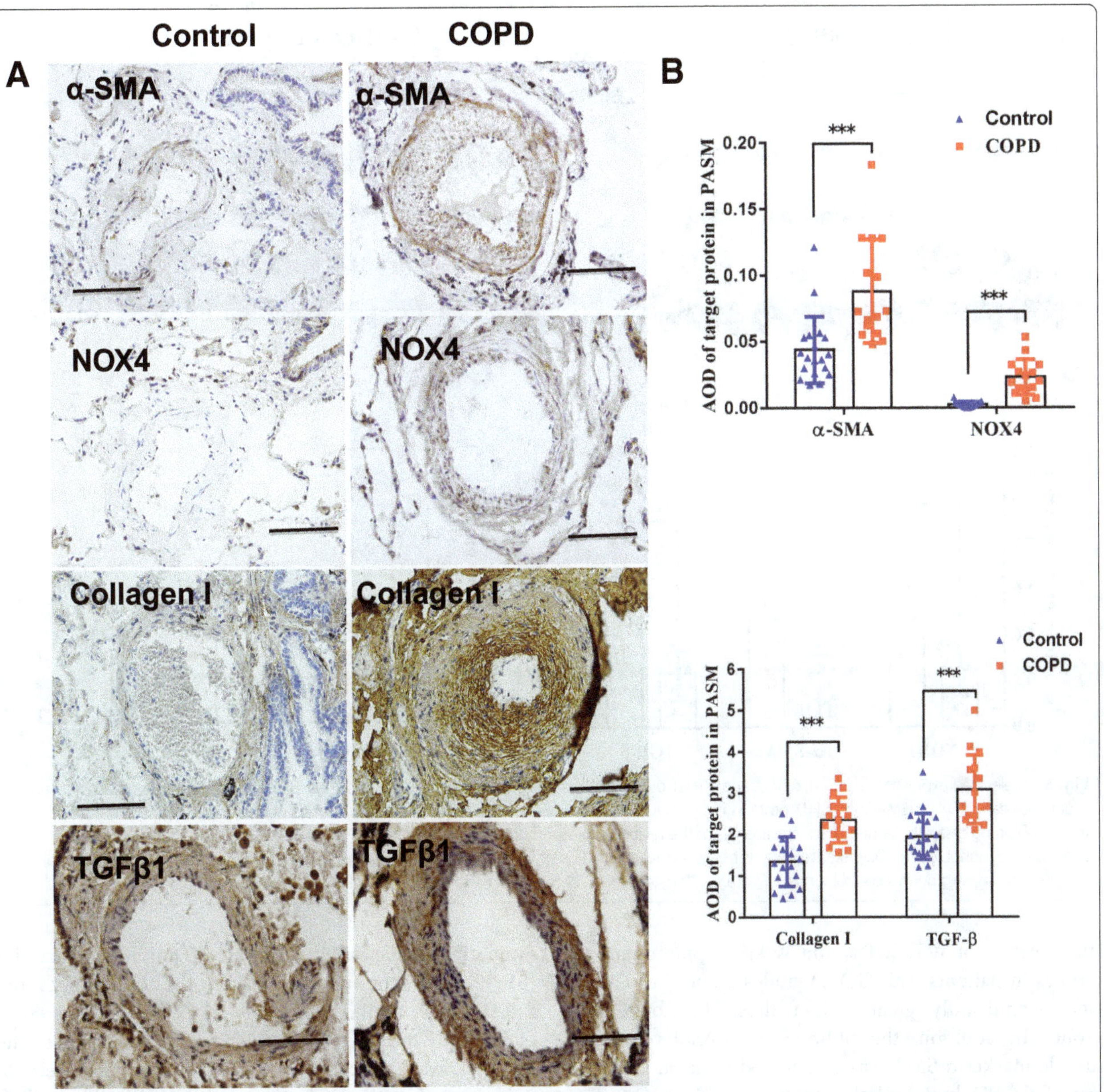

Fig. 4 An increased expression of NOX4, α-SMA, collage I and TGFβ1 in distal pulmonary arteries of COPD patients. **a** immunohistochemical (IHC) staining showed an elevated expression of NOX4, and collage I in the smooth muscle of small pulmonary artery of COPD lungs compared to normal control lungs; (**b**) The expression of NOX4 (top panel) and collage I (bottom panel) in non-COPD and COPD lungs determined by absorbance optical density (AOD) values of IHC. Compared to non-COPD lung, $^{*}P < 0.05$, *** $P < 0.01$ ($N = 19$ for non-COPD; $N = 15$ for COPD). Bars = 100 μm for all images in **a**

lead to the development of PH, an important negative prognostic factor in COPD patients [41, 42]. The 5-year survival rate of patients with COPD having mPAP> 25 mmHg is significantly lower compared to patients without PH [43, 44]. Previous studies found that the mPAP in stable COPD patients was usually 25–30 mmHg, which was significantly higher than that in patients with other chronic lung diseases [44, 45]. Therefore, an early diagnosis and intervention of COPD with PH is of paramount importance.

Pathologically, the abnormal proliferation of smooth muscle and extracellular matrix (ECM) deposition is a key part of the initiation and development of pulmonary vascular remodeling [46, 47]. Experimentally, mice exposed to chronic hypoxia showed a moderate membrane thickening and extracellular matrix deposition in pulmonary arteries (50-200 μm), along with a significantly increased WA% and WT% of pulmonary arteriole, RV hypertrophy index and RV systolic pressure, compared with mice exposed to normoxia [47]. In the present

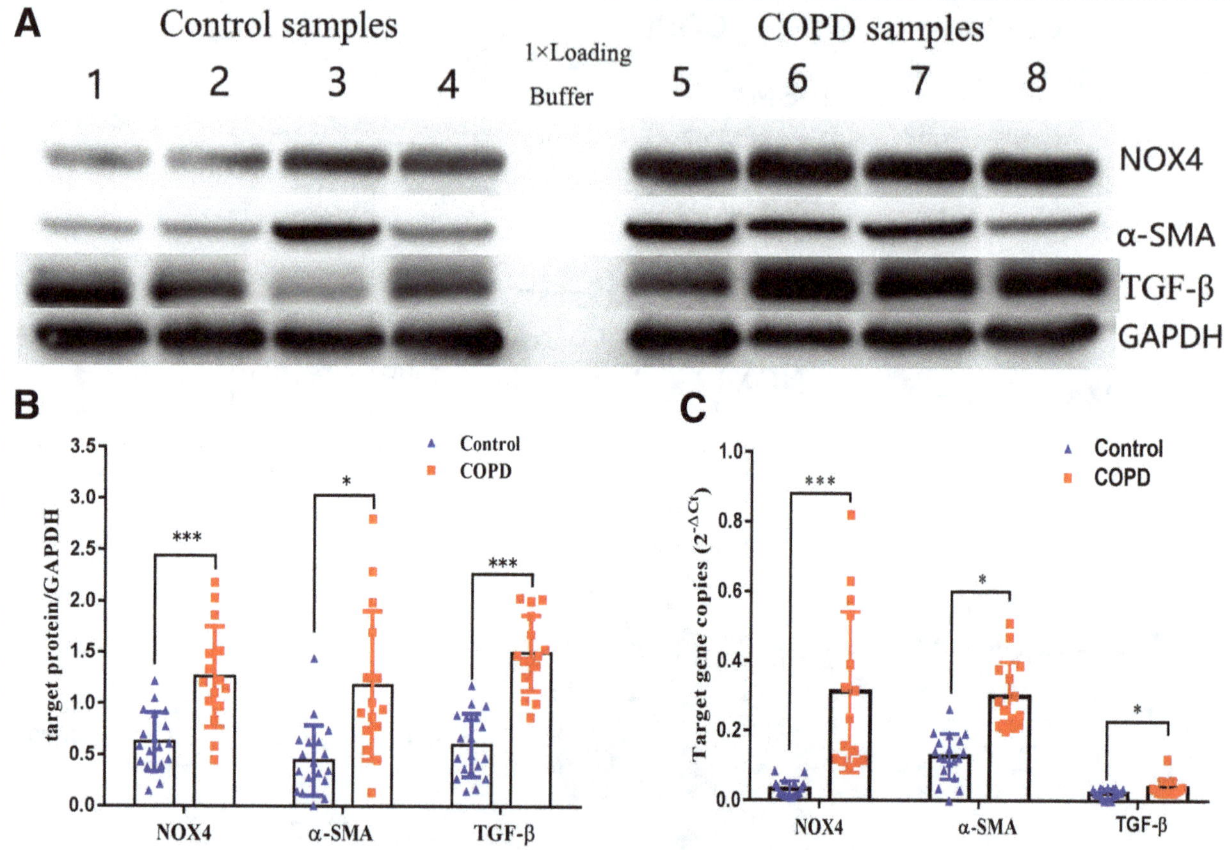

Fig. 5 An elevated expression of NOX4, α-SMA and TGFβ1 proteins in human COPD lung tissues. **a** Representative images of immunoblots showed more abundant NOX4, α-SMA and TGF**β**1 proteins in COPD lung specimens as compared with of normal lung controls as determined by an immunoblotting assay; (**b**) Semi-quantitative analysis of the relative expression of NOX4, α-SMA and TGF**β**1 proteins in COPD lungs by densometric analysis of immunoblots; (**c**) Quantitative analysis of the relative expression of NOX4 and α-SMA transcripts in COPD lung by reverse-transcriptional PCR. Compared with normal control lungs, *: $P < 0.05$, ***: $P < 0.01$ ($N = 19$ for non-COPD; $N = 15$ for COPD)

study, values of WT, WT%, and WA% of pulmonary arterioles in patients with GOLD grades 1 and 2 of COPD were significantly greater than those in non-COPD group. In addition, the pulmonary arteriolar smooth muscle marker α-SMA was augmented in distal pulmonary of COPD lungs relative to non-COPD lungs. The correlation analysis further demonstrated that both WA% and WT% in pulmonary arterioles were inversely correlated with parameters of pulmonary function of FEV_1/FVC and FEV_1%pred in these patients. These results clearly evidenced a pulmonary arteriolar remodeling that characterized by hyperplasia and smooth muscle thickening was developed, which was correlated with the obstruction degree of COPD airflow in patients with grade 1 and 2 COPD.

cMRI is a gold standard for measuring cardiac function, confirmed by extensive clinical trials [48, 49], which has been used to replace invasive angiography for the initial evaluation of COPD secondary pulmonary heart disease [50]. In this regard, previous studies revealed that the cMRI-measured mPAD% was a good index for evaluating the elasticity of wall of pulmonary arteries [51, 52]. In the present study, the cMRI-measured mPAD% was significantly lower in COPD patients compared with non-COPD individuals. In consistence, the mPAD% was positively correlated with parameters of pulmonary function in patients with COPD (FEV1/FVC and FEV1%pred). While the index of WA% and WT%, remodeling of pulmonary arterioles was inversely correlated with cMRI-measured mPAD%. Results in this study also showed that pulmonary vascular changes characterized by remodeling of distal pulmonary arteriolar smooth muscles and decreased dilatation of proximal main pulmonary arteries might have already occurred in COPD lungs before the definite manifestation of PH. Furthermore, the pulmonary vascular remodeling in COPD was related to the severity of airflow obstruction. These findings further indicate the existence of a common mechanism involved in pulmonary vascular remodeling and ASM remodeling in COPD lungs.

Alterations in the structure and function of RV usually occur in COPD and are characterized by ventricular

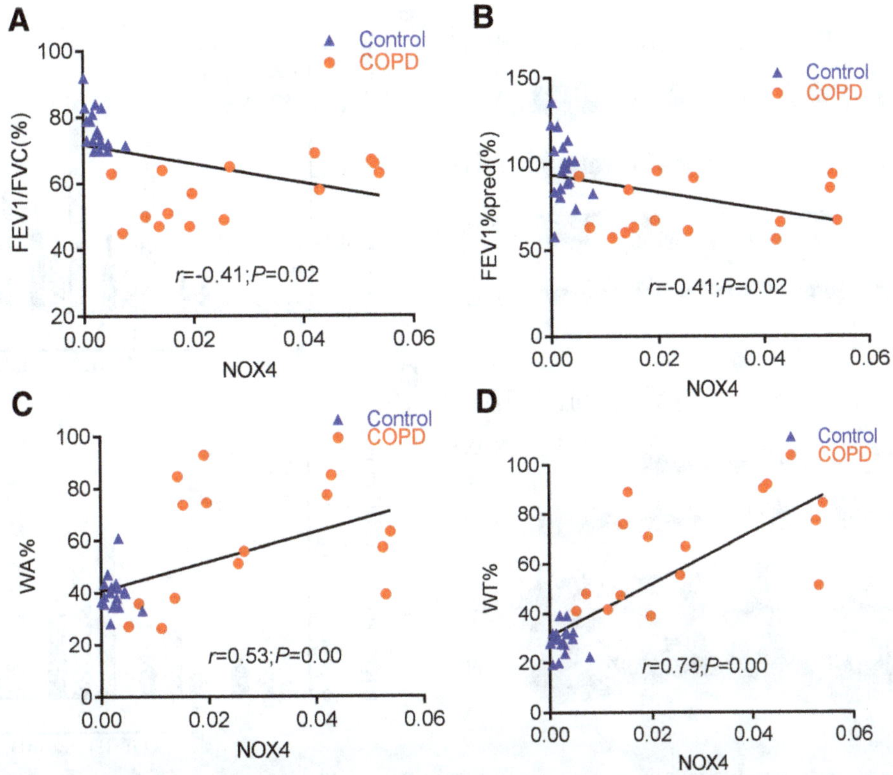

Fig. 6 Correlations of the abundance of NOX4 protein in pulmonary distal arteries with the volume of distal pulmonary arteries and pulmonary functions. **a** The correlation between the abundance of NOX4 protein in pulmonary distal arteries and FEV1/FVC ($r- = 0.411, P < 0.05$); (**b**) The correlation between the abundance of NOX4 protein in pulmonary distal arteries and FEV1%pred ($r = -0.407, P < 0.05$); (**c**) The correlation between the abundance of NOX4 protein in pulmonary distal arteries and WA% ($r = 0.53, P < 0.01$); (**d**) The correlation between the abundance of NOX4 protein in pulmonary distal arteries and WT% ($r = 0.79, P < 0.01$). FEV_1/FVC: forced expiratory volume in one second/ forced vital capacity; FEV1%pred: forced expiratory volume in one second total predicted value; WA%: the pulmonary artery smooth muscle area accounted for the percentage of total vascular area; WT%: the pulmonary artery smooth muscle thickness accounted for the percentage of vascular diameter

dilatation and cardiac hypertrophy. These changes of myocardium are adaptive to accommodate an increased pulmonary arterial pressure, and result in the impaired ventricular function, low cardiac output, and heart failure [53]. cMRI could be used for evaluating right ventricular functions, including RVMED, RVMES, RVMI, ANF, and RF% in patients with COPD. Of note, the aforementioned cMRI parameters were significantly increased in COPD patients in this study. Moreover, the value of RVMES, RVMED, and RF% was correlated with remodeling indexes of distal pulmonary arterioles such as WA% and WT%. These changes of pulmonary vessels and right ventricular morphology imply that the remodeling of distal pulmonary arteriolar smooth muscle and decreased dilatation of the proximal main pulmonary arteries may occur in COPD before a definite PH can be determined. In addition, such a structural change of distal pulmonary arterioles in patients with COPD may subsequently affect changes in the main pulmonary artery blood rheology, as well as the morphology and function of right ventricle.

Oxidative stresses have an important implication in the development and progression of the pulmonary disease-related hypertension. NADPH oxidases (NOXs) are an important source of intracellular ROS production, which recently gains an increased interest in the pathogenesis of COPD and PH. Several lines of evidence showed that an activation of NOX was an important mechanism in the pathogenesis of hypoxia-induced PH in mice [16, 17], in which the NOX-produced ROS participated in the development of chronic hypoxic pulmonary vascular remodeling [54]. In this regard, ROS has widely been recognized as an inducer of vascular wall cell proliferation and vasoconstriction [18]. Therefore, targeting mitochondria-derived ROS production may offer particularly effective in preventing hypoxia-induced PH [9, 55, 56]. Indeed, an inhibition of NOX/vascular peroxidase 1 (VPO1) pathway and inflammatory reaction showed a possibility to prevent cardiovascular remodeling in the hypoxia-induced pulmonary hypertensive rat model [57]. This notion was supported by evidences of that the NOX4 inhibitor GKT137831 could attenuate hypoxia-induced pulmonary

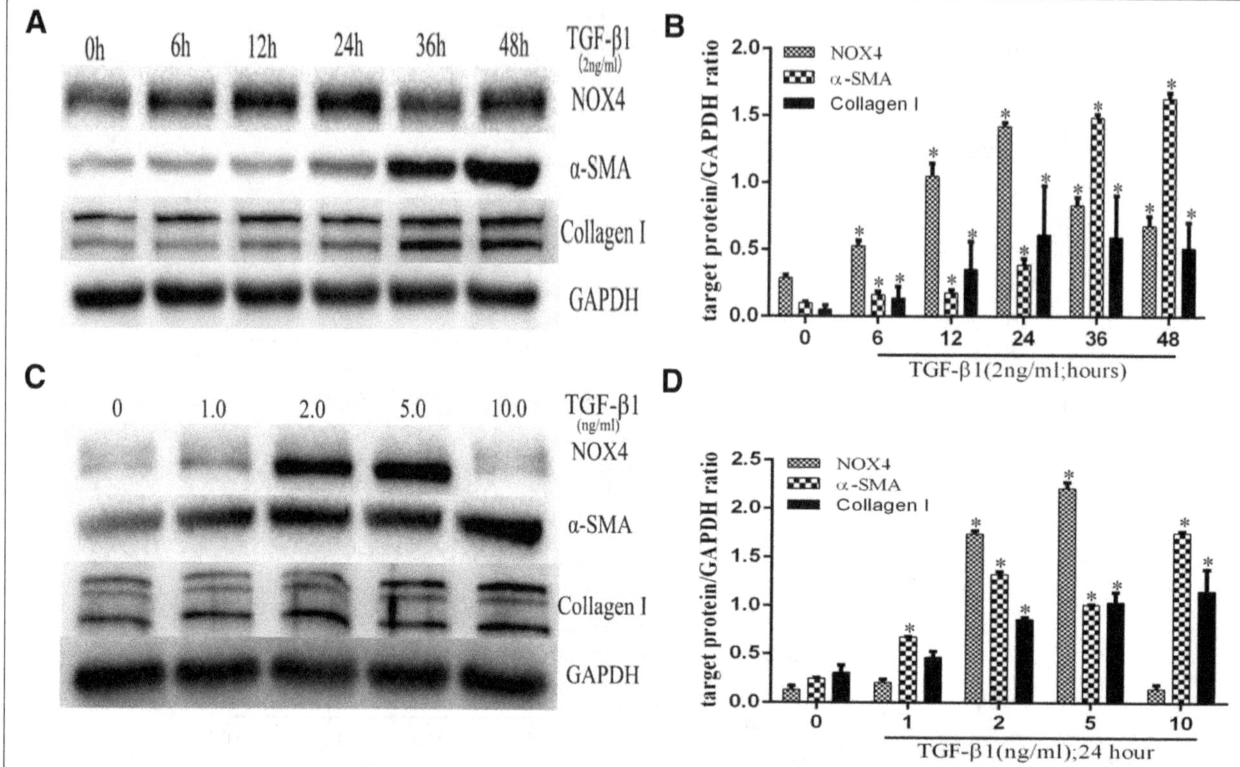

Fig. 7 A dynamic expression of NOX4, α-SMA, Collagen I induced by TGFβ1 in human primary artery smooth muscle cells (HPASMCs). HPASMCs were cultured in the presence of $TGFβ_1$ at various concentrations (0–10 ng/mL) for different time periods (0–48 h) before the cell lysates were used for analysis. **a** Representative images of immunoblots of NOX4, α-SMA and Collagen I in PASMCs exposed to 2.0 ng/ml of TGFβ1 for indicated time points (0–48 h); (**b**) relative expresions of NOX4, α-SMA and Collagen I determined by a densometric assay of immunoblots of (**a**). **c** Immunoblots of NOX4, α-SMA and Collagen I in PASMCs exposed to indicated concentrations of TGFβ1 (0-10 ng/mL) for 24 h; (**d**) relative expresions of NOX4, α-SMA and Collagen I determined by a densometric assay of immunoblots (**c**). Bar graphs represent mean ± SEM from three independent experiments. Compared with the TGFβ1 untreated group, *: $P < 0.05$ ($N = 3$)

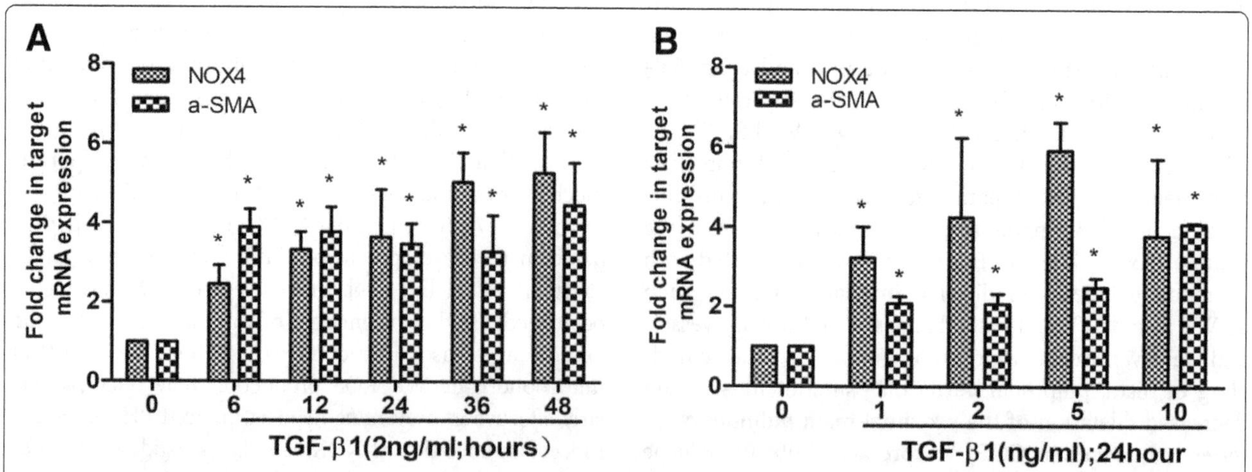

Fig. 8 A dynamic induction of NOX4 and α-SMA transcripts by TGF-β1 in human primary artery smooth muscle cells (HPASMCs) determined by RT-PCR assay. HPASMCs were cultured in the presence of $TGFβ_1$ at various concentrations (0–10 ng/mL) for different time periods (0–48 h) before the cell total RNA was used for RT-PCR analysis. **a** A dynamic induction of NOX4 and α-SMA transcripts in HPASMCs exposed to 2.0 ng/ml of TGFβ1 at indicated time points; (**b**) a dynamic induction of NOX4 and α-SMA transcripts in HPASMCs exposed to indicated concentration of TGFβ1 for 24 h. Data represent mean ± SEM from three independent experiments. Compared with the TGF-β1 untreated group, *: $P < 0.05$ ($N = 3$)

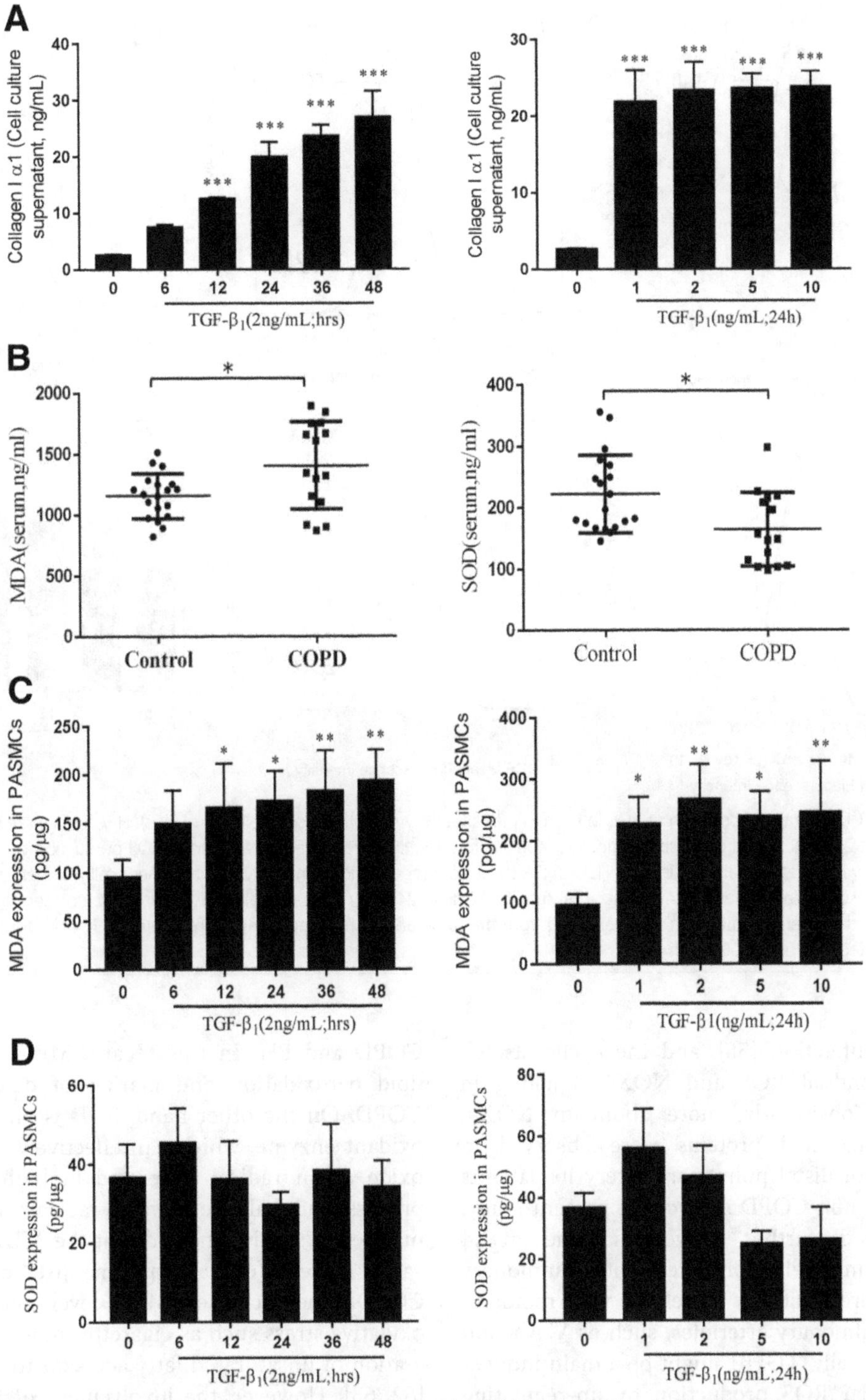

Fig. 9 Impacts of TGFβ1 on the production of Collagen type 1 alpha1, malondialdehyde (MDA) and superoxide dismutase (SOD) in human primary artery smooth muscle cells (HPASMCs). HPASMCs were cultured in the presence of $TGF\beta_1$ at various concentrations (0–10 ng/mL) for different time periods (0–48 h) before the supernatants were used for analysis. **a** The production of Collagen type 1 alpha1 in HPASMCs exposed to 2.0 ng/ml of TGF-β1 for indicated time (left panel) and to indicated concentration of TGFβ1 for 24 h (right panel); (**b**) A higher concentration of MDA (left panel) but a lower concentration of SOD (right panel) in sera of COPD patients relative to healthy subjects; (**c**) the production of MDA (left panel) and SOD (right panel) in HPASMCs exposed to 2.0 ng/ml of TGF-β1 for indicated time; (**d**) the production of MDA (left panel) and SOD (right panel) in HPASMCs exposed to indicated concentration of TGFβ1 for 24 h. Compared to untreated group, *: $P < 0.05$. Bar graphs represent mean ± SEM from three independent experiments. Compared to untreated group, *: $P < 0.05$; **: $P < 0.01$; ***: $P < 0.001$

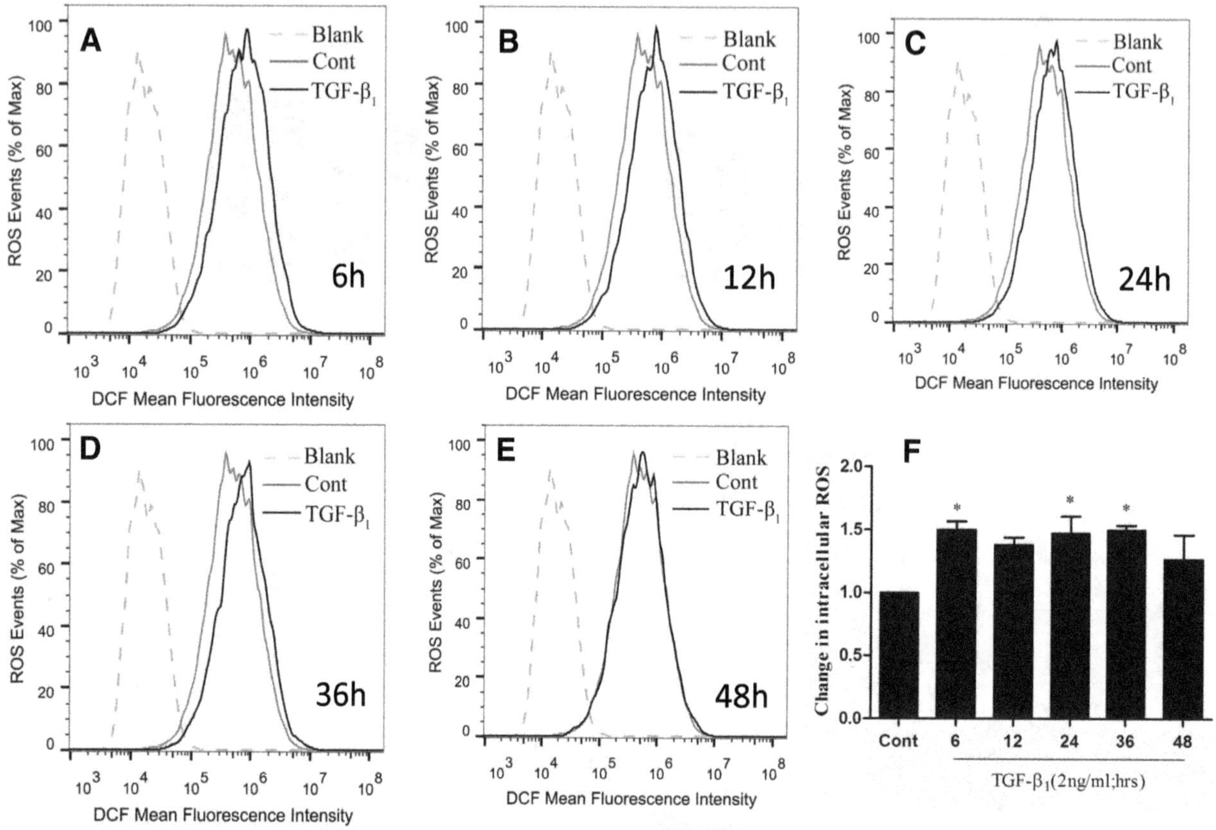

Fig. 10 Impacts of TGFβ1 on the production of ROS in human primary artery smooth muscle cells (HPASMCs). HPASMCs were cultured in the presence of $TGFβ_1$ at 2 ng/mL for different time periods (0–48 h) before the cells were used for analysis of ROS production by a cytometric assay. **a-e** Histogram of flow cytometric analysis using the H2DCF-DA dye to detect enhancement in ROS levels where cell numbers are plotted as a function of the fluorescence intensities at time point of (**a**) 6 h, (**b**) 12 h, (**c**) 24 h. (**d**) 36 h and (**e**) 48 h. (**f**) Bar chart representing the normalized relative ROS levels in the different time point as determined from the same analysisBar graphs represent mean ± SEM from three experiments. Compared to untreated group, *: $P < 0.05$ ($N = 3$).

vascular cell proliferation [58], and the cyclic stretch induced mitochondrial ROS and NOX4 signaling in PASMCs [59]. Consistently, more abundant NOX4, α-SMA, and collagen I proteins were observed in smooth muscles of distal pulmonary artery in patients with COPD than non-COPD subjects in present study. Correlation analysis further showed that the NOX4 expression was inversely correlated with pulmonary functions, but were positively correlated with remodeling indexes of pulmonary arterioles, such as WA% and WT%. Mechanistically, TGFβ1 might be a main inducer of the intracellular ROS production by up-regulating NOX4 in arteriolar smooth muscle cells, suggesting that TGFβ-induced NOX4 promotes cell transdifferentiation and ECM deposition (α-SMA and collagen I). These further indicate an involvement of NOX4 in the development of pulmonary artery remodeling and PAH in COPD (Fig. 11).

The imbalance of oxidant/antioxidants recently receives an increasing attention in the pathogenesis of COPD and PH. In this regard, MDA is a product of lipid peroxidation and marker of oxidative stress in COPD. On the other hand, SOD is an important antioxidant enzyme, which can effectively eliminate superoxide anion radical generated in biological oxidation process and balance oxygen radicals in the body. A number of studies showed that the MDA level was elevated in sera [60] and plasma [61] of patients with COPD. The increased MDA level might correlate to oxidative stress such as cigarette smoke-induced degeneration of unsaturated fatty acids on the cell membrane [62, 63]. However, the involvement of SOD activity in patients with COPD was inconsistent [60, 64]. In the present study a significant higher concentration of serum MDA was found in COPD patients relative to non-COPD individuals, but only moderate alteration of SOD level was observed between sera of COPD and non-COPD patients. In vitro study also demonstrated that TGFβ1 could induce the production of MDA and ROS, but suppress SOD production in HPASMCs.

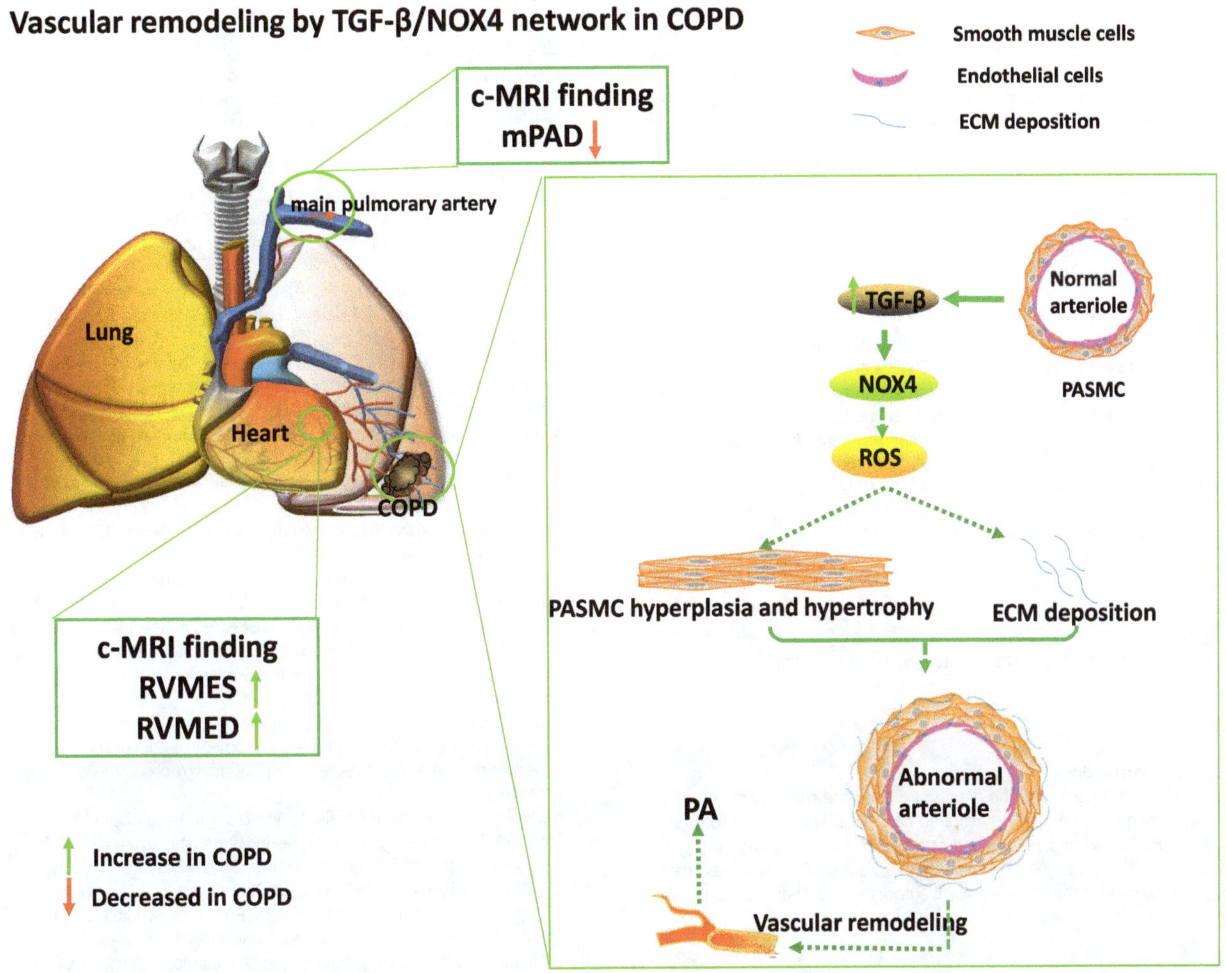

Fig. 11 A possible mechanism of distal pulmonary arteriolar remodeling and its role in pathogenesis of PH in COPD. The scheme illustrates the possible mechanism of NOX4 in distal pulmonary arteriolar remodeling and pathogenesis of PH in COPD. In an early stage of COPD, distal arteriolar remodeling distal arteriolar remodeling and changes in proximal pulmonary artery blood rheology, structure and function of the right heart, including the decreased mPAD, and increased RVMES and RVMED could be determined by cMRI before a definite PH in COPD patients. Pathogenically, the hyperactivated TGFβ signaling triggered the expression of NOX genes, particularly the NOX4 gene in PASMCs and endothelial cells of distal vascules, and smooth muscle cells and epithelial cells of distal airways in COPD lungs. The augmented expression of NOX4 could induce the production of ROS, which in turn led the hyperplasia and hypertrophy of PASMCs, and ECM deposition. As a consequence, these resulted in the distal pulmonary vascular remodeling, and eventually led PAH in patients with a late stage of COPD. Solid lines indicate previously confirmed mechanisms, and dished lines represent proposed mechanisms that need further investigations. mPAD: main pulmonary artery diameter; PAH: pulmonary arterial hypertension; RVMED: right ventricular myocardial mass end-diastolic; RVMES: right ventricular myocardial mass end-systolic

Therefore, it may be speculated that SOD is produced in response to an early stage of oxidative stress, whereas a long-term oxidative damage leads to the consumption of its antioxidant capacity in patients with COPD. This notion may suggest that oxidative stresses are a main pathogenic factor in pulmonary vascular remodeling of COPD.

Conclusion

In conclusion, two main findings were demonstrated in this study (1) distal arteriolar remodeling and changes in proximal pulmonary artery blood rheology, structure and function of the right heart might occur before a definite PH in COPD patients [65]; (2) TGFβ-triggered NADPH oxidase-ROS signaling cascade, particularly the NOX4/ROS signaling was involved in the development of pulmonary arteriole remodeling and PAH in COPD (Fig. 11).

Abbreviations

6MWD: 6-min walk distance; cMRI: Cardiac magnetic resonance imaging; COPD: Chronic obstructive pulmonary disease; ECM: Extracellular matrix; ED: External diameter of blood vessels; ELISA: Enzyme-linked immunosorbent assay; GOLD: Global Initiative on Obstructive Lung Disease; HE: Hematoxylin and eosin; HPASMCs: Human pulmonary artery smooth muscle cells; HPH: Hypoxic pulmonary hypertension; IPP6.0: Image-Pro Plus 6.0;

MDA: Malondialdehyde; mPAD%: Main pulmonary artery distensibility; ROS: Reactive oxygen species; RT-qPCR: Reverse-transcriptional quantitative PCR; RV: Right ventricle; RVEF: Right ventricular ejection fraction; RVMED: Right ventricular myocardial mass end-diastolic; RVMES: Right ventricular myocardial mass end-systolic; RVMI: Right ventricular mass index; RVMM: Right ventricular myocardial mass; SOD: Superoxide dismutase; VOP1: Vascular peroxidase 1; WA%: Pulmonary artery smooth muscle area accounting for the percentage of total vascular area; WT: Wall thickness of pulmonary artery smooth muscle); WT%: Pulmonary artery smooth muscle thickness accounting for the percentage of vascular diameter).

Funding
This study was supported by a grant from the National Natural Science Foundation of China (Nos. 81360004, 81760004 and 31472191); grants from the Ningxia Science and Technology Supporting Program to Juan Chen and Li Zhu (grant number 2015s); a grant from the Project of Postgraduate Education Innovation, Discipline Construction Program of Ningxia, China (grant number YXW 2017014), and a grant from Ningxia Medical University Scientific Research Project (grant number XY201702). These funding play no role in in the design of the study and collection, analysis, and interpretation of data and in writing the manuscript.

Images
All images presented in this study were generated by authors.

Authors' contributions
XG, YF, JC1 and BH analyzed the data and drafted the manuscript; XG, YF, JC1 performed experiments and acquired data; XS, LZ and YW performed cMRI analysis; JD, JH and JY collected samples; JY drew the image in Fig. 11; JC2 conceived and designed the experiments; XL and JC2 interpreted data and critically revised the manuscript. All authors read and approved the final version of the manuscript.

Consent for publication
Not applicable.

Competing interests
The authors declare that they have no competing interests. All authors certify that they have no affiliations with or involvement in any organization or entity with any financial interest, or non-financial interest in the subject matter or materials discussed in this manuscript.

Author details
[1]Department of Pulmonary and Critical Care Medicine, General Hospital of Ningxia Medical University, 804 Shengli South Street, Xingqing District, Yinchuan, Ningxia 750004, People's Republic of China. [2]Ningxia Medical University, Yinchuan 750004, Ningxia, China. [3]Department of Radiology, General Hospital of Ningxia Medical University, Yinchuan 750004, Ningxia, China. [4]Department of Thoracic Surgery, General Hospital of Ningxia Medical University, Yinchuan 750004, Ningxia, China. [5]Institute of Human Stem Cell Research, General Hospital of Ningxia Medical University, Yinchuan 750004, Ningxia, China. [6]Department of Radiotherapy, General Hospital of Ningxia Medical University, Yinchuan 750004, Ningxia, China. [7]Department of Pathology, Ningxia Medical University, Yinchuan 750004, Ningxia, China.

References
1. GOLD: Global Strategy for the Diagnosis,Management,and Prevention of COPD 2015. Global Initiative for Chronic Obstructive Lung Disease 2017, http://www.goldcopd.org. Accessed 3 Jan 2017.
2. Pruss-Ustun A, Wolf J, Corvalan C, Neville T, Bos R, Neira M. Diseases due to unhealthy environments: an updated estimate of the global burden of disease attributable to environmental determinants of health. J Public Health (Oxf). 2017;39(3):464-475.
3. Oswald-Mammosser M, Weitzenblum E, Quoix E, Moser G, Chaouat A, Charpentier C, Kessler R. Prognostic factors in COPD patients receiving long-term oxygen therapy. Importance of pulmonary artery pressure. Chest. 1995; 107(5):1193–8.
4. Zhou S, Li M, Zeng D, Sun G, Zhou J, Wang R. Effects of basic fibroblast growth factor and cyclin D1 on cigarette smoke-induced pulmonary vascular remodeling in rats. Exp Ther Med. 2015;9(1):33–8.
5. Wells JM, Iyer AS, Rahaghi FN, Bhatt SP, Gupta H, Denney TS, Lloyd SG, Dell'Italia LJ, Nath H, Estepar RS, et al. Pulmonary artery enlargement is associated with right ventricular dysfunction and loss of blood volume in small pulmonary vessels in chronic obstructive pulmonary disease. Circ Cardiovasc Imaging. 2015;8(4):e002546.
6. Kawut SM, Poor HD, Parikh MA, Hueper K, Smith BM, Bluemke DA, Lima JA, Prince MR, Hoffman EA, Austin JH, et al. Cor pulmonale parvus in chronic obstructive pulmonary disease and emphysema: the MESA COPD study. J Am Coll Cardiol. 2014;64(19):2000–9.
7. Barbera JA, Peinado VI, Santos S. Pulmonary hypertension in chronic obstructive pulmonary disease. Eur Respir J. 2003;21(5):892–905.
8. Wright JL, Lawson L, Pare PD, Hooper RO, Peretz DI, Nelems JM, Schulzer M, Hogg JC. The structure and function of the pulmonary vasculature in mild chronic obstructive pulmonary disease. The effect of oxygen and exercise. Am Rev Respir Dis. 1983;128(4):702–7.
9. Fulton DJR, Li X, Bordan Z, Haigh S, Bentley A, Chen F, Barman SA. Reactive oxygen and nitrogen species in the development of pulmonary hypertension. Antioxidants (Basel). 2017;6(3) https://doi.org/10.3390/antiox6030054.
10. Nozik-Grayck E, Suliman HB, Majka S, Albietz J, Van Rheen Z, Roush K, Stenmark KR. Lung EC-SOD overexpression attenuates hypoxic induction of Egr-1 and chronic hypoxic pulmonary vascular remodeling. Am J Physiol Lung Cell Mol Physiol. 2008;295(3):L422–30.
11. Wedgwood S, Lakshminrusimha S, Fukai T, Russell JA, Schumacker PT, Steinhorn RH. Hydrogen peroxide regulates extracellular superoxide dismutase activity and expression in neonatal pulmonary hypertension. Antioxid Redox Signal. 2011;15(6):1497–506.
12. Sturrock A, Cahill B, Norman K, Huecksteadt TP, Hill K, Sanders K, Karwande SV, Stringham JC, Bull DA, Gleich M, et al. Transforming growth factor-beta1 induces Nox4 NAD(P)H oxidase and reactive oxygen species-dependent proliferation in human pulmonary artery smooth muscle cells. Am J Physiol Lung Cell Mol Physiol. 2006;290(4):L661–73.
13. Mittal M, Roth M, Konig P, Hofmann S, Dony E, Goyal P, Selbitz AC, Schermuly RT, Ghofrani HA, Kwapiszewska G, et al. Hypoxia-dependent regulation of nonphagocytic NADPH oxidase subunit NOX4 in the pulmonary vasculature. Circ Res. 2007;101(3):258–67.
14. Wedgwood S, Lakshminrusimha S, Czech L, Schumacker PT, Steinhorn RH. Increased p22(phox)/Nox4 expression is involved in remodeling through hydrogen peroxide signaling in experimental persistent pulmonary hypertension of the newborn. Antioxid Redox Signal. 2013;18(14):1765–76.
15. Hood KY, Montezano AC, Harvey AP, Nilsen M, MacLean MR, Touyz RM. Nicotinamide adenine dinucleotide phosphate oxidase-mediated redox signaling and vascular remodeling by 16alpha-Hydroxyestrone in human pulmonary artery cells: implications in pulmonary arterial hypertension. Hypertension. 2016;68(3):796–808.
16. Fresquet F, Pourageaud F, Leblais V, Brandes RP, Savineau JP, Marthan R, Muller B. Role of reactive oxygen species and gp91phox in endothelial dysfunction of pulmonary arteries induced by chronic hypoxia. Br J Pharmacol. 2006;148(5):714–23.
17. Weissmann N, Zeller S, Schafer RU, Turowski C, Ay M, Quanz K, Ghofrani HA, Schermuly RT, Fink L, Seeger W, et al. Impact of mitochondria and NADPH oxidases on acute and sustained hypoxic pulmonary vasoconstriction. Am J Respir Cell Mol Biol. 2006;34(4):505–13.

18. Li JM, Shah AM. Endothelial cell superoxide generation: regulation and relevance for cardiovascular pathophysiology. Am J Physiol Regul Integr Comp Physiol. 2004;287(5):R1014–30.
19. Barman SA, Chen F, Su Y, Dimitropoulou C, Wang Y, Catravas JD, Han W, Orfi L, Szantai-Kis C, Keri G, et al. NADPH oxidase 4 is expressed in pulmonary artery adventitia and contributes to hypertensive vascular remodeling. Arterioscler Thromb Vasc Biol. 2014;34(8):1704–15.
20. Li Q, Mao M, Qiu Y, Liu G, Sheng T, Yu X, Wang S, Zhu D. Key role of ROS in the process of 15-lipoxygenase/15-Hydroxyeicosatetraenoiccid-induced pulmonary vascular remodeling in hypoxia pulmonary hypertension. PLoS One. 2016;11(2):e0149164.
21. Liu X, Hao B, Ma A, He J, Liu X, Chen J. The expression of NOX4 in smooth muscles of small airway correlates with the disease severity of COPD. Biomed Res Int. 2016;2016:2891810.
22. McLure LE, Peacock AJ. Cardiac magnetic resonance imaging for the assessment of the heart and pulmonary circulation in pulmonary hypertension. Eur Respir J. 2009;33(6):1454–66.
23. Swift AJ, Rajaram S, Condliffe R, Capener D, Hurdman J, Elliot CA, Wild JM, Kiely DG. Diagnostic accuracy of cardiovascular magnetic resonance imaging of right ventricular morphology and function in the assessment of suspected pulmonary hypertension results from the ASPIRE registry. J Cardiovasc Magn Reson. 2012;14:40.
24. Lungu A, Swift AJ, Capener D, Kiely D, Hose R, Wild JM. Diagnosis of pulmonary hypertension from magnetic resonance imaging-based computational models and decision tree analysis. Pulm Circ. 2016;6(2):181–90.
25. Hankinson JL, Odencrantz JR, Fedan KB. Spirometric reference values from a sample of the general U.S. population. Am J Respir Crit Care Med. 1999; 159(1):179–87.
26. Miller MR, Hankinson J, Brusasco V, Burgos F, Casaburi R, Coates A, Crapo R, Enright P, van der Grinten CP, Gustafsson P, et al. Standardisation of spirometry. Eur Respir J. 2005;26(2):319–38.
27. Lang RM, Badano LP, Mor-Avi V, Afilalo J, Armstrong A, Ernande L, Flachskampf FA, Foster E, Goldstein SA, Kuznetsova T, et al. Recommendations for cardiac chamber quantification by echocardiography in adults: an update from the American Society of Echocardiography and the European Association of Cardiovascular Imaging. Eur Heart J Cardiovasc Imaging. 2015;16(3):233–70.
28. ATS. Erratum: ATS statement: guidelines for the six-minute walk test. Am J Respir Crit Care Med. 2016;193(10):1185.
29. Sanz J, Kariisa M, Dellegrottaglie S, Prat-Gonzalez S, Garcia MJ, Fuster V, Rajagopalan S. Evaluation of pulmonary artery stiffness in pulmonary hypertension with cardiac magnetic resonance. JACC Cardiovasc Imaging. 2009;2(3):286–95.
30. Ibrahim el SH, White RD. Cardiovascular magnetic resonance for the assessment of pulmonary arterial hypertension: toward a comprehensive CMR exam. Magn Reson Imaging. 2012;30(8):1047–58.
31. Roeleveld RJ, Vonk-Noordegraaf A, Marcus JT, Bronzwaer JG, Marques KM, Postmus PE, Boonstra A. Effects of epoprostenol on right ventricular hypertrophy and dilatation in pulmonary hypertension. Chest. 2004;125(2):572–9.
32. Agathos EA, Shen M, Katsiboulas M, Koutsoukos P, Gloustianou G. In vivo calcification of glutaraldehyde-fixed cardiac valve and pericardium of Phoca groenlandica. ASAIO J. 2011;57(4):328–32.
33. Wang Q, Zeng YJ, Huo P, Hu JL, Zhang JH. A specialized plug-in software module for computer-aided quantitative measurement of medical images. Med Eng Phys. 2003;25(10):887–92.
34. Hale KA, Niewoehner DE, Cosio MG. Morphologic changes in the muscular pulmonary arteries: relationship to cigarette smoking, airway disease, and emphysema. Am Rev Respir Dis. 1980;122(2):273–8.
35. Santos S, Peinado VI, Ramirez J, Melgosa T, Roca J, Rodriguez-Roisin R, Barbera JA. Characterization of pulmonary vascular remodelling in smokers and patients with mild COPD. Eur Respir J. 2002;19(4):632–8.
36. Zhao L, Wang J, Wang L, Liang YT, Chen YQ, Lu WJ, Zhou WL. Remodeling of rat pulmonary artery induced by chronic smoking exposure. J Thorac Dis. 2014;6(6):818–28.
37. Zhou SJ, Li M, Zeng DX, Zhu ZM, Hu XW, Li YH, Wang R, Sun GY. Expression variations of connective tissue growth factor in pulmonary arteries from smokers with and without chronic obstructive pulmonary disease. Sci Rep. 2015;5:8564.
38. Xu P, Dai A, Zhou H, Shen H, Liu L, Song W. Expression and role of adrenomedullin and its receptor in patients with chronic obstructive pulmonary disease. Chin Med J. 2003;116(6):863–7.
39. Schmittgen TD, Livak KJ. Analyzing real-time PCR data by the comparative C(T) method. Nat Protoc. 2008;3(6):1101–8.
40. Li Y, Shi J, Yang J, Ma Y, Cheng L, Zeng J, Hao X, Ma C, Wang Y, Liu X. A Wnt/beta-catenin negative feedback loop represses TLR-triggered inflammatory responses in alveolar epithelial cells. Mol Immunol. 2014;59(2):128–35.
41. Jeffery PK. Remodeling in asthma and chronic obstructive lung disease. Am J Respir Crit Care Med. 2001;164(10 Pt 2):S28–38.
42. Tuder RM, Yun JH, Bhunia A, Fijalkowska I. Hypoxia and chronic lung disease. J Mol Med (Berl). 2007;85(12):1317–24.
43. Zychowski KE, Lucas SN, Sanchez B, Herbert G, Campen MJ. Hypoxia-induced pulmonary arterial hypertension augments lung injury and airway reactivity caused by ozone exposure. Toxicol Appl Pharmacol. 2016;305:40–5.
44. Coste F, Dournes G, Dromer C, Blanchard E, Freund-Michel V, Girodet PO, Montaudon M, Baldacci F, Picard F, Marthan R, et al. CT evaluation of small pulmonary vessels area in patients with COPD with severe pulmonary hypertension. Thorax. 2016;71(9):830–7.
45. Weitzenblum E, Chaouat A, Canuet M, Kessler R. Pulmonary hypertension in chronic obstructive pulmonary disease and interstitial lung diseases. Semin Respir Crit Care Med. 2009;30(4):458–70.
46. Galie N, Humbert M, Vachiery JL, Gibbs S, Lang I, Torbicki A, Simonneau G, Peacock A, Vonk Noordegraaf A, Beghetti M, et al. 2015 ESC/ERS guidelines for the diagnosis and treatment of pulmonary hypertension. Rev Esp Cardiol (Engl Ed). 2016;69(2):177.
47. Xu D, Li Y, Zhang B, Wang Y, Liu Y, Luo Y, Niu W, Dong M, Liu M, Dong H, et al. Resveratrol alleviate hypoxic pulmonary hypertension via anti-inflammation and anti-oxidant pathways in rats. Int J Med Sci. 2016;13(12):942–54.
48. Longmore DB, Klipstein RH, Underwood SR, Firmin DN, Hounsfield GN, Watanabe M, Bland C, Fox K, Poole-Wilson PA, Rees RS, et al. Dimensional accuracy of magnetic resonance in studies of the heart. Lancet. 1985; 1(8442):1360–2.
49. Miller S, Simonetti OP, Carr J, Kramer U, Finn JP. MR imaging of the heart with cine true fast imaging with steady-state precession: influence of spatial and temporal resolutions on left ventricular functional parameters. Radiology. 2002;223(1):263–9.
50. Lee-Chiong TL Jr, Matthay RA. Pulmonary hypertension and cor pulmonale in COPD. Semin Respir Crit Care Med. 2003;24(3):263–72.
51. Sanz J, Kuschnir P, Rius T, Salguero R, Sulica R, Einstein AJ, Dellegrottaglie S, Fuster V, Rajagopalan S, Poon M. Pulmonary arterial hypertension: noninvasive detection with phase-contrast MR imaging. Radiology. 2007; 243(1):70–9.
52. Swift AJ, Rajaram S, Condliffe R, Capener D, Hurdman J, Elliot C, Kiely DG, Wild JM. Pulmonary artery relative area change detects mild elevations in pulmonary vascular resistance and predicts adverse outcome in pulmonary hypertension. Investig Radiol. 2012;47(10):571–7.
53. Yoshibayashi M, Nishioka K, Nakao K, Saito Y, Matsumura M, Ueda T, Temma S, Shirakami G, Imura H, Mikawa H. Plasma endothelin concentrations in patients with pulmonary hypertension associated with congenital heart defects. Evidence for increased production of endothelin in pulmonary circulation. Circulation. 1991;84(6):2280–5.
54. Liu JQ, Zelko IN, Erbynn EM, Sham JS, Folz RJ. Hypoxic pulmonary hypertension: role of superoxide and NADPH oxidase (gp91phox). Am J Physiol Lung Cell Mol Physiol. 2006;290(1):L2–10.
55. Adesina SE, Kang BY, Bijli KM, Ma J, Cheng J, Murphy TC, Michael Hart C, Sutliff RL. Targeting mitochondrial reactive oxygen species to modulate hypoxia-induced pulmonary hypertension. Free Radic Biol Med. 2015;87:36–47.
56. Chen IC, Tan MS, Wu BN, Chai CY, Yeh JL, Chou SH, Chen IJ, Dai ZK. Statins ameliorate pulmonary hypertension secondary to left ventricular dysfunction through the rho-kinase pathway and NADPH oxidase. Pediatr Pulmonol. 2017;52(4):443–57.
57. Liu B, Luo XJ, Yang ZB, Zhang JJ, Li TB, Zhang XJ, Ma QL, Zhang GG, Hu CP, Peng J. Inhibition of NOX/VPO1 pathway and inflammatory reaction by trimethoxystilbene in prevention of cardiovascular remodeling in hypoxia-induced pulmonary hypertensive rats. J Cardiovasc Pharmacol. 2014;63(6):567–76.
58. Green DE, Murphy TC, Kang BY, Kleinhenz JM, Szyndralewiez C, Page P, Sutliff RL, Hart CM. The Nox4 inhibitor GKT137831 attenuates hypoxia-induced pulmonary vascular cell proliferation. Am J Respir Cell Mol Biol. 2012;47(5):718–26.
59. Wedgwood S, Lakshminrusimha S, Schumacker PT, Steinhorn RH. Cyclic stretch stimulates mitochondrial reactive oxygen species and Nox4 signaling in pulmonary artery smooth muscle cells. Am J Physiol Lung Cell Mol Physiol. 2015;309(2):L196–203.

60. Ismail M, Hossain MF, Tanu AR, Shekhar HU. Effect of spirulina intervention on oxidative stress, antioxidant status, and lipid profile in chronic obstructive pulmonary disease patients. Biomed Res Int. 2015;2015:486120.
61. Kuleci S, Hanta I, Kocabas A, Canacankatan N. The effect of different treatment modalities on oxidative stress in COPD. Adv Ther. 2008;25(7):710–7.
62. MacNee W. Oxidants/antioxidants and COPD. Chest. 2000;117(5 Suppl 1): 303S–17S.
63. Maskey-Warzechowska M, Nejman-Gryz P, Osinka K, Lis P, Malesa K, Gorska K, Krenke R. Acute response to cigarette smoking assessed in exhaled breath condensate in patients with chronic obstructive pulmonary disease and healthy smokers. Adv Exp Med Biol. 2017;944:73–80.
64. Wozniak A, Gorecki D, Szpinda M, Mila-Kierzenkowska C, Wozniak B. Oxidant-antioxidant balance in the blood of patients with chronic obstructive pulmonary disease after smoking cessation. Oxidative Med Cell Longev. 2013;2013:897075.
65. Poor HD, Kawut SM, Liu CY, Smith BM, Hoffman EA, Lima JA, Ambale-Venkatesh B, Michos ED, Prince MR, Barr RG. Pulmonary hyperinflation due to gas trapping and pulmonary artery size: the MESA COPD study. PLoS One. 2017;12(5):e0176812.

24

Predictors of one-year mortality after hospitalization for an exacerbation of COPD

Cristóbal Esteban[1,5*], Ady Castro-Acosta[2,3], Carlos Jose Alvarez-Martínez[2,3], Alberto Capelastegui[1], José Luis López-Campos[4] and Francisco Pozo-Rodriguez[2,3]

Abstract

Background: Hospitalization for a severe exacerbation of COPD (eCOPD) is an important event in the natural history of COPD. Identifying factors related to mortality 1 year after hospitalization could help determine interventions to reduce mortality.

Methods: In a prospective, observational, multicentre study, we evaluated data from two cohorts: the Spanish audit of hospital COPD exacerbation care (our derivation sample) and the Spanish cohort of the European audit of COPD exacerbation care (our validation sample). The endpoint was all-cause mortality. Mortality was determined by local research managers of the participating hospitals and matched the official national index records in Spain.

Results: In the multivariate analysis, factors independently related to an increase in mortality were older age, cardio-cerebro-vascular and/or dementia comorbidities, $PaCO2 > 55$ mmHg measured at emergency department arrival, hospitalizations for COPD exacerbations in the previous year, and hospital characteristics. The area under the receiver-operating curve for this model was 0.75 in the derivation cohort and 0.76 in the validation cohort.

Conclusion: One-year mortality following the index hospitalization for an exacerbation of COPD was related to clinical characteristics of the patient and of the index event, previous events of similar severity, and characteristics of the hospital where the patient was treated.

Keywords: Pulmonary disease, Chronic obstructive, Hospitalization, Mortality

Background

Hospitalization for a severe exacerbation of chronic obstructive pulmonary disease (eCOPD) is an important event in the natural history of this disease. Approximately half of the patients admitted for an eCOPD die within 4 years [1]. Identifying factors associated with mid-term mortality (1 year) after hospitalization for an eCOPD could provide tools for more targeted evaluation of these patients and interventions to prevent premature death.

Several studies designed for that purpose have yielded variable or conflicting results [2, 3]. These divergent results can largely be attributed to study methodology, such as the patient population (recruited from the medical ward or from intermediate or intensive care), source of the data (prospective studies, retrospective studies, or computerized databases), variables studied, duration of follow-up, and organizational and administrative distribution of hospital resources. Another source of uncertainty is whether indices used among patients with stable COPD have the same prognostic capacity when used in those admitted to the hospital [4, 5].

The aim of this study was to determine predictors of one-year mortality in patients hospitalized for an eCOPD following discharge for the index event.

Methods

The Cohorte Española de EPOC Avanzada (CEPA) is a prospective observational study designed to examine factors associated with one-year mortality among patients hospitalized for an eCOPD.

CEPA includes patients from two separate cohorts. One, defined as the derivation cohort, is a sample of patients from the Spanish COPD Audit [6]. The other, defined as the validation cohort, is from the Spanish sample of the

* Correspondence: cristobal.est@gmail.com
[1]Pulmonary Service, Galdakao-Usansolo Hospital, Galdakao, Bizkaia, Spain
[5]Network and Health Services Research Chronic Diseases (REDISSEC), Bilbao, Bizkaia, Spain
Full list of author information is available at the end of the article

European COPD Audit [7]. The methodology of both studies has been described in detail elsewhere [6, 7].

The Spanish COPD Audit was a cross-sectional study with prospective non-interventional case ascertainment of consecutive eCOPD hospital admissions for the 8-week period from November 1, 2008 to December 31, 2008. Patients were included in the cohort following a two-step process. Reports of all patients admitted to the hospital following an emergency department (ED) visit were reviewed daily to identify one or more of 13 clinical conditions compatible with the diagnosis of eCOPD. These patients were labelled as interim/possible eCOPD cases. They were assessed again at hospital discharge against a list of definite inclusion and exclusion criteria to identify patients with a clinical diagnosis of eCOPD. Those who qualified were labelled as definite eCOPD cases [6]. A total of 32 hospitals completed a one-year follow-up of their patients and were included in our study.

The European Respiratory Society COPD audit was designed as a pilot study to evaluate clinical practice variability as well as clinical and organizational factors associated with outcomes for COPD-related hospital admissions across Europe. This prospective, observational, non-interventional cohort trial was conducted during the 8-week period from January 1, 2011 and February 28, 2011 in 74 hospitals [7].

In both studies, all consecutive cases admitted to the participant hospitals due to an eCOPD were identified and information on clinical practice was gathered. Each patient was included only once in the study.

Comorbidities were standardized recorded from the clinical record of every patient, including any new one diagnosed during the index event. The Charlson index was used as a reference [8].

All the hospitals participating in the studies were asked to complete cross-sectional surveys of the resources and organization they devoted to COPD acute care. The survey included questions related both to the hospital and to the respiratory unit resources.

Mortality was determined by local research managers of the participating hospitals and matched the official national index records in Spain.

The study was approved by Instituto de Salud Carlos III CEI PI 30_2011-v4 and hospital participation in the two cohorts was approved by the ethics committees of the participating hospitals. All participants provided written informed consent. To allow for patient-level analyses, patient data was protected and dissociated.

Statistical analysis

Descriptive statistics of sociodemographic and clinical variables were calculated using means and standard deviations (SD) for quantitative data; frequencies and percentages were used for categorical variables. The Spanish cohort represented our derivation cohort and the European cohort the validation cohort.

A univariate analysis was undertaken in the derivation sample to determine variables that were predictors of one-year mortality (patients who died during the admission were excluded from the analysis). Student's t test (or the Wilcoxon test if normality was rejected) was used for continuous variables, while Chi-square and Fisher's exact tests were used for categorical variables. In the multivariate analysis, generalized linear mixed models were used so as to perform a multilevel multivariable analysis adjusted by hospital, with one-year mortality as the dependent dichotomous variable. The predictive accuracy of the model was determined by calculating the area under the receiver-operating curve (AUC).

The model developed in the derivation cohort was tested in the validation cohort to compare the predictive accuracy of the model by means of comparisons of their AUCs.

We also evaluated the independent influence of the hospital setting both models and determined which hospital characteristics were predictors of mortality.

All effects were deemed statistically significant at $p < 0.05$. All statistical analyses were performed using SAS System, version 9.2 (SAS Institute, Inc., Carey, NC).

Results

A sample of 1420 patients from the Spanish COPD Audit was included in the derivation cohort. Mean patient age was 73 years, 89% were men, 24.6% were current smokers, 43% had a Charlson Comorbidity Index higher than 3, and 74.6% had previously been admitted for an eCOPD (Table 1). The in-hospital mortality for that cohort was 5%.

The validation cohort included a sample of 3949 patients from the European COPD Audit. Compared to the derivation cohort, the validation cohort included more women (10.2 vs 14.5%), had a lower Charlson Comorbidity Index, and statistically significant differences were observed in the percentages of cardiovascular, cerebrovascular, and peripheral vascular disease between the two cohorts (Table 1). The in-hospital mortality for that cohort was 4.3%.

In the univariate analysis, statistically significant differences were observed between patients who had died within 1 year of the index hospitalization and those who had not, in age, smoking habit, Charlson Comorbidity Index, and presence of specific comorbidities such as cardiovascular disease, heart failure, peripheral vascular disease, cerebrovascular disease and dementia, previous eCOPD admissions, number of eCOPD admissions in the previous year, level of airway severity obstruction (FEV1% and Global Initiative for Chronic Obstructive Lung Disease [GOLD] stages of obstruction) and PaCO2

Table 1 Descriptive statistics of the COPD derivation and validation cohorts

	Derivation $n = 1420$	Validation $n = 3949$	p-value
Age[a]	73.4 (10.0)	72.7 (10.7)	0.07
Sex (% male)	1275 (89.8)	3375 (85.5)	< 0.0001
FEV1%	45.2 (16.2)	45.3 (16.6)	0.76
FEV1%/FVC	52.5 (13.4)	52.5 (12.9)	0.79
FEV1% categories			< 0.0001
≥ 80%	33 (3.8)	62 (2.5)	
< 80 - > 50	272 (31.2)	778 (31.0)	
< 50 - > 30	217 (24.3)	1187 (47.3)	
≤ 30	351 (40.2)	482 (19.2)	
Body Mass Index[a]	27.9 (5.3)	27.8 (5.7)	0.35
Smoking habit			0.34
- Ever smoker	52 (4.3)	182 (4.9)	
- Current smoker	343 (28.2)	977 (26.3)	
- Ex-smoker	822 (67.5)	2554 (68.8)	
Cigarette pack-years[a]	55,82 (29.0)	51,99 (30.3)	0.003
Charlson Comorbidity Index[a]	2,70 (1.8)	1,79 (1.7)	< 0.0001
1–2	795 (56.0)	2865 (72.5)	
≥ 3	625 (44.0)	1084 (27.4)	
Ischaemic heart disease	205 (15.7)	505 (12.8)	0.008
Cardiac failure	299 (23.0)	810 (20.5)	0.07
Peripheral vascular disease	221 (17.2)	494 (12.5)	< 0.0001
Cerebrovascular disease	146 (11.3)	380 (9.6)	0.09
Cardiac-Cerebro-Peripheral vascular disease	608 (46.2)	2217 (44.9)	0.41
Dementia	138 (3,49)	52 (4,04)	0.36
Diabetes mellitus	359 (26.2)	1032 (26.1)	0.95
Previous COPD hospitalization	1065 (76.7)	1881 (51.3)	< 0.0001
Mean of COPD-related admissions in the previous year	1.92 (2.0)	1.17 (1.8)	< 0.0001
pH at arrival	7.40 (0.1)	7.40 (0.1)	0.12
Acidaemia during admission	258 (19.3)	NA	
PaO2 at arrival[a]	59.1 (15.6)	60.4 (21.3)	0.79
PaCO2 at arrival[a]	47.2 (14.4)	48.4 (15.7)	0.074
Length of stay[a]	10.1 (6.9)	9.3 (7.0)	< 0.0001

[a]Represented as mean (std)

level upon ED arrival. At discharge, patients who died within 1 year were more likely to have been prescribed home oxygen therapy than those who did not die, while prescription of home mechanical ventilation support at discharge and length of stay were not different between these groups (Table 2).

In the multivariate analysis, independent variables related to one-year mortality were age, comorbidity (making reference to previous presence of cardiac, peripheral vascular or cerebral vascular diseases and dementia), admission for an eCOPD in the previous year, and PaCO2 at emergency department arrival, and the participant hospital. The hospital characteristics that influenced one-year mortality were the size of the hospital and whether they had a respiratory ward (Table 3).

The AUC for this model was 0.75 for the derivation cohort and 0.76 for the validation cohort (Tables 4 and 5).

A score based on the weight of the different variables included in the multivariate model was developed (Table 4). This score was stratified in 4 levels that showed a high rate of mortality at every risk level, especially in those patients having a score higher than 10 (Table 6).

Discussion

In this prospective cohort study, four groups of variables were associated with one-year mortality after an

Table 2 Univariate analysis performed in the derivation sample ($n = 1420$)

	Mortality		
	No 864	Yes 495	*p*-value
Age[a]	71.7 (10.2)	76.1 (9.1)	< 0.0001
Sex (% male)	763 (88.3)	453 (91.5)	0.06
FEV1%	46.6 (16.3)	43.2 (15.4)	0.004
FEV1%/FVC	53,0 (12.9)	51.6 (14.2)	0.18
FEV1% categories			< 0.0001
≥ 80%	24 (4.5)	7 (2.2)	
< 80 - > 50	183 (34.0)	85 (27.3)	
< 50 - > 30	144 (26.8)	62 (19.9)	
≤ 30	187 (34.8)	157 (50.5)	
Body Mass Index[a]	28.1 (5.3)	27.3 (5.4)	0.07
Smoking habit			0.0007
- Never smoker	29 (3.8)	19 (4.7)	
- Current smoker	246 (32.4)	89 (21.8)	
- Ex-smoker	485 (63.8)	300 (73.5)	
Cigarette pack-years[a]	53.2 (27.3)	60.9 (31.9)	0.002
Charlson Comorbidity Index[a]	2.5 (1.6)	3.1 (1.9)	< 0.0001
1–2	536 (62.0)	234 (47.3)	
≥ 3	328 (38.0)	261 (52.7)	
Ischaemic heart disease	111 (14.0)	84 (18.3)	0.04
Cardiac failure	148 (18.7)	129 (28.3)	< 0.0001
Peripheral arterial disease	113 (14.4)	94 (20.8)	0.004
Cerebrovascular disease	67 (8.5)	72 (15.9)	< 0.0001
Cardiac-Cerebro- Peripheral vascular disease	320 (40.1)	250 (54.2)	< 0.0001
Dementia	17 (2.18)	31 (6.84)	< 0.0001
Diabetes mellitus	208 (25.1)	129 (26.9)	0.46
Previous COPD hospitalization	610 (71.9)	404 (83.8)	< 0.0001
Mean of COPD-related admissions in the previous year	1.7 (1.9)	2.2 (2.2)	0.001
pH at arrival	7.40 (0.06)	7.40 (0.06)	0.49
Acidaemia during admission	150 (18.4)	84 (18.1)	0.89
PaO2 at arrival[a]	58.8 (15.0)	59.6 (16.2)	0.53
PaCO2 at arrival[a]	46.2 (13.0)	48.5 (15.2)	0.01
Length of stay[a]	10.4 (7.2)	9.7 (6.4)	0.11
Oxygen at discharge	329 (38.1)	276 (55.8)	< 0.0001
Noninvasive ventilation at discharge	48 (5.6)	29 (5.9)	0.81

[a]Represented as mean (std)

eCOPD hospitalization: general condition of the patient (older age, presence of cardiovascular, cerebrovascular, or peripheral vascular disease and dementia); clinical markers of the severity of the index event, (PaCO2 above the normal limit, at ED arrival); previous events of similar severity (hospitalization for an eCOPD in the previous year). The presence of any of these variables, added to the characteristics of the hospital where the patient was treated, were associated with higher mortality.

Patient's characteristics

Age, as a continuous variable, was an independent predictor of mortality. Age has been included, although controversially, as a variable in other multidimensional indexes for stable COPD [9, 10]. Among patients

Table 3 Univariate analysis. Hospital characteristics

	Dead *N* (%)	Alive *N* (%)	*p*-value
Hospital			< 0.0001
Total bed numbers[a]	601.0 (359.3)	627.3 (312.0)	0.005
Total bed numbers			< 0.0001
- < 300	115 (23.2)	134 (15.5)	
- 300–599	188 (38.0)	294 (34.0)	
- ≥ 600	192 (38.8)	436 (50.5)	
Population served by the hospital			0.01
- < 200,000	199 (40.2)	278 (32.2)	
- 200,000–299,999	167 (33.7)	338 (39.1)	
- ≥ 300,000	129 (26.1)	248 (28.7)	
Teaching Hospital			0.60
- No	241 (48.7)	407 (47.1)	
- Yes	254 (51.3)	457 (52.9)	
Intensive Care Unit			0.17
- No	30 (6.1)	38 (4.4)	
- Yes	465 (93.9)	826 (95.6)	
Spirometry available			0.47
- No	56 (11.3)	87 (10.1)	
- Yes	439 (88.7)	777 (89.9)	
Respiratory staff number[a]	9.43 (6.2)	9.49 (5.8)	0.44
Respiratory ward			0.04
- No	91 (18.4)	123 (14.2)	
- Yes	404 (81.6)	741 (85.8)	
Non-invasive ventilation available in the ward			0.47
- No	26 (5.2)	38 (4.4)	
- Yes	469 (94.7)	826 (95.6)	

[a]Represented as mean (std). *N* frequency, % percentage

experiencing severe exacerbations, age is a key predictive factor for in-hospital mortality [11] and long-term post-discharge mortality [12]. Data from 150 hospitals in the United Kingdom indicated that age was the main predictor of 30-day mortality following hospitalization for COPD (OR, 8.5; 95% CI, 7.7–9.4). Other predictive factors included comorbidities, and gender [13]. In other studies, age was an independent predictor of mortality during one-year of follow-up after hospitalization for an eCOPD [14, 15]. It must be noted, however, that age is a stronger predictor of long-term mortality following eCOPD hospitalization than it is as a predictor for in-hospital mortality [16].

Several reasons could explain our previously mentioned results, older COPD patients tend to have a low performance status, higher level of respiratory disability, and more comorbidities. Together with a diminished awareness of the signs of an exacerbation and poorer understanding of medication [17], these factors make older patients extremely vulnerable, with generally worse outcomes and increasing 90-day mortality [17]. Moreover, respiratory specialists usually find it more difficult to control COPD in older patients than in younger ones [17]. In the UK audit, hospital care varied with age, but the lower level of care given to older patients was not associated with mortality [18]. In sum, all of these circumstances could make age a key factor contributing to mortality after hospitalization for an eCOPD.

Although comorbidities are prevalent among hospitalized eCOPD patients [19], there is some controversy over their importance as a prognostic factor for mortality. In one study, non-respiratory organ failure was most closely related to in-hospital mortality while the overall level of respiratory severity was associated with long-term mortality [16].

Table 4 Derivation cohort. Multivariate analysis. Predicting factors of mortality in 1 year

	β (s.e.)	OR (95% CI)	*p*-value	Weight	AUC
Intercept	− 2.12 (0.56)		0.0002		0.672
Age[b]	0.46 (0.08)	1.581 (1.357–1.842)	< 0.0001	2	
COPD related previous admissions (Yes vs. No)	0.79 (0.18)	2.201 (1.541–3.144)	< 0.0001	4	
Cardio-cerebro-peripheral vascular disease[a] (Yes vs. No)	0.47 (0.15)	1.598 (1.189–2.148)	0.0019	2	
Dementia (Yes vs. No)	1.09 (0.39)	2.973 (1.394–6.340)	0.0048	5	
PaCO2					
45–55 (vs. < 45)	− 0.05 (0.18)	0.947 (0.663–1.353)	0.7631	0	
> 55 (vs. < 45)	0.47 (0.19)	1.601 (1.102–2.326)	0.0135	2	
Hospital characteristics					0.747

Hospital characteristics: defined by "total number of beds"

β parameter estimation, *s.e.* standard error, *OR* odds ratio, *CI* confidence interval, *AUC* area under the receiver operating characteristic Curve, *Weight* indicates the weight for each variable to create the risk score

[a]Include ischaemic heart disease, cardiac failure, peripheral vascular disease and cerebrovascular disease

[b]Estimation for increment of a decade with respect to patients with 50 years or less

p-value Hosmer y Lemeshow = 0.26 (including in the analysis hospital *p*-value = 0.19)

Table 5 Validation cohort. Multivariate analysis. Predicting factors of COPD mortality in 1 year

	β (s.e.)	OR (95% CI)	*p*-value	AUC
Intercept	− 3.08 (0.55)		< 0.0001	0.672
Age[b]	0.43 (0.06)	1.530 (1.367–1.712)	< 0.0001	
COPD related previous admissions (Yes vs. No)	0.72 (0.11)	2.045 (1.640–2.550)	< 0.0001	
Cardio-cerebro-peripheral vascular disease[a] (Yes vs. No)	0.31 (0.11)	1.367 (1.097–1.705)	0.0054	
Dementia (Yes vs. No)	0.50 (0.26)	1.648 (0.984–2.758)	0.0575	
PaCO2				
45–55 (vs. < 45)	0.22 (0.13)	1.245 (0.965–1.607)	0.0917	
> 55 (vs. < 45)	0.51 (0.13)	1.665 (1.280–2.165)	0.0001	
Hospital characteristics				0.763

Hospital characteristics: defined by "total number of beds"
β parameter estimation, *s.e.* standard error, *OR* odds ratio, *CI* confidence interval, *AUC* area under the receiver operating characteristic curve
[a]Include ischaemic heart disease, cardiac failure, peripheral arterial disease and cerebrovascular disease
[b]Estimation for increment of a decade. With respect to patients with 50 years or less
p-value Hosmer y Lemeshow = 0.25 (including in the analysis hospital *p*-value = 0,37)

In another study comorbidities—cor pulmonale, left ventricular failure, neurological conditions, and non-respiratory malignancies—were associated with in-hospital mortality while 90-day mortality was also increased by the presence of lung cancer or arrhythmias [19]. Almagro et al. showed that the Charlson Comorbidity Index score were associated with 90-day mortality [20]. Comorbidities such as cardiac failure [21], ischaemic heart disease [22], stroke, and diabetes [23] have also been identified as predictors of mortality after hospitalization for an eCOPD.

We did not observe an association between comorbidities evaluated by the Charlson index and mortality during the one-year follow-up, as in another study was [24]. In contrast, in our cohort specific comorbidities—cardiac disease (ischaemic heart disease, chronic heart failure), cerebrovascular disease, and peripheral vascular disease—were independently related to mortality. It seems that the impact of the different comorbidities is variable with respect to the outcome analysed [25] and is focused on the cardio-cerebro-vascular comorbidities, because not all the comorbidities have the same importance.

Apart from the cardio-cerebro-vascular comorbidities, it is worth mentioning dementia as a variable associated to mortality in our study. Prevalence of cognitive dysfunction is very variable in COPD patients, (up to 61%), depending on the place where the study was carried out [26].

COPD patients are prone to being affected by deterioration of their level of cognitive function, and there are several mechanisms involved, from the hypoxaemia, usually present in COPD, to smoking and some concurrent comorbidities, as cardiovascular [27].

Cognitive deterioration has been shown to have a great impact on important outcomes. In patients admitted to a general hospital those with dementia had a mortality rate of 48% after 1 year, higher than that of patients without dementia [28]. In COPD, those patients admitted suffering dementia had 38% and 69% higher risk of severe sepsis and hospital mortality respectively [29].

Our study adds that in COPD patients, dementia was a key point and the strongest variable associated to mortality in the mid term, after one hospitalization.

In sum, what our study showed was the important relationship between comorbidities and mortality, but not comorbidities in general, but some specific comorbidities such as cardio-cerebro-vascular and dementia.

Factors of the index event (hospitalization)

Several variables were registered from the hospitalization, however our study showed that only hypercapnia at the

Table 6 Description of the mortality rate at 1 year in the different risk groups

	Derivation sample			Validation sample		
	N (%)	Mortality 1 year	*p*-value	*N* (%)	Mortality 1 year	*p*-value
Risk groups			< 0.0001			< 0.0001
Low (0–5)	83 (8.03)	7 (8.43)		498 (15.39)	17 (3.41)	
Low-Medium (6–7)	112 (10.83)	22 (19.64)		513 (15.86)	38 (7.41)	
Medium-High (8–10)	412 (39.85)	134 (32.52)		1307 (40.40)	201 (15.38)	
High (>10)	427 (41.30)	206 (48.24)		917 (28.35)	236 (25.74)	
AUC (95% CI)	0.740 (0.709–0.771)			0.763 (0.741–0.784)		

N frequency, *%* percentage, *CI* confidence Interval

time of hospital admission was associated with one-year mortality.

PaCO2 has been recognized as a key predictor of in-hospital mortality [30] and one-year after admission mortality [14, 22] among eCOPD patients. A study that included COPD patients admitted to the intensive care unit established that the severity of the exacerbation reflected by respiratory physiology influenced one-year mortality but not in-hospital mortality [16]. Patients admitted with a PaCO2 > 50 mmHg—which would indicate the severity of the underlying respiratory disease, like ventilation/ perfusion mismatch or hypoventilation—had higher one-year mortality than those with PaCO2 < 50 mmHg. It is possible that in this study, the homogeneity of the cohort (ICU patients only) could have diluted the discriminative capacity of the analysis, limiting the possibility of finding any relationship between in-hospital mortality and variables (like PaCO2) that reflect the physiological respiratory impairment during an eCOPD.

We were not able to demonstrate if hypercapnia persisted at discharge, and if its persistence was related to mortality, as has been suggested by others [20]. Neither did we have any information on patient PaCO2 in a stable condition of our cohorts.

Previous hospitalizations

Previous eCOPD hospitalizations have been identified as an independent predictor of mortality in cohorts of stable and hospitalized patients. Soler-Cataluña et al., for example, demonstrated that mortality increases with the frequency of severe exacerbations requiring hospital evaluation [31]. Other researchers have observed that the number of severe eCOPD requiring hospitalization increases the risk of respiratory and all-cause mortality regardless of factors such as age, FEV_1, dyspnoea, cumulative pack-year smoking history, and health-related quality of life [32].

Across the lifespan of COPD patients, the addition of every new hospitalization significantly increases the rate of mortality, and the risk of other severe eCOPD peaks during the 3 months after the index event [1].

In cohorts derived from databases, episodes of previous COPD-related hospitalizations were an independent predictor of mortality [21, 33]. In fact, previous hospitalizations and comorbidities have been included as components of a multidimensional score predicting mortality in a cohort of hospitalized patients.

In our study having had one hospitalization the year before the index-event increased the probability of mortality the year after by 60%, which would be in accordance with the results of studies previously mentioned and outline more precisely the profile of the patient that should be carefully monitored after and eCOPD hospitalization.

Hospital characteristics

Hospital characteristics were reported as a predictor of mortality in the UK national audit 2003. Inpatient and 90-day mortality were lower in hospitals with more respiratory staff per 1000 beds. No other associations were found between other hospital resources and mortality.

The European COPD audit team evaluated adherence to 10 key management recommendations set forth by the GOLD standards in 13 European countries. It found great variability between hospitals and across countries, especially connected with the availability of the level of severity of the obstruction and the use of oxygen and non-invasive ventilation. The audit also showed that larger hospitals have more resources but this does not imply a better quality of care.

Walker et al. showed that 30-day mortality after hospitalization for an eCOPD was quite variable from 1 year to the following across various hospitals. Mortality in that period was independent of hospital size and of whether a respiratory specialist was responsible for the discharge of the patient [13].

In our study, hospital size, as measured by bed numbers and population served, was related to one-year mortality. Knowing the potential limitation of using data from one brief time point rather than data collected over several years we could speculate that having more resources provided not only better treatment of the index episode but better follow-up care afterward. We observed a significant influence of the hospital on one-year mortality since the AUC increases from 0.68 to 0.77 after including the variable hospital in the analysis. Nevertheless, we were not able to establish whether this is due exclusively to the hospital, or is also due to the primary care organization, the regional medical or social characteristics involved in the care of these patients, or all of these together. In any case including hospital size seems to be an important point in the final results.

Strengths and limitations

Strengths of our study included are the number of patients we were able to follow, the length of follow-up, and the fact that patients were recruited from multiple centres. The usage of multilevel models provides a better approach than ordinary logistic regression models when patients are clustered in different groups, as in our case, that we have patients clustered in different hospitals. In this way, the correlation effect among patients from the same hospitals is controlled, as we do not consider them independently.

Several limitations must also be noted, primarily related to the design of the study as an audit of care in eCOPD, which implies missing data. We used for the analysis only those variables with less than 15% of missing data. Another limitation is that we were not able to recover the whole cohort of the Spanish audit. Instead, we analysed only those hospitals that conducted a follow-up of 1 year. We checked our sample against the whole cohort and verified that there were no differences in the clinical characteristics of the patients. Patients who died during the admission were not included in this analysis, only discharged patients. We were not able to pinpoint the cause of death because it is not accurately registered in death records, but this was not the objective of this study. As an audit of general practice some variables currently used as part of predictive mortality scores were not collected. Thus, a comparison with others mortality scores was not possible. The low percentage of women in both cohorts of the study limited the possibility of carrying out an analysis about potential differences with respect to men in the main outcomes studied.

Conclusions

In a cohort of patients hospitalized for an eCOPD, predictors of mortality in the year following the index hospitalization were patient characteristic age, characteristics of the disease (admission for an eCOPD in the previous year and specific comorbidities), aspects of the index event (PaCO2), and the characteristics of the hospitals in which the patients were treated. Some of these aspect are potentially adjustable to impact in the care and outcomes of severe eCOPD.

In conclusion our study provides the patient profile with the highest probability of mortality during the year after an eCOPD hospitalization. We should pay attention to a man in his seventies, with cardio-vascular and/or dementia, with a previous eCOPD hospitalization the year before the index event and with hypercapnia > 50 mmHg during the admission. In those patients with these characteristics a more personalized follow-up is mandatory.

Abbreviations

AUC: Area under the receiver-operating curve; COPD: Chronic obstructive pulmonary disease; eCOPD: Exacerbation of COPD; ED: Emergency department

Acknowledgements

We are grateful for the support of the participating hospitals.

Grupo AUDIPOC España-CEPA Subproyecto 1

COMITÉ COORDINADOR: ESTEBAN, Cristóbal. Neumología, Hospital de Galdakao. Vizcaya. POZO RODRIGUEZ, Francisco. Neumología, Hospital 12 de Octubre. Madrid. CASTRO ACOSTA, Ady Angélica. Médico Investigador CIBERES Unidad de Epidemiología Clínica, Hospital Universitario 12 de octubre. Madrid. BOUKICHOU ABDELKADER, Nisa Lic. CC y TT. Estadísticas. Investigador CIBERES Unidad de Epidemiología Clínica, Hospital Universitario 12 de octubre. Madrid. ESTEBAN GARCIA-NAVAS, Sara Investigador CIBERES Unidad de Epidemiología Clínica, Hospital Universitario 12 de octubre. Madrid. **COMITÉ CIENTÍFICO**: POZO RODRÍGUEZ, Francisco. AGUSTÍ, Alvar. Neumología, Instituto Cardiotorácico Hospital Clinic, Barcelona. ÁLVAREZ MARTÍNEZ, Carlos José. Neumología, Hospital 12 de Octubre. Madrid. CAPELASTEGUI SAIZ, Alberto. Neumología, Barakaldo. Bilbao. HERNÁNDEZ CARCERENY, Carme. Neumología, Hospital Clinic. Barcelona. IZQUIERDO ALONSO, José Luis. Neumología, Hospital de Guadalajara. LOPEZ CAMPOS, José Luís. Neumología, Hospital Universitario Virgen del Rocío. Sevilla. MELERO MORENO, Carlos. Neumología, Hospital Universitario 12 de octubre. Madrid. **ANDALUCIA:** RESPONSABLE REGIONAL: José Luís López Campos. Neumología, Hospital Universitario Virgen del Rocío. RESPONSABLES LOCALES: Almería, Complejo Hospitalario Torrecárdenas: José Calvo Bonachera. Cádiz, Hospital de La Línea de la Concepción: Armando Falces Sierra, Hospital General de Jerez de la Frontera: Gregorio Soto Campos, Hospital Puerta del Mar: Fernando Romero Valero y Isidro Blasco, Hospital Puerto Real: Jesús Sánchez Gómez. Hospital Universitario Reina Sofía: Marisol Arenas de la Riva y María Jesús Cobos Ceballos. Granada: Hospital Universitario San Cecilio: Alicia Conde Valero. Huelva: Hospital Infanta Elena: Rosa Vázquez Oliva y Fernando Hernández Utrera. Hospital Juan Ramón Jiménez: Rut Ayerbe García. Jaén: Centro Hospitalario Ciudad de Jaén: Bernardino Alcázar Navarrete. E.P.H.A.G. Alto Guadalquivir (Andujar): Juan Manuel Bravo Santervás. Málaga: Hospital Costa del Sol: José Fernández Guerra. Hospital Comarcal de Vélez Málaga: Carlos Rueda, Hospital Regional Carlos Haya: José Luís de la Cruz Ríos. Hospital Serranía de Ronda: Francisco José Cabello Rueda. Hospital Virgen de la Victoria: Francisco Marín Sánchez. Sevilla: Hospital de la Merced – Osuna: José Pérez Ronchel. Hospital Universitario Virgen del Rocío: José Luís López Campos. Hospital Universitario Valme: Inmaculada Alfageme Michavila. **ARAGÓN**: RESPONSABLE REGIONAL: Luis Borderías. Neumología, Hospital San Jorge de Huesca, José Manuel Gascón Pelegrín. Neumología, Hospital Miguel Servert. Zaragoza, Instituto Aragonés de Salud: Anselmo López y Mónica Torrijos RESPONSABLES LOCALES: Hospital Clínico Universitario Lozano Bleza: Joaquín Carlos Costan Galicia. Hospital Miguel Servert: Salvador Bello Dronda, Andrés Sánchez Barón y José Manuel Gascón Pelegrín. Hospital San Jorge de Huesca: Luis Borderías. **CANARIAS**: RESPONSABLE REGIONAL Ana Velázquez Benítez. H Ntra Señora de la Candelaria. José Gabriel Julia. Neumología, Hospital Dr. Negrín RESPONSABLES LOCALES: Las Palmas: Hospital Dr. Negrín: Carlos Cabrera López. Lanzarote: Hospital Dr. José Molina Orosa, Lanzarote: Javier Navarro Esteva. Santa Cruz de Tenerife: HM Nuestra Señora de Candelaria: Magdalena Alonso, Ruth Pitti, José Batista y Orlando Acosta Fernández. Hospital Universitario de Tenerife: José Antonio Gullón. **CANTABRIA**: RESPONSABLE REGIONAL Ramón Agüero Balbín. Neumología, Hospital Marqués de Valdecilla. Cantabria: Hospital de Laredo: Miguel Zabaleta Murguiondo. Hospital Marqués de Valdecilla: Beatriz Abascal Bolado y Ramón Agüero Balbín. Hospital Sierrallana: Mar García Pérez. **CASTILLA LA MANCHA**: RESPONSABLE REGIONAL Jose Celdran Gil. Neumología, Hospital Nuestra Señora del Prado de Talavera. Jesús Fernández Francés. Neumología, Hospital de Guadalajara. RESPONSABLES LOCALES: Albacete: Hospital de Albacete: Ana Isabel Tornero. Ciudad Real: Hospital La Mancha Centro (ALCAZAR): Gloria Francisco. Hospital Manzanares. Fernando Pedraza y Marisi Verdugo. Cuenca: Hospital Virgen de la Luz de Cuenca: María José Peirón. Guadalajara: Hospital de Guadalajara: Jesús Fernández Francés y JL Izquierdo. Soria: Complejo Asistencial de Soria, H Santa Bárbara: José Luis Orcastegui Candial Toledo: Hospital Nuestra Señora del Prado de Talavera: José Celdrán. Hospital Virgen de la Luz de Toledo: Encarnación López Gabaldón. **CASTILLA Y LEÓN**: RESPONSABLE REGIONAL Jesús Reyes Hernández Hernández. Neumología, Hospital Nuestra señora de Sonsoles. RESPONSABLES LOCALES: Ávila: H Nuestra señora de Sonsoles: José Eugenio Alonso Muñoz y Eugenio Trujillo Santos. Burgos: Complejo Hospitalario de Burgos: Luís Rodríguez Pascual. Hospital Santiago Apóstol de Miranda de Ebro: Esteban Pascual Pablo. Hospital Santos Reyes Aranda de Duero: Pedro Cancelo Suárez. León: Complejo Asistencial de León: Ana José Seco García. Hospital del Bierzo: Juan Ortiz De Saracho y Bobo. Palencia: Complejo Asistencial de Palencia: María Ángeles Fernández Jorge. Salamanca: Complejo hospitalario de Salamanca: Rosa Cordovilla Pérez. Segovia: Hospital General de Segovia: Graciliano Estrada Trigueras. Soria: Complejo Asistencial de Soria, Hospital Santa Bárbara: José Luís Orcastegui Candial. Valladolid: Hospital Clínico Universitario: Carlos Disdier y Enrique Macías Fernández. Hospital Río Hortera: Félix del Campo Matías. Zamora: Complejo Hospitalario de Zamora. Hospital de Benavente: Carmen Fernández García, Cecilia Alonso Medievilla y María Victoria Domínguez Rodríguez. **CATALUÑA**: RESPONSABLE REGIONAL Carlos Martínez Rivera. Neumología, Hospital Universitari Germans Trias i Pujol. Eduard Monsó Molas. Neumología, Hospital Universitari Germans Trias i Pujol. RESPONSABLES LOCALES: Barcelona: Hospital Clinic Barcelona: Néstor Soler Porcar, Carmen Hernández. Hospital Comarcal de L'alt Penedés,Vilefrance de Penedés: Nuria Rodríguez Lázaro. Hospital del Mar: Joaquim Gea, Roser Pedreny y Sergi Pascual. Hospital General de Vic: Fernando Ruiz Mori. Hospital San Pau: Antonio Antón y

Virginia Pajares Ruiz. Virginia Pajares Ruiz. Hospital Universitari Germans Trias i Pujol: Eduard Monsó Molas y Ignasi Garcia Olivé. Hospital Vall d'Hebron: Esther Rodríguez González, Eva Lozano, Eva Tapia Melechon, Mª Angeles Barrio, Mª Antonia Roman, Mieria Guzman Perez, Milagros Gandara Sanz y Xavier Pérez. Hospital Viladecans: Joan Anton Lloret Queraltó, Mercedes Palau Benavent y Nuria Celorrio Jiménez. Gerona (Girona): Hospital Universitario Doctor Josep Trueta: Manuel Haro Estarriol. Lérida (Lleida): Hospital Arnau: Ferrán Barbé. H General Par Sanitari Sant Joan de Déu: Luis Lores Obradors, H Parc Taulí de Sabadell: Eduard Monso, H Joan XXIII de Tarragona: Leonardo Esteban **MADRID**: RESPONSABLE REGIONAL. Julio Ancoechea Bermúdez. Neumología, Hospital de la Princesa. Carlos Melero Moreno y Carlos José Álvarez Martínez. Neumología, Hospital Universitario 12 de Octubre. RESPONSABLES LOCALES: Madrid. H. 12 OCTUBRE: Virginia Pérez González. Hospital Clínico San Carlos: Gema Rodríguez Trigo. Hospital de la Princesa: Enrique Zamora García. Hospital de Tajo, Aranjuez: José. Fernando González Torralba. Hospital de Valdemoro: Rocío García García. Hospital El Escorial: Francisco Gómez Rico. Hospital Fundación Alcorcón: Barbara Steen. Eva De Higes Martínez. Mercedes Izquierdo Patrón y Ángela Ramos Pinedo. Hospital Gómez Ulla: Javier Jareño, Ignacio Granda Uribe y Sergio Campos Tellez. Hospital Gregorio Marañón: Jorge García, José De Miguel Rodríguez González Moro. Hospital Infanta Cristina, Parla: Beatriz Jara Chinarro, María Teresa Rio. Ramírez. Hospital Infanta Sofía: Raúl Moreno Zabaleta, Maria Teresa Ramirez Prieto y Blas Rojo Moreno Arrones. Hospital La Paz: Francisco García Río y Sergio Alcolea Batres. Hospital Puerta de Hierro: Rosa Malo de Molina Ruíz, Antolin López Viña y Pietat Ussetti. Hospital Ramón y Cajal: Esteban Pérez Rodríguez y Salvador Díaz Lobato. Hospital Infanta Leonor: Carmen Matesanz Ruíz, Maria Jesus Buendia. Hospital Sureste Arganda del Rey: Sergio Salgado Aranda. Fundación Jiménez Díaz: German Peces Barba. Hospital de Getafe: Mª Antonia Juretschke Moragues. Hospital Príncipe de Asturias Alcalá Henares: Soledad Alonso Viteri. Hospital de Móstoles: Dolores Álvaro. Hospital Severo Ochoa de Leganés: Asunción Perpina. Hospital del Henares: Mª Ángeles Ruíz-Cobos. **C.F.NAVARRA**: RESPONSABLE REGIONAL. Javier Hueto Perez de Heredia. Neumología, Complejo Hospitalario de Navarra. RESPONSABLES LOCALES: Navarra: Complejo hospitalario de Navarra: José Javier Lorza Blasco, José Antonio Cascante Rodrigo, Jalil Abú-Shams, Victor Manuel Eguía Astibia, Idoya Pascal Martínez, Joan Boldú Mitgans y Pilar Cebollero Rivas. Hospital García Orcoyen De Estella: Idoya Pascal Martínez. Hospital Reina Sofía De Tudela: José Antonio Cascante Rodrigo y José Javier Lorza Blasco. Hospital Virgen Del Camino De Pamplona:. **C. VALENCIANA**: RESPONSABLE REGIONAL Pablo Catalán Serra y Juan José Soler Cataluña. Neumología, Hospital de Requena. RESPONSABLES LOCALES: Alicante: Hospital de Elda: Alejandro Muñoz. Hospital de Orihuela: José Manuel Querol. Hospital de San Joan: Eusebi Chiner Vives y Adaluz Andreu Rodríguez. Hospital de Torrevieja: Esther Pastor. Castellón de la Plana: Hospital de la Magdalena: Khaled Bdeir Egnayem Hospital de La Plana: Luis Miravet. Hospital General de Castellón: Margarita Marín Royo. Valencia: Hospital Clínico Valencia: María Cruz González Villaescusa. Hospital de Requena: Pablo Catalán Serra y Juan José Soler Cataluña. Hospital Dr. Peset: Estrella Fernández Fabrellas, Ángela Cervera Juan, Alberto Herreron Silvestre y Alfonso Martinez Martinez. Hospital Francés de Borja, Gandia: Concha Pellicer Ciscar. Hospital de la Rivera: Elsa Naval Sendra. Hospital Sagunto: Eva Martínez Moragon. Hospital Universitario la Fe: Montserrat Leon Fabregas. **EXTREMADURA**: RESPONSABLE REGIONAL Juan Antonio Riesco Miranda. Neumología, Hospital de Cáceres. RESPONSABLES LOCALES: Badajoz: Hospital Infanta Cristina de Badajoz: José Antonio Gutierrez Lara, Fernando Fuentes. Cáceres: Hospital de Cáceres: Juan Antonio Riesco Miranda. Hospital de Plasencia: Miguel Ángel Hernández Mezquita. Mérida: Hospital de Mérida: Germán García Vinuesa. **GALICIA**: RESPONSABLE REGIONAL Alberto Fernández Villar. Neumología, Complejo hospitalario de Vigo. Juan Suárez Antelo. Neumología, Complejo Hospitalario Universitario A Coruña. RESPONSABLES LOCALES: La Coruña (A Coruña): Complejo Hospitalario Universitario A Coruña: Juan Suarez Antelo. FPH Barbanza: Emilio Manuel Padin Paz. Hospital de Conxo - Santiago de Compostela: Jesús Suarez Martinez. Lugo: Hospital Comarcal Burela: Sonia Paredes Vila. Hospital Xeral, Lugo: Rafael Golpe Gomez y Luis Pérez de Llano. Orense (Ourense): CH Ourense: Pedro Marcos, Carlos Vilariño Pombo y Jose Manuel García Pazos. Pontevedra: Hospital provincial de Pontevedra: Adolfo Baloira. Hospital Xeral, Vigo: Alberto Fernández Villar y Cristina Represas Represas. Hospital do Meixoero, Vigo: Manuel Nuñez Delgado. Hospital Povisa: Maria Dolores Corbacho Abelaira. Hospital Xeral, Vigo: Marta Nuñez Fernandez. **ISLAS BALEARES**: RESPONSABLE REGIONAL Borja García Cosio. Neumología, Hospital Son Espases. RESPONSABLES LOCALES: Palma de Mallorca: Hospital Comarcal de Inca: Elena Laserna Martinez. Hospital de Manacor: Rosa Maria Irigaray Canals. Hospital de San Llatzer: Salvador Pons Vivas. Hospital Son Espases: Borja Garcia Cosio. Menorca: Hospital Mateu Orfila: Jordi Guerrero. Ibiza: Hospital Can Misses, Ibiza: Alvaro De Astorza y Antonio Cascales García. **LA RIOJA**: RESPONSABLE REGIONAL Manuel Barrón Medrano. Neumología, Hospital de la Rioja. RESPONSABLES LOCALES: La Rioja: Fundación Hospital de Calahorra: Susana Chic Palacin y Manuel Barron Medrano. Hospital De La Rioja: Carlos Ruiz Martínez y Manuel Barron Medrano. **PAIS VASCO**: RESPONSABLE REGIONAL Cristóbal Esteban. Neumología, Hospital de Galdakao. RESPONSABLES LOCALES: Álava: H de Santiago: Mª Ines Carrascosa. H Txagorritxu: Laura Tomas. Gipuzcoa (Guipuzkoa): H Bidasoa: Jose Antonio Miguel Arce, Mª Asunción Celaya y Silvia Dorronsoro. H Donostia: Mª Rosa Berdejo, Mónica Rayón y Gabriel Zubillaga Garmendia. Hospital de Mendaro: Jose Ignacion Royo, Susana Chic Palacin y Nicolás Gurrutxaga. H de Mondragón: Iñaki Peña y Mikel Temprano Gogenola. H Zumarraga: Silvia Dorronsoro, Cristina Estirado y Raquel Sanchez. Vizcaya (Bizkaia): H Basurto: Miren Begoña Salinas y Igor Iturbe. H Cruces: José Mª Antoñana y Pilar Marin. H Galdakao: Cristóbal Esteban, Mikel Egurrola y Alberto Capelastegui. H San Eloy: Juan Manuel Nuñez, Jesús Caminos y Luis Alberto Ruiz Iturriaga. **PRINCIPADO DE ASTURIAS**: RESPONSABLE REGIONAL Cristina Martinez. Neumología, Hospital Universitario Central de Asturias. RESPONSABLES LOCALES: Hospital Universitario Central de Asturias: Marta García Clemente, Hospital de Cabueñes Gijón: Teresa Pascual Pascual y Concepción Diaz Sanchez. Hospital del Oriente-Arriondas: Blanca Requejo Mañana. Hospital Fundación Jove: Benigno Del Busto Lorenzo. Hospital San Agustín, Avilés: Fernando Álvarez Navascues y Marta García Clemente. Hospital Universitario Central de Asturias: Aida Quero Martínez y Cristina Martínez. Hospital Valle del Nalón Langreo: Hortencia Canto Argiz. **REGION DE MURCIA**: RESPONSABLE REGIONAL. Juan Miguel Sánchez Nieto. Neumología, Hospital General Universitario Morales Meseguer. RESPONSABLES LOCALES: Hospital de los Arcos: Damián Melia Alvarado, Jose A Ros Lucas y Nuria Castejon Piña. Hospital General Universitario Morales Meseguer: Roberto Bernabeu Mora, Juan Miguel Sanchez Nieto y Maria Loreto Alemany Frances. Hospital Universitario Santa Lucía: Ines Bernal Belijar, Jose Javier Martinez Garceran, Mercedes Guillamon Sanchez y Pilar Berlinches Acin. Hospital U Reina Sofía: Carlos Orts Arqueros, Maria Jesus Aviles Ingles y Pedro Mendez Martinez.

Funding

This work was supported in part by grants from the Fondo de Investigación Sanitaria PI 06\10.

Authors' contributions

Conception and design: FPR; Analysis and interpretation: CE, ACA, FPR; Drafting the manuscript for important intellectual content: CE, ACA, CJAM, AC, JLLP, FPR. All authors have read and approved the final version of this manuscript.

Consent for publication

Not applicable

Competing interests

The authors declare that they have no competing interests.

Author details

[1]Pulmonary Service, Galdakao-Usansolo Hospital, Galdakao, Bizkaia, Spain. [2]Pulmonary Service and Research Institute, Doce de Octubre University Hospital, Madrid, Spain. [3]CIBER Enfermedades Respiratorias (CIBERES), Madrid, Spain. [4]Hospital Universitario Virgen del Rocío, Medical- Surgical Unit of Respiratory Diseases, Seville, Spain. [5]Network and Health Services Research Chronic Diseases (REDISSEC), Bilbao, Bizkaia, Spain.

References

1. Suissa S, Dell'Aniello S, Ernst P. Long-term natural history of chronic obstructive pulmonary disease: severe exacerbations and mortality. Thorax. 2012;67:957–63.
2. Steer J, Gibson GJ, Bourke SC. Predicting outcomes following hospitalization for acute exacerbations of COPD. QJM. 2010;103:817–29.
3. Singanayagam A, Schembri S, Chalmers JD. Predictors of mortality in hospitalized adults with acute exacerbation of chronic obstructive pulmonary disease. Ann Am Thorac Soc. 2013;10:81–9.
4. Celli BC, Cote CG, Marín JM, Casanova C, Montes de Oca M, Mendez RA, Pinto Plata V, Cabral HJ. The body-mass index, airflow obstruction, dyspnea, and exercise capacity index in chronic obstructive pulmonary disease. NEJM. 2004;350:1005–12.
5. Puhan MA, Garcia-Aymerich J, Frey M, ter Riet G, Antó JM, Agustí AG, Gómez FP, Rodríguez-Roisín R, Moons KG, Kessels AG, Held U. Expansion of the prognostic assessment of patients with chronic obstructive pulmonary disease: the updated BODE index and the ADO index. Lancet. 2009;374:704–11.
6. Pozo-Rodríguez F, Alvarez CJ, Castro-Acosta A, Melero Moreno C, Capelastegui A, Esteban C, Hernández Carcereny C, López-Campos JL, Izquierdo Alonso JL, López Quílez A, Agustí A, por el Grupo AUDIPOC España. Clinical audit of patients admitted to hospital in Spain due to exacerbation of COPD (AUDIPOC study): method and organisation. Arch Bronconeumol. 2010;46:349–57.
7. Lopez-Campos JL, Hartl S, Pozo-Rodriguez F, et al. European COPD Audit: design, organisation of work and methodology. Eur Respir J. 2013;41:270–6.
8. Puhan MA, Hansel NN, Sobradillo P, Enright P, Lange P, Hickson D, Menezes AM, Riet GT, Held U, Domingo-Salvany A, Mosenifar Z, Antó JM, Moons KG, Kessels A, Garcia-Aymerich J, International COPD Cohorts Collaboration Working Group. Large-scale international validation of the ADO index in subjects with COPD: an individual subject data analysis of 10 cohorts. BMJ Open. 2012;2:e002152.
9. Esteban C, Quintana JM, Aburto M, Moraza J, Arostegui I, España PP, Aizpiri S, Capelastegui A. The health, activity, dyspnea, obstruction, age, and hospitalization: prognostic score for stable COPD patients. Respir Med. 2011; 105:1662–70.
10. Patil SP, Krishnan JA, Lechtzin N, Diette GB. In-hospital mortality following acute exacerbations of chronic obstructive pulmonary disease. Arch Intern Med. 2003;163:1180–6.
11. Piquet J, Chavaillon JM, David P, Martin F, Blanchon F, Roche N, French College of General Hospital Respiratory Physicians (CPHG). High-risk patients following hospitalisation for an acute exacerbation of COPD. Eur Respir J. 2013;42:946–55.
12. Walker PP, Thompson E, Crone H, Flatt G, Holton K, Hill SL, Pearson MG. Use of mortality within 30 days of a COPD hospitalisation as a measure of COPD care in UK hospitals. Thorax. 2013;68:968–70.
13. Groenewegen KH, Schols AM, Wouters EF. Mortality and mortality-related factors after hospitalization for acute exacerbation of COPD. Chest. 2003;124:459–67.
14. Connors AF Jr, Dawson NV, Thomas C, Harrell FE Jr, Desbiens N, Fulkerson WJ, Kussin P, Bellamy P, Goldman L, Knaus WA. Outcomes following acute exacerbation of severe chronic obstructive lung disease. The SUPPORT investigators (Study to Understand Prognoses and Preferences for Outcomes and Risks of Treatments). Am J Respir Crit Care Med. 1996;154:959–67.
15. Seneff MG, Wagner DP, Wagner RP, Zimmerman JE, Knaus WA. Hospital and 1-year survival of patients admitted to intensive care units with acute exacerbation of chronic obstructive pulmonary disease. JAMA. 1995;274:1852–7.
16. Stone RA, Lowe D, Potter JM, Buckingham RJ, Roberts CM, Pursey NJ. Managing patients with COPD exacerbation: does age matter? Age Ageing. 2012;41:461–8.
17. Connolly MJ, Lowe D, Anstey K, Hosker HS, Pearson MG, Roberts CM, Society BT, the Royal College of Physicians Clinical Effectiveness Evaluation Unit (CEEu). Admissions to hospital with exacerbations of chronic obstructive pulmonary disease: Effect of age related factors and service organisation. Thorax. 2006;61:843–8.
18. Roberts CM, Stone RA, Lowe D, Pursey NA, Buckingham RJ. Co-morbidities and 90-day outcomes in hospitalized COPD exacerbations. COPD. 2011;8:354–61.
19. Almagro P, Calbo E, Ochoa de Echagüen A, Barreiro B, Quintana S, Heredia JL, Garau J. Mortality after hospitalization for COPD. Chest. 2002;121:1441–8.
20. McGhan R, Radcliff T, Fish R, Sutherland ER, Welsh C, Make B. Predictors of rehospitalization and death after a severe exacerbation of COPD. Chest. 2007;132:1748–55.
21. Fruchter O, Yigla M. Predictors of long-term survival in elderly patients hospitalized for acute exacerbations of chronic obstructive pulmonary disease. Respirology. 2008;13:851–5.
22. Gudmundsson G, Ulrik CS, Gislason T, Lindberg E, Brøndum E, Bakke P, Janson C. Long-term survival in patients hospitalized for chronic obstructive pulmonary disease: a prospective observational study in the Nordic countries. Int J Chron Obstruct Pulmon Dis. 2012;7:571–6.
23. Ranieri P, Bianchetti A, Margiotta A, Virgillo A, Clini EM, Trabucchi M. Predictors of 6-month mortality in elderly patients with mild chronic obstructive pulmonary disease discharged from a medical ward after acute nonacidotic exacerbation. J Am Geriatr Soc. 2008;56:909–13.
24. Cheng Y, Han X, Luo Y, Xu W. Deaths of obstructive lung disease in the Yangpu district of Shanghai from 2003 through 2011: a multiple cause analysis. Chin Med J. 2014;127:1619–25.
25. Steer J, Gibson J, Bourke SC. The DECAF Score: predicting hospital mortality in exacerbations of chronic obstructive pulmonary disease. Thorax. 2012;67:970–6.
26. Gunen H, Hacievliyagil SS, Kosar F, Mutlu LC, Gulbas G, Pehlivan E, Sahin I, Kizkin O. Factors affecting survival of hospitalised patients with COPD. Eur Respir J. 2005;26:234–41.
27. Soler-Cataluña JJ, Martinez-Garcia MA, Román Sánchez P, et al. Severe acute exacerbations and mortality in patients with chronic obstructive pulmonary disease. Thorax. 2005;60:925–31.
28. Esteban C, Quintana JM, Aburto M, Moraza J, Egurrola M, España PP, Pérez-Izquierdo J, Capelastegui A. Predictors of mortality in patients with stable COPD. J Gen Intern Med. 2008;23:1829–34.
29. Slenter RH, Sprooten RT, Kotz D, Wesseling G, Wouters EF, Rohde GG. Predictors of 1-year mortality at hospital admission for acute exacerbations of chronic obstructive pulmonary disease. Respiration. 2013;85:15–26.
30. Almagro P, Soriano J, Cabrera F, Boixeda R, Alonso M, Barreiro B, Diez-Manglano J, Murio C, Heredia J, Working Group on COPD, Spanish Society of Internal Medicine. Short- and medium-term prognosis in patients hospitalized for COPD exacerbation: the CODEX index. Chest. 2014;145:972–80.
31. Price LC, Lowe D, Hosker HS, Anstey K, Pearson MG, Roberts CM, Society BT, the Royal College of Physicians Clinical Effectiveness Evaluation Unit (CEEu). UK National COPD Audit 2003: Impact of hospital resources and organisation of care on patient outcome following admission for acute COPD exacerbation. Thorax. 2006;61:837–42.
32. Roberts CM, Lopez-Campos JL, Pozo-Rodriguez F, Hartl S, on behalf of the European COPD Audit team. European hospital adherence to GOLD recommendations for chronic obstructive pulmonary disease (COPD) exacerbation admissions. Thorax. 2013;68:1169–71.
33. López-Campos JL, Hartl S, Pozo-Rodriguez F, Roberts CM, on behalf of the European COPD Audit team. Variability of hospital resources for acute care of COPD patients: European COPD audit. Eur Respir J. 2013;41:270–6.

Burden of asthma and COPD overlap (ACO) in Taiwan: a nationwide population-based study

Sumitra Shantakumar[1], Raoh-Fang Pwu[2,6], Liesel D'Silva[3], Keele Wurst[4], Yao-Wen Kuo[5], Yen-Yun Yang[2], Yi-Chen Juan[2*] and K. Arnold Chan[2,5]

Abstract

Background: Patients with symptoms of both asthma and chronic obstructive pulmonary disease (COPD) may be classified with the term asthma-COPD overlap (ACO). ACO is of considerable interest as it is currently poorly characterised and has been associated with worse health outcomes and higher healthcare costs compared with COPD or asthma alone. Patients with ACO in Asia remain poorly described, and there is limited information regarding their resource utilisation compared with patients with asthma or COPD only. This study investigated the characteristics, disease burden and medical resource utilisation of patients with ACO in Taiwan.

Methods: This was a retrospective cohort study of patients identified from National Health Insurance (NHI) claims data in Taiwan in 2009–2011. Patients were classified into incident ACO, COPD or asthma cohorts according to International Classification of Disease, ninth revision, clinical modification codes in claims. Eligible patients were ≥40 years of age with 12 months' continuous enrolment in the NHI programme pre- and post-index date (date of the first relevant medical claim).

Results: Patients with ACO ($N = 22{,}328$) and COPD ($N = 69{,}648$) were older and more likely to be male than those with asthma ($N = 50{,}293$). Patients with ACO had more comorbidities and exacerbations, with higher medication use: short-acting β_2-agonist prescriptions ranged from 30.4% of patients (asthma cohort) to 43.6% (ACO cohort), and inhaled corticosteroid/long-acting β_2-agonist combination prescriptions ranged from 11.1% (COPD cohort) to 35.0% (ACO cohort) in the 12 months following index. Patients with ACO generally had the highest medication costs of any cohort (long-acting muscarinic antagonist costs ranged from $227/patient [asthma cohort] to $349/patient [ACO cohort]); they also experienced more respiratory-related hospital visits than patients with asthma or COPD (mean outpatient/inpatient visits per patient post-index: 9.1/1.9 [ACO cohort] vs 5.7/1.4 [asthma cohort] and 6.4/1.7 [COPD cohort]).

Conclusions: Patients with ACO in Taiwan experience a greater disease burden with greater healthcare resource utilisation, and higher costs, than patients with asthma or COPD alone.

Keywords: Asthma-chronic obstructive pulmonary disease overlap, Asthma, Chronic obstructive pulmonary disease, Epidemiology, Medical resource utilisation, Taiwan

* Correspondence: d49306002@ym.edu.tw
[2]Health Data Research Center, National Taiwan University, No.33, Linsen South Road, Suite 526, Taipei 10051, Taiwan
Full list of author information is available at the end of the article

Background

Patients presenting with overlapping clinical features of asthma and chronic obstructive pulmonary disease (COPD) may be described with the term asthma-COPD overlap (ACO). ACO has been recognised in the Global Initiative for Chronic Obstructive Lung Disease (GOLD) and Global Initiative for Asthma (GINA) guidelines since 2014, when the existence of ACO syndrome (ACOS) was proposed; [1, 2] however, more recent guidance has suggested that, since ACOS cannot be considered to be a single disease entity, the term ACO is more appropriate [3]. ACO is of considerable interest worldwide as it is currently poorly characterised with no clear diagnostic definition, yet it has been associated with worse health outcomes and higher healthcare costs compared with COPD or asthma alone [4, 5]. Most large-scale studies investigating the prevalence of ACO and the characteristics of patients have examined populations outside of Asia [4, 6–11]. Within Asia, several studies have examined Korean, [12–14] Japanese [15–18] and Chinese patients [19, 20]. However, since some studies in Asian patients involved small populations or examined only particular aspects of the disease, patients with ACO in Asia remain poorly described, and there is limited information regarding their resource utilisation compared with patients with asthma or COPD only.

The ACO population in Taiwan is particularly poorly described; one study assessed the prevalence of ACO and compared the incidence of acute respiratory events in patients with ACO and COPD; [21] a second study examined the association between ACO and tuberculosis [22]. However, both studies used only a sample of data from the Taiwanese population and therefore may not capture the full clinical picture. Healthcare in Taiwan is provided through the National Health Insurance (NHI) programme. This single-payer, universal programme provides medical coverage to >99% of the population; [23] therefore, Taiwan is an ideal setting for quantification of the country-level incidence of ACO and its associated healthcare utilisation and costs.

This study aimed to characterise patients with ACO in Taiwan and compare them with patients with asthma or COPD only, examining demographics at diagnosis, disease burden, healthcare and medication resource utilisation and associated costs using recent national administrative health insurance data from the entire Taiwanese population. Additionally, an exploratory analysis of different ACO definitions was performed.

Methods

Study design

This was a retrospective cohort study (GSK study number PRJ2356; National Taiwan University grant number 105R104012) of patients meeting criteria for ACO, COPD, or asthma based on NHI claims data for 2009–2011 (patients were followed through 2012). NHI claims were based on International Classification of Disease, ninth revision, clinical modification (ICD-9-CM) codes. Data were obtained through the Health and Welfare Data Science Center, Department of Statistics, Ministry of Health and Welfare in Taiwan.

Patients

Eligibility criteria

Eligible patients were ≥40 years of age with incident NHI disease claims relevant to COPD or asthma (COPD, ICD-9-CM codes: 491 [chronic bronchitis], 492 [emphysema] or 496 [chronic airway obstruction, not elsewhere classified]; asthma, ICD-9-CM code: 493 [asthma]). A disease was considered to be incident when there were no prior relevant claims in the study period, including a look-back period from 2006 to 2008. Patients were also required to have at least 12 months of continuous enrolment in the NHI programme both prior to and following the index date (defined below), and at least three outpatient claims or one inpatient claim in the year that followed. Patients were also required to have at least one dispensing claim for a relevant respiratory treatment (specified below) in the year following the index date.

Exclusion criteria included the presence of conditions (based on ICD-9-CM codes used for claims) related to lung or bronchial developmental anomalies, degenerative processes, bronchiectasis, pulmonary resection or other significant respiratory disorders (excluding cancer) that could interfere with clinical diagnosis of COPD or its natural history (ICD-9-CM codes 490, 494 or 495).

Disease cohorts

Three mutually exclusive incident disease cohorts (asthma, COPD and ACO) were defined for analysis based on a combination of ICD-9-CM diagnosis codes and respiratory drug use. The asthma cohort included patients with claims related to asthma (ICD-9-CM code 493) and a prescription for an asthma-specific treatment (specified below), while the COPD cohort included patients with claims related to COPD (ICD-9-CM codes 491, 492 or 496) and a prescription for a COPD-specific treatment. However, patients were excluded from these cohorts if they fulfilled any of the necessary criteria for the ACO cohort, while patients with claims for both asthma and COPD who did not fulfil any of the criteria for the ACO cohort were excluded from the study.

For the ACO cohort, patients conforming to any of four operational definitions of ACO were included. These definitions were not mutually exclusive, but patients conforming to multiple definitions were counted only once in the overall ACO cohort. The four operational definitions explored were as follows:

1) ACO-I: patients with a claim related to chronic obstructive asthma (ICD-9-CM code: 493.2×) at the index date and at least 3 outpatient claims and/or at least 1 inpatient claim with this code in the year post-index, with or without additional asthma or COPD codes;
2) ACO-II: patients with ICD-9-CM codes for both asthma and COPD in a single claim at the index date and at least 3 outpatient claims and/or at least 1 inpatient claim with codes for both asthma and COPD in the year post-index;
3) ACO-III: patients with incident COPD, as defined for the COPD cohort above, with at least 3 outpatient claims and/or at least 1 inpatient claim for asthma in the 12 months pre-index;
4) ACO-IV: patients with incident asthma, as defined for the asthma cohort above, with at least 3 outpatient claims and/or at least 1 inpatient claim for COPD in the 12 months pre-index.

Index date definition

The index date for the COPD and asthma cohorts was the date of the first relevant medical claim in the study time frame (encompassing the look-back period from 2006 to 2008) (Fig. 1). For the ACO cohort, the index date was the date of the first medical claim for the related diagnosis: the date of the first claim with the 493.2× ICD-9-CM code [ACO-I definition]; the date of the first claim with both asthma and COPD codes [ACO-II]; the date of the first claim with a COPD code [ACO-III]; or the date of the first claim with an asthma code [ACO-IV]. Where patients met the criteria for more than one ACO definition with different possible index dates, the earlier index date was used.

Relevant respiratory treatments

Relevant respiratory treatments for COPD included: short- or long-acting muscarinic antagonists (SAMAs or LAMAs), short- or long-acting β_2-agonists (SABAs or LABAs), inhaled corticosteroids (ICS), ICS/LABA combinations, systemic corticosteroids, xanthine or systemic β_2-agonists. Relevant treatments for asthma or ACO comprised all of these classes, plus leukotriene receptor antagonists (LTRAs) or anti-immunoglobulin E (anti-IgE) therapy. Each prescription was assumed to be of 30 days' duration with the exception of systemic corticosteroids, which were classified as being prescribed for either 14 days or fewer, or more than 14 days. Monotherapies were those that did not overlap with prescriptions of other therapies, while multiple therapies in combination or separate inhalers had to be prescribed together or overlap by one day to be considered part of a combination.

Outcomes

The following parameters were characterised and compared between cohorts: patient demographics and comorbidities (at index date); treatment with respiratory medication and medication costs (in the 12 months post-index); incidence of exacerbations (post-index); and healthcare utilisation (post-index, including: frequency of outpatient, inpatient, emergency room [ER] and intensive care unit [ICU] hospital visits; and use of X-rays, computed tomography [CT] and pulmonary function tests).

Three definitions of exacerbations were employed based on ICD-9-CM codes, and the requirement for a prescription of systemic corticosteroids for <14 days. Definition 1 required: ICD-9-CM codes 491, 492 or 496 for COPD; ICD-9-CM code 493 for asthma; and a

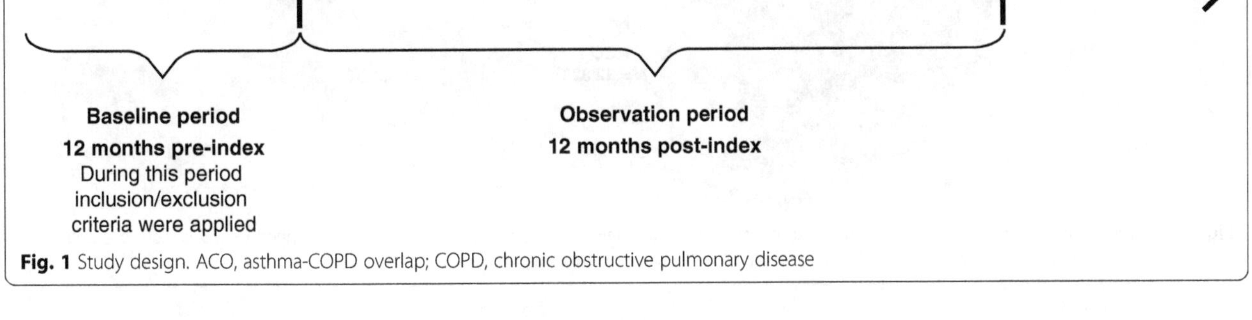

Fig. 1 Study design. ACO, asthma-COPD overlap; COPD, chronic obstructive pulmonary disease

combination of these events for ACO. Definition 2 was the same as for Definition 1, with the addition of ICD-9-CM codes 480–486 for the COPD and asthma cohorts. Definition 3 required: ICD-9-CM code 491.21 for COPD; ICD-9-CM code 493.92 for asthma; and a combination of these events for ACO.

All cost data were measured in New Taiwan Dollars and converted to US dollars (USD) using the exchange rate at the end of the data collection period (31 December, 2012) [24].

Statistical analysis

Differences between variables were assessed using the chi-squared test for categorical variables, and the student's t-test for continuous variables. All tests were two-sided and p-values < 0.05 were considered statistically significant. Analyses were performed using SAS software version 9.4 (SAS Institute, Inc., Cary, NC).

Results

Patient demographics

Of 480,900 patients with claims involving COPD codes, 69,648 patients met the criteria for the 'COPD only' cohort (Additional file 1: Figure S1). Of 621,670 patients with claims involving asthma codes, 50,293 patients met the criteria for the 'asthma only' cohort (Additional file 1: Figure S2). The ACO cohort comprised 22,328 patients (ACO-I, 7711 patients; ACO-II, 5572 patients; ACO-III, 5458 patients; ACO-IV, 8765 patients; some patients met the criteria for more than one definition) (Additional file 1: Figure S3). Using this figure, it can be estimated that the incidence of ACO among adults of ≥40 years of age in Taiwan during the study period (2009–2011) is approximately 7.0 per 10,000, based on the average mid-year populations in this period. There were 1865 patients with claims with both asthma and COPD codes, but who did not meet any of the four pre-defined criteria for ACO (the COPD/asthma cohort) and were excluded from the analysis. The overall distribution of the patient cohorts is shown in Fig. 2.

Patients in the ACO and COPD cohorts had similar mean ages and were more likely to be male, while patients in the asthma cohort were younger and more likely to be female (Table 1). Patients in the ACO cohort had the highest mean Charlson comorbidity index (CCI) score ($p < 0.0001$ vs asthma and COPD), while patients with asthma had the lowest score. In particular, patients with ACO had a significantly higher presence of cardiovascular comorbidities (cerebrovascular disease, congestive heart failure and hypertension) than patients with COPD or asthma ($p < 0.0001$, all comparisons).

Across the four groups with different ACO definitions (Additional file 1: Table S1) the percentage of male patients ranged from 52.5% (ACO-III) to 66.2% (ACO-I) versus 60.4% for the ACO cohort overall; the mean age ranged from 65.8 years (ACO-II) to 72.0 years (ACO-IV) versus 68.7 years for the ACO cohort overall; and the mean CCI score ranged from 0.66 (ACO-II) to 1.13 (ACO-IV) versus 0.91 for the ACO cohort overall.

Respiratory-related medication use and costs

In all cohorts, the most commonly prescribed medication in the 12 months post-index was oral xanthine, followed by oral systemic β_2-agonists and oral systemic corticosteroids (≤14 days) (Fig. 3). SABAs were among the most commonly prescribed medications (30.4–43.6% of patients), while SAMAs were less frequently prescribed (7.8–13.3% of patients). All short-acting therapies (SABAs, SAMAs and SABA/SAMA combinations) were more commonly prescribed than long-acting

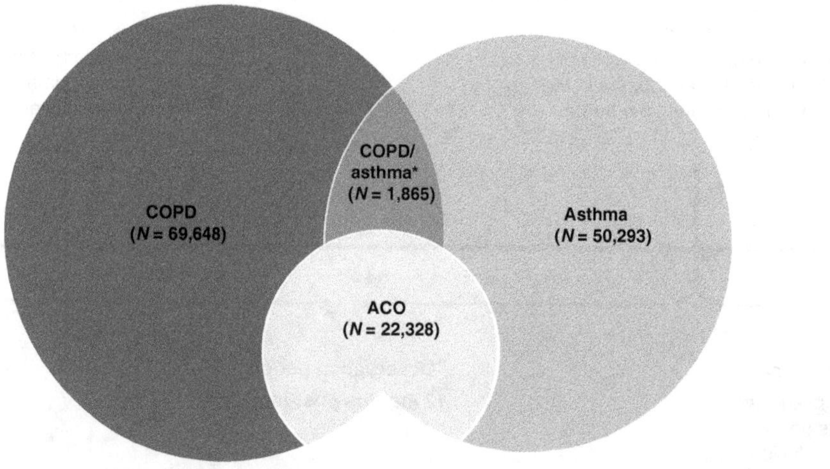

Fig. 2 Diagram of the four cohorts identified in the study. *Patients with claims for both COPD and asthma not meeting any of four pre-defined criteria for ACO. ACO, asthma-COPD overlap; COPD, chronic obstructive pulmonary disease

Table 1 Demographics of the ACO, COPD and asthma cohorts at index date

Characteristics	ACO cohort (*N* = 22,328)	COPD cohort (*N* = 69,648)	Asthma cohort (*N* = 50,293)	*p*-value (ACO vs COPD)	*p*-value (ACO vs asthma)	*p*-value (3 groups)
Gender, *n* (%)						
Male	13,477 (60.4)	45,165 (64.9)	19,499 (38.8)	< 0.0001	< 0.0001	< 0.0001
Age						
Mean (SD), years	68.7 (13.3)	68.1 (13.4)	60.6 (13.3)	< 0.0001	< 0.0001	< 0.0001
Socioeconomic status (monthly income), *n* (%)						
High: ≥$1035	5118 (22.9)	15,144 (21.7)	16,013 (31.8)	< 0.0001	< 0.0001	< 0.0001
Medium: $690–$1035	9110 (40.8)	29,832 (42.8)	19,922 (39.6)			
Low: <$690	7558 (33.9)	22,430 (32.2)	13,838 (27.5)			
Unknown	542 (2.4)	2242 (3.2)	520 (1.0)			
Charlson comorbidity index, mean (SD)	0.91 (1.49)	0.85 (1.57)	0.51 (1.17)	< 0.0001	< 0.0001	< 0.0001
Comorbidities[a], *n* (%)						
Anaemia	1136 (5.1)	3086 (4.4)	1144 (2.3)	< 0.0001	< 0.0001	< 0.0001
Anxiety	1576 (7.1)	3612 (5.2)	3351 (6.7)	< 0.0001	0.0505	< 0.0001
Cancer	1272 (5.7)	4200 (6.0)	1764 (3.5)	0.0668	< 0.0001	< 0.0001
Cerebrovascular disease	3337 (15.0)	9372 (13.5)	2846 (5.7)	< 0.0001	< 0.0001	< 0.0001
Congestive heart failure	1566 (7.0)	2817 (4.0)	1267 (2.5)	< 0.0001	< 0.0001	< 0.0001
Dementia	1283 (5.8)	3577 (5.1)	977 (1.9)	0.0004	< 0.0001	< 0.0001
Diabetes mellitus	3442 (15.4)	10,386 (14.9)	5947 (11.8)	0.0670	< 0.0001	< 0.0001
Hypertension	8950 (40.1)	22,136 (31.8)	13,802 (27.4)	< 0.0001	< 0.0001	< 0.0001
Peptic ulcer	2698 (12.1)	6119 (8.8)	3393 (6.8)	< 0.0001	< 0.0001	< 0.0001

Differences between variables were assessed using the chi-squared test (categorical variables) or the student's t-test (continuous variables). All tests were two-sided and *p*-values < 0.05 were considered statistically significant
ACO asthma-COPD overlap, *COPD* chronic obstructive pulmonary disease, *SD* standard deviation
[a]Only comorbidities occurring at rates >5% in any cohort are presented

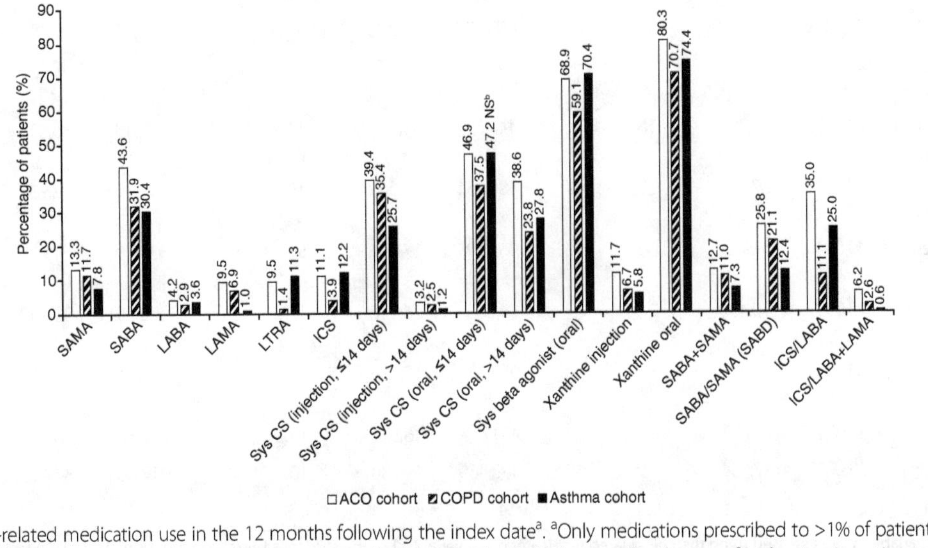

Fig. 3 Respiratory-related medication use in the 12 months following the index date[a]. [a]Only medications prescribed to >1% of patients in at least two cohorts are presented. [b]All comparisons with ACO were statistically significant ($p \leq 0.001$) except for the use of oral systemic corticosteroids (≤14 days) between the ACO and COPD cohorts ($p = 0.500$). ACO, asthma-COPD overlap; COPD, chronic obstructive pulmonary disease; CS, corticosteroid; ICS, inhaled corticosteroid; IgE, immunoglobulin E; LABA, long-acting $β_2$-agonist; LAMA, long-acting muscarinic antagonist; LTRA, leukotriene receptor antagonist; NS, not significant; SABA, short-acting $β_2$-agonist; SABD, short-acting bronchodilator; SAMA, short-acting muscarinic antagonist; Sys, systemic

bronchodilator monotherapies (LAMAs or LABAs) in all cohorts. ICS/LABA combinations were also prescribed more commonly than LAMAs or LABAs alone. Oral systemic corticosteroids and ≤14-day courses of injected systemic corticosteroids were prescribed more frequently than ICS.

For most medications, the prescription rate was highest in the ACO cohort (Fig. 3); however, prescription of ICS, LTRAs and oral systemic β_2-agonists was higher in patients with asthma than patients with ACO ($p < 0.0001$) or COPD. Some differences in prescription frequencies between cohorts were considerable: ICS and ICS/LABA combinations were prescribed approximately three times more frequently in patients with ACO than COPD (ICS: 11.1% vs 3.9%; ICS/LABA: 35.0% vs 11.1%), while LTRAs were prescribed over six times more frequently (9.5% vs 1.4%). LAMA monotherapy and ICS/LABA + LAMA open triple therapy were prescribed almost ten times more frequently in patients with ACO than asthma (LAMA: 9.5% vs 1.0%; ICS/LABA + LAMA: 6.2% vs 0.6%). In patients with COPD, LAMA monotherapy was prescribed approximately seven times more frequently as in patients with asthma (6.9% vs 1.0%; Fig. 3).

The total cost of each medication in the 12 months post-index was generally highest in the COPD cohort, although the asthma cohort had the highest total cost for anti-IgE, ICS, LTRA and ICS/LABA medications (Table 2). However, when assessed as the mean cost per patient, the costs of most medications were highest in the ACO cohort.

When comparing the different medications, ICS/LABA therapy contributed the most to the total medication costs in all cohorts. This was followed by LAMA monotherapy

Table 2 Respiratory-related medication costs in the 12 months post-index date

Medication type[a]	ACO cohort ($N = 22,328$)			COPD only ($N = 69,648$)			Asthma only ($N = 50,293$)		
	Total cost (USD)	Number of patients	Mean cost/ person (USD)	Total cost (USD)	Number of patients	Mean cost/ person (USD)	Total cost (USD)	Number of patients	Mean cost/ person (USD)
Anti-IgE	28,993	< 5[b]		2842	< 5[b]		61,397	6	10,233
ICS	132,777	2482	53	116,536	2710	43	283,766	6136	46
LTRA	329,286	2119	155	81,646	993	82	738,900	5659	131
LABA	16,242	944	17	35,013	2023	17	16,909	1832	9
ICS/LABA	2,224,844	7820	285	1,582,052	7732	205	2,465,128	12,579	196
LAMA	742,647	2125	349	1,497,123	4826	310	110,641	488	227
SABA	276,888	9731	28	461,267	22,227	21	222,497	15,299	15
SAMA	86,336	2974	29	181,629	8179	22	54,971	3900	14
SABA/SAMA (SABD)	319,419	5758	55	653,839	14,720	44	181,868	6228	29
Systemic β_2-agonist injection	6	20	0.3	34	62	1	15	48	0.3
Systemic β_2-agonist oral	241,131	15,384	16	444,653	41,179	11	194,135	35,419	5
Systemic corticosteroids injection (≤14 days)	223,498	8794	25	480,051	24,662	19	197,142	12,936	15
Systemic corticosteroids injection (>14 days)	43,054	719	60	96,799	1745	55	33,618	619	54
Systemic corticosteroids oral (≤14 days)	18,951	10,480	2	34,385	26,126	1	30,325	23,742	1
Systemic corticosteroids oral (>14 days)	62,043	8620	7	97,912	16,564	6	61,374	13,994	4
Xanthine injection	3469	2611	1	4517	4629	1	2102	2894	1
Xanthine oral	295,758	17,934	16	483,469	49,230	10	217,083	37,405	6
Xanthine unknown	2	6	0.3	0.4	8	0.1	0	5	0.0

Differences between variables were assessed using the chi-squared test (categorical variables) or the student's t-test (continuous variables). All tests were two-sided and p-values < 0.05 were considered statistically significant

ACO asthma-COPD overlap, *COPD* chronic obstructive pulmonary disease, *ICS* inhaled corticosteroid, *IgE* immunoglobulin E, *LABA* long-acting β_2-agonist, *LAMA* long-acting muscarinic antagonist, *LTRA* leukotriene receptor antagonist, *SABA* short-acting β_2-agonist, *SABD* short-acting bronchodilator, *SAMA* short-acting muscarinic antagonist, *USD* US dollars

[a]Categories were not mutually exclusive

[b]Numbers <5 could not be retrieved from the Health and Welfare Data Science Center

in the ACO and COPD cohorts, while the second greatest contributor in the asthma cohort was LTRA therapy. Other medications were minor contributors to the overall medication cost for each cohort, contributing <11% of the total. Despite the high use of oral xanthine and oral systemic β_2-agonists, their costs contributed <8% of the total medication cost in any cohort. Although anti-IgE therapy had the highest cost per patient in all cohorts, it was rarely prescribed (≤6 patients in any cohort). Of the other medications, LAMA monotherapy had the highest cost per patient in all cohorts, followed by ICS/LABA therapy.

As in the overall ACO cohort, oral xanthine and oral systemic β_2-agonists were the most commonly prescribed medications in each of the groups with different ACO definitions, while prescription rates of ICS, LAMAs, LTRAs and ICS/LABA + LAMA combinations were among the lowest of the medications (Additional file 1: Table S2).

There were significant differences in the use of most medications between the groups with different ACO definitions (p-values for each ACO group vs the overall ACO cohort were < 0.05 for ≥8 of the 15 medications prescribed to >5% of patients in the ACO cohort; Additional file 1: Table S2). However, the magnitudes of the differences in medication use between the different ACO groups were <12% for all medications except for ICS/LABA, which had a difference of 16.3% between the ACO-I and ACO-II groups (31.4% vs 47.7% of patients). The medications with the next largest differences between groups were systemic corticosteroid injections for ≤14 days (prescription rates ranged from 33.3% [ACO-II] to 44.9% [ACO-IV]), and SABAs (prescription rates ranged from 41.5% [ACO-II] to 49.2% [ACO-IV]) (Additional file 1: Table S2).

All-cause medical utilisation

In the 12 months post-index, patients with ACO had a significantly higher mean number of all-cause outpatient visits, ER visits and ICU admissions than patients with asthma or COPD ($p < 0.05$, all comparisons) (Additional file 1: Table S3). However, patients with COPD had the highest mean number of inpatient visits ($p < 0.05$, all comparisons). Pulmonary function tests were used most commonly in the ACO cohort, while use of CT was highest in the COPD cohort. X-ray use was similar in the ACO and COPD cohorts and higher than in the asthma cohort (Additional file 1: Table S3).

Respiratory-related medical utilisation

In the 12 months post-index, patients in the ACO cohort had the highest mean numbers of respiratory-related outpatient and ER visits (Table 3). Patients with ACO also had a significantly higher mean number of hospitalisations and ICU admissions than patients with asthma or COPD ($p < 0.0001$). A higher percentage of patients with ACO experienced all types of hospital visit than patients with asthma or COPD (data not shown).

Use of X-ray and pulmonary function tests was significantly higher in the ACO cohort (X-ray: 51.0%; pulmonary function tests: 21.2%) than in the asthma (X-ray: 25.9%; pulmonary function tests: 14.4%) or COPD cohorts (X-ray: 43.1%; pulmonary function tests: 14.6%) (Table 3). Use of CT was similar between the ACO and COPD cohorts (both 9.0% [$p = 0.8800$]) and higher than in the asthma cohort (3.5%).

Of the groups with different ACO definitions, patients in the ACO-IV group generally had the highest resource use, with the highest mean number of outpatient visits and the highest use of X-ray and CT scans (Additional file 1: Table S4). Patients in the ACO-II group had the lowest resource use with the lowest percentages of patients experiencing ER visits, hospitalisations and ICU admissions (data not shown).

Exacerbations

In the 12 months post-index, more patients with ACO experienced exacerbations (35.3%) than patients with asthma (29.0%, $p < 0.0001$ vs ACO) or COPD (18.6%, $p < 0.0001$ vs ACO) based on Definition 1. The same pattern was observed for the other two definitions (Table 3). The higher rate of exacerbations in the ACO cohort was reflected in the higher use of injected systemic corticosteroids (≤14 days) in this cohort; however, the use of oral systemic corticosteroids (≤14 days) was similar between the ACO and COPD cohorts. More exacerbations required outpatient than inpatient treatment in each cohort (outpatient vs inpatient visits: ACO: 28.0% vs 15.2%; asthma: 26.7% vs 3.7%; COPD: 12.1% vs 8.8%). Patients with ACO had considerably higher rates of exacerbations requiring ER visits (8.2% vs 2.7% for the COPD cohort [$p < 0.0001$] and vs 2.3% for the asthma cohort [$p < 0.0001$]) and ICU treatment (4.3% vs 2.7% for the COPD cohort [$p < 0.0001$] and vs 0.5% for the asthma cohort [$p < 0.0001$]) than patients with COPD or asthma. The same pattern was observed for the other two definitions of exacerbations.

Of the groups with different ACO definitions, the percentage of patients experiencing exacerbations in the 12 months post-index was highest in the ACO-IV group (38.5% using Definition 1) and lowest in the ACO-II group (33.4% using Definition 1) (Additional file 1: Table S4).

Discussion

Overall, these findings suggest that patients with ACO in Taiwan experience a considerably higher disease burden than patients with asthma or COPD alone, as evidenced by patterns of healthcare and medication

Table 3 Respiratory-related medical utilisation in the 12 months post-index date

Utilisation type	ACO cohort (*N* = 22,328)	COPD cohort (*N* = 69,648)	Asthma cohort (*N* = 50,293)	*p*-value (ACO vs COPD)	*p*-value (ACO vs asthma)	*p*-value (3 groups)
Medical utilisation (outpatient)						
Mean number of outpatient visits (SD)	9.14 (7.48)	6.43 (5.39)	5.68 (4.36)	< 0.0001	< 0.0001	< 0.0001
Mean number of ER visits (SD)	2.01 (3.20)	1.43 (1.00)	1.42 (1.22)	< 0.0001	< 0.0001	< 0.0001
Medical utilisation (inpatient)						
Mean number of inpatient visits (SD)	1.93 (1.54)	1.68 (1.38)	1.38 (0.95)	< 0.0001	< 0.0001	< 0.0001
Mean number of ICU admissions (SD)	1.31 (0.70)	1.20 (0.53)	1.14 (0.42)	< 0.0001	< 0.0001	< 0.0001
X-rays, *n* (%)	11,390 (51.0)	30,044 (43.1)	13,046 (25.9)	< 0.0001	< 0.0001	< 0.0001
Computed tomography, *n* (%)	2010 (9.0)	6293 (9.0)	1737 (3.5)	0.8800	< 0.0001	< 0.0001
Pulmonary function tests, *n* (%)	4724 (21.2)	10,157 (14.6)	7243 (14.4)	< 0.0001	< 0.0001	< 0.0001
Exacerbations, *n* (%)						
Event 1[a]	7883 (35.3)	12,934 (18.6)	14,583 (29.0)	< 0.0001	< 0.0001	< 0.0001
Event 2[b]	2207 (9.9)	3658 (5.3)	1876 (3.7)	< 0.0001	< 0.0001	< 0.0001
Event 3[c]	3083 (13.8)	5068 (7.3)	2577 (5.1)	< 0.0001	< 0.0001	< 0.0001

Differences between variables were assessed using the chi-squared test (categorical variables) or the student's t-test (continuous variables). All tests were two-sided and *p*-values < 0.05 were considered statistically significant

ACO asthma-COPD overlap, *COPD* chronic obstructive pulmonary disease, *ER* emergency room, *ICD-9-CM* International Classification of Disease, ninth revision, clinical modification, *ICU* intensive care unit, *SD* standard deviation

[a]Event 1 for:
- COPD: visits with ICD-9 code of 491, 492 or 496 with prescription of systemic corticosteroids for <14 days
- Asthma: visits with ICD-9 code of 493 with prescription of systemic corticosteroids for <14 days
- ACO: combination of COPD and asthma event

[b]Event 2 for:
- COPD: visits with ICD-9 code of 491, 492 or 496, and 480–486, with prescription of systemic corticosteroids for <14 days
- Asthma: visits with ICD-9 code of 493 and 480–486, with prescription of systemic corticosteroids for <14 days
- ACO: combination of COPD and asthma event

[c]Event 3 for:
- COPD: visits with ICD-9 code of 491.21 with prescription of systemic corticosteroids for <14 days
- Asthma: visits with ICD-9-CM code of 493.92 with prescription of systemic corticosteroids for <14 days
- ACO: combination of COPD and asthma event

utilisation. These results are consistent with findings from studies in other Asian countries (Korea, [12, 13] Japan [16] and China [19]) and Western countries [4–6, 8, 9].

Several studies have investigated the prevalence of ACO, with estimates ranging from 1.6% to 4.5% across studies in Italy, Latin America, South Korea, and the United States [25]. However, few estimates of incidence have been made; one study reported an estimated incidence of ACO in a Danish population sample of 0.64 per 1000 person-years, [26] while another study reported an estimated incidence in the Ontario population of 1.9 per 1000 people in 2012 [27]. As with prevalence estimates, some degree of variation might be expected due to differences in populations and definitions of ACO used between studies. However, further research is required to corroborate the estimated incidence in this study.

The similarity in age and gender between patients with ACO and COPD, and the lower age and higher proportion of females in patients with asthma, observed here are consistent with studies in Korea [14] and Japan [18]. The mean age and gender distribution in patients with ACO here are also consistent with smaller studies in Taiwan; [21, 22] however, studies outside Asia mostly found that patients with ACO were younger [10, 28] and more likely to be female [8, 10, 11] than those with COPD. These differences may relate to the requirement for patients in this study to be ≥40 years of age, thereby pre-selecting an older population.

The higher presence of comorbidities in patients with ACO than COPD or asthma found here is consistent with studies in Korea, [12] Spain [11] and the USA, [10] although other studies have reported a similar or lower presence of comorbidities in patients with ACO compared with COPD [14, 18]. These inconsistencies may be related to varying procedures for recruiting and categorising patients, and varying inclusion and exclusion criteria [25].

The higher medication use and higher associated costs in patients with ACO compared with asthma or COPD has been observed in several other studies [8, 10, 12]. The higher use of LTRA and ICS in patients with asthma compared with patients with COPD, and higher use of LAMA-containing agents in patients with COPD compared with patients with asthma, are consistent with the GINA [29, 30] and GOLD [31, 32] guideline recommendations available during the study and the differences in asthma and COPD phenotypes.

The high use of xanthine oral therapy in all cohorts is perhaps surprising given its reported poorer efficacy compared with alternative therapies, higher risk of side effects [33–35] and resultant low priority in the GINA [29, 30] and GOLD [31, 32] guidelines available during this study (this is maintained in the current guidelines [3, 36]). Inhaled β_2-agonists have a quicker onset of action and reduced risk of side effects compared with their oral counterparts, [29–32] but here, use of oral β_2-agonists was higher than inhaled β_2-agonists in all cohorts. This is consistent with studies of COPD therapy in the Taiwanese population [37] and other Asian countries, [38] which attributed the higher relative use of oral bronchodilators to lower costs and less clinical evidence being required for their prescription; patients may also find oral medication easier to take. European studies suggest that the use of xanthines and oral bronchodilators for COPD treatment is considerably lower than reported in Asia, while use of LAMA, ICS and ICS/LABA combinations tends to be higher [39–42].

Patients in the ACO cohort were often treated with short-term (≤14 days) systemic corticosteroids, SABAs and ICS/LABA combinations. Although guidelines specific to ACO were not available at the time of this study, more recent GOLD and GINA guidelines recommended ICS therapy with the possible addition of a LABA and/or LAMA [3, 43]. The use of short-term corticosteroids and SABAs observed here may relate to the higher exacerbation frequency in patients with ACO, which could potentially be reduced with longer-term use of guideline-recommended therapy.

The higher rate of hospital visits for patients with ACO compared with COPD was consistent with studies in Korea [12, 13] and China [19]. Reported rates of hospital visits may vary between Asian and other countries as specialists are more commonly located in public hospitals in Asia, while more outpatient or private care options may be available in other countries due to variations in reimbursement systems. An Asian study examining medical costs found that patients with ACO had higher medical costs than patients with COPD, [12] as seen here. Outside Asia, several studies report similar findings, with patients with ACO having a higher presence of comorbidities and exacerbations than patients with COPD or asthma (the higher rate of exacerbations in patients with ACO found here is consistent with other studies within Asia [19] and elsewhere [4, 8, 11, 28]). Patients with ACO experienced more hospitalisations and ER visits [6, 8, 10, 44] than patients with asthma or COPD, with higher resulting medical costs [10, 44, 45].

As there is no consensus on a formal definition of ACO, an exploratory analysis was performed to examine the impact of different definitions, using four different algorithms to define patients with ACO (ACO groups I-IV). Out of these different groups, patients in the ACO-IV group (incident asthma and a previous history of COPD) tended to have the highest resource use. Due to their history of COPD, these patients tended to be older and may have progressed further in the course of their disease (they also had a higher presence of comorbidities) than patients in the ACO-I and ACO-II groups, who were newly diagnosed with chronic obstructive asthma, or with concurrent asthma and COPD. These newly diagnosed patients had lower resource use in the 12 months post-index, suggesting that earlier diagnosis and intervention may reduce medical costs; alternatively, as these patients were younger, they may have progressed less far in the course of their disease and so would not be directly comparable with the older patients. These differences demonstrate that varying definitions of ACO can affect patient outcome measures; ultimately, greater consistency between definitions used in different studies would enable clearer comparisons to be made and overall trends to be identified. The lack of a clear definition makes it challenging to characterise patients and their outcomes, but also demonstrates the heterogeneity of patients described as having ACO, suggesting a spectrum of pathophysiology between COPD and asthma that cannot necessarily be split into well-defined groups [46, 47]. Further follow-up of these different patient groups could provide more evidence to assess the value of earlier diagnosis and intervention, and to compare the values of the different ACO definitions.

A possible consequence of the higher disease burden observed in patients with ACO compared with those with asthma and COPD alone is that patients with ACO may have a poorer long-term prognosis. However, studies assessing long-term outcomes in patients with ACO have shown mixed results: a study in the USA reported a higher mortality risk in patients with ACO compared with patients with asthma or COPD, [7] while an Italian study reported that the long-term prognosis of patients with ACO was poorer than that of patients with asthma, but similar to that of patients with COPD [48]. Studies in Spain [49] and Sweden [50] reported lower mortality rates in patients with ACO than in patients with COPD alone, while a Canadian study reported a lower all-cause mortality rate, but a higher respiratory-cause mortality rate, in patients with ACO compared with COPD or asthma [51]. Similarly mixed results have been reported in Asian populations, although fewer studies have been undertaken: studies in China [52] and Japan [18, 53] have reported lower mortality rates in patients with ACO compared with COPD, while a study in Korea reported a higher mortality rate in patients with ACO [13]. To the best of our knowledge, the long-term prognosis and mortality rates of patients with ACO have not been assessed in the Taiwanese population; this would be an interesting extension to the current study. The conflicting nature of these results can be at least partly attributed to the considerable variations between studies in characteristics and sizes of patient populations, type of data sources used, factors adjusted for in models and follow-up period duration, as well as the definition of ACO employed. The differences in long-term prognosis between COPD, asthma and ACO cannot therefore be established; further research with consistent, systematic methodology is required to confirm whether the higher disease burden in patients with ACO translates to a poorer long-term prognosis.

A strength of this study was that the patients were from a population-based data source without any sampling, and that the data source had near-total population coverage; therefore, the data are representative of the entire Taiwanese population. A limitation was the potential risk of patient misclassification, as classification was dependent on ICD-9-CM codes and how accurately the codes were applied, rather than spirometric or other clinical data, which were unavailable. Patients may have received both asthma and COPD-related ICD-9-CM codes in claims to access certain medications, rather than due to a definitive classification of ACO. Data on smoking status were also unavailable for analysis, so it was not possible to take smoking history into account when assigning disease classifications. There appears to be a growing consensus that tobacco exposure is a requirement for a classification of ACO, while patients with asthma and non-fully reversible airflow obstruction, but without a history of tobacco exposure, should be classified as having obstructive asthma and not ACO [54–56]. Without smoking history data, it was not possible to distinguish between such patients in this study. A further limitation of this study was the requirement for patients to have at least three relevant outpatient claims or one relevant inpatient claim in the year following index date, which reflects a relatively high level of patient contact with healthcare providers that may not be generalisable to other countries and healthcare systems.

Conclusions

Patients with ACO in Taiwan experience a higher disease burden than patients with asthma or COPD alone, as evidenced by their higher presence of comorbidities and exacerbations, and their increased healthcare and medication utilisation. Healthcare costs associated with ACO also appear to be higher than those for asthma or COPD alone. Further research into how to define and diagnose patients with ACO will help to further characterise this important and diverse patient population.

Additional file

Additional file 1: Figure S1. Patient flow diagram for the COPD cohort. **Figure S2.** Patient flow diagram for the asthma cohort. **Figure S3.** Patient flow diagram for the ACO cohort and groups with different ACO definitions. **Table S1.** Characteristics of the ACO cohort and groups with different ACO definitions at index date. **Table S2.** Respiratory-related medication use in the 12 months post-index date for the ACO cohort and groups with different ACO definitions. **Table S3.** All-cause medical utilisation in the asthma, COPD and ACO cohorts in the 12 months post-index date. **Table S4.** Respiratory-related medical utilisation in the 12 months post-index date for the ACO cohort and groups with different ACO definitions.

Abbreviations

ACO: Asthma COPD overlap; anti-IgE: Anti-immunoglobulin E; CCI: Charlson comorbidity index; COPD: Chronic obstructive pulmonary disease; CT: Computed tomography; ER: Emergency room; GINA: Global Initiative for Asthma; GOLD: Global Initiative for Chronic Obstructive Lung Disease; ICD-9-CM: International Classification of Disease, ninth revision, clinical modification; ICS: Inhaled corticosteroid; ICU: Intensive care unit; LABA: Long-acting β_2-agonist; LAMA: Long-acting muscarinic antagonist; LTRA: Leukotriene receptor antagonist; NHI: National Health Insurance; NS: Not significant; SABA: Short-acting β_2-agonist; SABD: Short-acting bronchodilator; SAMA: Short-acting muscarinic antagonist; SD: Standard deviation; USD: US dollars

Acknowledgements

This study was a collaboration between the Health Data Research Center at National Taiwan University (NTU) and GSK. Source data were obtained from the Health and Welfare Data Science Center, Ministry of Health and Welfare, Taiwan. The authors wish to acknowledge Hui-Min Diana Lin, RPh, for developing the list of Taiwan-specific drug codes according to the Anatomical and Therapeutic Classification System. Editorial assistance in the preparation of this manuscript was provided by Elizabeth Jameson, PhD, and Natasha Thomas, PhD, of Fishawack Indicia Ltd., and was funded by GSK.

Funding

This study was a collaboration between the Health Data Research Center at National Taiwan University (NTU) and GSK, and was funded by both NTU and GSK (NTU grant number: 105R104012; GSK study number: PRJ2356). GSK and NTU employees both contributed to the study design, data analysis, data interpretation, and writing of the manuscript. The corresponding author had access to the aggregated results and the final responsibility to submit results for publication.

Authors' contributions

SS and LD'S contributed to the study conception and design and were involved in data analysis or interpretation. R-FP and Y-CJ were involved in data analysis or interpretation. KW contributed to the study conception and design. Y-WK and KAC contributed to the study conception and design and were involved in data acquisition and data analysis or interpretation. Y-YY was involved in data acquisition and data analysis or interpretation. All authors were involved in preparation and review of the manuscript and approved the final version to be submitted.

Consent for publication

Not applicable.

Competing interests

SS, LD'S and KW are employees of GSK and hold stocks/shares in GSK. R-FP, Y-WK, Y-YY, Y-CJ and KAC declare that they have no competing interests.

Author details

[1]R&D, Real World Evidence & Epidemiology, GSK, 50 Beach Road, #21-00 Gateway West, Singapore 189720, Singapore. [2]Health Data Research Center, National Taiwan University, No.33, Linsen South Road, Suite 526, Taipei 10051, Taiwan. [3]National Respiratory Physician Lead, GSK, 7333 Mississauga Road, Mississauga, ON L5N 6L4, Canada. [4]R&D, Real World Evidence & Epidemiology, GSK, 1250 South Collegeville Road, Collegeville, PA 19426, USA. [5]National Taiwan University Hospital, No.7, Zhongshan S. Road, Zhongzheng District, Taipei City 10002, Taiwan. [6]Present Address: Ministry of Health and Welfare, Taipei City, Taiwan.

References

1. Global Initiative for Asthma. Global strategy for asthma management and prevention, updated 2014. http://ginasthma.org/. Accessed 6 Oct 2014.
2. Global Initiative for Chronic Obstructive Lung Disease. Global strategy for the diagnosis, management, and prevention of chronic obstructive pulmonary disease, updated 2014. www.goldcopd.org. Accessed 6 Oct 2014.
3. Global Initiative for Asthma. Global strategy for asthma management and prevention, updated 2017. http://ginasthma.org/. Accessed 15 May 2017.
4. Alshabanat A, Zafari Z, Albanyan O, Dairi M, FitzGerald JM. Asthma and COPD overlap syndrome (ACOS): a systematic review and meta analysis. PLoS One. 2015;10:e0136065.
5. Tho NV, Park HY, Nakano Y. Asthma-COPD overlap syndrome (ACOS): a diagnostic challenge. Respirology. 2016;21:410–8.
6. de Marco R, Pesce G, Marcon A, Accordini S, Antonicelli L, Bugiani M, et al. The coexistence of asthma and chronic obstructive pulmonary disease (COPD): prevalence and risk factors in young, middle-aged and elderly people from the general population. PLoS One. 2013;8:e62985.
7. Diaz-Guzman E, Khosravi M, Mannino DM. Asthma, chronic obstructive pulmonary disease, and mortality in the U.S. population. COPD. 2011;8: 400–7.
8. Menezes AM, Montes de Oca M, Perez-Padilla R, Nadeau G, Wehrmeister FC, Lopez-Varela MV, et al. Increased risk of exacerbation and hospitalization in subjects with an overlap phenotype: COPD-asthma. Chest. 2014;145:297–304.
9. Pleasants RA, Ohar JA, Croft JB, Liu Y, Kraft M, Mannino DM, et al. Chronic obstructive pulmonary disease and asthma-patient characteristics and health impairment. COPD. 2014;11:256–66.
10. Blanchette CM, Gutierrez B, Ory C, Chang E, Akazawa M. Economic burden in direct costs of concomitant chronic obstructive pulmonary disease and asthma in a Medicare advantage population. J Manag Care Pharm. 2008;14: 176–85.
11. Miravitlles M, Soriano JB, Ancochea J, Munoz L, Duran-Tauleria E, Sanchez G, et al. Characterisation of the overlap COPD-asthma phenotype. Focus on physical activity and health status. Respir Med. 2013;107:1053–60.
12. Rhee CK, Yoon HK, Yoo KH, Kim YS, Lee SW, Park YB, et al. Medical utilization and cost in patients with overlap syndrome of chronic obstructive pulmonary disease and asthma. COPD. 2014;11:163–70.
13. Kim MA, Noh CS, Chang YJ, Hong YK, Lee JS, Lee SW, et al. Asthma and COPD overlap syndrome is associated with increased risk of hospitalisation. Int J Tuberc Lung Dis. 2015;19:864–9.
14. Chung JW, Kong KA, Lee JH, Lee SJ, Ryu YJ, Chang JH. Characteristics and self-rated health of overlap syndrome. Int J Chron Obstruct Pulmon Dis. 2014;9:795–804.
15. Kitaguchi Y, Komatsu Y, Fujimoto K, Hanaoka M, Kubo K. Sputum eosinophilia can predict responsiveness to inhaled corticosteroid treatment in patients with overlap syndrome of COPD and asthma. Int J COPD. 2012;7: 283–9.
16. Kurashima K, Takaku Y, Ohta C, Takayanagi N, Yanagisawa T, Sugita Y. COPD assessment test and severity of airflow limitation in patients with asthma, COPD, and asthma-COPD overlap syndrome. Int J Chron Obstruct Pulmon Dis. 2016;11:479–87.
17. Tamada T, Sugiura H, Takahashi T, Matsunaga K, Kimura K, Katsumata U, et al. Biomarker-based detection of asthma-COPD overlap syndrome in COPD populations. Int J Chron Obstruct Pulmon Dis. 2015;10:2169–76.
18. Yamauchi Y, Yasunaga H, Matsui H, Hasegawa W, Jo T, Takami K, et al. Comparison of in-hospital mortality in patients with COPD, asthma and asthma-COPD overlap exacerbations. Respirology. 2015;20:940–6.
19. Ding B, DiBonaventura M, Karlsson N, Ling X. Asthma-chronic obstructive pulmonary disease overlap syndrome in the urban Chinese population: prevalence and disease burden using the 2010, 2012, and 2013 China National Health and wellness surveys. Int J Chron Obstruct Pulmon Dis. 2016;11:1139–50.
20. Xie M, Wang W, Dou S, Cui L, Xiao W. Quantitative computed tomography measurements of emphysema for diagnosing asthma-chronic obstructive pulmonary disease overlap syndrome. Int J Chron Obstruct Pulmon Dis. 2016;11:953–61.
21. Chung WS, Lin CL, Kao CH. Comparison of acute respiratory events between asthma-COPD overlap syndrome and COPD patients: a population-based cohort study. Medicine (Baltimore). 2015;94:e755.
22. Yeh JJ, Wang YC, Kao CH. Asthma-chronic obstructive pulmonary diseases overlap syndrome increases the risk of incident tuberculosis: a national cohort study. PLoS One. 2016;11:e0159012.
23. Bureau of National Health Insurance of Taiwan. Universal Health Coverage in Taiwan. http://www.nhi.gov.tw/English/index.aspx. Accessed 22 Aug 2016.
24. ExchangeRates.org.uk. US Dollar to New Taiwan Dollar conversion at 31 December 2012 (1 New Taiwan Dollar = 0.0345 USD). http://www.exchangerates.org.uk/USD-TWD-31_12_2012-exchange-rate-history.html. Accessed 11 Oct 2016.
25. Wurst KE, Kelly-Reif K, Bushnell GA, Pascoe S, Barnes N. Understanding asthma-chronic obstructive pulmonary disease overlap syndrome. Respir Med. 2016;110:1–11.
26. Barnes CB, Andersen ZJ, Overvad K, Tjonneland A, Ulrik CS. Prevalence and mortality of the asthma-COPD overlap syndrome (ACOS) in Denmark: a long-term follow-up study of a large random population sample. Am J Respir Crit Care Med. 2016;193:A6161.
27. Kendzerska T, Sadatsafavi M, Aaron SD, To T, Lougheed M, FitzGerald JM, et al. Trends in asthma-COPD overlap syndrome prevalence, incidence and mortality in Ontario, Canada: a population study. Am J Respir Crit Care Med. 2015;191:A6165.
28. Hardin M, Silverman EK, Barr RG, Hansel NN, Schroeder JD, Make BJ, et al. The clinical features of the overlap between COPD and asthma. Respir Res. 2011;12:127.
29. Global Initiative for Asthma. Global strategy for asthma management and prevention, updated 2008. http://ginasthma.org/. Accessed 26 Aug 2008.
30. Global Initiative for Asthma. Global strategy for asthma management and prevention, updated 2011. http://ginasthma.org/. Accessed 26 Oct 2011.
31. Global Initiative for Chronic Obstructive Lung Disease. Global strategy for the diagnosis, management, and prevention of chronic obstructive pulmonary disease, updated 2006. http://goldcopd.org/. Accessed 28 Aug 2006.
32. Global Initiative for Chronic Obstructive Lung Disease. Global strategy for the diagnosis, management, and prevention of chronic obstructive pulmonary disease, updated 2011. http://goldcopd.org/. Accessed 27 Oct 2011.
33. Dahl R, Larsen BB, Venge P. Effect of long-term treatment with inhaled budesonide or theophylline on lung function, airway reactivity and asthma symptoms. Respir Med. 2002;96:432–8.
34. Ram FS. Use of theophylline in chronic obstructive pulmonary disease: examining the evidence. Curr Opin Pulm Med. 2006;12:132–9.
35. Ram FS, Jones P, Jardim JR, Castro AA, Alatallah AN, Lacasse Y, et al. Oral theophylline for chronic obstructive pulmonary disease (review). Cochrane Database Syst Rev. 2002:(4)CD003902.
36. Global Initiative for Chronic Obstructive Lung Disease. Global strategy for the diagnosis, management, and prevention of chronic obstructive pulmonary disease, updated 2017. www.goldcopd.org. Accessed 28 Nov 2016.
37. Dong YH, Hsu CL, Li YY, Chang CH, Lai MS. Bronchodilators use in patients with COPD. Int J Chron Obstruct Pulmon Dis. 2015;10:1769–79.

38. Tan WC. Chapter 5: Chronic Obstructive Pulmonary Disease: Pharmacological Treatment. In Respiratory Medicine: an Asian Perspective. Edited by Ip M, Chan-Yeung M, Lam W, Zhong N. Hong Kong: Hong Kong University Press; 2005.
39. Corrado A, Rossi A. How far is real life from COPD therapy guidelines? An Italian observational study. Respir Med. 2012;106:989–97.
40. Franssen FM, Spruit MA, Wouters EF. Determinants of polypharmacy and compliance with GOLD guidelines in patients with chronic obstructive pulmonary disease. Int J Chron Obstruct Pulmon Dis. 2011;6:493–501.
41. Glaab T, Banik N, Rutschmann OT, Wencker M. National survey of guideline-compliant COPD management among pneumologists and primary care physicians. COPD. 2006;3:141–8.
42. Roche N, Lepage T, Bourcereau J, Terrioux P. Guidelines versus clinical practice in the treatment of chronic obstructive pulmonary disease. Eur Respir J. 2001;18:903–8.
43. Global Initiative for Chronic Obstructive Lung Disease. Global strategy for the diagnosis, management, and prevention of chronic obstructive pulmonary disease, updated 2016. www.goldcopd.org. Accessed 15 Nov 2016.
44. Gerhardsson de Verdier M, Andersson M, Kern DM, Zhou S, Tunceli O. Asthma and chronic obstructive pulmonary disease overlap syndrome: doubled costs compared with patients with asthma alone. Value Health. 2015;18:759–66.
45. Sadatsafavi M, Tavakoli H, Kendzerska T, Gershon A, To T, Aaron SD, et al. History of asthma in patients with chronic obstructive pulmonary disease. A comparative study of economic burden. Ann Am Thorac Soc. 2016;13:188–96.
46. Gibson PG, Simpson JL. The overlap syndrome of asthma and COPD: what are its features and how important is it? Thorax. 2009;64:728–35.
47. Lenz PH, Panos RJ. Chapter 2: Asthma and COPD - overlapping disorders or distinct processes? In COPD Clinical Perspectives. Croatia: Edited by Panos RJ. InTech; 2014.
48. Sorino C, Pedone C, Scichilone N. Fifteen-year mortality of patients with asthma-COPD overlap syndrome. Eur J Intern Med. 2016;34:72–7.
49. Cosio BG, Soriano JB, Lopez-Campos JL, Calle-Rubio M, Soler-Cataluna JJ, de- Torres JP, et al. Defining the asthma-COPD overlap syndrome in a COPD cohort. Chest. 2016;149:45–52.
50. Lundbäck B, Eriksson B, Lindberg A, Ekerljung L, Muellerova H, Larsson LG, et al. A 20-year follow-up of a population study-based COPD cohort-report from the obstructive lung disease in Northern Sweden studies. COPD. 2009; 6:263–71.
51. Kendzerska T, Sadatsafavi M, Aaron SD, To TM, Lougheed MD, FitzGerald JM, et al. Concurrent physician-diagnosed asthma and chronic obstructive pulmonary disease: a population study of prevalence, incidence and mortality. PLoS One. 2017;12:e0173830.
52. Bai JW, Mao B, Yang WL, Liang S, HW L, Xu JF. Asthma-COPD overlap syndrome showed more exacerbations however lower mortality than COPD. QJM. 2017;110:431–6.
53. Suzuki M, Makita H, Konno S, Shimizu K, Kimura H, Kimura H, et al. Asthma-like features and clinical course of chronic obstructive pulmonary disease. An analysis from the Hokkaido COPD cohort study. Am J Respir Crit Care Med. 2016;194:1358–65.
54. Louie S, Zeki AA, Schivo M, Chan AL, Yoneda KY, Avdalovic M, et al. The asthma-chronic obstructive pulmonary disease overlap syndrome: pharmacotherapeutic considerations. Expert Rev Clin Pharmacol. 2013;6: 197–219.
55. Miravitlles M. Diagnosis of asthma-COPD overlap: the five commandments. Eur Respir J. 2017;49:1700506. https://doi.org/10.1183/13993003.00506-2017
56. Sin DD, Miravitlles M, Mannino DM, Soriano JB, Price D, Celli BR, et al. What is asthma-COPD overlap syndrome? Towards a consensus definition from a round table discussion. Eur Respir J. 2016;48:664–73.

Risk factors of postoperative pulmonary complications in patients with asthma and COPD

Takanori Numata*, Katsutoshi Nakayama, Satoko Fujii, Yoko Yumino, Nayuta Saito, Masahiro Yoshida, Yusuke Kurita, Kenji Kobayashi, Saburo Ito, Hirofumi Utsumi, Haruhiko Yanagisawa, Mitsuo Hashimoto, Hiroshi Wakui, Shunsuke Minagawa, Takeo Ishikawa, Hiromichi Hara, Jun Araya, Yumi Kaneko and Kazuyoshi Kuwano

Abstract

Background: Postoperative pulmonary complications (PPC) in patients with pulmonary diseases remain to be resolved clinical issue. However, most evidence regarding PPC has been established more than 10 years ago. Therefore, it is necessary to evaluate perioperative management using new inhalant drugs in patients with obstructive pulmonary diseases.

Methods: April 2014 through March 2015, 346 adult patients with pulmonary diseases (257 asthma, 89 chronic obstructive pulmonary disease (COPD)) underwent non-pulmonary surgery except cataract surgery in our university hospital. To analyze the risk factors for PPC, we retrospectively evaluated physiological backgrounds, surgical factors and perioperative specific treatment for asthma and COPD.

Results: Finally, 29 patients with pulmonary diseases (22 asthma, 7 COPD) had PPC. In patients with asthma, smoking index (≥ 20 pack-years), peripheral blood eosinophil count (≥ 200/mm^3) and severity (Global INitiative for Asthma(GINA) STEP ≥ 3) were significantly associated with PPC in the multivariate logistic regression analysis [odds ratio (95% confidence interval) = 5.4(1.4–20.8), 0.31 (0.11–0.84) and 3.2 (1.04–9.9), respectively]. In patients with COPD, age, introducing treatment for COPD, upper abdominal surgery and operation time (≥ 5 h) were significantly associated with PPC [1.18 (1.00–1.40), 0.09 (0.01–0.81), 21.2 (1.3–349) and 9.5 (1.2–77.4), respectively].

Conclusions: History of smoking or severe asthma is a risk factor of PPC in patients with asthma, and age, upper abdominal surgery, or long operation time is a risk factor of PPC in patients with COPD. Adequate inhaled corticosteroids treatment in patients with eosinophilic asthma and introducing treatment for COPD in patients with COPD could reduce PPCs.

Keywords: Risk factors, Postoperative pulmonary complication, Asthma, COPD, Eosinophils

Background

Postoperative pulmonary complications (PPCs) and their management are clinically important in patients with asthma and chronic obstructive pulmonary disease (COPD). PPCs include bronchospasm, atelectasis, pulmonary infection, respiratory failure and exacerbation of chronic pulmonary disease [1]. The prevalence of PPCs in all surgeries was reported to be 2 to 19% [1, 2]. Because PPCs contribute to mortality and longer stays in the hospital [3], it is necessary to appropriately evaluate relevant risk factors and establish perioperative management strategies. There are two types of risk factors for PPCs. One is patient-related risk factors, such as aging and pulmonary function, and the other is procedure-related risk factors, such as anesthetic techniques and operating time [1].

Although Global INitiative for Asthma (GINA) [4] and Global initiative for chronic Obstructive Lung Diseases

* Correspondence: t-numata@jikei.ac.jp
Division of Respiratory Diseases, Department of Internal Medicine, Jikei University School of Medicine, 3-25-8, Nishi-Shimbashi, Minato-ku, Tokyo, Japan

(GOLD) [5] documents describe the perioperative management, most of the evidence presented in these documents was reported from 1990 to 2000. More recent progress in treatments for pulmonary diseases, especially new inhalants and devices, has significantly improved patient quality of life. It has been reported that some video-associated surgeries could decrease the prevalence of postoperative complications [6, 7].

To reduce PPC, we implemented the preoperative pulmonary management program in our hospital over 10 years ago. In our management program, all surgical patients with an abnormal pulmonary function test undergo a medical examination performed by pulmonologists and are administered medical treatment and evaluated for risk factors for PPC development. However, most evidence regarding the risk factors for PPC was established more than 10 years ago, and recent advances in inhalant drugs have changed the clinical course in affected patients, especially those with asthma and COPD. It is therefore critically important to precisely evaluate the risk factors for PPC development during perioperative management and to use recently available inhalant drugs in patients with both asthma and COPD.

Methods

Definition of asthma

All patients with asthma were diagnosed by physicians or self-reported, when the patients had past medical histories of asthma, typical symptoms (cough, wheezing, circadian variation and seasonal episodes) and pulmonary function compatible with asthma. Severity at baseline and during exacerbation was defined according to the GINA document [4]. Recently, a category called asthma-COPD overlap (ACO) was proposed. However, the definition of ACO has not yet been confirmed. Furthermore, patients with asthma, including those potentially in the ACO category, are at high risk of intraoperative asthma attacks, and they therefore receive inhaled or systemic corticosteroid therapy to prevent bronchospasm as a serious PPC of asthma. Therefore, in the present study, we classified asthma patients with any smoking history, including ACO, as the asthma group.

Definition of COPD

All patients were diagnosed with COPD by the physicians, based on a smoking history (smoking index >10 pack-years), post-bronchodilator forced expiratory volume in one second [(FEV_1)/ forced volume capacity(FVC)] < 0.7 and the exclusion of other diseases [5].

Study subjects

Between April 2014 and March 2015, a total of 14,194 surgeries were performed in Jikei University hospital (Tokyo, Japan). We excluded 3782 cases of cataract surgery, 1081 pediatric surgeries (under 15 years old) and 223 cases of lung resection surgery from these cases. We excluded cataract surgery because of very short operation time, and also, we excluded lung resection surgery, because of a crucial risk factor for PPC by itself. The criteria for preoperative consultation by pulmonologists were as follows: (1) patients with any past or present pulmonary diseases, (2) patients with an abnormal pulmonary function test (spirometry) prior to general anesthesia, or (3) patients with abnormal chest images. After preoperative examinations, 421 patients met one or more of these criteria. The participants in the present study included 346 adult patients who consulted pulmonologists for asthma or COPD (Fig. 1). Patients with other pulmonary diseases were excluded from this study. Therefore, the operations covered in this study included those performed in the head, neck, limbs, abdomen, pelvis and cardiovascular system. This study was approved by the Ethical Committee of Jikei University (28–260(8503)).

Data collection

We retrospectively examined the gender, age, underlying pulmonary diseases, medication, smoking index, peripheral blood eosinophil counts, pulmonary function test (volume capacity(VC), forced expiratory volume in one second (FEV_1), FEV_1/FVC, and %FEV_1), Asthma Control Test (ACT), surgery-related factors (anesthetic technique, American Society of Anesthesiologists (ASA) physical status (PS), duration of operation time, and surgery site) and PPCs of all included patients. We defined PPC as bronchospasm, pneumonia, atelectasis, respiratory failure with oxygen therapy, and exacerbation of chronic pulmonary diseases within the first seven postoperative days [1, 8, 9]. We defined bronchospasm as symptoms (wheezing, shortness of breath, and cough) requiring additional medications, and we defined respiratory failure as hypoxia requiring more than oxygen therapy or prolonged oxygen therapy. We reviewed all medical records to measure these outcomes.

Intervention

Patients consulted a pulmonologist four weeks before surgery. All smokers among the included patients were instructed to quit smoking. Our standard baseline therapy for bronchial asthma is based on the GINA stepwise approach [4]. We primarily targeted safe surgeries and referred to this document. To prevent perioperative bronchospasm, we increased the dose of inhaled corticosteroids(ICS) administered to most patients. After the first visit to our department, patients with severe/uncontrolled asthma revisited the department for a final decision regarding whether surgery was advisable. In patients with GINA STEP ≥ 3,

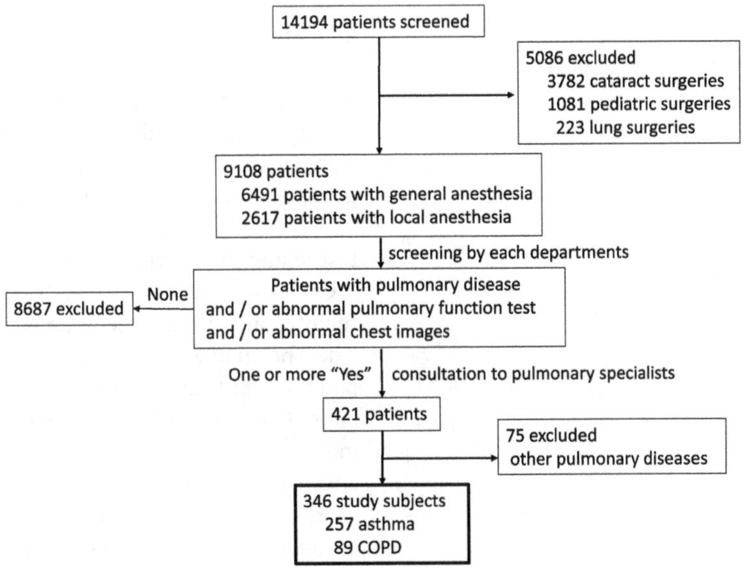

Fig. 1 Study flow

neurosurgery, emergency surgery, PPC history, or low ACT scores (approximately <22) after ICS dose escalation, we introduced systemic corticosteroids, such as prednisolone (e.g., 20 mg/day, p.o.) for several days before surgery and a short-acting corticosteroid, such as hydrocortisone (e.g., 100 mg i.v. every 8 h) on the day of the surgery [10]. We recommended postponing the scheduled surgery in patients who had asthma exacerbation within two months. In patients with COPD, we introduced a long-acting muscarinic antagonist (LAMA), a long-acting beta 2 agonist (LABA) and a combination of ICS/LABA in accordance with the GOLD document [5]. Furthermore, in patients with very low pulmonary function, we recommended local anesthesia when possible.

Statistical analysis

All statistical analyses were performed using StatView version 5 (SAS Institute Inc., Cary, NC, USA). All values are expressed as the mean ± standard deviation (SD). A p-value of <0.05 was considered statistically significant. The factors associated with patient characteristics were examined using a Mann-Whitney U test, Student's t test, Fisher's exact test, or chi-squared test (univariate model). Then, a logistic regression analysis was performed to evaluate the identified PPC risk factors (multivariate model), including age, gender (male), and other variables that achieved $p < 0.20$ in the univariate models. In patients with asthma, we selected age, gender (male), smoking index (≥20), peripheral blood eosinophil count (≥200/mm^3), GINA STEP (≥3), %FEV_1, upper abdominal surgery, perioperative systemic steroid therapy and operation time (minutes) for the multivariate analysis. On the other hand, in patients with COPD, we selected age, gender (male), COPD treatment, upper abdominal surgery and operation time (≥5 h) for the multivariate analysis.

Results

Of the 421 patients who consulted pulmonologists for perioperative management, 257 had asthma and 89 had COPD. These patients included 186 males and 160 females. The mean age was 58.1 years old (range, 20–89 years old). The remaining 75 patients who met the consultation criteria had conditions including interstitial pneumonia, bronchiectasis, pulmonary infection, and malignant diseases.

We recommended changing the anesthetic to local anesthesia in 5 patients, because these patients had exacerbated chronic respiratory diseases or very low pulmonary functions. Furthermore, we recommended cancelling 19 surgeries, which were excluded from the analysis.

Medical departments/services

A list of medical departments or services that performed surgical operations is provided in Table 1. Otolaryngology surgeries were the most frequent (177 patients) and 146 (82%) of these patients suffered from bronchial asthma.

Patients' characteristics associated with asthma and COPD

Patient characteristics associated with asthma and COPD are shown in Table 2. The mean age of the patients was younger in those with asthma than those with COPD. The mean FEV_1/FVC was higher in the patients with asthma was than in the patients with COPD. In patients with asthma, disease severity at baseline was significantly

Table 1 Medical departments that underwent surgical operations ($n = 346$)

Department	male	female	total
Otolaryngologic surgery	98	79	177 (51)
Orthopedic surgery	19	18	37 (11)
Gastrointestinal surgery	23	10	33 (9.5)
Urological surgery	22	7	29 (8.4)
Gynecological surgery	0	27	27 (7.8)
Hepatic surgery	7	4	11 (3.2)
Vascular surgery	6	3	9 (2.6)
Neurosurgery	4	5	9 (2.6)
Plastic surgery	5	3	8 (2.3)
Dermatological surgery	1	2	3 (0.9)
Breast surgery	0	2	2 (0.6)
Cardiac surgery	1	0	1 (0.3)

Data are presented as *n*, *n* (%)

associated with perioperative systemic corticosteroids treatment, and patients with severer asthma were treated with systemic corticosteroids ($p < 0.0001$, chi-square test, data not shown). A symptom questionnaire was performed at enrolment and completed by 77% of patients with asthma. The results revealed that there was a significant difference in ACT scores according to the GINA STEP ($p < 0.0001$, chi-square test, Table 3). Furthermore, there was a significant difference in ACT scores between the groups with and without perioperative corticosteroid treatment (22.3 ± 3.5 ($n = 106$) and 23.2 ± 2.2 ($n = 92$), respectively, $p = 0.023$, Student's t test, data not shown).

Postoperative pulmonary complications

In our study, 29 of 346 patients with asthma or COPD had PPCs. The details related to the PPCs and the clinical characteristics of the patients with asthma and COPD are shown in Tables 4, 5 and 6, respectively. Of the 257 patients with asthma, 18 (7.0%) had the PPC mild/moderate bronchospasm, and their symptoms promptly improved with additional treatment. There was a significant difference in ACT scores between the groups with and without PPCs (21.2 ± 4.8 ($n = 16$) vs 22.9 ± 2.8 ($n = 182$), respectively; $p = 0.032$, Student's t test, data not shown).

Of the 89 patients with COPD, seven (7.9%) had PPCs, mainly pneumonia accompanied by respiratory failure. The hospitalization period was extended in these patients, but all of them survived. Nineteen of the patients underwent surgery with local anesthesia, including three in whom general was changed to local anesthesia. Of these 19 patients, no one had a PPC, but there was no difference in the prevalence of PPCs between patients treated with general and local anesthesia ($p = 0.39$, Fisher's exact test). There was no significant difference in the prevalence of PPCs between patients who underwent laparoscopic surgery and those who did not ($p = 0.94$, chi-square test).

Table 2 Clinical characteristics in asthma and COPD patients

	asthma ($n = 257$)	COPD ($n = 89$)
gender, male / female	111 / 146	75 / 14
age, years(range)	53.8 ± 16.0 (20–88)	70.6 ± 8.3 (49–89)
BMI, kg/m^2	23.3 ± 4.5	23.0 ± 23.0
Smoking index, pack-years	9.4 ± 16.7	47.7 ± 33.6
(never/former/current)	(130 / 104 / 23)	(3 / 61 / 25)
%VC, %	110.5 ± 18.2	104.1 ± 20.5
FEV$_1$/FVC, %	70.5 ± 12.2	59.3 ± 7.7
%FEV$_1$, %	91.7 ± 19.6	84.5 ± 21.1
GINA STEP, 1/2/3/4/5	67 / 58 / 94 / 34 / 4	NA
CS (+), $n_1/n_2/n_3/n_4/n_5$	25 / 19 / 60 / 25 / 4	NA
GOLD stage, 1/2/3/4	NA	47 / 35 / 6 / 1

Data are presented as n or mean ± SD (range)
NA not available
CS systemic corticosteroids
"nx" means that the number of patients whose GINA STEP is "x"

Risk factors

We performed a univariate analysis to assess PPC risk factors in asthma (Table 5) and COPD (Table 6) patients. Regarding procedure-related risk factors in the univariate analysis, a longer operation time was a risk factor for PPCs. However, laparoscopic surgery did not decrease the prevalence of PPCs in the present study. We then evaluated PPC risk factors in a multivariate logistic regression analysis using the extracted variables shown in Table 7. Accordingly, the following were PPC risk factors in asthma patients: smoking history ≥20 pack-years [odds ratio (OR) 5.4, 95% confidence interval (CI) (1.4–20.8), $p = 0.014$], peripheral blood eosinophil count ≥200/mm^3 [0.31, (0.11–0.84), $p = 0.021$], GINA STEP ≥3 [3.2, (1.04–9.9), $p = 0.043$]. However, there was no significant difference between former and current smokers in the incidence of PPCs in the univariate analysis ($p = 0.28$, Fisher's exact test, data not shown).

The following PPC risk factors associated with COPD were identified in the multivariate logistic regression analysis: age [1.18, (1.00–1.40), $p = 0.046$], the introduction of COPD treatment [0.09, (0.01–0.81), $p = 0.032$], upper abdominal surgery [21.2, (1.3–349), $p = 0.033$], and an operation time ≥ 5 h [9.5, (1.2–77.4), $p = 0.035$] (Table 7).

Discussion

In the present study, we show that treating asthma with perioperative systemic corticosteroids seemed to significantly increase the risk of PPCs in the univariate analysis. However, no significant risk of PPCs was detected for systemic corticosteroids in the multivariate logistic

Table 3 ACT scores and GINA STEP

GINA STEP (n = 257)	1 (*n* = 67)	2 (*n* = 58)	3 (*n* = 94)	4 (n = 34)	5 (n = 4)	*p* value
ACT score (*n* = 198)	24.5 ± 1.0 (*n* = 45)	23.3 ± 1.9 (*n* = 43)	22.0 ± 3.0 (*n* = 81)	21.2 ± 4.5 (n = 25)	20.3 ± 5.5 (n = 4)	<0.0001*

Data are presented as n or mean ± SD
*chi-square test

analysis. Does treatment with systemic corticosteroids increase the risk of PPCs? Previous studies reported that the incidence of PPCs in untreated patients with asthma was 24% [11], whereas it was 4.5% in patients with asthma who received perioperative systemic corticosteroids [12]. In the present study, the incidence of bronchospasm in patients with treated asthma was 7.0%, similar to the results observed in later studies. As described in the methods and the results section, all of the patients with asthma were treated with ICS, and some with more severe and unstable asthma were also treated with systemic corticosteroids. The patients with severe/uncontrolled asthma were more likely to experience PPC events. Accordingly, treatment with systemic corticosteroids behaved like a risk factor in the univariate analysis. However, in the multivariate analysis of factors associated with disease severity, this potential disadvantage was cancelled out. The results of our study suggest that increasing the ICS dose is sufficient to prevent bronchospasm in patients with mild and stable asthma. Because most of bronchospasms that present as PPCs are mild, we propose that in clinical practice, systemic corticosteroids effectively minimize the severity of PPCs in patients with severe asthma.

According to the multivariate logistic analysis of patients with asthma, peripheral blood eosinophilia and a history of heavy smoking were significantly associated with PPCs. Both of these variables are implicated in steroid responsiveness. Interestingly, the result of the present study demonstrated that a peripheral blood eosinophil count ≥200/mm^3 decreased the risk of PPCs to one-third. There are several phenotypes of bronchial asthma [13]. The eosinophilic asthma phenotype that presents with a higher eosinophil count in the blood and sputum responded better to inhaled or systemic corticosteroid therapy [14–16]. Hence, perioperative intervention could effectively reduce PPC risk in eosinophilic asthma. We also found that a blood eosinophil count of approximately 200/mm^3 was correlated with both sputum eosinophil count and the efficacy of ICS [14, 16, 17]. Our result is compatible with those reported in other studies.

Table 4 Details of postoperative pulmonary complications

PPC	asthma patients (*n* = 257)	COPD patients (*n* = 89)
Total patients with PPC	22 (8.6)	7 (7.9)
Bronchospasm	18 (7.0)	0 (0.0)
Pneumonia/atelectasis	4 (1.6)	7 (7.9)
Respiratory failure[a]	2[b] (0.8)	1[b] (1.1)

Data are presented as n (%)
[a]All patients complicated with respiratory failure had pneumonia and/or atelectasis
[b]One patient in each group required mechanical ventilation

A smoking history of ≥20 pack-years was associated a five-fold increased risk of PPCs. However, Chaudhuri et al. [18] demonstrated that the efficacy of treatment with oral corticosteroids was impaired even in former smokers with asthma. Çolak et al. [19] also found that in patients with asthma, the risk of exacerbations and pneumonia was higher in current/former smokers vs never smokers, perhaps because the efficacy of inhaled corticosteroids is reduced by smoking. The reason for this phenomenon could be that cigarette smoking inactivated histone deacetylase activity, which is important for the corticosteroid-mediated repression of anti-inflammatory gene expression [20]. Therefore, smoking could be an important PPC risk factor, even in patients with asthma who receive appropriate treatments. Again, eosinophilia and a history of heavy smoking are associated with sensitivity and resistance, respectively, to corticosteroids, and both are therefore related to steroid responsiveness in a broad sense. Hence, in the present study, steroid responsiveness was viewed as a crucial factor that influenced PPC risks.

Patients with ACO were included in the asthma group in the present study. There were three reasons for this. First, no standardized definition has yet been established for ACO. Recently, a new definition, including a post-bronchodilator $FEV_1/FVC < 0.7$ and a peripheral blood eosinophil count >400/mm^3, was proposed [21] that requires verification. Second, patients with ACO are more responsive to corticosteroids than are patients with COPD alone [22]. Because inhaled and systemic corticosteroids are required to treat bronchospasm and wheezing, symptoms that are caused by eosinophilic airway inflammation, we emphasized this fact. The latest GINA document recommends starting treatment for asthma in affected patients [23]. Third, asthma patients with a smoking history and irreversible air flow obstruction, including patients with ACO, were treated with ICS/LABA therapy to prevent bronchospasm, which was the most considerable complication of asthma. We therefore included the patients with ACO

Table 5 Clinical characteristics of asthma patients with PPCs (+) or (−)

Variables	PPC (+) $n = 22$	PPC (−) $n = 235$	p-value
gender, male/female	10 / 12	101 / 134	0.82*
age, years	56.5 ± 15.4	53.5 ± 16.1	0.43†
BMI, kg/m^2	23.1 ± 3.0	23.3 ± 4.7	0.95†
Smoking Index, pack-years	18.3 ± 23.8	8.6 ± 15.9	0.15†
%VC, %	107.8 ± 22.1	110.7 ± 17.8	0.61†
%FEV$_1$, %	96.5 ± 22.8	91.3 ± 19.3	0.15†
Peripheral blood eosinophil, /mm^3	245 ± 183	337 ± 271	0.085†
GINA STEP ≥ 3, y/n	16 / 6	116 / 119	0.061*
Perioperative CS (+), y/n	17 / 5	116 / 119	0.022*
ASA-PS, 1/2/3-	1 / 19 / 2	13 / 201 / 19	0.97*
Upper abdominal surgery, y/n	4 / 18	15 / 220	0.11‡
Laparoscopic surgery, y/n	4 / 18	32 / 203	0.52‡
Operation time, min	200 ± 150	141 ± 86	0.023†

Data are presented as n or mean ± SD, unless otherwise stated
CS systemic corticosteroids
ASA-PS American Society of Anesthesiologists physical status
*chi-square test, †Mann-Whitney *U* test, ‡Fisher's exact test

Table 6 Clinical characteristics of COPD patients with PPCs (+) or (−)

Variables	PPC (+) $n = 7$	PPC (−) $n = 82$	p-value
gender, male / female	7 / 0	68 / 14	0.59‡
age, years	77.3 ± 7.9	70.0 ± 8.1	0.034†
BMI, kg/m^2	23.8 ± 2.6	23.0 ± 3.0	0.66†
Smoking Index, pack-years	40.7 ± 8.6	48.2 ± 34.7	0.88†
%VC, %	104.8 ± 15.5	104.0 ± 21.0	0.99†
%FEV$_1$, %	89.5 ± 11.0	84.1 ± 21.7	0.34†
GOLD stage (1/2/3/4)	6/1/0/0	41/34/6/1	0.39*
Peripheral blood eosinophil, /mm^3	210 ± 97	187 ± 135	0.38†
COPD treatment, y/n	3 / 4	63 / 19	0.07‡
ASA-PS, 1/2/3-	1 / 5 / 1	7 / 62 / 13	0.88*
Upper abdominal surgery, y/n	2 / 5	5 / 75	0.14‡
Laparoscopic surgery, y/n	1 / 6	15 / 67	>0.99‡
Operation time, min	393 ± 149	196 ± 131	0.002†

Data are presented as n or mean ± SD, unless otherwise stated
*chi-square test, †Mann-Whitney *U* test, ‡Fisher's exact test
ASA-PS American Society of Anesthesiologists physical status

Table 7 Risk factors of PPCs in asthma and COPD patients

	Variables	OR(95%CI)	*p*-value
asthma	Smoking index ≥20 pack-years	5.4 (1.4–20.8)	0.014
	Eosinophil ≥200/mm^3	0.31 (0.11–0.84)	0.021
	GINA STEP ≥3	3.2 (1.04–9.9)	0.043
COPD	age, years	1.18 (1.00–1.40)	0.046
	COPD treatments, yes	0.09 (0.01–0.81)	0.032
	Upper abdominal surgery, yes	21.2 (1.3–349)	0.033
	Operation time ≥ 5 h	9.5 (1.2–77.4)	0.035

These data were analyzed by multivariate logistic regression test

in the asthma group in our analysis of risk factors for PPC. It will be important to perform comparisons among these three types of obstructive pulmonary disease (bronchial asthma, ACO and COPD) in the future after a consensus is reached regarding the definition of ACO.

Next, regarding patients with COPD, previous studies have found that aging, upper abdominal surgery and operation time are risk factors for PPCs [1, 8]. Canet et al. [24] found that an operation time longer than 2 h was a predictor of PPCs, and in the present study, a multivariate analysis showed that an operation time longer than 5 h was a risk factor of PPCs. Hence, the threshold at which operation time increases the risk of PPCs was longer. The reason for this difference might be that perioperative management and anesthetic techniques have progressed over the last decade. In particular, non-invasive ventilation and high-flow therapy are effective in preventing post-extubation respiratory failure and reintubation in some patients [25–29]. To determinate whether the progress made in recent years has reduce the risk of PPCs was one of the purposes of this study. Laparoscopic surgery was not found to reduce PPC risk. We found that operation times were significantly longer in patients with COPD who underwent laparoscopic surgery than in those who underwent non-laparoscopic surgery (288 ± 139 min vs 195 ± 141 min, $p < 0.01$, Mann-Whitney *U* test, data not shown). The merit of using laparoscopic surgery to reduce the risk of PPC was masked by its intrinsically longer operation time. In addition to these risk factors, in the present study, we provide the newly evidence demonstrating that introducing treatment for COPD, including LAMA and LABA, reduced the risk of PPC. These inhaled drugs were recently developed and are much more effective in preventing COPD exacerbation. The mechanisms underlying their actions involve their ability to decrease hyperinflation and mechanical stress, to modulate mucus production and mucociliary clearance and to improve symptoms [30]. Low pulmonary function was not identified as a risk factor in this study. We changed the anesthetic techniques from general to local or cancelled the surgery in patients with advanced low pulmonary function. These adjustments reduced the risk of PPC in patients with low pulmonary function, but the difference was not significant.

Limitations

The present study has some limitations. First, this study is a retrospective case-control study performed at a single institution. Because early reports have demonstrated that systemic corticosteroid is effective as a precaution against PPC in patients with asthma, we believe that it may not be ethical to perform a prospective study using a control group consisting of untreated patients. The number of patients with asthma or COPD analyzed in the present study may depend on the proportion of surgical cases per department. Otolaryngology patients comprised approximately 20% of all patients treated with general anesthesia, and these patients often had asthma. However, the number of cases in which cardiovascular diseases, esophageal cancer or laryngopharyngeal cancer coexisted with COPD was small. Hence, multicenter cohort studies are desirable for collecting balanced data.

Second, although the total number of patients was 346, it would be preferable to register more patients. In addition, fewer PPC events in patients with COPD were observed than expected in this study. However, the reason for the small number of PPC events could be that we managed our patients in a manner aimed at reducing PPCs. Third, we excluded patients who underwent lung resection, because it is a direct risk factor for pulmonary complications. In the future, these concerns should be addressed in separate studies.

Conclusions

In summary, our results demonstrate that asthma patients with a history of smoking or severe asthma had an increased risk of PPCs. Sufficiently and aggressively increasing ICS can reduce the risk of PPCs in asthma patients with eosinophilia. Although aging, upper abdominal surgery and long operation times are risk factors for pneumonia and respiratory failure in COPD patients, introducing treatment for COPD significantly reduces the risk of PPC by improving pulmonary function.

Abbreviations

ACO: Asthma-COPD overlap; ACT: Asthma Control Test; ASA-PS: American Society of Anesthesiologists physical status; CI: Confidence interval; COPD: Chronic obstructive pulmonary disease; FEV_1: Forced expiratory volume in one second; FVC: Forced volume capacity; GINA: Global Initiative for Asthma; GOLD: Global initiative for chronic Obstructive Lung Diseases; ICS: Inhaled corticosteroids; LABA: Long-acting beta 2 agonist; LAMA: Long-acting muscarinic antagonist; OR: Odds ratio; PPC: Postoperative pulmonary complication; SD: Standard deviation; VC: Volume capacity

Funding

None

Authors' contributions

Concept and design: TN, SF, YY, data interpretation, writing of manuscript, revision of manuscript: TN, KN, SF, YY, HH, JA, Data Analysis and interpretation: TN, KN, Original data collection and revision of manuscript: TN, NS, MY, HU, HY, MH, KK, YK, SI, HW, SM, TI. KN and KK assisted in the writing of the manuscript and provided helpful discussion. All authors read and approved the final manuscript.

Consent for publication

Not applicable.

Competing interests

The authors declare that they have no competing interests.

References

1. Smetana GW. Preoperative pulmonary evaluation. N Engl J Med. 1999; 340:937–44.
2. Kroenke K, Lawrence VA, Theroux JF, Tuley MR, Hilsenbeck S. Postoperative complications after thoracic and major abdominal surgery in patients with and without obstructive lung disease. Chest. 1993;104:1445–51.
3. Smetana GW, Lawrence VA, Cornell JE. Preoperative pulmonary risk stratification for noncardiothoracic surgery: systematic review for the American College of Physicians. Ann Intern Med. 2006;144:581–95.
4. Global Initiative for Asthma. Global Strategy For Asthma Management and Prevention. revised 2014. http://www.ginasthma.org. Accessed 21 May 2014.
5. Vestbo J, Hurd SS, Agusti AG, Jones PW, Vogelmeier C, Anzueto A, Barnes PJ, Fabbri LM, Martinez FJ, Nishimura M, Stockley RA, Sin DD, Rodriguez-Roisin R. Global strategy for the diagnosis, management, and prevention of chronic obstructive pulmonary disease GOLD executive summary. Am J Respir Crit Care Med. 2013;187:347–65.
6. Swanson SJ, Meyers BF, Gunnarsson CL, Moore M, Howington JA, Maddaus MA, McKenna RJ, Miller DL. Video-assisted thoracoscopic lobectomy is less costly and morbid than open lobectomy: a retrospective multiinstitutional database analysis. Ann Thorac Surg. 2012;93:1027–32.
7. Wang J-f, Zhang S-z, Zhang N-y, Wu Z-y, Feng J-y, Ying LP, Zhang JJ. Laparoscopic gastrectomy versus open gastrectomy for elderly patients with gastric cancer : a systematic review and. World J Surg Oncol. 2016;14:90–9.
8. Qaseem A, Snow V, Fitterman N, Hornbake ER, Lawrence VA, Smetana GW, Weiss K, Owens DK, Aronson M, Barry P, Casey DE Jr, Cross JT Jr, Sherif KD, Weiss KB. Risk assessment for and strategies to reduce perioperative pulmonary complications for patients undergoing noncardiothoracic surgery: a guideline from the American College of Physicians. Ann Intern Med. 2006;144:575–80.
9. McAlister FA, Bertsch K, Man J, Bradley J, Jacka M. Incidence of and risk factors for pulmonary complications after nonthoracic surgery. Am J Respir Crit Care Med. 2005;171:514–7.
10. National Asthma Education and Prevention Program. Expert panel report 3 (EPR-3): guidelines for the diagnosis and Management of Asthma-Summary Report 2007. J Allergy Clin Immunol. 2007;120:S94–138.
11. Palmer KN. Post-operative pulmonary complications. Postgrad Med J. 1955;31:25–9.
12. Kabalin CS, Yarnold PR, Grammer LC. Low complication rate of corticosteroid-treated asthmatics undergoing surgical procedures. Arch Intern Med. 1995;155:1379–84.
13. Haldar P, Pavord ID, Shaw DE, Berry MA, Thomas M, Brightling CE, Wardlaw AJ, Green RH. Cluster analysis and clinical asthma phenotypes. Am J Respir Crit Care Med. 2008;178:218–24.
14. Green RH, Brightling CE, Woltmann G, Parker D, Wardlaw AJ, Pavord ID. Analysis of induced sputum in adults with asthma: identification of subgroup with isolated sputum neutrophilia and poor response to inhaled corticosteroids. Thorax. 2002;57:875–9.
15. Pavord ID, Brightling CE, Woltmann G, Wardlaw AJ. Non-eosinophilic cor ticosteroid unresponsive asthma. Lancet. 1999;353:2213–4.
16. Schleich FN, Manise M, Sele J, Henket M, Seidel L, Louis R. Distribution of sputum cellular phenotype in a large asthma cohort: predicting factors for eosinophilic vs neutrophilic inflammation. BMC Pulm Med. 2013;13:1–8.
17. McGrath KW, Icitovic N, Boushey HA, Lazarus SC, Sutherland ER, Chinchilli VM, Fahy JVA. Large subgroup of mild-to-moderate asthma is persistently noneosinophilic. Am J Respir Crit Care Med. 2012;185:612–9.
18. Chaudhuri R, Livingston E, McMahon AD, Thomson L, Borland W, Thomson NC. Cigarette smoking impairs the therapeutic response to oral corticosteroids in chronic asthma. Am J Respir Crit Care Med. 2003;168:1308–11.
19. Colak Y, Afzal S, Nordestgaard BG, Lange P. Characteristics and prognosis of never-smokers and smokers with asthma in the copenhagen general population study: a prospective cohort study. Am J Respir Crit Care Med. 2015;192:172–81.
20. Barnes PJ, Adcock IM, Ito K. Histone acetylation and deacetylation: importance in inflammatory lung diseases. Eur Respir J. 2005;25:552–63.
21. Miravitlles M, Alvarez-Gutierrez FJ, Calle M, Casanova C, Cosio BG, López-Viña A, Pérez de Llano L, Quirce S, Roman-Rodríguez M, Soler-Cataluña JJ, Plaza V. Algorithm for identification of asthma–COPD overlap: consensus between the Spanish COPD and asthma guidelines. Eur Respir J. 2017; https://doi.org/10.1183/13993003.00068-2017.
22. Sin DD, Miravitlles M, Mannino DM, Soriano JB, Price D, Celli BR, Leung JM, Nakano Y, Park HY, Wark PA, Wechsler ME. What is asthma?COPD overlap syndrome? Towards a consensus definition from a round table discussion. Eur Respir J. 2016;48:664–73.
23. Global Initiative for Asthma. Global Strategy for Asthma Management and Prevention, 2017 update. http://ginasthma.org. Accessed: 1 June 2017.
24. Canet J, Gallart L, Gomar C, Paluzie G, Vallès J, Castillo J, Sabaté S, Mazo V, Briones Z, Sanchis J, ARISCAT Group. Prediction of postoperative pulmonary complications in a population-based surgical cohort. Anesthesiology. 2010; 113:1338–50.
25. Faria DA, da Silva EM, Atallah ÁN, Vital FM. Noninvasive positive pressure ventilation for acute respiratory failure following upper abdominal surgery. Cochrane Database Syst Rev. 2015; https://doi.org/10.1002/14651858.CD009134.pub2.
26. Futier E, Burtz CP, Godet T, Ear LK, Rozencwajg S, Delay JM, Verzilli D, Dupuis J, Chanques G, Bazin JE, Constantin JM, Pereira B, Jaber S. Effect of early postextubation high - flow nasal cannula vs conventional oxygen therapy on hypoxaemia in patients after major abdominal surgery: a French multicentre randomised controlled trial (OPERA). Intensive Care Med. 2016; 42:1888–98.
27. Glossop AJ, Shepherd N, Bryden DC, Mills GH. Non-invasive ventilation for weaning, avoiding reintubation after extubation and in the postoperative period: a meta-analysis. Br J Anaesth. 2012;109:305–14.
28. Hernández G, Vaquero C, González P, Subira C, Fernando Frutos-Vivar M, Rialp G, Laborda C, Colinas L, Cuena R, Fernández R. Effect of Postextubation high-flow nasal cannula vs conventional oxygen therapy on reintubation in low-risk patients a randomized clinical trial. JAMA. 2016;315:1354–61.
29. Hernández G, Vaquero C, Colinas L, Cuena R, González P, Canabal A, Sanchez S, Rodriguez ML, Villasclaras A, Fernández R. Effect of Postextubation high-flow nasal cannula vs noninvasive ventilation on reintubation and Postextubation respiratory failure in high-risk patients a randomized clinical trial. JAMA. 2016;316:1565–74.
30. Beeh KM, Burgel PR, Franssen FM, Lopez-Campos JL, Loukides S, Hurst JR, Fležar M, Ulrik CS, Di Marco F, Stolz D, Valipour A, Casserly B, Ställberg B, Kostikas K, Wedzicha JA. How do dual long-acting bronchodilators prevent exacerbations of chronic obstructive pulmonary disease? Am J Respir Crit Care Med. 2017;196:139–49.

27

Management and attitudes about IPF (Idiopathic Pulmonary Fibrosis) among physicians from Latin America

Iván Cherrez-Ojeda[1*], Vincent Cottin[3], Juan Carlos Calderón[1,2], César Delgado[4], Erick Calero[1,2], Daniel Simanca-Racines[5], Silvia Quadrelli[6,7] and Annia Cherrez[2,8]

Abstract

Background: The aim of our study was to assess current practice patterns and attitudes towards diagnosis and management of idiopathic pulmonary fibrosis (IPF) patients in Latin America.

Methods: A Cross-sectional survey was developed and up to 455 physicians were enrolled. We used a rigorous method of validation using the translated version of the AIR Survey.

Results: Mean age was 47.5 years (SD 12.6) with 20.4 years (SD 12.3) of practice. In around 30% of physicians were reported access to radiologist, pathologist and multidisciplinary team. Despite almost all physicians reported that (ATS/ERS/JRS/ALAT) guidelines are useful, half of them prescribed corticoids for treatment of disease. Most respondents (69.9%) reported cough as the presenting symptom. Around 80% considered IPF to be an important clinical disorder, and felt that identifying patients at risk for IPF was important or extremely important. However, only 59.7% felt confident in managing patients with IPF, and similar numbers (60.8%) felt confident about their knowledge. Pulmonologist have more confidence and management of IPF that no pulmonologist.

Conclusion: The results of this survey of Latin American physicians could help to fill gaps regarding awareness, management and treatment of IPF and improve earlier diagnosis of IPF.

Keywords: Idiopathic pulmonary fibrosis, Health knowledge, Attitudes, Practice, Surveys and questionnaires, Latin America, Physicians

Background

Idiopathic Pulmonary Fibrosis (IPF) is characterised by chronic, progressive and irreversible decline in pulmonary function. Clinical symptoms and natural history are unpredictable and vary in severity [1]. Because of the complex nature and variable course of IPF, diagnosis and treatment are difficult. New data have been published on the safety and efficacy of treatments proposed to slow the progression of the disease, to relieve symptoms, and to improve quality of life [2, 3].

Using narrow case definitions, the annual incidence of IPF in the US is estimated to be 6.8–8.8 per 100,000. IPF incidence increases with age and is higher among males. In recent years the incidence appears to be increasing [4].

A retrospective longitudinal study suggested that median survival of IPF patients is 3–5 years following diagnosis [5].

Confirmation of the diagnosis requires exclusion of other causes of interstitial lung disease (ILD), along with the presence of the characteristic usual interstitial pneumonia (UIP) indicated by honeycombing on high resolution computed tomography (HRCT). In those without definitive radiological UIP, a surgical lung biopsy revealing characteristic findings of UIP is necessary for conclusive diagnosis [6, 7].

The 2011 American Thoracic Society/ Japanese Respiratory Society/ Latin American Thoracic Society (ATS/ERS/JRS/ALAT) guidelines call for a multidisciplinary team (MDT) approach to IPF, in which

* Correspondence: ivancherrez@gmail.com
[1]Universidad de Especialidades Espíritu Santo, Samborondón, Ecuador
Full list of author information is available at the end of the article

information from several sources is combined and evaluated [1]. MDT discussion is now considered the gold standard for distinguishing IPF from other ILDs disease [6]. In practice, MDT discussion may not always be possible [8]. Consequently, there is a degree of variability in clinical practice among physicians, both in terms of diagnosis and treatment of IPF [9].

A European survey of IPF management suggested that physicians may benefit from periodic education and update regarding IPF management [10]. In some countries there is a lack of uniformity regarding the diagnosis and management of IPF [11]. On the other hand more of a half trainees physician felt that their ILD training was inadequate [12].

In Latin America, where information is scarce, there is a clear need to standardise the approach to diagnosis and treatment of IPF patients.

The aim of our study was to assess current practice patterns and attitudes towards diagnosis and management of IPF patients in Latin America, to compare specifically pulmonologists and non-pulmonologists related to IPF management.

Methods

Study design

We conducted an anonymous cross-sectional survey, in which physicians evaluated themselves regarding idiopathic pulmonary fibrosis. The original questionnaire (AIR Survey, written in English) consisted of 28 questions relating to the clinical management of patients with IPF [8]. We included questions designed to assess physician attitude toward the disease. We used a rigorous method of validation using the translated version of the AIR Survey which we briefly described in the following paragraph.

Two of the investigators translated the AIR survey to Spanish. After that, the Spanish-language version was translated to English by a third investigator who did not know the original version of the AIR Survey. The back-translated English-language version of the new Spanish-language questionnaire was compared with the original English-language version. Each item on the back-translated English-language version was ranked by 30 individuals who were bilingual and independent of the study team for comparability and similarity of interpretability with the same item on the original English-language version. Any translated item with a mean score > 3 (seven was the worst agreement and one was the best agreement) was formally reviewed and corrected. The revised item was then translated back to English and compared again with the original English-language version of that item. This process continued until the mean scores for each item indicated a valid version (63 on each of the comparability and interpretability rankings, and preferably <2.5 on the interpretability rankings) [13].

Recruitment

The target population included physicians from Ecuador and elsewhere in Latin America who attended the following meetings between November 2015 and October 2016: the VII-VIIIth International Meeting of Allergy and Respiratory Medicine, Guayaquil, Ecuador; and the XIIth Latin-American Expert Forum Santiago, Chile. The inclusion criterion was having received a diploma as a medical doctor. Potential candidates were asked if they often managed patients with IPF. If they answered in the affirmative, they were eligible for the study, and a self-administered survey was delivered. This study was performed in accordance with the Declaration of Helsinki. This human study was approved by Comité de Ética en Investigación en Seres Humanos - Clínica Kennedy. All adult participants provided verbal consent to participate in this study and this was approved by our IRB and was because survey was anonymous and no interventions were conducted. The verbal consent process was recorded/documented by the moment in which physician completed the questionnaire.

Assessment

The first 28 questions of the AIR survey assessed the current diagnostic and management of IPF, including pharmacological therapy by physicians experienced in IPF and management of comorbidities. Furthermore, we included two "attitude questions" regarding the importance of IPF as a clinical disorder and IPF diagnosis, and three attitude questions regarding the physician's confidence in diagnosing, managing and knowledge about IPF. These "attitudes and confidence questions" were scored on a five-point Likert scale.

Statistical analysis

We used mean and standard deviation (SD) for age, years of practice, and for number of patients with IPF attended according to their age and forced vital capacity (FVC). Percentages (%) were calculated for gender, nationality, location of medical's office, pulmonologist, access to pathologist, radiologist, multidisciplinary team, perception of IPF guidelines, risk factors and onset of disease, treatment, monitoring progression of IPF and managing comorbidities, and attitudes towards disease. Attitudes towards disease were summarized as very important (very important and extremely important) and very confident (agree and strongly agree). Mann-Whitney U tests and chi square were used for comparisons among pulmonologists and non-pulmonologists and number of patients with IPF attended according to their age and FVC. Crude logistic analysis were performed among pulmonologists (non-pulmonologist as reference category) and access to pathologist, radiologist, multidisciplinary team, perception of IPF guidelines, risk factors and onset of disease, treatment, monitoring progression of IPF and managing comorbidities, and attitudes towards disease. Statistical tests were performed using SPSS version 13 (SPSS, Inc., Chicago, IL, 2000). A p-value <0.05 was significant.

Results

Up to 455 physicians were enrolled. The majority were male (55.4%). In total, 23.7% reported being a pulmonologist. Mean age was 47.5 years (SD 12.6) with 20.4 years (SD 12.3) of practice.

Most physicians (74.7%, $n = 340$) reported having cared for an IPF patient in previous year. Among these physicians, 38.6% were female, attending in private settings (48.4%), and one third (29.7%) were pulmonologists. Most of participants were from Ecuador (67.9%), followed by Chile (9.7%) and Peru (8.8%) (Additional file 1: Table S1).

On average, 13.8 (SD 21.4) IPF patients were cared for in the previous year. Physicians reported the highest average number of IPF patients in the age group 66–80 years old (3.6 patients, SD 12.1), with a forced vital capacity (FVC) ranging from 50%–70% (3.3 patients, SD 9.8) (Table 1). Pulmonologist reported the highest number of IPF patients with a FVC ≥50% ($p < 0.001$).

Access to pathologists, radiologists and multidisciplinary teams

Approximately one third of survey respondents reported access to pathologists (27.8%), radiologists (39.4%), and multidisciplinary teams (26.9%). Pulmonologists reported greater access to radiologists (OR 1.59, CI 95% 0.91–2.78) and pathologists (OR 1.80, CI 95% 1.09–2.96). Access to multidisciplinary teams was more common in pulmonologists (41.1% vs 20.8%) compared with non-pulmonologists ($p < 0.001$).

Perception regarding IPF guidelines, risk factors and disease onset

ATS/ERS 2011 guidelines were considered useful by almost all respondents (93.7%). No differences were found among among physician specialties (OR 0.44, CI 95% 0.12–1.56). A total of 18.9% of respondents reported that 0–10% of their IPF patients smoke. Pulmonologists reported higher rates of attending patients who smoking (21.3% vs 17.8%, $p < 0.05$). Up to 49.5% were aware that average time between symptom onset and diagnosis was ≤6 months, with no differences among specialties.

Almost one third (39.3%) of respondents reported that their patients had visited one or two physicians prior to diagnosis, with no differences among specialties.

Most respondents (69.9%) reported cough as the presenting symptom. This result held with pulmonologists and non-pulmonologists (OR 1.29, CI 95% 0.75–2.23), and was similar among countries. In addition, dyspnoea was frequently reported (54.6%), more often by pulmonologists (OR 5.22, CI 95% 2.92–9.34)). "Velcro" breath sounds were considered to be the first sign of IPF in 27.9% of respondents, more frequently in pulmonologists (OR 7.93, CI 95% 4.53–13.90).

Up to 92.8% of respondents reported obtaining family history. In total, 97.9% inquired about occupation, while 18.4% pursued genetic causes. Up to 22.3% of respondents reported managing mild and moderate IPF patients themselves, without collaboration. This finding was more frequent among pulmonologists (35.0% vs 17.2%) ($p < 0.001$).

Regarding diagnosis and treatment of patients with mild to moderate IPF, greater than 80% of physicians reported that it was somewhat important (> 3 points) to make and confirm the diagnosis, to manage comorbidities, to develop a monitoring plan, and to monitor efficacy and tolerability of medication. Differences were not found among physician specialties.

Treatment of IPF

Supplemental oxygen was prescribed most often (71.2%), followed by corticosteroids alone (48.0%), N-acetylcysteine

Table 1 Comparisons among pulmonologist and non-pulmonologist physicians according to FVC value of IPF patients attended by them

Amount of patients	Pulmonologists						
	Yes $n = 91$ (29.7%)		No $n = 215$ (70.3%)		Total		MW-U*
	Mean	SD	Mean	SD	Mean	SD	p value
FVC < 50%	2.75	7.36	1.54	5.10	1.90	5.88	0.214
FVC 50%–70%	7.13	15.40	1.74	5.22	3.35	9.76	0.000
FVC 71%–80%	2.99	8.44	1.10	5.44	1.66	6.52	0.000
FVC > 80%	1.47	5.89	.63	4.67	.88	5.07	0.001

*MW-U: Mann–Whitney U test

(NAC) alone (29.1%), and pirfenidone (17.0%). Higher chances of supplemental oxygen prescription (OR 2.89; CI 95% 1.53–5.45) and pirfenidone (OR 10.29, CI 95% 5.20–20.39) were observed in pulmonologists (Table 2). Participation in studies with pirfenidone were reported by 10.5% of respondents, with higher chances among pulmonologists (OR 6.54, CI 95% 2.95–14.48) .

Monitoring progression of disease

The most common metrics for assessing progression of disease were dyspnoea (63.7%), followed by FVC (62.1%). Diffusing capacity (DLCO) was used less commonly (24.8%). Similarly, only 28.4% of respondents reported using the 6-min-walk test (6MWT). Pulmonologists reported higher chances of employing for most of these tests ($p < 0.001$) (Table 3).

Managing comorbidities

In total, 64.1% of respondents reported always investigating for gastroesophageal reflux disease (GERD) (69.7% in pulmonologists vs 61.7% in non-pulmonologists, $p < 0.05$). GERD was considered very important to manage by 48.5% of respondents, but was treated systematically by only 32.3% (37.8% by pulmonologists vs 29.8% by non-pulmonologists). Non-pulmonologists considered managing GERD as very important (55.6%) more frequently than pulmonologists (45.3%).

Diet and lifestyle modifications were commonly recommended (75.7%), followed by proton pump inhibitors (PPI) (69.3%) for treatment of GERD. PPI was more commonly prescribed by pulmonologists (OR 2.67, CI 95% 1.45–4.90)). H2 blockers were prescribed by one quarter of respondents (23.9%). This non-recommended treatment was recommended more commonly by non-pulmonologists (OR 0.53, CI 95% 0.28–1.00)).

The most frequent assessed comorbidity was cardiovascular disease (9.1%), followed by GERD (8.6%), and lung cancer (7.4%). Lung cancer was assessed more frequently among pulmonologists (10.0% vs 6.2%, $p < 0.05$).

Pulmonary Hypertension (PH) was treated in 55.0% of patients. Sildenafil was used by half of respondents (52.5%), more frequently by pulmonologists (OR 2.01, CI 95% 1.22–3.34)).

Attitudes about IPF

Among respondents that saw at least one IPF patient per year, 77.2% considered IPF to be an important clinical disorder, and 83.5% felt that identifying patients at risk for IPF was important or extremely important. Of these, 65.9% felt confident in identifying patients at risk for IPF. However, only 59.7% felt confident in managing patients with IPF, and similar numbers (60.8%) felt confident about their knowledge (regarding diagnosis and management) of IPF. Pulmonologists reported highest rates of importance and confidence ($p < 0.001$) (Table 4).

Discussion

In our study, approximately one quarter of Latin American respondents reported access to a pathologist or a multidisciplinary team in their professional network, as compared with European participants (74% and 56%, respectively). Meanwhile, European physicians reported greater access to a radiologist (85%), in our continent this access is only available in one third of physicians [8]. In contrast, pulmonologist have more access to

Table 2 Comparisons among pulmonologist and non-pulmonologist physicians, according to progressionassessment of disease

Treatment	Pulmonologist					Total		
	Yes $N = 91$ (29.7%)		No $N = 215$ (70.3%)					
	n	%	n	%	OR (CI 95%)	n	%	p value*
Supplemental oxygen	77	84.6	141	65.6	2.89 (1.53–5.45)	218	71.2	0.001
Corticosteroids (CS)	39	42.9	108	50.2	0.74 (0.45–1.22)	147	48.0	0.238
Azatioprine	5	5.5	13	6.0	0.90 (0.31–2.61)	18	5.9	0.851
CS + immunosupressors (IS)	6	6.6	26	12.1	0.51 (0.20–1.29)	32	10.5	0.151
N-acetylcisteine (NAC)	30	33.0	59	27.4	1.30 (0.77–2.21)	89	29.1	0.331
Corticosteroids + NAC + IS	14	15.4	45	20.9	0.69 (0.36–1.33)	59	19.3	0.261
Corticosteroids + NAC	17	18.7	46	21.4	0.84 (0.45–1.57)	63	20.6	0.591
Colchicine	3	3.3	11	5.1	0.63 (0.17–2.32)	14	4.6	0.486
Ciclosporine	0	0.0	2	0.9	NS	2	0.7	0.356
Anti-blotting	1	1.1	15	7.0	0.15 (0.02–1.14)	16	5.2	0.035
Pirfenidona	38	41.8	14	6.5	10.29 (5.20–20.39)	52	17.0	0.000
Pirferidona + NAC	18	19.8	7	3.3	7.33 (2.94–18.25)	25	8.2	0.000

*Chi square

Table 3 Comparisons among pulmonologist and non-pulmonologist physicians, according to progression assessment of disease.

Progression assesment	Pulmonologist							
	Yes n = 91 (29.7%)		No n = 215 (70.3%)			Total		
	n	%	n	%	OR (CI 95%)	n	%	*p* value*
Dyspnea Scale	60	65.9	135	62.8	1.15 (0.69–1.92)	195	63.7	0.601
FVC lowering	75	82.4	115	53.5	4.08 (2.23–7.45)	190	62.1	0.000
DLCO lowering	50	54.9	26	12.1	8.87 (4.95–15.86)	76	24.8	0.000
CT	51	56.0	73	34.0	2.48 (1.50–4.09)	124	40.5	0.000
Exacerbation	28	30.8	65	30.2	1.03 (0.60–1.75)	93	30.4	0.926
6MWT	49	53.8	38	17.7	5.43 (3.16–9.33)	87	28.4	0.000
patient's feedback	22	24.2	19	8.8	3.29 (1.68–6.44)	41	13.4	0.000

*Chi square test

pathologist, radiologist and multidisciplinary teams. Approximately 20% of respondents determine IPF management on their own, compared with 7% reported in the European survey [8].

Earlier diagnosis of IPF has become more relevant since controlled clinical trials have demonstrated a reduction in the rate of decline of FVC [14, 15]. Almost half of respondents reported that the average time between symptoms and diagnosis was ≤6 months, this result differs from European surveys in which the range was 9–12 months. It is possible that our Latin-American IPF patients were actually diagnosed earlier. Alternatively, our result may reflect projection bias.

Our respondents reported that the most common presenting symptom was cough (69.9%). This result was similar across specialties. This result differs from European reports [8], because physician reported that dyspnoea was the most common symptom (99%). However, pulmonologist reported more dyspnoea and that velcro breath sounds were the first sign of IPF. All this could indicate that pulmonologists have more clinical suspicion of IPF. It is possible that our IPFß patients present with a different IPF phenotype.

Our respondents reported that 22% of their patients smoked, a substantially smaller percentage than reported in the European survey (60%) [8]. This finding suggests that there may be other risk factors associated with IPF in our countries. Due to pulmonologists reported higher rates of smoking, it could be possible that non-pulmonologists attend patients with other causes of IPF. Despite of our patients smoke less, they reported cough as the primary onset symptom, and in general present with more aggressive symptoms. Few physicians pursued genetic causes, probably owing to the difficulty of performing this kind of test in our countries.

Because IPF is a disease with a variable clinical course, it is important to identify factors that may help predict prognosis. Published guidelines recommended such tests as FVC, DLCO and 6MWT [16, 17]. The high variability associated with IPF makes predicting prognosis difficult, and this in turn complicates treatment planning. Less than one quarter of respondents employ DLCO and 6MWT, both of which could aid assessment and treatment planning. Is known that physician have low confidence interpreting result investigations in IPF [12]. In our study, the pulmonologists reported higher chances of usage for most of these tests.

Only 10% reported assessing GERD in IPF patients. Half of respondents treated PH patients with sildenafil, in contrast to the AIR survey, in which only a small

Table 4 Comparisons among pulmonologist (n = 91, 29.7%) and non-pulmonologist physicians (n = 215; 70.3%) according to attitudes toward disease

Attitudes	Pulmonologist						
	Yes N = 91 (29.7%)		No N = 215 (70.3%)		Total		
	n	%	no	%	n	%	*p* value*
As a clinical disorder, IPF is important	76	86.4	148	73.3	224	77.2	0.014
IPF diagnosis is important	82	93.2	161	79.3	243	83.5	0.003
Confidence about diagnosing IPF	73	83.0	118	58.4	191	65.9	0.000
Confidence about maging IPF	68	77.3	105	52.0	173	59.7	0.000
Confidence about knowledge of IPF	69	78.4	106	53.0	175	60.8	0.000

*Chi square test

proportion of respondents (4%) would regularly treat PH. [8].

We predicted that IPF recommendations would be followed by our respondent group because almost half of participants reported they felt IPF guidelines were useful. This was not necessarily the case. First, corticosteroids were frequently prescribed, in combination with immunosuppressive therapy or NAC, contrary to guidelines. A similar discrepancy was found in an Australasian study [11]. However, pulmonologist have higher rates of supplemental oxygen prescription and use of pirfenidone.

Approximately one third of respondents prescribed no specific treatment for IPF, similar to the result found in European surveys [3, 9]. Pirfenidone, a recommended medication according to guidelines, was variably prescribed, possibly because of limited availability in some countries.

There are some disagreements between IPF guideline recommendations and confidence in managing patients with IPF. These discrepancies may reflect a degree of self-protection among respondents.

Our results are comparable to the AIR study because respondents manage IPF patients with similar levels of severity [11]. Establishment of earlier diagnosis in both studies suggests that we may be optimistic regarding the future of IPF. Pulmonologists reported better confidence and manage of IPF.

We suggest that optimal physician management of IPF helps to identify factors that substantially affect patient outcomes. Updated IPF guidelines in local languages could lead to improved collaboration among primary care physicians, pulmonologists, specialised centres, pharmacists and other stakeholders involved in IPF management.

Our study has several limitations. First, this was a cross-sectional survey of physicians attending conferences. Therefore, we cannot infer causation from any of the associations we observed. We cannot generalise our results to all Spanish-speaking physicians because medical education regarding IPF might differ in other Spanish-speaking countries in important ways. Furthermore we have few physician from other Latin-American countries and we cannot generalize our result from all Latinamerica. Physicians who travel to medical meetings are likely to attend educational programs routinely, and therefore these physicians might have access to more updated medical knowledge than the larger group of general practice physicians practicing in the community who do not attend continuing medical education meetings. Thus, management of IPF in the larger population of general practice physicians and pulmonologists is likely to be less optimal than was reported in our survey. Furthermore, survey was self-administered with subjective answers, that could reflect some protection bias. Finally, our study didn't include radiologists and pathologist, who are members of MDT in diagnosis of IPF.

The results of this survey of Latin American physicians could help to fill gaps regarding awareness, management and treatment of IPF especially in GP. Future studies are needed to validate this survey in Latin America and other Spanish-speaking physician populations. Also, IPF guidelines in clinical practice in Latin America could be implemented according to clinical scenario in our region. Incorporating IPF-focused educational interventions during medical school and residency training programs could help to improve management of the disease. Latin American pulmonology societies could offer more IPF sessions at continuing medical education conferences. They could also create IPF education programs for general physicians such as those that currently exist for asthma and chronic obstructive pulmonary disease.

Conclusions

Despite high rates of awareness of international IPF guidelines, most IPF recommendations are not followed. To achieve better outcomes for our patients, we recommend improving IPF education in Latin America. Better knowledge of the disease and improved skills in generating a differential diagnosis may contribute to earlier diagnosis and treatment of IPF.

Abbreviations

6MWT: Six-minute walking test; AIR: Advanced IPF Research; ATS/ERS/JRS/ALAT: American Thoracic Society/European Respiratory Society/Japanese Respiratory Society/Asociación Latinoamericana del Tórax; DLCO: Diffusing capacity of Co; FVC: Forced Vital Capacity; GERD: Gastro-Esophageal Reflux Disease; HRCT: High Resolution Computed Tomography; IPF: Idiopathic Pulmonary Fibrosis; PH: Pulmonary Hipertension; SD: Standard Deviation; UIP: Usual Interstitial Pneumonia

Acknowledgements

We appreciate the guidance and knowledge imparted by the MECOR Program; specially to Sonia Buist, MD and Ana Menezes, MD. We are also very grateful for all the support provided by Martin Sivori, Boehringer-Ingelheim's Medical Director. Finally, we express our congratulation to José Cano, Karin Plaza, as well as all others members of the RespiraLab Research Group.

Funding

This study was not funded.

Authors' contributions

COI, CV, CJC, CE, SRD, and CA designed the study. COI, CJC, DC, CE, SRD, and QS acquired the data. All authors interpreted the data, drafted the article, revised it critically and approved the final version to be published.

Consent for publication
Not applicable.

Competing interests
C.V. reports personal fees from Actelion, Bayer, Biogen Idec, Boehringer Ingelheim, Gilead, GSK, MSD, Novartis, Pfizer, Roche, Sanofi, grants from Actelion, Boehringer Ingelheim, GSK, Pfizer, Roche, personal fees from Boehringer Ingelheim, outside the submitted work.

Author details
[1]Universidad de Especialidades Espíritu Santo, Samborondón, Ecuador. [2]Respiralab, Respiralab Research Group, Guayaquil, Ecuador. [3]Louis Pradel Hospital, Reference center for rare pulmonary diseases, Auvernia-Ródano-Alpes, Lyon, France. [4]Hospital Metropolitano, Quito, Ecuador. [5]Centro de Investigación en Salud Pública y Epidemiología Clínica. Facultad de Ciencias de la Salud Eugenio Espejo. Universidad Tecnológica Equinoccial., Quito, Ecuador. [6]Hospital Británico, Buenos Aires, Argentina. [7]Sanatorio Güemes, Buenos Aires, Argentina. [8]University of Heidelberg, Heidelberg, Germany.

References
1. Raghu G, Collard HR, Egan JJ, Martinez FJ, Behr J, Brown KK, Colby TV, Cordier J-F, Flaherty KR, Lasky JA, et al. An official ATS/ERS/JRS/ALAT statement: idiopathic pulmonary fibrosis: evidence-based guidelines for diagnosis and management. Am J Respir Crit Care Med. 2011;183:788–824.
2. Fregonese L, Eichler I. The future of the development of medicines in idiopathic pulmonary fibrosis. BMC Med. 2015;13:239.
3. Cottin V, Maher T. Long-term clinical and real-world experience with pirfenidone in the treatment of idiopathic pulmonary fibrosis. Eur Respir Rev. 2015;24:58–64.
4. Nalysnyk L, Cid-Ruzafa J, Rotella P, Esser D. Incidence and prevalence of idiopathic pulmonary fibrosis: review of the literature. Eur Respir Rev. 2012; 21:355–61.
5. Ley B, Collard HR, King TE Jr. Clinical course and prediction of survival in idiopathic pulmonary fibrosis. Am J Respir Crit Care Med. 2011;183:431–40.
6. Travis WD, Costabel U, Hansell DM, King TE Jr, Lynch DA, Nicholson AG, Ryerson CJ, Ryu JH, Selman M, Wells AU, et al. An official American Thoracic Society/European Respiratory Society statement: update of the international multidisciplinary classification of the idiopathic interstitial pneumonias. Am J Respir Crit Care Med. 2013;188:733–48.
7. Flaherty KR, King TE, Jr., Raghu G, Lynch JP, 3rd, Colby TV, Travis WD, Gross BH, Kazerooni EA, Toews GB, Long Q, et al: Idiopathic interstitial pneumonia: what is the effect of a multidisciplinary approach to diagnosis? Am J Respir Crit Care Med 2004, 170:904–910.
8. Cottin V. Current approaches to the diagnosis and treatment of idiopathic pulmonary fibrosis in Europe: the AIR survey. Eur Respir Rev. 2014;23:225–30.
9. Cottin V, Cadranel J, Crestani B, Dalphin JC, Delaval P, Israel-Biet D, Kessler R, Reynaud-Gaubert M, Valeyre D, Wallaert B, et al. Management of idiopathic pulmonary fibrosis in France: a survey of 1244 pulmonologists. Respir Med. 2014;108:195–202.
10. Cottin V, Bergot E, Bourdin A, Cadranel J, Camus P, Crestani B, Dalphin JC, Delaval P, Dromer C, Israel-Biet D, et al. Adherence to guidelines in idiopathic pulmonary fibrosis: a follow-up national survey. ERJ Open Res. 2015;1
11. Troy LK, Chapman SA, Lake F, Wilsher ML, Honeysett LB, Macansh S, Corte TJ. Current Australasian practice for diagnosis and management of idiopathic pulmonary fibrosis: where are we now? Respirology. 2015;20:647–53.
12. Sharp C, Maher TM, Welham S, Gibbons M: UK trainee experience in interstitial lung disease: results from a British Thoracic Society survey. Thorax 2014:thoraxjnl-2014-206397.
13. Sperber AD. Translation and validation of study instruments for cross-cultural research. Gastroenterology. 2004;126:S124–8.
14. Noble PW, Albera C, Bradford WZ, Costabel U, Glassberg MK, Kardatzke D, King TE Jr, Lancaster L, Sahn SA, Szwarcberg J, et al. Pirfenidone in patients with idiopathic pulmonary fibrosis (CAPACITY): two randomised trials. Lancet. 2011;377:1760–9.
15. Richeldi L, du Bois RM, Raghu G, Azuma A, Brown KK, Costabel U, Cottin V, Flaherty KR, Hansell DM, Inoue Y, et al. Efficacy and safety of nintedanib in idiopathic pulmonary fibrosis. N Engl J Med. 2014;370:2071–82.
16. Xaubet A, Ancochea J, Bollo E, Fernandez-Fabrellas E, Franquet T, Molina-Molina M, Montero MA, Serrano-Mollar A, Sociedad Espanola de Neumologia y Cirugia Toracica research group on diffuse pulmonary D: Guidelines for the diagnosis and treatment of idiopathic pulmonary fibrosis. Sociedad Espanola de Neumologia y Cirugia Toracica (SEPAR) research group on diffuse pulmonary diseases. Arch Bronconeumol 2013, 49:343–353.
17. Selman M, Undarraga A: Recomendaciones para el diagnóstico y tratamiento de la Fibrosis Pulmonar Idiopática. RESPIRAR 2015:e24.

Permissions

All chapters in this book were first published in PM, by BioMed Central; hereby published with permission under the Creative Commons Attribution License or equivalent. Every chapter published in this book has been scrutinized by our experts. Their significance has been extensively debated. The topics covered herein carry significant findings which will fuel the growth of the discipline. They may even be implemented as practical applications or may be referred to as a beginning point for another development.

The contributors of this book come from diverse backgrounds, making this book a truly international effort. This book will bring forth new frontiers with its revolutionizing research information and detailed analysis of the nascent developments around the world.

We would like to thank all the contributing authors for lending their expertise to make the book truly unique. They have played a crucial role in the development of this book. Without their invaluable contributions this book wouldn't have been possible. They have made vital efforts to compile up to date information on the varied aspects of this subject to make this book a valuable addition to the collection of many professionals and students.

This book was conceptualized with the vision of imparting up-to-date information and advanced data in this field. To ensure the same, a matchless editorial board was set up. Every individual on the board went through rigorous rounds of assessment to prove their worth. After which they invested a large part of their time researching and compiling the most relevant data for our readers.

The editorial board has been involved in producing this book since its inception. They have spent rigorous hours researching and exploring the diverse topics which have resulted in the successful publishing of this book. They have passed on their knowledge of decades through this book. To expedite this challenging task, the publisher supported the team at every step. A small team of assistant editors was also appointed to further simplify the editing procedure and attain best results for the readers.

Apart from the editorial board, the designing team has also invested a significant amount of their time in understanding the subject and creating the most relevant covers. They scrutinized every image to scout for the most suitable representation of the subject and create an appropriate cover for the book.

The publishing team has been an ardent support to the editorial, designing and production team. Their endless efforts to recruit the best for this project, has resulted in the accomplishment of this book. They are a veteran in the field of academics and their pool of knowledge is as vast as their experience in printing. Their expertise and guidance has proved useful at every step. Their uncompromising quality standards have made this book an exceptional effort. Their encouragement from time to time has been an inspiration for everyone.

The publisher and the editorial board hope that this book will prove to be a valuable piece of knowledge for researchers, students, practitioners and scholars across the globe.

List of Contributors

Michael S. Broder and Eunice Chang
Partnership for Health Analytic Research, LLC, 280 S. Beverly Dr. Ste. 404, Beverly Hills, CA, USA

Maureen P. Neary and Beilei Cai
Novartis Pharmaceuticals Corporation, One Health Plaza, East Hanover, New Jersey, USA

Helen E. Jo, Annabelle Mahar, Wendy Cooper, and Tamera J. Corte
Royal Prince Alfred Hospital, Missenden Road, Camperdown, NSW 2050, Australia

Wendy Cooper, Tamera J. Corte and Helen E. Jo
University of Sydney, Camperdown, NSW, Australia

Samantha Ellis, Ian Glaspole and Nicole Goh
The Alfred Hospital, Melbourne, VIC, Australia

Yuben Moodley
Fiona Stanley Hospital, Murdoch, WA, Australia

Paul Reynolds and Sally Chapman
Royal Adelaide Hospital, Adelaide, SA, Australia

Nicole Goh
The Austin Hospital, Heidelberg, VIC, Australia

Peter Hopkins
Prince Charles Hospital, Chermside West, QLD, Australia

Greg Keir
Princess Alexandria Hospital, Woolloongabba, QLD, Australia

Wendy Cooper
School of Medicine, Western Sydney University, Parramatta, NSW, Australia

E. Haydn Walters
School of Medicine, University of Tasmania, Hobart, TAS, Australia
University of Tasmania, Hobart, TAS, Australia

Christopher Zappala
Royal Brisbane and Women's Hospital, Herston, QLD, Australia

Christopher Grainge
John Hunter Hospital, New Lambton Heights, NSW, Australia

Heather Allan and Sacha Macansh
Lung Foundation Australia, Milton, QLD, Australia

Jens Bräunlich, Friederike Mauersberger and Hubert Wirtz
Department of Respiratory Medicine, University of Leipzig, Liebigstrasse 20, 04103 Leipzig, Germany

Thomas Zoller, David Wimmersberger, Frederick Haraka and Klaus Reither
Swiss Tropical and Public Health Institute, Basel, Switzerland

Francis Mhimbira, Elirehema H. Mfinanga, Tresphory B. Zumba, Peter J. Asilia, Edwin M. Mutabazi, Frederick Haraka and Thomas Zoller
Ifakara Health Institute, Dar es Salaam, Tanzania

Florian Kurth and Thomas Zoller
Charité - Universitätsmedizin Berlin, corporate member of Freie Universität Berlin, Humboldt-Universität zu Berlin, and Berlin Institute of Health, Berlin, Germany
Department of Infectious Diseases and Respiratory Medicine, Charité - Universitätsmedizin Berlin, Berlin, Germany

Klaus Reither, Frederick Haraka, David Wimmersberger and Thomas Zoller
University of Basel, Basel, Switzerland

Klaus Reither
Clinical Research Unit, Schweizerisches Tropen- und Public Health Institut, Socinstr. 57, 4051 Basel, Switzerland

Alexis A. Tazinya, Lawrence T. Mbuagbaw and Martin Abanda
Department of Internal Medicine and Pediatrics, Faculty of Health Sciences University of Buea, Buea, Cameroon

Gregory E. Halle-Ekane
Department of Surgery and Obstetrics/Gynecology, Faculty of Health Sciences, University of Buea, Buea, Cameroon

Julius Atashili
Department of Public Health and Hygiene, Faculty of Health Sciences, University of BueaCameroon

Marie Therese Obama
Faculty of Medicine and Biomedical Sciences, University of Yaoundé 1, Yaoundé, Cameroon

Yating Peng, Shan Cai, Yan Chen, Zijing Zhou, Jiaxi Duan and Ping Chen
Department of Respiratory Medicine, The Second Xiangya Hospital, Central South University, Changsha, Hunan 410011, China
Research Unit of Respiratory Diseases, Central South University, Changsha, Hunan 410011, China
Diagnosis and Treatment Center of Respiratory Disease, Central South University, Changsha, Hunan 410011, China

Weirong Dai, Wenfeng Liu and Xin Li
Hunan Institute of Occupational Disease Prevention, Hunan Provincial Center for Disease Control and Prevention, 410011 Changsha, People's Republic of China

Jussi Lampi, Sari Ung-Lanki and Juha Pekkanen
Department of Health Security, Environmental Health, National Institute for Health and Welfare, Finland
Social and Health, City of Kuopio, Kuopio, Finland

Päivi Santalahti
Department of Health, Mental Health Unit, National Institute for Health and Welfare, Helsinki, Finland

Juha Pekkanen
Department of Public Health, University of Helsinki, Helsinki, Finland

Liang Dong, Jingwen Xia, Jing Zhang, Yuanyuan Zhang, Ning Zhu, Peng Zhang, Youzhi Zhang, Xiujuan Zhang and Shengqing Li
Department of Pulmonary and Critical Care Medicine, Huashan Hospital, Fudan University, #12, Urumqi middle Road, Shanghai 200040, China

Alexander Kiefer and Volker O. Melichar
Department of Pediatrics and Adolescent Medicine, Clinic for Cystic Fibrosis, Universitätsklinikum Erlangen, Loschgestraße 15, 91054 Erlangen, Germany

Christian Bogdan
Microbiology Institute - Clinical Microbiology, Immunology and Hygiene, Universitätsklinikum Erlangen, Friedrich-Alexander-Universität (FAU) Erlangen-Nürnberg, Wasserturmstraße 3/5, 91054 Erlangen, Germany

Damilya Nugmanova and Nadezhda Nurkina
Semey State Medical University, Almaty, Kazakhstan

Yuriy Feshchenko and Liudmyla Iashyna
National Institute of Phthisiology and Pulmonology F.G. Yanovsky of NAMS, Kiev, Ukraine

Olga Gyrina
National Medical University n.a. O.O. Bogomoletz, Kiev, Ukraine

Averyan Vasylyev and Kateryna Malynovska
Glaxo Smith Kline, Kiev, Ukraine

Eljan Mammadbayov and Irada Akhundova
Scientific Research Institute of Lung Diseases, Baku, Azerbaijan

Luqman Tariq
Glaxo Smith Kline, Dubai, UAE

Janina Makarova
Glaxo Smith Kline, Moscow, Russia
GSK Russia Business Park "Krylatsky Hills", 17, Krylatskaya Street, Building 3 ("Air"), 121614 Moscow, Russia

Dongmei Zhang, Xinlun Tian, Xiaobei Guo, Yi Xiao and Kai-Feng Xu
Department of Respiratory Medicine, Peking Union Medical College Hospital, Chinese Academy of Medical Sciences & Peking Union Medical College, Beijing, China

Ruie Feng
Department of Pathology, Peking Union Medical College Hospital, Chinese Academy of Medical Sciences & Peking Union Medical College, Beijing, China

Peng Wang
Laboratory Department, Peking Union Medical College Hospital, Chinese Academy of Medical Sciences & Peking Union Medical College, Beijing, China

Yusen Situ
Department of Biochemistry, Faculty of Medicine and Dentistry, University of Alberta, Edmonton, Canada

Dongmei Zhang
Department of Respiratory and Critical Care Medicine, Beijing Institute of Respiratory Medicine and Beijing Chaoyang Hospital, Capital Medical University, Beijing, China

Hideaki Yamakawa, Yumie Yamanaka, Satoshi Ikeda, Akimasa Sekine, Hideya Kitamura, Tomohisa Baba and Takashi Ogura
Department of Respiratory Medicine, Kanagawa Cardiovascular and Respiratory Center, 6-16-1 Tomioka-higashi, Kanazawa-ku, Yokohama 236-0051, Japan

Tamiko Takemura
Department of Pathology, Japanese Red Cross Medical Center, Tokyo, Japan

Tae Iwasawa
Department of Radiology, Kanagawa Cardiovascular and Respiratory Center, Yokohama, Japan

Shinichiro Iso
Department of Radiology, Yokohama Rousai Hospital for Labour Welfare Corporation, Yokohama, Japan

Koji Okudela
Department of Pathobiology, Yokohama City University Graduate School of Medicine, Yokohama, Japan

Kazuyoshi Kuwano, Hideaki Yamakawa, Yumie Yamanaka and Hideya Kitamura
Department of Respiratory Medicine, Tokyo Jikei University Hospital, Tokyo, Japan

Bryan A. Garcia, Jacque L. Carden, Dana L. Goodwin, Tim A. Smith, Amit Gaggar, Kevin Leon, Veena B. Antony, Steven M. Rowe and George M. Solomon
Department of Medicine, Division of Allergy, Pulmonary and Critical Care Medicine, 1900 University Blvd, THT 422, Birmingham, AL 35294, USA

Gaggar, Kevin Leon, Veena B. Antony, Steven M. Rowe and George M. Solomon
Gregory Fleming James Cystic Fibrosis Research Center, Birmingham, AL, USA

Yong Suk Jo, Chul-Gyu Yoo and Chang-Hoon Lee
Division of Pulmonary and Critical Care Medicine, Department of Internal Medicine, Seoul National University Hospital, 101 Daehak-Ro Jongno-Gu, Seoul 03080, Republic of Korea

Sangshin Park
Center for International Health Research, Rhode Island Hospital, The Warren Alpert Medical School of Brown University, Providence, RI 02903, USA
Department of Pediatrics, The Warren Alpert Medical School of Brown University, Providence, RI 02903, USA

Deog Kyeom Kim
Division of Pulmonary and Critical Care Medicine, Department of Internal Medicine, Seoul Metropolitan Government-Seoul National University Boramae Medical Center, Seoul, Republic of Korea

Munemasa Nagao, Akihisa Fukuda and Hiroshi Seno
Department of Gastroenterology and Hepatology, Graduate School of Medicine, Kyoto University, 54 Kawahara-cho, Syogoin, Sakyo-ku, Kyoto 606-8507, Japan

Takeshi Matsumura and Toshiyuki Kimura
Department of Gastroenterology and Hepatology, HyogoPrefectural Amagasaki General Medical Center, Amagasaki, Japan

Xunliang Tong
Department of Geriatrics, Beijing Hospital, National Center of Gerontology, Beijing 100730, People's Republic of China

Anqi Cheng
Tobacco Medicine and Tobacco Cessation Centre, Center of Respiratory Medicine, China-Japan Friendship Hospital; WHO Collaborating Centre for Tobacco Cessation and Respiratory Diseases Prevention; National Clinical Research Center for Respiratory Diseases, Beijing 100029, People's Republic of China

Hongtao Xu
Department of Laboratory Medicine, Beijing Hospital, Beijing 100730, People's Republic of China

Jin Jin, Yimeng Yang and Yanming Li
Department of Respiratory and Critical Care Medicine, Beijing Hospital, Beijing 100730, People's Republic of China

Sainan Zhu
Statistics Department, First Hospital of Peking University, Beijing 100034, People's Republic of China

Johannes Träger, Renate Meyer, Christian Bogdan and Jürgen Held
Mikrobiologisches Institut - Klinische Mikrobiologie, Immunologie und Hygiene, Universitätsklinikum Erlangen und Friedrich-Alexander-Universität (FAU) Erlangen-Nürnberg, Wasserturmstr. 3/5, 91054 Erlangen, Germany

Manfred Rauh and Volker Otto Melichar
Kinder- und Jugendklinik, Universitätsklinikum Erlangen und Friedrich-Alexander-Universität (FAU) Erlangen-Nürnberg, Erlangen, Germany

Adrian Egli
Applied Microbiology Research, Department of Medicine, University of Basel, Basel, Switzerland
Clinical Microbiology, University Hospital Basel, Basel, Switzerland

Jyotshna Mandal, Desiree M. Schumann, Michael Roth and Michael Tamm
Clinic of Pneumology and Pulmonary Cell Research, University Hospital Basel, Petersgraben 4, 4031 Basel, Switzerland

Brad Thomas and D. Lorne Tyrrell
Li Ka Shing Institute for Virology, University of Alberta, Edmonton, Canada

Renaud Louis
Department of Pneumology, CHU Liege, University of Liege, GIGAI Research Group, Liege, Belgium

Joachim G. Aerts
Department of Pneumology, Amphia Hospital/ Erasmus MC, Breda, The Netherlands

Tobias Welte
Department of Pneumology, Medizinische Hochschule Hannover, Hannover, Germany

Antoni Torres
Department of Pneumology, Hospital Clinic, Barcelona, Spain

Nina F. Caspersen, Helge Røsjø, Anna Randby, Torbjørn Omland and Gunnar Einvik
Division of Medicine, Akershus University Hospital, Lørenskog, Norway
Institute of Clinical Medicine, University of Oslo, Oslo, Norway

Allan Flyvbjerg
Steno Diabetes Center Copenhagen (SDCC), the Capital Region of Denmark and University of Copenhagen, Copenhagen, Denmark

Mette Bjerre
Medical Research Laboratory, Department of Clinical Medicine, Aarhus University, Aarhus, Denmark

Harald Hrubos-Strøm
Department of Otorhinolaryngology, Division of Surgery, Akershus University Hospital, Lørenskog, Norway

Safi Alqatari
Royal College of Physicians of Ireland, Rheumatology Department, Cork University Hospital, Wilton, Cork, IrelandT12 DC4A

Peter Riddell, Michael Henry and Grainne Murphy
Rheumatology Department, Cork University Hospital, Wilton, Cork, Ireland

Sinead Harney
Internal Medicine and Rheumatology Consultant Rheumatology Department, Cork University Hospital, Wilton, Cork, Ireland

Daniela Savi, Marcello Di Paolo and Paolo Palange
Department of Public Health and Infectious Diseases, Adult Cystic Fibrosis Center, Sapienza University of Rome, 00185 Rome, Italy
Cystic Fibrosis Unit, Bambino Gesù Children's Hospital, Rome, Italy

Nicholas J. Simmonds
Department of Cystic Fibrosis, Royal Brompton Hospital and Imperial College, London SW3 6NP, UK

Chiara Pascucci
Department of Experimental Medicine, Sapienza University of Rome, 00185 Rome, Italy

Serena Quattrucci
Department of Pediatrics, Cystic Fibrosis Center, Sapienza University of Rome, 00185 Rome, Italy

Paolo Palange
Eleonora Lorrillard-Spencer Cenci Foundation, 00185 Rome, Italy

Adrien Tissot, Matthew F. Thomas, Paul A. Corris and Malcolm Brodlie
Institute of Cellular Medicine, Newcastle University, Medical School, Framlington Place, Newcastle upon Tyne NE2 4HH, UK
Institute of Transplantation, Freeman Hospital, Newcastle upon Tyne Hospitals NHS Foundation Trust, Newcastle upon Tyne NE7 7DN, UK
Centre Hospitalier Universitaire de Nantes, Nantes, France

Malcolm Brodlie and Matthew F. Thomas
Great North Children's Hospital, Newcastle upon Tyne Hospitals NHS Foundation Trust, Level 3, Clinical Resource Building, Queen Victoria Road, Newcastle upon Tyne NE1 4LP, UK

Xiaotong Guo, Yuchun Fan, Jieda Cui, Binwei Hao, Xiaoming Liu and Juan Chen
Department of Pulmonary and Critical Care Medicine, General Hospital of Ningxia Medical University, 804 Shengli South Street, Xingqing District, Yinchuan, Ningxia 750004, People's Republic of China
Ningxia Medical University, Yinchuan 750004, Ningxia, China

Li Zhu and Xiao Sun
Department of Radiology, General Hospital of Ningxia Medical University, Yinchuan 750004, Ningxia, China

Jinxi He
Department of Thoracic Surgery, General Hospital of Ningxia Medical University, Yinchuan 750004, Ningxia, China

Jiali Yang and Xiaoming Liu
Institute of Human Stem Cell Research, General Hospital of Ningxia Medical University, Yinchuan 750004, Ningxia, China

Yanyang Wang
Department of Radiotherapy, General Hospital of Ningxia Medical University, Yinchuan 750004, Ningxia, China

Jianda Dong
Department of Pathology, Ningxia Medical University, Yinchuan 750004, Ningxia, China

Cristóbal Esteban and Alberto Capelastegui
Pulmonary Service, Galdakao-Usansolo Hospital, Galdakao, Bizkaia, Spain

Francisco Pozo-Rodriguez, Ady Castro-Acosta and Carlos Jose Alvarez-Martínez
Pulmonary Service and Research Institute, Doce de Octubre University Hospital, Madrid, Spain
CIBER Enfermedades Respiratorias (CIBERES), Madrid, Spain

José Luis López-Campos
Hospital Universitario Virgen del Rocío, Medical-Surgical Unit of Respiratory Diseases, Seville, Spain

Cristóbal Esteban
Network and Health Services Research Chronic Diseases (REDISSEC), Bilbao, Bizkaia, Spain

Sumitra Shantakumar
R&D, Real World Evidence & Epidemiology, GSK, 50 Beach Road, #21-00 Gateway West, Singapore 189720, Singapore

Yen-Yun Yang, Raoh-Fang Pwu K. Arnold Chan and Yi-Chen Juan
Health Data Research Center, National Taiwan University, No.33, Linsen South Road, Suite 526, Taipei 10051, Taiwan

Liesel D'Silva
National Respiratory Physician Lead, GSK, 7333 Mississauga Road, Mississauga, ON L5N 6L4, Canada

Keele Wurst
R&D, Real World Evidence & Epidemiology, GSK, 1250 South Collegeville Road, Collegeville, PA 19426, USA

Yao-Wen Kuo and K. Arnold Chan
National Taiwan University Hospital, No.7, Zhongshan S. Road, Zhongzheng District, Taipei City 10002, Taiwan

Raoh-Fang Pwu
Present Address: Ministry of Health and Welfare, Taipei City, Taiwan

Takanori Numata, Katsutoshi Nakayama, Satoko Fujii, Yoko Yumino, Nayuta Saito, Masahiro Yoshida, Yusuke Kurita, Kenji Kobayashi, Saburo Ito, Hirofumi Utsumi, Haruhiko Yanagisawa, Mitsuo Hashimoto, Hiroshi Wakui, Shunsuke Minagawa, Takeo Ishikawa, Hiromichi Hara, Jun Araya, Yumi Kaneko and Kazuyoshi Kuwano
Division of Respiratory Diseases, Department of Internal Medicine, Jikei University School of Medicine, 3-25-8, Nishi-Shimbashi, Minato-ku, Tokyo, Japan

Iván Cherrez-Ojeda, Juan Carlos Calderón and Erick Calero
Universidad de Especialidades Espíritu Santo, Samborondón, Ecuador

Annia Cherrez, Juan Carlos Calderón and Erick Calero
Respiralab, Respiralab Research Group, Guayaquil, Ecuador

Vincent Cottin
Louis Pradel Hospital, Reference center for rare pulmonary diseases, Auvernia-Ródano-Alpes, Lyon, France

César Delgado
Hospital Metropolitano, Quito, Ecuador

Daniel Simanca-Racines
Centro de Investigación en Salud Pública y Epidemiología Clínica. Facultad de Ciencias de la Salud Eugenio Espejo. Universidad Tecnológica Equinoccial., Quito, Ecuador

Silvia Quadrelli
Hospital Británico, Buenos Aires, Argentina
Sanatorio Güemes, Buenos Aires, Argentina. 8University of Heidelberg, Heidelberg, Germany

Index

www.ingramcontent.com/pod-product-compliance
Lightning Source LLC
LaVergne TN
LVHW080905210926
848485LV00004B/594